Medical Knowledge Self-Assessment Program®

MKSAP®
for
Students
5

Developed by
American College of Physicians
Clerkship Directors in Internal Medicine

Editorial Production: Helen Kitzmiller
Design: Michael E. Ripca
Composition: ACP Graphic Services

Printed in the United States of America by Sheridan Books

American College of Physicians
190 N. Independence Mall West
Philadelphia, PA 19106-1572
215-351-2600

ISBN: 978-1-934465-54-7

Acknowledgments

MKSAP for Students 5 Editorial Board

Eyad Al-Hihi, MD, MBA, FACP
Associate Professor of Medicine
Chief, Division of General Internal & Hospital Medicine
Director, Internal Medicine Ambulatory Clerkship
University of Missouri-Kansas City School of Medicine
Medical Director, Medicine Clinics, Truman Med Center
Kansas City, Missouri

Irene Alexandraki, MD, MPH, FACP
Assistant Professor, Department of Medicine
Medicine Clerkship Director
University of Florida College of Medicine
Jacksonville, Florida

Mark Allee, MD, FACP
Associate Professor, Department of Medicine
Medicine Clerkship Director
University of Oklahoma School of Medicine
Oklahoma City, Oklahoma

Saad Alvi, MD, FACP
Assistant Professor of Clinical Medicine
M3 Clerkship Director
University of Illinois College of Medicine at Peoria
(UICOMP)
Peoria, Illinois

Alpesh Amin, MD, MBA, FACP
Professor of Medicine
Medicine Clerkship Director
University of California, Irvine
Orange, California

Lisa M. Antes, MD
Associate Professor
Department of Internal Medicine/Division of Nephrology
Inpatient Internal Medicine Clerkship Co-Director
Carver College of Medicine/University of Iowa Hospitals
    and Clinics
Iowa City, Iowa

Joel Appel, DO
Director Ambulatory and Student Programs
Wayne State University School of Medicine
Chief Hematology/Oncology
Sinai-Grace Hospital
Detroit Medical Center
Detroit, Michigan

Jonathan S. Appelbaum, MD, FACP
Associate Professor, Clinical Sciences
Director, Internal Medicine Education
Florida State University College of Medicine
Tallahassee, Florida

Scott Arnold, MD, FACP
Associate Professor, Department of Medicine
Medicine Clerkship Director
University of Alabama School of Medicine
Tuscaloosa Campus
Tuscaloosa, Alabama

Emily Chism Barker, MD
Assistant Professor of Medicine
Senior Associate Program Director for Internal Medicine
University of Texas Houston Medical School
Houston, Texas

Jennifer Bierman, MD, FACP
Primary Care Clerkship Director
Northwestern University Feinberg School of Medicine
Chicago, Illinois

Susan Crouch Brewer, MD, FACP
Assistant Dean for Clinical Education
Associate Chair for Student Programs
College of Medicine
University of Tennessee Health Science Center
Memphis, Tennessee

Cynthia A. Burns, MD, FACP
Assistant Professor
Internal Medicine Clerkship Director
Department of Internal Medicine
Section on Endocrinology & Metabolism
Wake Forest University School of Medicine
Winston-Salem, North Carolina

Maria L. Cannarozzi, MD, FACP, FAAP
Associate Professor of Internal Medicine & Pediatrics
Clerkship Director, Internal/Family Medicine
University of Central Florida College of Medicine
Orlando, Florida

Danelle Cayea, MD, MS
Assistant Professor of Medicine
Medicine Clerkship Director
Johns Hopkins University School of Medicine
Baltimore, Maryland

J. Charles, MD, FACP, FHM
Assistant Professor of Medicine
Division Education Coordinator
Mayo Clinic Hospital
Phoenix, Arizona

Brian J. Costello, DO
Co-Clerkship Director Ambulatory Medicine
Lehigh Valley Health Network
Allentown, Pennsylvania

Camilla Curren, MD
Assistant Clinical Professor of Internal Medicine
Ohio State University Medical Center
Clinical Assistant Professor of Pediatrics
Nationwide Childrens Hospital
Assistant Clerkship Director, Ambulatory Medicine
Ohio State University College of Medicine
Columbus, Ohio

Thomas M. DeFer, MD, FACP
Clerkship Director
Division of Medical Education
Department of Internal Medicine
Washington University School of Medicine
St. Louis, Missouri

Stephanie A. Detterline, MD, FACP
Associate Program Director, Internal Medicine
Union Memorial Hospital
Medicine Clerkship Site Director
University of Maryland School of Medicine
Baltimore, Maryland

Gurpreet Dhaliwal, MD
Site Director, Internal Medicine Clerkships
San Francisco VA Medical Center
Associate Professor of Clinical Medicine
University of California San Francisco
San Francisco, California

Gretchen Diemer, MD, FACP
Assistant Professor of Medicine
Director of Undergraduate Medical Education
Clerkship Director Internal Medicine
Assistant Program Director Internal Medicine
Thomas Jefferson University
Philadelphia, Pennsylvania

Anne Eacker, MD, FACP
Associate Professor, Department of Medicine
Medical Director, General Internal Medicine Center
University of Washington
Seattle, Washington

Mark J Fagan, MD, FACP
Clerkship Director
Department of Medicine
Alpert Medical School of Brown University
Providence, Rhode Island

Pamela J. Fall, MD, FACP, FASH
Professor of Medicine
Section of Nephrology, Hypertension and Transplantation
Clerkship Director, Internal Medicine
Medical College of Georgia
Augusta, Georgia

L. Christine Faulk, MD
Medicine Clerkship Co-Director
University of Kansas School of Medicine-Wichita
Wichita, Kansas

Sara B. Fazio, MD, FACP
Associate Professor, Harvard Medical School
Director, Core I Medicine Clerkship
Division of General Internal Medicine
Beth Israel Deaconess Medical Center
Boston, Massachusetts

J. Michael Finley, DO, FACP, FACOI
Associate Professor of Medicine
Chief, Division of Rheumatology
Associate Dean for Graduate Medical Education
Western University College of Osteopathic Medicine
Pomona, California

Jose Franco, MD, AGAF
Professor of Medicine and Pediatrics
Director of Hepatology
Medicine Clerkship Director
Medical College of Wisconsin
Milwaukee, Wisconsin

Erica Friedman, MD, FACP
Associate Dean
Associate Professor of Medicine and Medical Education
Mount Sinai School of Medicine
New York, New York

Peter Gliatto, MD, FACP
Assistant Professor of Medicine and Medical Education
Co-Director, Medicine-Geriatrics Clerkship
Director, Medicine Subinternship
Mount Sinai School of Medicine
New York, New York

Susan A. Glod, MD
Assistant Professor of Medicine
Associate Clerkship Director, Internal Medicine
Penn State College of Medicine
Hershey, Pennsylvania

Gabrielle R. Goldberg, MD
Education Director
The Hertzberg Palliative Care Institute
Assistant Professor
Department of Geriatrics and Palliative Medicine
Department of Medicine
Mount Sinai School of Medicine
New York, New York

Eric Goren, MD
Medicine Sub-Internship Course Co-Director
Assistant Professor of Clinical Medicine
University of Pennsylvania School of Medicine
Philadelphia, Pennsylvania

Cyril M. Grum, MD, FACP
Professor and Senior Associate Chair
for Undergraduate Medical Education
Department of Internal Medicine
Internal Medicine Clerkship Director
University of Michigan
Ann Arbor, Michigan

Heather Harrell, MD, FACP
Associate Professor, Department of Medicine
Medicine Clerkship Director
Director of Fourth Year Programs
University of Florida College of Medicine
Gainesville, Florida

Dan A. Henry, MD, FACP
Professor of Medicine
Director of Clinical Education
Medicine Clerkship Director
University of Connecticut School of Medicine
Farmington, Connecticut

Susan Thompson Hingle, MD, FACP
Associate Professor of Medicine
Internal Medicine Clerkship Director
Internal Medicine Residency Associate Program Director
Southern Illinois University School of Medicine
Springfield, Illinois

William Howell, MBChB
Clinical Instructor of Medicine
Medicine Clerkship Co-Director
University of Utah School of Medicine
Salt Lake City, Utah

Eric Hsieh, MD
Director, Internal Medicine Clerkship
Senior Associate Director, Internal Medicine Residency
Department of Medicine
Keck School of Medicine
University of Southern California
Los Angeles, California

Hugh F. Huizenga, MD, MPH
Assistant Professor of Medicine
Clerkship Director-Inpatient Medicine
Dartmouth Medical School
Hanover, New Hampshire

T.J. Hundley, MD, FACP
Director, Internal Medicine Clerkship
Assistant Professor of Medicine
Department of Internal Medicine
University of South Alabama College of Medicine
Mobile, Alabama

Nadia J. Ismail, MD, MPH, Med, FACP
Director, Internal Medicine Core Clerkship
Assistant Professor of Medicine
Baylor College of Medicine
Houston, Texas

Harish Iyer, MD, MRCP (UK)
Chief Medical Resident
Department of Medicine
Albert Einstein Medical Center
Philadelphia, Pennsylvania

Robert Jablonover, MD
Assistant Professor in Internal Medicine
Clerkship Director in Internal Medicine
George Washington University School of Medicine
Washington, District of Columbia

Janet A. Jokela, MD, MPH, FACP
Associate Professor of Clinical Medicine
Department of Medicine
University of Illinois at Urbana-Champaign
Urbana, Illinois

Jason Kahn, MD, FACP
Internal Medicine Clerkship Site Director
St. Joseph Mercy Hospital
Ann Arbor, Michigan

Christopher A. Klipstein, MD
Associate Professor of Medicine
Director, Internal Medicine Clerkship
University of North Carolina School of Medicine
Chapel Hill, North Carolina

Mary Ann Kuzma, MD, FACP
Associate Professor of Medicine
Medicine Clerkship Director
Drexel University College of Medicine
Philadelphia, Pennsylvania

Rosa Lee, MD
Medicine Clerkship Site Leader,
Montefiore Medical Center
Assistant Professor, Department of Medicine
Albert Einstein College of Medicine
Bronx, New York

Beth W. Liston, MD, PhD, FACP
Assistant Professor of Clinical Medicine/Pediatrics
Sub-internship Clerkship Director
The Ohio State University College of Medicine
Columbus, Ohio

Mai A Mahmoud, MBBS, FACP
Assistant Professor of Medicine
Medicine Clerkship Co-Director
Weill Cornell Medical College in Qatar
Doha, Qatar

Lianne Marks, MD, PhD, FACP
Division Director, Internal Medicine
Scott & White Healthcare
Assistant Professor and Internal Medicine
Clerkship Director for 3rd Year Medical Students
Texas A&M College of Medicine
Round Rock, Texas

Kevin M. McKown, MD
Associate Professor and Head, Division of Rheumatology
Co-Director M3 and M4 Student Programs
Department of Medicine
University of Wisconsin
School of Medicine & Public Health
Madison, Wisconsin

Laura Meinke, MD
Assistant Professor of Medicine
Medicine Clerkship Director
Section of Pulmonary & Critical Care Medicine
University of Arizona College of Medicine
Tucson, Arizona

James L. Meisel, MD, FACP
Clerkship Director/Evans Student Educator
Assistant Professor of Medicine
Boston University School of Medicine
Boston, Massachusetts

Chad S. Miller, MD, FACP
Internal Medicine Clerkship Director
Associate Program Director, Residency
Tulane University Health Sciences Center
New Orleans, Louisiana

Nina Mingioni, MD FACP
Associate Program Director, Internal Medicine
Clerkship Site Director, Internal Medicine
Albert Einstein Medical Center
Philadelphia, Pennsylvania

Alita Mishra, MD, FACP
Clerkship Director, Department of Medicine
Hospitalist, Inova Fairfax Hospital
Clinical Assistant Professor of Medicine
Virginia Commonwealth University School of Medicine
Inova Campus
Falls Church, Virginia

Archana Mishra, MD, MS, FACP, FCCP
Associate Professor of Medicine
Associate Clerkship Director
SUNY Buffalo School of Medicine and Biomedical Sciences
Buffalo, New York

Lynda Misra, DO, FACP, MA Ed
Director of Students - William Beaumont Hospital
Medicine Clerkship Director
Oakland University William Beaumont School of Medicine
Royal Oak, Michigan

Neha Mittal, MD
Assistant Professor
Year 4 Clerkship Director
Department of Internal Medicine
Texas Tech University Health Science Center
Lubbock, Texas

Justin B. Moore, MD
Division Chief, Endocrinology
Assistant Professor, Department of Medicine
Medicine Clerkship Co-Director
University of Kansas School of Medicine-Wichita
Wichita, Kansas

Mark T. Munekata, MD, MPH, FACP
Associate Clinical Professor of Medicine
Co-Director, Ambulatory Internal Medicine Clerkship
David Geffen School of Medicine at UCLA
Medical Director, Utilization Management
Director, Urgent Care Clinic
Harbor-UCLA Medical Center
Torrance, California

Marty Muntz, MD
Assistant Professor of Medicine
Division of General Internal Medicine
Ambulatory Medicine Clerkship Director
Medicine Subinternship Director
Medical College of Wisconsin
Milwaukee, Wisconsin

David G. Naylor, MD
Assistant Clerkship Director
University of Kansas Medical Center
Kansas City, Kansas

Adesoji E. Oderinde, MD, MSCR, FACP
Associate Program Director
Associate Director Student Education
Department of Medicine
Morehouse School of Medicine
Atlanta, Georgia

Thomas D. Painter MD
Inpatient Internal Medicine Clerkship Director
University of Pittsburgh School of Medicine
Pittsburgh, Pennsylvania

Carlos Palacio, MD, MPH, FACP
Associate Professor of Medicine, Department of Medicine
Clerkship Director
University of Florida College of Medicine-Jacksonville
Jacksonville, Florida

Robert I. Pargament, MD, FACP
Internal Medicine Clerkship Director
York Hospital
York, Pennsylvania

Alisa Peet, MD
Assistant Professor of Medicine
Medicine Clerkship Director
Temple University School of Medicine
Philadelphia, Pennsylvania

Roshini C. Pinto-Powell, MD
Associate Professor of Medicine
Dartmouth Medical School
Lebanon, New Hampshire

Suma Pokala, MD, FACP
Associate Professor, Department of Medicine
Texas A&M Health Sciences Center
Central Texas Veterans Health Care System
Temple, Texas

Hari Raja, MD, FACP
Professor of Medicine
Clerkship Director
Department of Internal Medicine
UT Southwestern Medical Center
Dallas, Texas

Temple A. Ratcliffe, MD
Assistant Professor of Medicine
Assistant Clerkship Director
F. Edward Hébert School of Medicine
Uniformed Services University of the Health Sciences
Bethesda, Maryland

Emran Rouf, MD, FACP
Assistant Professor, Department of Medicine
Scott & White Healthcare
Texas A & M Health Science Center College of Medicine
Temple, Texas

Gary M. Rull, MD, FACP
Associate Professor of Clinical Internal Medicine
Doctoring Director
Department of Internal Medicine
Southern Illinois University School of Medicine
Springfield, Illinois

James L. Sebastian, MD, FACP
Professor of Medicine
Division of General Internal Medicine
Medical College of Wisconsin
Milwaukee, Wisconsin

Thomas K. Schulz, MD
Associate Program Director,
Internal Medicine Residency Program
Associate Professor
University of Kansas School of Medicine-Wichita
Wichita, Kansas

Monica Ann Shaw, MD, FACP
Associate Professor of Medicine
Chief, Division of General Internal Medicine
Director, Internal Medicine Clerkships
University of Louisville School of Medicine
Louisville, Kentucky

Leigh H. Simmons, MD
Assistant in Medicine
Associate Medicine Clerkship Director
Massachusetts General Hospital
Harvard Medical School
Boston, Massachusetts

Harold M. Szerlip, MD, FACP, FCCP, FASN
Professor and Vice-Chair, Department of Medicine
Chief, Medical Service, UPH Hospital
University of Arizona College of Medicine
Tucson, Arizona

Heather Tarantino, MD
Assistant Professor
Medicine Clerkship Director
West Virginia University School of Medicine
Charleston Division
Charleston, West Virginia

Robert L. Trowbridge, MD, FACP
Assistant Professor of Medicine
Tufts University School of Medicine
Director of Undergraduate Medical Education
Department of Medicine
Maine Medical Center
Portland, Maine

John Varras, MD
Associate Professor
Interim Chair
Clerkship Director
Department of Internal Medicine
University of Nevada School of Medicine
Las Vegas, Nevada

T. Robert Vu, MD, FACP
Associate Professor of Clinical Medicine
Director, Internal Medicine Clerkship
Indiana University School of Medicine
Indianapolis, Indiana

Joseph T. Wayne, MD, MPH, FACP
Internal Medicine Clerkship Director
Department of Internal Medicine
Albany Medical College
Albany, New York

Barry J. Wu, MD, FACP
Associate Program Director of Internal Medicine
Hospital of Saint Raphael
Clinical Professor of Medicine
Yale University School of Medicine
New Haven, Connecticut

Parekha Yedla, MBBS, FACP
Assistant Professor, Department of Medicine
Medicine Clerkship Director
University of Alabama, Huntsville Campus
Huntsville, Alabama

MKSAP for Students 5 Contributors

Arlina Ahluwalia, MD, FACP
Associate Professor of Medicine
Medicine Clerkship Site Director, Palo Alto VAHCS
Stanford University School of Medicine
Palo Alto, California

Erik K. Alexander, MD, FACP
Director, Medical Student Education
Brigham & Women's Hospital
Associate Professor of Medicine
Harvard Medical School
Boston, Massachusetts

Irene Alexandraki, MD, MPH, FACP
Assistant Professor, Department of Medicine
Medicine Clerkship Director
University of Florida College of Medicine
Jacksonville, Florida

Mark Allee, MD, FACP
Associate Professor of Medicine
Clerkship Director
Department of Internal Medicine
University of Oklahoma College of Medicine
Oklahoma City, Oklahoma

Alpesh Amin, MD, MBA, FACP
Professor of Medicine
Medicine Clerkship Director
University of California, Irvine
Orange, California

Joel Appel, DO
Director, Ambulatory and Subinternship Programs
Wayne State University School of Medicine
Detroit, Michigan

Jonathan S. Appelbaum, MD, FACP
Associate Professor, Clinical Sciences Department
Director, Internal Medicine Education
Florida State University College of Medicine
Tallahassee, Florida

MJ Barchman, MD, FACP, FASN
Professor of Medicine
Internal Medicine Clerkship Director
Section of Nephrology and Hypertension
Brody School of Medicine at East Carolina University
Greenville, North Carolina

Gonzalo Bearman, MD, MPH
Associate Professor of Medicine
Associate Hospital Epidemiologist
Medicine Clerkship Director
Virginia Commonwealth University
Richmond, Virginia

Seth Mark Berney, MD, FACP
Professor of Medicine
Chief, Section of Rheumatology
Director, Center of Excellence for Arthritis and
    Rheumatology
Louisiana State University Health Sciences Center School of
    Medicine in Shreveport
Shreveport, Louisiana

Jennifer Bierman, MD, FACP
Primary Care Clerkship Director
Northwestern University Feinberg School of Medicine
Chicago, Illinois

Cynthia A. Burns, MD, FACP
Assistant Professor
Internal Medicine Clerkship Director
Department of Internal Medicine
Section on Endocrinology & Metabolism
Wake Forest University School of Medicine
Winston Salem, North Carolina

Danelle Cayea, MD, MS
Assistant Professor of Medicine
Medicine Clerkship Director
Johns Hopkins University School of Medicine
Baltimore, Maryland

J. Charles MD, FACP, FHM
Assistant Professor of Medicine
Division Education Coordinator
Mayo Clinic Hospital
Phoenix, Arizona

Amanda Cooper, MD
Assistant Professor of Medicine
University of Pittsburgh Medical Center
University of Pittsburgh School of Medicine
Pittsburgh, Pennsylvania

Mark D. Corriere, MD, FACP
Associate Clerkship Director, Department of Medicine
Uniformed Services University of the Health Sciences
Bethesda, Maryland

Gretchen Diemer, MD, FACP
Assistant Professor of Internal Medicine
Clerkship Director Internal Medicine
Director of Undergraduate Medical Education
Associate Program Director Internal Medicine
Thomas Jefferson University
Philadelphia, Pennsylvania

Reed E. Drews, MD, FACP
Associate Professor
Harvard Medical School
Program Director, Hematology-Oncology Fellowship
Beth Israel Deaconess Medical Center
Boston, Massachusetts

D. Michael Elnicki, MD, FACP
Professor and Chief, Section of General Internal Medicine,
    UPMC Shadyside
Ambulatory Clerkship Director
University of Pittsburgh
Pittsburgh, Pennsylvania

Mark J. Fagan, MD, FACP
Clerkship Director
Department of Medicine
Alpert Medical School of Brown University
Providence, Rhode Island

Sara B. Fazio, MD, FACP
Associate Professor, Harvard Medical School
Director, Core I Medicine Clerkship
Division of General Internal Medicine
Beth Israel Deaconess Medical Center
Boston, Massachusetts

J. Michael Finley, DO, FACP, FACOI
Associate Professor of Medicine
Chief, Division of Rheumatology
Associate Dean for Graduate Medical Education
Western University College of Osteopathic Medicine
Pomona, California

Jane P. Gagliardi, MD, MHS
Assistant Professor of Psychiatry & Behavioral Sciences
Assistant Professor of Medicine
Director of UME, Department of Medicine
Medicine Clerkship and Subinternship Director
Duke University School of Medicine
Durham, North Carolina

Peter Gliatto, MD, FACP
Associate Dean for Undergraduate Medical Education
    and Student Affairs
Mount Sinai School of Medicine
New York, New York

Eric H. Green MD, MSc, FACP
Clinical Associate Professor of Medicine
Drexel University College of Medicine
Associate Program Director
Mercy Catholic Medical Center
Darby, Pennsylvania

Heather Harrell, MD, FACP
Associate Professor, Department of Medicine
Medicine Clerkship Director
Director of Fourth Year Programs
University of Florida College of Medicine
Gainesville, Florida

Warren Hershman, MD, MPH
Director of Student Education
Boston University School of Medicine
Department of Medicine
Boston, Massachusetts

Susan Thompson Hingle, MD, FACP
Associate Professor of Medicine
Internal Medicine Clerkship Director
Internal Medicine Residency Associate Program Director
Southern Illinois University School of Medicine
Springfield, Illinois

Bryan Ho, MD
Assistant Professor, Department of Neurology
Neurology Clerkship Director
Tufts University School of Medicine
Boston, Massachusetts

Mark D. Holden, MD, FACP
Vice-Chair for Undergraduate Education
Department of Internal Medicine
University of Texas Medical Branch
Galveston, Texas

Jeffrey Guy House, DO, FACP
Assistant Professor of Medicine
Program Director Internal Medicine Residency
University of Florida Health Science Center-Jacksonville
Jacksonville, Florida

Eric Hsieh, MD
Director, Internal Medicine Clerkship
Senior Associate Director, Internal Medicine Residency
Department of Medicine
Keck School of Medicine
University of Southern California
Los Angeles, California

Robert Jablonover, MD
Assistant Professor in Internal Medicine
Clerkship Director in Internal Medicine
George Washington University School of Medicine
Washington, District of Columbia

Saba Khan, MD
Fellow, Section of Rheumatology
Louisiana State University Health Sciences Center
School of Medicine in Shreveport
Shreveport, Louisiana

Sarang Kim, MD, FACP
Assistant Professor of Medicine
Division of General Internal Medicine
University of Medicine and Dentistry of New Jersey,
    Robert Wood Johnson Medical School
New Brunswick, New Jersey

Valerie J. Lang, MD, FACP
Director, Inpatient Medicine Clerkship
University of Rochester School of Medicine & Dentistry
Hospital Medicine Division
Rochester, New York

Rosa Lee, MD
Clinical Assistant Professor, Department of Medicine
Albert Einstein College of Medicine
Site Leader, Medicine Clerkship
Montefiore Medical Center
Bronx, New York

Bruce Leff, MD, FACP
Professor of Medicine
Co-Director, Basic Medicine Clerkship
Johns Hopkins University School of Medicine
Baltimore, Maryland

Kyle L. Lokitz, MD
Fellow, Section of Rheumatology
Louisiana State University Health Sciences Center
School of Medicine in Shreveport
Shreveport, Louisiana

Fred A. Lopez, MD, FACP
Richard Vial Professor and Vice Chair
Department of Medicine
Louisiana State University Health Sciences Center
New Orleans, Louisiana

Kevin M. McKown, MD, FACP
Associate Professor and Head, Division of Rheumatology
Co-Director M3 and M4 Student Programs
Department of Medicine
University of Wisconsin
School of Medicine & Public Health
Madison, Wisconsin

Chad S. Miller, MD, FACP
Director, Student Programs
Associate Program Director, Residency
Department of Internal Medicine
Tulane University Health Sciences Center
New Orleans, Louisiana

Katherine Nickerson, MD
Professor of Clinical Medicine
Vice Chair, Department of Medicine
Clerkship Director, Internal Medicine
College of Physicians & Surgeons
Columbia University
New York, New York

L. James Nixon, MD
Vice Chair for Education, Department of Medicine
Medicine Clerkship Director
University of Minnesota Medical School
Minneapolis, Minnesota

Isaac O. Opole, MD, PhD, FACP
Assistant Dean for Student Affairs
Internal Medicine Clerkship Director
Kansas University Medical Center
Kansas City, Kansas

Carlos Palacio, MD, MPH, FACP
Associate Professor of Medicine, Department of Medicine
Clerkship Director
University of Florida College of Medicine-Jacksonville
Jacksonville, Florida

Suma Pokala, MD, FACP
Associate Professor, Department of Medicine
Texas A&M Health Sciences Center
Central Texas Veterans Health Care System
Temple, Texas

Nora L. Porter, MD, MPH, FACP
Co-director, Internal Medicine Clerkship
Saint Louis University School of Medicine
St. Louis, Missouri

Shalini Reddy, MD
Associate Dean
Student Programs and Professional Development
The University of Chicago Pritzker School of Medicine
Chicago, Illinois

Klara J. Rosenquist, MD
Clinical/Research Fellow
Division of Endocrinology, Diabetes and Hypertension
Brigham & Women's Hospital
Harvard Medical School
Boston, Massachusetts

Kathleen F. Ryan, MD, FACP
Associate Professor of Medicine
Department of Medicine
Drexel University College of Medicine
Philadelphia, Pennsylvania

Mysti D. W. Schott, MD, FACP
Associate Professor of Medicine
Course Director, Advanced Clinical Evaluation Skills
Department of Medicine, Division of General Medicine
     & Office of Educational Programs
University of Texas Health Science Center San Antonio
San Antonio, Texas

Amy Wiegner Shaheen, MD
Ambulatory Medicine Clerkship Director
University of North Carolina School of Medicine
Chapel Hill, North Carolina

Monica Ann Shaw, MD, FACP
Associate Professor and Chief
Division of General Internal Medicine, Palliative
Medicine and Medical Education
Medicine Clerkship Director
University of Louisville
Louisville, Kentucky

Patricia Short, MD, FACP
Assistant Professor of Medicine
Associate Clerkship Director
Uniformed Services University of the Health Sciences
Madigan Army Medical Center
Tacoma, Washington

Karen Szauter, MD, FACP
Professor
Department of Internal Medicine and Office of
     Educational Development
Co-Director, Internal Medicine Clerkship
University of Texas Medical Branch
Galveston, Texas

Harold M. Szerlip, MD, FACP, FCCP, FASN
Professor and Vice-Chair, Department of Medicine
Chief, Medical Service, UPH Hospital
University of Arizona College of Medicine
Tucson, Arizona

Gary Tabas, MD, FACP
Associate Professor of Medicine
University of Pittsburgh School of Medicine
Pittsburgh, Pennsylvania

Dario M. Torre, MD, MPH, PhD, FACP
Associate Professor of Medicine
Associate Program Director Internal Medicine University
    of Pittsburgh-Shadyside
University of Pittsburgh School of Medicine
Pittsburgh, Pennsylvania

John Varras, MD
Associate Professor
Interim Chair
Clerkship Director
Department of Internal Medicine
University of Nevada School of Medicine
Las Vegas, Nevada

H. Douglas Walden, MD, MPH, FACP
Professor of Medicine
Co-Director, Internal Medicine Clerkship
Saint Louis University School of Medicine
St. Louis, Missouri

John A. Walker, MD, FACP
Professor and Vice-Chair for Education
Department of Medicine
Medicine Clerkship Director
University of Medicine and Dentistry of New Jersey
Robert Wood Johnson Medical School
New Brunswick, New Jersey

Joseph T. Wayne, MD, MPH, FACP
Internal Medicine Clerkship Director
Department of Internal Medicine
Albany Medical College
Albany, New York

John Jason White, MD, FASN
Associate Professor of Medicine
Section of Nephrology, Hypertension & Transplantation
Georgia Health Sciences University
Augusta, Georgia

The American College of Physicians gratefully acknowledges the contributions to *MKSAP for Students* 5 of Scott Hurd (production systems), Lisa Rockey (editorial production support), Rosemarie Houton (editorial production support) and the Self-Assessment editorial staff. The College also wishes to acknowledge that many other persons, too numerous to mention, have contributed to the production of this product. Without their dedicated efforts, the publication would not have been possible.

Foreword

Dear Student:

    As the national organization for internal medicine specialists and subspecialists, the American College of Physicians is committed to providing the highest quality educational materials and resources throughout the continuum of training and practice in internal medicine. Early in that continuum are the clinical clerkships in internal medicine for students during their third and fourth years of medical school. Recognizing the critical importance of these clerkships for all students – whether or not they plan to enter the specialty of internal medicine – the College has been collaborating with the Clerkship Directors in Internal Medicine to develop and produce two publications specifically targeted to medical students on their internal medicine clerkships.

    This publication, *MKSAP for Students,* now in its 5th edition, employs an interactive, case-based model of topic-based questions (with accompanying answers and critiques) to teach students about the major clinical problems in internal medicine. The companion publication, *Internal Medicine Essentials for Medical Students,* nicely complements *MKSAP for Students,* providing a concise text that can be read from cover to cover during an internal medicine clerkship. Both *MKSAP for Students* and *Internal Medicine Essentials* are modeled after the much larger *Medical Knowledge Self-Assessment Program (MKSAP),* which has served for the past 43 years (and through 15 editions) as the gold standard for residents preparing for the certifying examination in internal medicine and for practicing physicians who wish to refresh, update, and assess their knowledge.

    Internal medicine is an exciting and intellectually stimulating specialty. We hope that *MKSAP for Students* will reinforce that feeling for you, enriching your clinical experiences and serving as a useful companion as you learn the fundamental concepts of the specialty and apply them in clinical settings. Remember, the knowledge we gain is not just abstract learning – it provides the foundation for the care of our patients, who deserve only the best!

    Best of luck to you in your studies and in your future career.

Steven E. Weinberger, MD, FACP
Executive Vice President and Chief Operating Officer
American College of Physicians

Preface

Welcome to the newest edition of *MKSAP for Students*. The fifth edition of this popular series contains over **450 completely new** multiple-choice questions, updated references, more color photographs and ECG tracings than ever before. *MKSAP for Students* is intended primarily for third-year students participating in their required internal medicine clerkship. Other audiences include fourth-year students on an advanced medicine clerkship; second-year students involved in problem-based learning; and physician assistant students.

MKSAP for Students 5 is supported by its companion textbook, *Internal Medicine Essentials for Students*. Authors who contributed to the *Essentials* textbook also wrote questions for *MKSAP for Students*. Additional questions were written by internal medicine clerkship directors. Like *Essentials*, *MKSAP for Students 5* is organized into 11 chapters that correspond to the traditional subspecialty disciplines of internal medicine and general internal medicine. The editors and authors have made every effort to ensure that all questions in *MKSAP for Students* are associated with relevant content in the textbook that can directly answer the question. This allows a one-to-one correspondence between the textbook and the self-assessment questions.

As in previous issues, the questions are formatted as clinical vignettes that resemble the types of questions you will encounter at the end of the clerkship subject examination and the internal medicine component of the USMLE licensing examination. Each question has a detailed answer critique that identifies the correct answer and explains why that answer is correct and the other options are incorrect, an educational objective, and a short bibliography. Succinct "Key Points" summarize the important "take-home messages" for each question. We anticipate that reviewing the "Key Points" will be an efficient way to prepare for upcoming examinations. We recommend that students read the clinical vignette, select an answer, and then read the associated answer critique. Each question has been specifically reviewed by at least three clerkship directors to ensure that it meets the learning needs of students participating in the medicine clerkship.

New to this edition is a categorization scheme for the self-assessment questions. All questions are categorized as either Advanced (A) or Basic (B) by the *MKSAP for Students* Editorial Board, which consists entirely of clerkship directors. Advanced questions are difficult and assess knowledge expected of an honors-level student or beginning first-year internal medicine resident. Basic questions assess knowledge expected of all third-year students completing the basic internal medicine clerkship. It is our expectation that clerkship students will be able to answer most of the Basic questions and approximately half of the Advanced questions. We hope that this new system will provide students with a better measure of their knowledge acquisition.

The fifth edition of *MKSAP for Students* would have been impossible without the valuable and entirely voluntary contributions of many people, some of whom are named in the Acknowledgments section. Others, not specifically named, were representatives of a wide spectrum of constituencies and organizations, such as the Clerkship Directors in Internal Medicine and various committees within the American College of Physicians, including the Education and Publication Committee and the Council of Student Members.

As in the past, we hope to receive more excellent feedback from students to improve future editions. Thank you for making *MKSAP for Students* such a success!

Patrick C. Alguire, MD, FACP
Editor-in-Chief
Senior Vice President for Medical Education
American College of Physicians

Note: The drug dosage schedules contained in this publication are, we believe, accurate and in accordance with current standards. However, please ensure that the recommended dosages concur with information provided in the product information material, especially for new, infrequently used, or highly toxic drugs.

Contents

Section 1

Cardiovascular Medicine

Questions

Item 1 [Basic]

A 66-year-old man is evaluated in the emergency department for left-sided chest pain that began at rest, lasted for 15 minutes, and has since resolved. A similar episode occurred at rest yesterday. Pertinent medical history includes hypertension and type 2 diabetes mellitus. Current medications are amlodipine, glyburide, and aspirin.

On physical examination, blood pressure is 125/65 mm Hg, heart rate is 70/min, and respiratory rate is 12/min. Estimated central venous pressure is 6 cm H_2O, carotid upstroke is normal, there are no cardiac murmurs, and the lung fields are clear.

Laboratory findings include an elevated serum troponin I level. Electrocardiogram is shown. Chest radiograph is normal.

Which of the following is the most likely diagnosis?

(A) Chronic stable angina
(B) Non–ST-elevation myocardial infarction
(C) ST-elevation myocardial infarction
(D) Unstable angina

Item 2 [Basic]

A 63-year-old woman is admitted to the hospital with pleuritic chest pain, diaphoresis, and dyspnea of 1 hour's duration. The pain is not affected by food, antacids, or exertion. It may be worse when supine and with deep breathing. She has a 10-year history of hypertension and hyperlipidemia. Her medications are chlorthalidone and lovastatin.

On physical examination, temperature is 37.8°C (100.0°F), blood pressure is 145/90 mm Hg (both arms), heart rate is 108/min, and respiration rate is 22/min. Cardiovascular examination reveals a regular rhythm and a biphasic, scratchy sound best heard at the lower left sternal border. No murmur, S_3, or S_4 is heard. The lungs are clear to auscultation. The jugular venous pressure is normal and no peripheral edema is noted.

The electrocardiogram shows sinus tachycardia with diffuse ST elevation. Troponin level and chest radiograph findings are normal.

Which of the following is the most likely diagnosis?

(A) Acute myocardial infarction
(B) Acute pericarditis
(C) Aortic dissection
(D) Pulmonary embolism

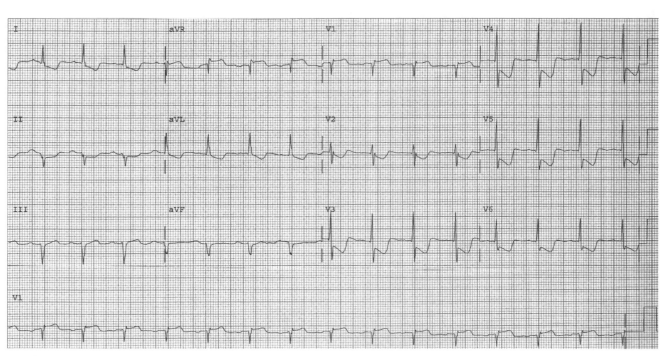

Item 1

1

Item 3 [Basic]

A 78-year-old man is evaluated in the emergency department for new-onset chest pain. He describes a crushing pain that is located in the left substernal area and has been present for 10 hours. He has had no prior episodes of chest pain. His medical history is notable for hypertension and hyperlipidemia. Current medications are aspirin, hydrochlorothiazide, and atorvastatin.

On physical examination, blood pressure is 100/70 mm Hg in both arms, pulse is 100/min, and respiration rate is 16/min. There is no jugular venous distention and no cardiac murmurs or rubs. The lungs are clear.

Laboratory results are notable for elevated levels of serum creatine kinase and troponin I. The initial electrocardiogram is shown. Chest radiograph is normal.

Which of the following is the best management for this patient?

(A) Chest CT with contrast
(B) Echocardiogram
(C) Percutaneous coronary intervention
(D) Thrombolytic therapy

Item 4 [Basic]

A 50-year-old man is evaluated for a 2-hour episode of epigastric discomfort and dyspnea during exercise that is relieved by rest. He is now pain free. The patient states a similar episode occurred on three previous occasions, but he did not seek medical advice. He has been using antacids for the past 6 weeks with partial relief. He reports no fever, chills, nausea, vomiting, diaphoresis, or postprandial abdominal pain. He has a 15-year history of hypertension and hyperlipidemia; his only medication is chlorthalidone.

On physical examination, he is afebrile, blood pressure is 150/85 mm Hg, pulse rate is 88/min, and respiration rate is 14/min. BMI is 28. Estimated central venous pressure is normal. Cardiac examination reveals a regular rhythm. The S_2 is normal, and an S_4 is heard at the apex; no murmurs or other extracardiac sounds are heard. The lungs are clear to auscultation. The abdomen is not tender to palpation.

Complete blood count and troponin level are normal as are the electrocardiogram and chest radiograph.

Which of the following is the most likely diagnosis?

(A) Acute pericarditis
(B) Aortic dissection
(C) Ischemic heart disease
(D) Peptic ulcer disease

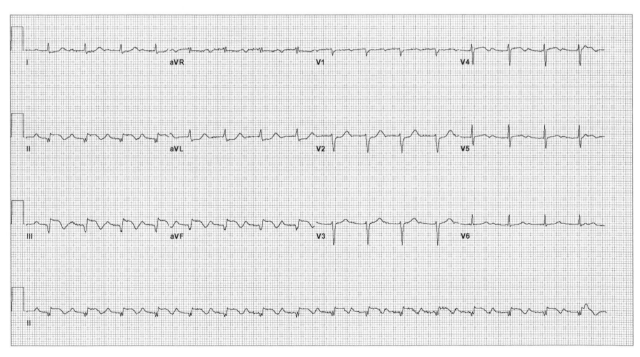

Item 3

Item 5 [Advanced]

A 52-year-old woman is evaluated in the emergency department for ongoing substernal chest pressure associated with nausea, diaphoresis, and lightheadedness. Her symptoms began 3 hours ago. She has hypertension and hypercholesterolemia. Her medications are hydrochlorothiazide, pravastatin, and aspirin.

On physical examination, her blood pressure is 84/62 mm Hg, pulse is 68/min, and respiration rate is 20/min. Cardiac auscultation reveals distant heart sounds with an S_4. The lungs are clear bilaterally; estimated central venous pressure is elevated at 11 cm H_2O.

Electrocardiogram with right-sided precordial leads is shown. (Leads V_1 through V_6 are recorded from the right side of the chest.)

Which of the following should be given next in the treatment of this patient?

(A) Dobutamine intravenously
(B) Metoprolol intravenously
(C) Nitroglycerin sublingually
(D) 0.9% saline intravenous bolus

Item 6 [Basic]

A 58-year-old woman is evaluated in the emergency department for substernal chest pain of 18 hours' duration. She describes the pain as a tightening that is not associated with eating or exertion and that radiates to the neck. The pain is not accompanied by dyspnea, nausea, or diaphoresis and is not associated with exertion. She also reports symptoms of occasional heartburn and acid regurgitation. She had a similar episode of substernal chest pain 1 month ago, and an exercise stress test that achieved 90% her predicted maximal heart rate showed no ischemia. The patient's medical history is otherwise unremarkable.

On physical examination, temperature is 37.2°C (99.0°F), blood pressure is 130/74 mm Hg, pulse rate is 88/min, and respiration rate is 16/min; BMI is 32. The cardiopulmonary examination is normal. Electrocardiography shows nonspecific ST-segment and T-wave abnormalities, which are unchanged from several previous examinations.

Which of the following is the most appropriate management for this patient?

(A) Ambulatory esophageal pH monitoring
(B) Coronary angiography
(C) Esophagogastroduodenoscopy
(D) Oral proton pump inhibitor therapy
(E) Repeat exercise stress test

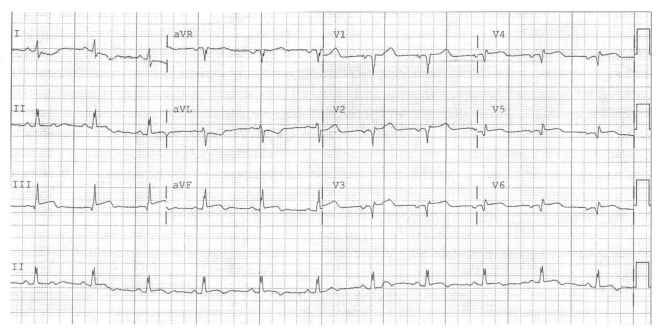

Item 5

Item 7 [Advanced]

A 22-year-old man is evaluated during the month of June in the emergency department for intermittent palpitations and dizziness for the past week. He has not experienced chest pain, dyspnea, or orthopnea. He has no prior medical history and is healthy and active. He reports being ill 6 to 8 weeks ago with fever, fatigue, myalgia, and a gradually expanding, flat, erythematous rash on his abdomen measuring a minimum of 5 cm at widest point. He works as a forester in Massachusetts and has not traveled out of the area recently.

On physical examination, his temperature is normal, blood pressure is 120/70 mm Hg, and pulse is 45/min. There are cannon waves in the jugular pulsation. There is no rash, and results of cardiac and pulmonary auscultation are normal.

The electrocardiogram is shown.

Which of the following is the most likely diagnosis?

(A) First-degree atrioventricular block
(B) Mobitz type I atrioventricular block
(C) Mobitz type II atrioventricular block
(D) Third-degree atrioventricular heart block

Item 8 [Basic]

A 46-year-old man is evaluated for an 8-year history of episodic chest pain associated with dyspnea, tachycardia, diaphoresis, and dizziness that occurs several times each week. The symptoms develop suddenly, are often so severe that he feels that he is going to die, and improve significantly within 20 to 30 minutes. The patient does not know what precipitates these episodes or whether anything makes the symptoms better or worse.

Previous medical evaluations have been unremarkable. Studies have included electrocardiographic exercise stress testing, 24-hour electrocardiographic monitoring, echocardiography, cardiac catheterization, and upper endoscopy. The patient takes no medications. Findings on physical examination are unremarkable. Medical records reveal that during these episodes, hypertension or tachycardia have never been documented.

Which of the following is the most likely diagnosis?

(A) Acute coronary syndrome
(B) Panic disorder
(C) Pheochromocytoma
(D) Pneumothorax
(E) Pulmonary embolism

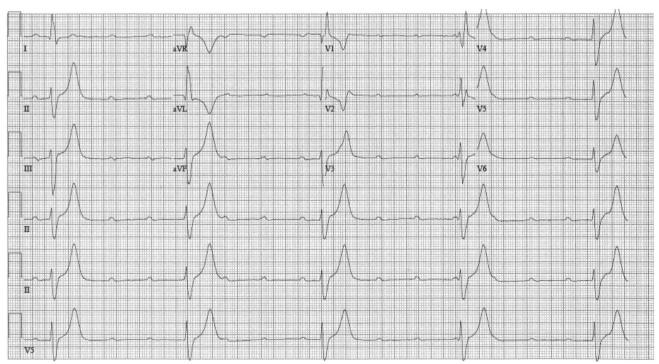

Item 7

Item 9 [Basic]

A 65-year-old woman is hospitalized for chest pain secondary to an acute coronary syndrome. Her immediate treatment consists of metoprolol, heparin, nitroglycerin, and aspirin, which results in immediate relief of her chest discomfort. A rhythm strip is shown.

Which of the following is the most likely electrocardiographic diagnosis?

(A) First-degree atrioventricular block
(B) Mobitz type I second-degree atrioventricular block
(C) Mobitz type II second-degree atrioventricular block
(D) Third-degree atrioventricular block (complete heart block)

Item 11 [Advanced]

A 48-year-old woman is evaluated in the emergency department 3 hours after the sudden onset of central anterior chest pain and dyspnea. There is constant chest pressure, tightness, and dyspnea. She is not on any medications.

On physical examination, the patient is afebrile. Blood pressure is 144/76 mm Hg bilaterally, pulse is 118/min, and respiration rate is 18/min. Estimated central venous pressure is 15 cm H_2O. There are no murmurs, rubs, or gallops on cardiac auscultation. Her lungs are clear. There is mild pedal and lower leg edema that is more pronounced on the right side.

The electrocardiogram shows ST-segment depression in the lateral leads. The chest radiograph is normal. Handheld echocardiography shows a small, hyperdynamic left ventricle with normal regional wall motion.

Which of the following tests should be performed next?

(A) CT pulmonary angiography
(B) Coronary angiography
(C) Radionuclide perfusion imaging
(D) Transesophageal echocardiography

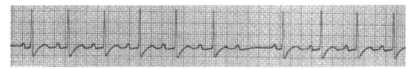

Item 9

Item 10 [Advanced]

A 65-year-old man is evaluated during a routine follow-up examination for coronary artery disease. He was diagnosed with a myocardial infarction 5 years ago, and was started on aspirin, metoprolol, atorvastatin, lisinopril, and sublingual nitroglycerin. He was asymptomatic until 3 months ago, when he noted exertional angina after walking two blocks. He now uses sublingual nitroglycerin on a daily basis. He has not had any episodes of pain at rest or prolonged chest pain that were not relieved by sublingual nitroglycerin.

On physical examination, blood pressure is 146/94 mm Hg and heart rate is 87/min. Carotid upstrokes are normal with no bruits. Cardiac examination is normal. The lungs are clear.

His electrocardiogram is unchanged since the last visit, with no evidence of acute changes.

In addition to adding a long-acting nitrate, which of the following is the most appropriate management for this patient?

(A) Add ranolazine
(B) Coronary angiography
(C) Exercise treadmill stress testing
(D) Increase metoprolol

Item 12 [Basic]

A 68-year-old woman is evaluated for chest pain of 3 months' duration. She describes the pain as a left-sided burning that occurs both at rest and when she exercises. It lasts for about 10 minutes, and is relieved by eating and by rest. She has hypertension, for which she takes hydrochlorothiazide. She has asthma, for which she takes inhaled corticosteroids and inhaled albuterol as needed. If she pretreats herself with the inhaled bronchodilator, she can walk long distances at a brisk pace without dyspnea. She continues to smoke cigarettes and has smoked 1 pack per day for 40 years.

On physical examination, she is afebrile. Blood pressure is 138/84 mm Hg, pulse is 64/min, and respiration rate is 18/min. Cardiopulmonary examination is normal. The results of an electrocardiogram are normal.

Which of the following is the most appropriate diagnostic test for this patient?

(A) Adenosine nuclear perfusion stress test
(B) Coronary angiography
(C) Dobutamine stress echocardiography
(D) Exercise stress test

Item 13 [Basic]

A 54-year-old man is evaluated for 2 days of fatigue and dyspnea on exertion. He denies chest pain and lightheadedness. He has no other medical problems, and his only medication is aspirin.

On physical examination, his blood pressure is 123/65 mm Hg and his pulse is 100/min. Cardiac examination reveals a normal S_1 and S_2 and no murmurs or gallops. Lungs are clear to auscultation.

The electrocardiogram is shown.

Which of the following is the most likely diagnosis?

(A) Atrial fibrillation
(B) Atrial flutter
(C) Sinoatrial node dysfunction
(D) Ventricular tachycardia

Item 14 [Basic]

A 75-year-old man with chronic stable angina is evaluated during a routine appointment. He had a myocardial infarction 5 years ago treated medically and has had no complications. He only gets chest pain with significant exertion, typically occurring less than once a week. The pain is relieved by one sublingual nitroglycerin tablet or resting. He reports no shortness of breath or edema. Medications are lisinopril, carvedilol, simvastatin, aspirin, and nitroglycerin, as needed.

On examination, temperature is 37.0°C (98.6°F), blood pressure is 118/70 mm Hg, pulse rate is 60/min, and respiration rate is 14/min. BMI is 22. Cardiovascular examination reveals normal heart sounds without murmurs, gallops, or rubs. Lungs are clear to auscultation. The remainder of the examination is normal.

Total cholesterol	140 mg/dL (3.6 mmol/L)
Triglycerides	100 mg/dL (1.1 mmol/L)
HDL cholesterol	44 mg/dL (1.1 mmol/L)
LDL cholesterol	76 mg/dL (2.0 mmol/L)

Which of the following is the best management for this patient?

(A) Add clopidogrel
(B) Add ranolazine
(C) Coronary angiography
(D) No changes

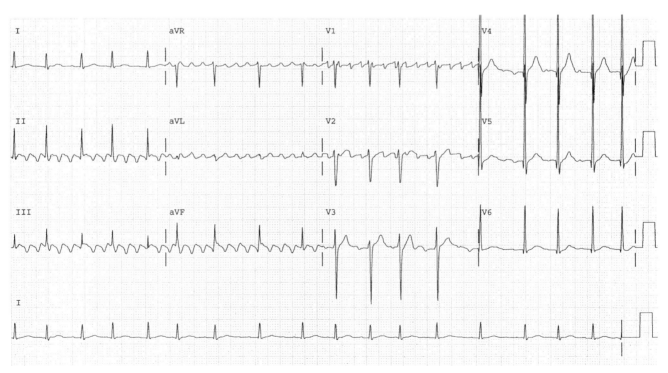

Item 13

Item 15 [Basic]

A 43-year-old man is evaluated in the emergency department for dyspnea. He has no prior personal or family history of cardiovascular disease, diabetes mellitus, or hypertension. On physical examination, the lungs are clear. Cardiovascular examination is unremarkable with the exception of a rapid heart rate.

The chest radiograph is normal. The electrocardiogram is shown.

Which of the following is the most likely diagnosis?

(A) Atrial fibrillation
(B) Atrial flutter
(C) Sinus tachycardia
(D) Ventricular tachycardia

Item 16 [Basic]

A 48-year-old man is evaluated after a coworker had a myocardial infarction; he is worried about having a heart attack. He reports no episodes of chest pain or shortness of breath. He jogs on a treadmill 30 minutes a day four times a week. He does not smoke. He has hypertension for which he takes hydrochlorothiazide. Family history is negative for coronary artery disease.

On physical examination his vital signs are normal. The cardiopulmonary examination is normal, as is the remainder of the physical examination.

The most recent lipid panel shows: total cholesterol 208 mg/dL (5.4 mmol/L), HDL cholesterol 70 mg/dL (1.8 mmol/L), and LDL cholesterol 114 mg/dL (3.0 mmol/L).

The patient's Framingham Risk Score for a major cardiac event is calculated as 4% over the next 10 years.

Which of the following is the best diagnostic test for this patient?

(A) Coronary angiography
(B) Coronary calcium scoring
(C) CT angiography
(D) Exercise stress test
(E) No additional testing

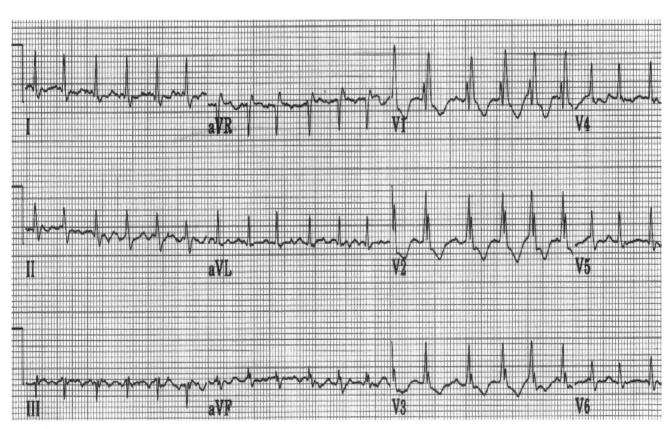

Item 15

Item 17 [Advanced]

A 26-year-old nurse is evaluated in the emergency department after an episode of syncope. While working in the intensive care unit, she developed tachycardia and then lost consciousness. She has had brief episodes of rapid palpitations in the past but no prior syncope.

Physical examination is unremarkable and the patient is in sinus rhythm. The chest radiograph is unremarkable. The electrocardiogram is shown.

Which of the following is the most likely diagnosis?

(A) Accelerated idioventricular tachycardia
(B) Atrial flutter
(C) Atrioventricular reentrant tachycardia
(D) Multifocal atrial tachycardia

Item 18 [Basic]

A 62-year-old man with coronary artery disease is evaluated for angina. He was diagnosed with coronary artery disease 4 years ago. Medical therapy was started with aspirin, metoprolol, isosorbide mononitrate, pravastatin, and sublingual nitroglycerin. He was asymptomatic until 8 months ago, when he noted exertional angina; his dosages of metoprolol and isosorbide mononitrate were increased and long-acting diltiazem was added, resulting in control of his symptoms. Over the past 2 months, however, he has had gradually increasing symptoms, and currently he requires daily nitroglycerin for angina relief during exercise. He has not had any episodes of angina at rest.

On physical examination, blood pressure is 100/60 mm Hg and heart rate is 48/min. Carotid upstroke is normal with no bruits. Cardiac examination reveals no murmurs, and the lungs are clear.

An electrocardiogram shows no acute ischemic changes.

Which of the following should be the next step in this patient's management?

(A) Coronary angiography
(B) Exercise treadmill stress testing
(C) Increase metoprolol
(D) Intravenous heparin and nitroglycerin

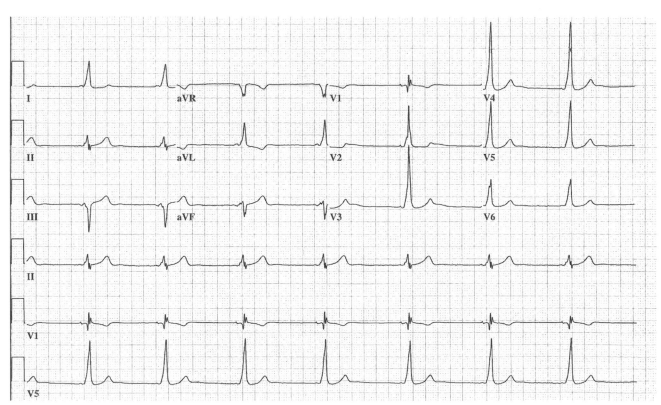

Item 17

Item 19 [Basic]

A 62-year old man with a history of a myocardial infarction 1 year ago is evaluated in the emergency department for sudden episodes of dyspnea and weakness. He is diaphoretic, cool, clammy, and pale; cannon waves are noted in the jugular pulsations. An electrocardiogram taken at the beginning of a typical episode is shown.

Which of the following is the most likely diagnosis?

(A) Atrial fibrillation with left bundle branch block
(B) Atrial fibrillation with preexcitation (Wolf-Parkinson-White syndrome)
(C) Supraventricular tachycardia with right bundle branch block
(D) Ventricular tachycardia

Item 20 [Basic]

A 54-year-old woman is evaluated in the emergency department for jaw and shoulder pain that has occurred intermittently for the past week. The symptoms occur with activity and are relieved by rest. Medical and family history is unremarkable. She is not taking any medications.

Physical examination shows a blood pressure of 150/68 mm Hg and a pulse of 90/min. There is no jugular venous distention and carotid upstrokes are normal. There are no cardiac murmurs and the lung fields are clear. Extremities show no edema and peripheral pulses are normal bilaterally. The troponin I level is elevated.

Electrocardiogram shows 1.0-mm ST-segment depression in leads V_1 through V_4 with T-wave inversions.

The patient is given aspirin, intravenous nitroglycerin, low-molecular-weight heparin, clopidogrel, and atorvastatin.

Which of the following is the most appropriate additional immediate treatment for this patient?

(A) Intra-aortic balloon pump
(B) Metoprolol
(C) Verapamil
(D) Warfarin

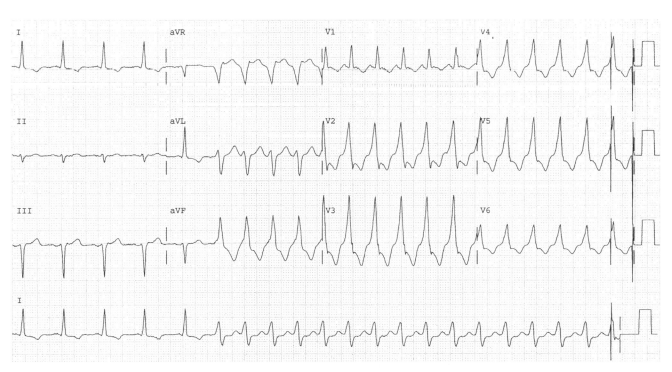

Item 19

Item 21 [Advanced]

A 72-year-old man is evaluated in the emergency department for dyspnea. One week ago, an episode of severe chest pain and dyspnea awoke him from sleep. Over the next several days his dyspnea stabilized. On the morning of admission, the patient noted a sudden increase in dyspnea. His medical history is significant for hypertension and hyperlipidemia. He has no history of heart murmur. He currently takes simvastatin, aspirin, and lisinopril.

On physical examination, the patient is sitting up with labored breathing. Blood pressure is 86/52 mm Hg, pulse is regular at 110/min, and respiration rate is 24/min. Oxygen saturation is 92% on 6 L of oxygen. Jugular veins are distended to the angle of the jaw while sitting upright. Cardiac examination reveals a grade 3/6 holosystolic murmur at the cardiac apex radiating toward the left axilla. Bibasilar crackles are present.

An electrocardiogram is shown. A chest radiograph shows pulmonary vascular congestion.

Which of the following is the most likely diagnosis?

(A) Acute mitral regurgitation
(B) Left ventricular aneurysm
(C) Pulmonary embolism
(D) Ventricular free wall rupture

Item 22 [Advanced]

A 62-year-old woman is brought to the emergency department for chest pain that has been present for 5 hours. Medical history is notable for type 2 diabetes mellitus, hyperlipidemia, and hypertension. Medications are glyburide, lisinopril, atorvastatin, and aspirin.

On physical examination, blood pressure is 160/80 mm Hg, pulse rate is 88/min, and respiration rate is 16/min. Cardiac examination shows no murmurs, extra sounds, or rubs. The lungs are clear. Neurologic examination is normal.

The electrocardiogram shows 2-mm ST-segment elevation in leads II, III, and aVF.

A coronary catheterization laboratory is not available, and the nearest hospital with percutaneous intervention capability is 3 hours away.

Which of the following is the best management option for this patient?

(A) Aggressive medical therapy without reperfusion attempt
(B) Immediate thrombolytic therapy
(C) Transfer for coronary artery bypass graft surgery
(D) Transfer for percutaneous coronary intervention

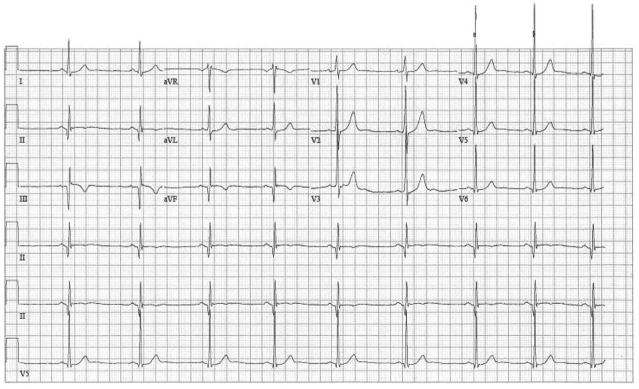

Item 21

Item 23 [Basic]

A 65-year-old man is evaluated before beginning an exercise program. He is asymptomatic and his only medical problem is chronic hypertension that is well controlled on hydrochlorothiazide. He takes no other medications.

On physical examination, blood pressure is 138/76 mm Hg, and pulse is 80/min and regular. Physical examination is normal, except for a soft S_1. His electrocardiogram is shown.

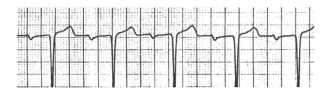

Which of the following best describes the electrocardiographic findings?

(A) First-degree atrioventricular block
(B) Second-degree atrioventricular block
(C) Third-degree (complete) atrioventricular block
(D) Ventricular preexcitation (Wolff-Parkinson-White) syndrome

Item 24 [Advanced]

A 56-year-old man is evaluated in the emergency department for chest discomfort that began 3 hours ago. He describes the pain, which is well localized to the left chest, as pressure. He denies prior episodes. Medical history is notable for type 2 diabetes mellitus and hyperlipidemia. Medications are aspirin, metformin, and atorvastatin.

On physical examination, he is diaphoretic. Blood pressure is 95/60 mm Hg and heart rate is 110/min. There is jugular venous distention, with an estimated central venous pressure of 14 cm H_2O. An S_3 is heard on cardiac auscultation, but no murmurs are present. The lung fields are clear and there is no peripheral edema.

The electrocardiogram shows sinus tachycardia, 2-mm ST-segment elevation in leads II, III, and aVF, and 0.5-mm ST-segment elevation in lead V_1. The chest radiograph is normal.

Which of the following is the most likely cause of hypotension in this patient?

(A) Increased vagal tone
(B) Pericardial tamponade
(C) Right ventricular infarction
(D) Ventricular septal defect

Item 25 [Basic]

An 85-year-old woman is admitted to the coronary care unit following successful thrombolytic therapy for an acute anteroseptal ST-elevation myocardial infarction. Blood pressure is 120/70 mm Hg and heart rate is 90/min. There is no jugular venous distention and no cardiac murmurs. The lung fields are clear. Medications started in the hospital are aspirin, low-molecular-weight heparin, intravenous nitroglycerin, and metoprolol.

On hospital day 3, the patient experiences acute onset of respiratory distress and her systolic blood pressure falls to 80 mm Hg. Her oxygen saturation remains at 80% despite the administration of 100% oxygen by face mask. On physical examination, blood pressure is 96/40 mm Hg, pulse rate is 100/min, and respiration rate is 28/min. Findings include jugular venous distention, crackles throughout both lung fields, and a grade 4/6 systolic murmur associated with a thrill.

Which of the following is the most likely diagnosis?

(A) Aortic dissection
(B) Pericardial tamponade
(C) Pulmonary embolism
(D) Ventricular septal defect

Item 26 [Advanced]

A 77-year-old woman is admitted to the hospital for intermittent dizziness over the past few days. She has hypertension, hyperlipidemia, and paroxysmal atrial fibrillation with a history of rapid ventricular response. Medications are metoprolol, hydrochlorothiazide, pravastatin, lisinopril, aspirin, and warfarin.

On physical examination, blood pressure is 137/88 mm Hg and pulse is 52/min. Estimated central venous pressure is 7 cm H_2O. Cardiac auscultation reveals bradycardia with regular S_1 and S_2, as well as an S_4. The lungs are clear to auscultation.

On telemetry, she has sinus bradycardia with rates between 40/min and 50/min, with two symptomatic sinus pauses of 3 to 5 seconds each.

Which of the following is the most likely diagnosis?

(A) Mobitz I atrioventricular block
(B) Mobitz II atrioventricular block
(C) Third-degree atrioventricular block
(D) Sinoatrial node dysfunction

Item 27 [Advanced]

A 70-year-old man is evaluated in the emergency department for bradycardia that was detected in the nursing home and is found to have second-degree atrioventricular block. The patient has Alzheimer dementia. His medications are donepezil (dosage recently increased); memantine (recently started); vitamin E; and trazodone for agitation.

Which of the patient's medications is likely to explain the bradycardia?

(A) Donepezil
(B) Memantine
(C) Trazodone
(D) Vitamin E

Item 28 [Basic]

A 67-year-old man is brought to the emergency department after he lost consciousness. His wife reports he had been experiencing palpitations and lightheadedness earlier in the day. He has hypertension, dyslipidemia, and chronic obstructive pulmonary disease. His medications are lisinopril, hydrochlorothiazide, pravastatin, and a fluticasone-salmeterol inhaler.

On physical examination, the patient is awake but confused and in respiratory distress. He is afebrile, blood pressure is 80/45 mm Hg, pulse rate is 167/min, and respiration rate is 24/min and labored. Oxygen saturation is 86% on ambient air. The cardiac rhythm is irregular, and bibasilar crackles are present on pulmonary examination.

An electrocardiogram shows atrial fibrillation.

Which of the following is the most appropriate immediate management for this patient?

(A) Bedside echocardiography
(B) CT pulmonary angiography
(C) Coronary angiography
(D) Electrical cardioversion

Item 29 [Basic]

A 62-year-old-woman is evaluated for a 6-month history of difficulty falling asleep and an unexplained 4.5-kg (10 lb) weight loss. She is active and rides her bicycle 5 miles a day. She does not drink alcohol, smoke cigarettes, or use recreational drugs. She has no other medical problems and takes no medications.

On physical examination, she is afebrile, blood pressure is 125/75 mm Hg, pulse rate is 108/min, and respiration rate is 14/min. On cardiac examination, a regular rhythm without murmurs or extra cardiac sounds is heard. The remainder of the physical examination is normal.

A metabolic profile and complete blood count are normal.

An electrocardiogram shows only sinus tachycardia.

Which of the following is the most appropriate management for this patient?

(A) Administer adenosine intravenously
(B) Measure serum thyroid-stimulating hormone level (TSH)
(C) Obtain an exercise stress test
(D) Radiofrequency ablation of the sinoatrial node

Item 30 [Advanced]

A 79-year-old man is evaluated in the emergency department for a 1-week history of dyspnea and weakness. He has had several such episodes over the past 5 years but has never sought medical attention. He reports that 1 year ago, he had a 10-minute episode of left arm weakness that resolved spontaneously. He was never evaluated for this problem. He has hypertension treated with lisinopril and hydrochlorothiazide.

On physical examination, blood pressure is 135/80 mm Hg and heart rate is 143/min. Other than a rapid heart rate, the cardiopulmonary examination is normal, as is the remainder of the physical examination.

Electrocardiogram shows atrial fibrillation with a rapid ventricular rate without evidence of ischemic changes. Cardiac enzyme values are normal. Following the administration of metoprolol, he converts to sinus rhythm, with a heart rate of 74/min.

Which of the following is the most appropriate long-term treatment for this patient?

(A) Amiodarone
(B) Low-molecular-weight heparin followed by warfarin
(C) Metoprolol
(D) Metoprolol and warfarin

Item 31 [Basic]

A 28-year-old man is evaluated for a pre-employment physical examination and electrocardiogram before entering the police academy. He has no medical problems, describes no worrisome symptoms, and does not take any medications. He does not smoke cigarettes, has one alcoholic drink or less each week, and rarely consumes caffeine. He runs 4 miles a day 3 days a week and bikes 25 to 50 miles on the weekends. His parents are both alive and in good health as are his two older brothers.

On physical examination, vital signs are normal. The cardiopulmonary examination is normal as is the remainder of the examination.

The resting 12-lead electrocardiogram shows 3 unifocal premature ventricular contractions.

Which of the following is the best management plan for this patient?

(A) Begin amiodarone
(B) Begin metoprolol
(C) Exercise stress test
(D) No further investigation or therapy
(E) Order 24-hour ambulatory electrocardiography

Item 32 [Advanced]

A 55-year-old man is evaluated for fatigue, dyspnea with modest exertion, occasional lightheadedness, and palpitations. He has a history of ischemic cardiomyopathy following a large anterolateral myocardial infarction 6 weeks ago. He does not have chest pain, and a postdischarge adenosine stress test with nuclear imaging demonstrated no inducible ischemia. His medications are lisinopril, carvedilol, furosemide, spironolactone, digoxin, and aspirin.

On physical examination, he is afebrile, blood pressure is 130/83 mm Hg, pulse rate is 50/min, and respiration rate is 12/min. He has no jugular venous distension. S_1 and S_2 are soft, and S_3 and S_4 are present. A grade 2/6 holosystolic murmur at the cardiac apex is present. The lungs are clear. No peripheral edema is noted.

An electrocardiogram shows an episode of nonsustained ventricular tachycardia. Echocardiography shows diminished anterior wall motion with an ejection fraction of 25%.

Which of the following is the most appropriate treatment for this patient?

(A) Amiodarone
(B) Flecainide
(C) Procainamide
(D) Implantable cardioverter-defibrillator (ICD)

Item 33 [Advanced]

A 67-year-old man presented to the emergency department 2 days ago with an acute ST-elevation myocardial infarction. During the initial evaluation, he became unresponsive due to ventricular fibrillation. He was successfully resuscitated and taken to the cardiac catheterization lab, where a 100% occlusion of his proximal left anterior descending artery was stented. His postinfarction course was notable for mild heart failure, which has now resolved. He is now stable on aspirin, metoprolol, atorvastatin, clopidogrel, and lisinopril.

On physical examination, blood pressure is 115/72 mm Hg, pulse is 65/min, and respiration rate is 12/min. There is no jugular venous distention, crackles, murmur, or S_3. The electrocardiogram shows ST-segment changes consistent with a resolving anterior myocardial infarction but is otherwise unremarkable. Transthoracic echocardiogram reveals mild hypokinesis of the anterior wall and a left ventricular ejection fraction of 42%.

Which of the following is the best management option at this time?

(A) Add amiodarone
(B) Continue medical management
(C) Implantable cardioverter-defibrillator placement
(D) Pacemaker placement

Item 34 [Advanced]

An 18-year-old woman is evaluated for recurrent syncope. She has experienced four syncopal episodes in her lifetime, all of which occurred during activity. Episodes have no prodrome, and she has had no dizziness. She is healthy and active, without cardiopulmonary complaints, and takes no medications. Her maternal cousin drowned at age 10 years, and her mother has been evaluated for recurrent episodes of loss of consciousness.

On physical examination, blood pressure is 112/65 mm Hg, and pulse is 67/min and regular. The cardiopulmonary and general physical examinations are normal. An echocardiogram examination is normal. An electrocardiogram is ordered.

Which of the following electrocardiographic findings is most likely to provide a diagnosis?

(A) Left bundle branch block
(B) Long PR interval
(C) Long QT interval
(D) Right bundle branch block

Item 35 [Basic]

A 50-year-man with a 6-month history of New York Heart Association class IV heart failure secondary to idiopathic dilated cardiomyopathy is evaluated following a recent hospitalization for worsening heart failure symptoms. The patient is adherent to his medications and his fluid and sodium restrictions. His medications are lisinopril, carvedilol, spironolactone, and furosemide.

On physical examination, vital signs are normal. He has no jugular venous distention. The cardiac rhythm is regular. Cardiac auscultation reveals an S3 and holosystolic murmur at the cardiac apex. The chest is clear, and no peripheral edema is noted.

In the hospital, no evidence of ischemia, infection, arrhythmia, or thyroid disease was present. An echocardiogram demonstrated global hypokinesis of the left ventricle, moderate mitral regurgitation, and an ejection fraction of 25%

Which of the following medications should be initiated for this patient?

(A) Digoxin
(B) Metolazone
(C) Valsartan
(D) Warfarin

Item 36 [Basic]

A 35-year-old woman is evaluated for progressive dyspnea 3 weeks after delivery of her first child. The pregnancy and delivery were uncomplicated. She has no history of cardiovascular disease.

On physical examination, blood pressure is 110/70 mm Hg in both arms, heart rate is 105/min and regular, and respiratory rate is 28/min. The estimated central venous pressure is 10 cm H_2O and there are no carotid bruits. The apical impulse is displaced and diffuse. There is a grade 2/6 holosystolic murmur at the apex. Third and fourth heart sounds are present. There is dullness to percussion at the posterior lung bases bilaterally, and there are crackles extending up half of the lung fields. Lower extremity pulses are normal and without delay. Pedal edema is present.

The electrocardiogram demonstrates sinus tachycardia. There are no ST-segment or T-wave changes. The chest radiograph demonstrates bilateral pleural effusions and interstitial infiltrates. The aortic contour is unremarkable.

Which of the following is the most likely cause of the patient's current symptoms?

(A) Acute myocardial infarction
(B) Aortic dissection
(C) Coarctation of the aorta
(D) Heart failure

Item 37 [Advanced]

A 65-year-old man is evaluated for 2 months of central chest pain with exertion and relief with rest, exertional dyspnea, orthopnea, and lower-extremity edema. The chest discomfort is increasing in frequency and severity. He has a 25-year history of hypertension and a 44-year history of smoking. His only medication is hydrochlorothiazide.

On physical examination, blood pressure is 118/80 mm Hg, pulse is 95/min, and respiration rate is 16/min. There is jugular venous distention. Cardiac examination reveals a regular rhythm. S_1 and S_2 are normal, and an S_3 and S_4 are present. Crackles are heard at both lung bases. There is edema at the ankles. Laboratory studies show a normal serum troponin T level. Electrocardiogram is normal. Echocardiogram shows an ejection fraction of 40%, global hypokinesis, and left ventricular hypertrophy.

Which of the following is the most appropriate diagnostic test?

(A) Cardiac angiography
(B) Nuclear medicine stress test
(C) Radionuclide ventriculography
(D) Standard exercise stress test

Item 38 [Basic]

A 40-year-old woman is evaluated for 2 months of progressive dyspnea on exertion, orthopnea, and lower extremity edema. She denies chest discomfort and has no other medical problems and takes no medications. She does not smoke cigarettes and rarely drinks alcohol. There is no family history of heart disease.

On physical examination, she is afebrile. Blood pressure is 120/80 mm Hg and pulse is 80/min. Estimated central venous pressure is 10 cm H_2O. The lungs are clear. Cardiac examination reveals a regular rhythm, an S_3, and no murmurs. There is ankle edema. Chest radiograph shows vascular congestion. Electrocardiogram is normal. Initial laboratory evaluation reveals a normal hemoglobin level and metabolic profile, including thyroid studies.

Which of the following is the most appropriate initial diagnostic test?

(A) B-type natriuretic peptide level
(B) Echocardiography
(C) Radionuclide ventriculography
(D) Stress test

Item 39 [Basic]

A 70-year-old woman is evaluated for a 1-month history of dyspnea on exertion and fatigue. She can still perform activities of daily living, including vacuuming, grocery shopping, and ascending two flights of stairs carrying laundry. She has a history of hypertension. Her medications are lisinopril and hydrochlorothiazide.

On physical examination, blood pressure is 110/80 mm Hg and pulse is 70/min. Jugular veins are not distended. S_1 and S_2 are normal, and there is no S_3 or murmur. The pulmonary examination is normal and there is no edema. Laboratory studies show normal hemoglobin and thyroid-stimulating hormone levels. Electrocardiogram shows low voltage and left axis deviation. Echocardiogram shows a left ventricular ejection fraction of 45% and global hypokinesis. Chest radiograph is normal.

Which of the following is the most appropriate additional treatment?

(A) Amlodipine
(B) Carvedilol
(C) Digoxin
(D) Losartan
(E) Spironolactone

Item 40 [Basic]

A 60-year-old woman is diagnosed with heart failure due to nonischemic cardiomyopathy. Her ejection fraction is 40%. She currently has mild shortness of breath with moderate exertion but no orthopnea or lightheadedness. She has a history of hypertension treated with hydrochlorothiazide and metoprolol.

On physical examination, she is afebrile. Blood pressure is 120/80 mm Hg and pulse is 65/min. The jugular veins are not distended, and the lungs are clear. Cardiac examination discloses a regular rate and rhythm with no S_3 or murmurs. There is no edema.

Which of the following agents should be added to her regimen?

(A) Digoxin
(B) Eplerenone
(C) Hydralazine and a nitrate
(D) Lisinopril

Item 41 [Basic]

A 60-year-old woman is evaluated for dyspnea with mild activity (ascending less than one flight of stairs, walking less than one block on level ground) that has been stable for the past year. She has a history of nonischemic cardiomyopathy (most recent left ventricular ejection fraction, 20%). Her current medications are lisinopril, carvedilol, digoxin, and furosemide. She had an implantable cardioverter-defibrillator placed 1 year ago.

On physical examination, blood pressure is 115/75 mm Hg and pulse rate is 70/min. Jugular veins are not distended, and the lungs are clear. Cardiac examination discloses a regular rhythm, no murmurs, normal S_1 and S_2, and no S_3. There is no edema. Laboratory studies show normal serum creatinine and potassium levels.

Which of the following is the most appropriate addition to this patient's treatment?

(A) Losartan
(B) Metolazone
(C) Nifedipine
(D) Spironolactone

Item 42 [Basic]

An 81-year-old woman with aortic stenosis is evaluated for increased shortness of breath and exercise intolerance. She was asymptomatic until 2 weeks ago when she noted increased shortness of breath with exertion. She reports no chest pain, orthopnea, paroxysmal nocturnal dyspnea, or palpitations. She has had no fever, chills, or recent procedures that might increase the risk for infective endocarditis. She has no other medical problems and takes no medications.

On physical examination, she is afebrile, blood pressure is 116/72 mm Hg, pulse rate is irregularly irregular at 112/min, and respiration rate is 12/min. No jugular venous distention is present. Cardiac auscultation reveals an irregular rhythm with a grade 3/6 crescendo-decrescendo systolic murmur loudest at the second left intercostal space with radiation to the carotid arteries. Bibasilar pulmonary crackles are present, as is 1+ bilateral lower extremity edema.

Which of the following is most likely responsible for the new symptoms?

(A) Atrial fibrillation
(B) Infective endocarditis
(C) Development of mitral stenosis
(D) Development of mitral regurgitation

Item 43 [Basic]

A 54-year-old man is evaluated for increased shortness of breath of 3 weeks' duration. He has dyspnea on exertion, orthopnea, and occasional paroxysmal nocturnal dyspnea. He reports no chest pain, fever, or chills. He had an aortic bio-prosthetic valve replacement for bicuspid valve aortic stenosis 15 years ago. He takes no medications.

On physical examination, he is afebrile, blood pressure is 140/50 mm Hg, pulse rate is 100/min, and respiration rate is 14/min. The carotid pulse is hyperdynamic. The S_2 is diminished. Cardiac auscultation reveals a grade 2/6 diastolic murmur, heard loudest at the third left intercostal space. A few scattered crackles can be heard at the lung bases. No peripheral edema is present.

Which of the following is the most likely diagnosis?

(A) Aortic regurgitation
(B) Atrial septal defect
(C) Coarctation of the aorta
(D) Mitral stenosis
(E) Ventricular septal defect

Item 44 [Basic]

A 65-year-old woman is evaluated as a new patient during a routine office visit. She is healthy and active and swims laps three or four times per week. She does not smoke and she takes no medications.

On physical examination, blood pressure is 118/60 mm Hg. There are no carotid bruits. There is a normal S_1 and a physiologically split S_2. There is a grade 2/6 midsystolic murmur that does not radiate and is heard best at the second right intercostal space. The rest of the physical examination is unrevealing.

Which of the following is the most appropriate management?

(A) Antibiotic endocarditis prophylaxis
(B) Transthoracic echocardiography
(C) Treadmill stress echocardiography
(D) No further intervention

Item 45 [Advanced]

A 30-year-old woman is evaluated in the emergency department for shortness of breath, palpitations, and pedal edema. She is gravida 1, para 0, and she is 30 weeks pregnant. She has not received prenatal care until this point.

On physical examination, the patient is sitting upright to breathe. Blood pressure is 112/80 mm Hg, and pulse is 96/min. There is jugular venous distention to her jaw line while sitting upright. Cardiac auscultation demonstrates an irregularly irregular rhythm, a loud P_2, and an opening snap followed by a low-pitched diastolic murmur heard best at the cardiac apex. Bibasilar crackles are present.

Which of the following is the most likely diagnosis?

(A) Acute aortic regurgitation
(B) Atrial septal defect
(C) Mitral stenosis
(D) Tricuspid regurgitation

Item 46 [Advanced]

An 18-year-old woman is evaluated during a routine examination prior to entering college. She has had no major medical problems and there is no family history of cardiovascular disease.

On physical examination, blood pressure is 110/60 mm Hg and pulse is 70/min. S_1 and S_2 are normal and there is an S_4 present. There is a harsh grade 2/6 midsystolic murmur heard best at the lower left sternal border. The murmur does not radiate to the carotid arteries. A Valsalva maneuver increases the intensity of the murmur; moving from a standing position to a squatting position decreases the intensity. Rapid upstrokes of the carotid pulses are present. Blood pressures in the upper and lower extremities are equal.

Which of the following is the most likely diagnosis?

(A) Aortic coarctation
(B) Bicuspid aortic valve
(C) Hypertrophic cardiomyopathy
(D) Ventricular septal defect

Item 47 [Basic]

A 25-year-old asymptomatic man is evaluated during a routine examination. His blood pressure is 150/40 mm Hg and his heart rate is 90/min. Estimated central venous pressure is normal. The carotid upstroke is brisk and collapses quickly. The apical impulse is displaced. A grade 3/6 high-pitched decrescendo diastolic murmur is heard at the second right intercostal space with radiation down the left sternal border. The murmur is heard best with the patient leaning forward and in end-expiration. There is evidence of nailbed pulsation. Femoral pulsations are full and collapse quickly. There is no change in the murmur with inspiration.

Which of the following is the most likely diagnosis?

(A) Aortic valve regurgitation
(B) Mitral valve stenosis
(C) Patent ductus arteriosus
(D) Tricuspid regurgitation

Item 48 [Basic]

A 35-year-old woman is evaluated during a routine examination. She has no cardiovascular risk factors and no family history of cardiovascular disease. She is not currently on any medications.

On physical examination, vital signs are normal. There is a midsystolic click and a grade 2/6 late systolic murmur at the cardiac apex that radiates toward the left axilla. Following squat-to-stand maneuvers, the midsystolic click moves closer to the S_1, and murmur duration and intensity are increased. Carotid upstrokes are normal. The rest of the examination is unremarkable.

Which of the following is the most likely diagnosis?

(A) Aortic stenosis
(B) Coarctation of the aorta
(C) Hypertrophic cardiomyopathy
(D) Mitral valve prolapse

Item 49 [Advanced]

A 43-year-old man is evaluated during a routine examination. He has a history of a cardiac murmur diagnosed during childhood. He exercises regularly without restriction to activity and has no history of syncope, palpitations, or edema. He takes no medications.

On physical examination, blood pressure is 120/64 mm Hg, pulse is 80/min and regular, and respiration rate is 16/min. Cardiac examination reveals a normal S_1 and a physiologically split S_2. There is a grade 2/6 decrescendo diastolic murmur at the upper left sternal border. Distal pulses are brisk. There is no pedal edema.

A transthoracic echocardiogram demonstrates normal ventricular size and function, with ejection fraction of 60% to 65%. There is a bicuspid aortic valve with moderate regurgitation. Pulmonary pressure estimates are in the normal range.

Which of the following is the most appropriate management option for this patient?

(A) Antibiotic endocarditis prophylaxis
(B) Aortic valve replacement
(C) Begin metoprolol
(D) Clinical follow-up in 1 year

Section 1

Cardiovascular Medicine
Answers and Critiques

Item 1   **Answer: B**

Educational Objective: *Diagnose non–ST-elevation myocardial infarction.*

The most likely diagnosis is a non–ST-elevation myocardial infarction (NSTEMI). This patient has had chest pain at rest, an elevated serum troponin I level, and an electrocardiogram that shows ST-segment depression that is particularly prominent in leads V_2 through V_6. These features indicate a NSTEMI.

In an acute coronary syndrome, obstruction to coronary blood flow results in either transient or prolonged episodes of severe myocardial ischemia. ST-elevation myocardial infarction (STEMI) is diagnosed in patients with a clinical presentation consistent with acute myocardial infarction together with electrocardiographic evidence of ST segment elevation. Although most patients with STEMI ultimately develop Q waves on electrocardiogram, some exhibit diagnostic ST segment elevation and cardiac enzyme elevations without Q waves.

Patients who present with ischemic chest pain but without diagnostic ST-segment elevation are categorized as having unstable angina or NSTEMI. These two conditions are closely related and have similar pathophysiology and clinical presentations, but they differ in the severity of the myocardial ischemia. Patients with either condition typically present with angina at rest; however, some patients describe a pattern of new-onset or increasing angina. In NSTEMI, ischemia is severe and results in a detectable release of biomarkers of myocardial injury hours after the onset of ischemic chest pain, most commonly cardiac troponin I, troponin T, and the MB isoenzyme of creatine kinase. In unstable angina, there is no detectable increase in these enzymes.

Chronic stable angina refers to a coronary artery syndrome that is characterized by chest discomfort that occurs predictably and reproducibly at a certain level of exertion and is relieved with rest or nitroglycerin. Ischemic pain that occurs with rest is not compatible with the diagnosis of chronic stable angina, and the presence of positive serum biomarkers for myocardial necrosis also excludes this diagnosis.

KEY POINT

Non–ST-elevation myocardial infarction is characterized by chest pain at rest, absence of ST-elevation on the electrocardiogram, and elevated biomarkers of myocardial injury.

Bibliography

Hillis LD, Lange RA. Optimal management of acute coronary syndromes. N Engl J Med. 2009;360(21):2237-2240. [PMID: 19458369]

Item 2   **Answer: B**

Educational Objective: *Diagnose acute pericarditis*

The most likely diagnosis is acute pericarditis. Chest pain from acute pericarditis is sharp and pleuritic and worsened by assuming a supine position. Acute pericarditis is diagnosed by the presence of at least two of the three classic features: (1) pleuritic chest pain; (2) friction rub; and (3) diffuse concordant ST-segment elevation on electrocardiography, often with depression of the PR segment. The classic pericardial friction rub has three components (not all components may be heard) related to cardiac motion and occurs during atrial systole, ventricular contraction, and rapid ventricular filling. The sound of the rub can be squeaky, scratchy, and high-pitched.

Patients with an acute aortic dissection present with the abrupt onset of severe pain in the thorax. Blood pressure is variable. Pain described as "ripping" or "tearing" occurs in only about 50% of patients. The physical finding of a pulse deficit is uncommon. At least one third of patients have no electrocardiographic abnormality, and at least 40% of patients lack widening of the mediastinum on plain chest radiograph. However, pleuritic chest pain, pericardial friction rub, and diffuse ST elevations are not compatible with aortic dissection.

The pain of an acute myocardial infarction is usually retrosternal in location, may radiate to the shoulders or arms, and may be associated with nausea and vomiting, diaphoresis, or shortness of breath. Although the initial electrocardiogram is nondiagnostic in up to 50% of patients, compatible changes would include focal ST elevations with reciprocal ST depression associated with elevation of cardiac biomarkers such as troponin.

Patients with pulmonary embolism may present with the classic symptoms of dyspnea, chest pain, hemoptysis, or syncope, but the presentation is often more subtle. At times, only nonspecific respiratory or hemodynamic manifestations may occur. Pulmonary embolism is not associated with a pericardial friction rub or diffuse ST-segment changes.

KEY POINT

Diagnosis of acute pericarditis is made by the presence of at least two of the three classic features: (1) pleuritic chest pain; (2) friction rub; and (3) diffuse concordant ST-segment elevation on electrocardiography.

Bibliography

Lee TH, Goldman L. Evaluation of the patient with acute chest pain. N Engl J Med. 2000;20;342(16):1187-95. [PMID: 10770985]

Item 3   Answer: C

Educational Objective: *Treat a patient with ST-elevation myocardial infarction with percutaneous coronary intervention.*

The best management for this patient is percutaneous coronary intervention (PCI). This patient is presenting with an ST-elevation inferior wall myocardial infarction (STEMI). The diagnosis is based upon the presence of chest pain, elevated cardiac biomarkers, and ST-segment elevations in the inferior leads (II, III, and aVF). Reperfusion strategies for STEMI patients include either thrombolytic therapy or PCI. Percutaneous angioplasty and stent placement is the preferred therapy for most patients with STEMI because it is associated with a lower 30-day mortality rate compared to thrombolytic therapy. PCI is also indicated in patients with a contraindication to thrombolytic therapy and in patients with cardiogenic shock. Contraindications to thrombolytic therapy include prior intracerebral hemorrhage, ischemic stroke within 3 months, suspected aortic dissection, or active bleeding. PCI is most effective if completed within 12 hours of the onset of chest pain; the earlier the intervention, the better the outcome.

A chest CT can be a useful diagnostic tool in patients being evaluated for chest pain if there is a high clinical suspicion for an aortic dissection. This patient does not have any characteristics of ascending aortic dissection—back pain, unequal blood pressures or pulses, or a widened mediastinum on chest radiograph. Given these factors, the possibility of an acute aortic dissection is extremely low, and further imaging with a chest CT would likely further delay treatment for the STEMI.

An echocardiogram is occasionally useful in the management of patients presenting with chest pain and a nondiagnostic electrocardiogram (ECG). A focal wall motion abnormality suggests a cardiac basis to the symptoms. In this patient presenting with a markedly abnormal ECG with ST-segment elevation and elevated cardiac biomarkers, echocardiography would not add to the management.

KEY POINT

Percutaneous angioplasty and stent placement is the preferred therapy for most patients with ST-elevation myocardial infarction.

Bibliography

Hillis LD, Lange RA. Optimal management of acute coronary syndromes. N Engl J Med. 2009;360(21):2237-2240. [PMID: 19458369]

Item 4   Answer: C

Educational Objective: *Diagnose angina pectoris.*

Symptoms of ischemic heart disease are fairly predictable for an individual patient, but great heterogeneity exists between patients. Patients may have a difficult time describing the pain and may use words such as discomfort, pressure, or heaviness. Although the location of the pain is classically substernal, it may be difficult for patients to localize the pain; they may indicate the entire chest or upper abdomen is involved. Sharp pain, well-localized pain, and back pain are infrequently associated with ischemic heart disease. Ischemic cardiac pain has a predictable relation to exercise and relief with rest or nitroglycerin. In some patients, exertional dyspnea may be the only manifestation of cardiac ischemia (angina equivalent). A normal electrocardiogram at rest does not exclude ischemic heart disease nor does a normal troponin level.

The pain of acute pericarditis is often pleuritic, may radiate to the top of the shoulder, and is often worse when the patient is supine. Fever and a pericardial friction rub are usually evident. Characteristic electrocardiographic changes include diffuse ST elevations and PR depression.

The classic presentation of aortic dissection consists of sudden-onset severe chest pain radiating to the back. Other findings may include a blood pressure differential between the right and left arms, murmur of aortic regurgitation, and a widened mediastinum on chest x-ray. Aortic dissection should always be considered in the differential diagnosis of acute chest pain, but this patient's pain is not consistent with this diagnosis.

Most patients with peptic ulcer disease do not have pain at diagnosis; ulcers are usually detected during an evaluation for potential ulcer-related complications such as overt or obscure bleeding. When symptoms are present, they include dyspepsia or a nonspecific, gnawing epigastric pain. Other presentations include bleeding, perforation (sometimes with penetration into adjacent organs), and gastric outlet obstruction. Finally, discomfort caused by a duodenal ulcer is not typically relieved by rest, worsened by exertion, or accompanied by shortness of breath.

KEY POINT

Ischemic cardiac pain has a predicable relation to exercise and relief with rest or nitroglycerin.

Bibliography

Lee TH, Goldman L. Evaluation of the patient with acute chest pain. N Engl J Med. 2000;342(16):1187-95. [PMID: 10770985]

Item 5   Answer: D

Educational Objective: *Treat right ventricular myocardial infarction with normal saline infusion.*

Volume expansion with normal saline is the primary supportive treatment for the hemodynamic abnormalities of a right ventricular myocardial infarction. The physical examination findings of hypotension, clear lung fields, and elevated estimated central venous pressure represent the classic triad of right ventricular myocardial infarction. However, the most predictive finding is ST-segment elevation on right-sided electrocardiographic lead V_4R. Therefore, all patients with an inferior ST-elevation myocardial infarction (STEMI) should have a right-sided electrocardiogram performed at the time of presentation. This patient's electrocardiogram shows ST-segment elevation in frontal inferior leads II, III, and aVF, and 1-mm

ST-segment elevation in right-sided precordial lead V$_4$R. These findings indicate inferior and right ventricular injury in the setting of an inferior STEMI, likely related to a right coronary artery occlusion.

In the setting of right ventricular myocardial infarction, right ventricular contractility is reduced, resulting in higher right ventricular diastolic pressure, lower right ventricular systolic pressure, and reduced preload or filling of the left ventricle. Volume expansion improves the hemodynamic abnormalities of right ventricular myocardial infarction because the gradient of pressure from the right atrium to the left atrium maintains filling of the left ventricle. In addition to reperfusion therapy for STEMI, the acute treatment of right ventricular myocardial infarction is supportive.

Inotropic support, specifically using intravenous dobutamine, is appropriate treatment in patients with right ventricular myocardial infarction whose hypotension is not corrected after 1 L of saline infusion. However, volume expansion should be tried before giving inotropic agents. By increasing cardiac contractility, inotropic agents increase myocardial oxygen demand and potentially extend the infarction.

Bradycardia, potentially caused by increased vagal activity or sinoatrial node ischemia, exacerbates the hemodynamic abnormalities of right ventricular myocardial infarction, so β-blocker therapy with metoprolol is contraindicated in this patient.

Nitroglycerin is contraindicated in patients with hypotension and patients with the potential for hypotension, particularly right ventricular myocardial infarction. In right ventricular infarction, nitrate-induced venodilation impairs right ventricular filling and thereby cardiac output.

KEY POINT

Volume expansion is the primary supportive treatment for the hemodynamic abnormalities of a right ventricular myocardial infarction.

Bibliography

Reynolds HR, Hochman JS. Cardiogenic shock: current concepts and improving outcomes. Circulation. 2008;117(5):686-697. [PMID: 18250279]

Item 6   Answer: D

Educational Objective: *Manage noncardiac chest pain caused by gastroesophageal reflux disease with an oral proton pump inhibitor.*

The most appropriate management for this patient is empiric treatment with a proton pump inhibitor. Esophageal disease is the most common cause of noncardiac chest pain. Gastroesophageal reflux disease (GERD) is caused by reflux of gastric contents into the esophagus. Symptoms of GERD can mimic cardiac ischemia, with substernal squeezing or burning that may radiate widely, including to the back, neck, jaw, or arms. Chest pain due to GERD may last minutes to hours and can resolve spontaneously or with antacids. Most patients

with GERD-induced chest pain also have typical reflux symptoms, including regurgitation and heartburn. The recommended approach in patients with suspected esophageal chest pain is to rule out cardiac ischemia and then treat the patient empirically with a proton pump inhibitor.

Ambulatory esophageal pH monitoring can be used if the patient's condition does not respond to empiric therapy or if the patient has atypical symptoms. Esophagogastroduodenoscopy is indicated in patients with long-standing reflux disease to screen for Barrett esophagus and in patients with such alarm symptoms as anemia, weight loss, or dysphagia, but not as the initial screening test for GERD.

This patient's previous normal stress test makes cardiac disease very unlikely and a repeat exercise stress test or coronary angiography is unlikely to provide additional diagnostic information. Because ischemic heart disease has been ruled out, it is reasonable in this patient to attempt empiric acid suppression therapy with a proton pump inhibitor. A complete response to empiric therapy is considered diagnostic of GERD.

KEY POINT

Empiric proton pump inhibitor therapy is the first step in the management of esophageal noncardiac chest pain.

Bibliography

Fass R. Evaluation and diagnosis of noncardiac chest pain. Dis Mon. 2008;54(9):627-641. [PMID: 18725005]

Item 7   Answer: D

Educational Objective: *Diagnose third-degree atrioventricular heart block.*

This patient most likely has third-degree (complete) atrioventricular heart block due to Lyme carditis. The presence of the characteristic skin rash (erythema migrans) with or without a history of tick bite in an endemic region, has a probability greater than 80% of being caused by *Borrelia burgdorferi* infection. Lyme carditis is manifested by acute-onset, high-grade atrioventricular conduction defects that may occasionally be associated with myocarditis.

Atrioventricular block is classified as first, second, or third degree. First-degree block is characterized by prolongation of the PR interval to greater than 0.2 sec and usually is not associated with alterations in heart rate. There are two types of second-degree block, both recognized electrocardiographically by the presence of a P wave that is not followed by a ventricular complex. Mobitz type I block (Wenckebach block) manifests as progressive prolongation of the PR interval until there is a dropped beat, whereas Mobitz type II block manifests as a dropped beat without progressive PR-interval prolongation. Mobitz type I block usually does not progress to complete heart block, but Mobitz type II block, which is usually associated with a bundle branch block, typically progresses to third-degree block. Second-degree block may be associated with bradycardia, depending upon the frequency of blocked atrial impulses. Third-degree block is the complete absence of conduction of atrial impulses to the ventricle and is the most common cause of marked bradycardia; ventricular rates are usually 30-50/min. Patients with atrioventricular block may be asymptomatic or have severe bradycardia-related symptoms (weakness, presyncope, syncope) and ventricular arrhythmias.

KEY POINT

Third-degree block is the complete absence of conduction of atrial impulses to the ventricle and is the most common cause of marked bradycardia.

Bibliography

Barold SS. Atrioventricular block revisited. Compr Ther. 2002;28(1):74-78. [PMID: 11894446]

Item 8   Answer: B

Educational Objective: *Diagnose panic disorder.*

This patient's presentation is characteristic of panic disorder. Panic disorder is characterized by recurrent, unexpected panic attacks that feature the abrupt onset of numerous somatic symptoms, such as palpitations, sweating, tremulousness, dyspnea, chest pain, nausea, dizziness, and numbness. Symptoms typically peak within 10 minutes of onset, and attacks usually last from 15 to 60 minutes. The most appropriate treatment for panic disorder is cognitive-behavioral therapy and a selective serotonin reuptake inhibitor, such as paroxetine.

Because the symptoms of panic disorder are primarily physical, most patients with this disorder present to their primary care physicians or to emergency departments for evaluation. Patients with panic disorder are evaluated, on average, by 10 clinicians before the diagnosis is established. The alarming nature of their symptoms prompts patients with panic disorder to seek medical attention; consequently, they have very high health care utilization rates.

The clinical manifestations of pheochromocytomas are variable, with hypertension (episodic or sustained) observed in more than 90% of patients. Other major symptoms include diaphoresis, pallor, palpitations, and headaches; the classic triad of sudden severe headache, diaphoresis, and palpitations is highly suggestive of pheochromocytoma. Other manifestations include hyperglycemia, weight loss, arrhythmias (atrial and ventricular fibrillation), and catecholamine-induced cardiomyopathy. The absence of hypertension and the long duration of symptoms make this diagnosis unlikely.

The diagnosis of acute coronary syndrome is unlikely in a patient with recurrent, self-limited attacks and previous normal results of coronary angiography. The current nature of the symptoms and normal physical examination findings are not compatible with the diagnosis of pneumothorax. Symptoms that resolve after 20 minutes or recur frequently over many years are not compatible with the diagnosis of pulmonary embolism.

KEY POINT

Panic disorder is characterized by recurrent, unexpected panic attacks that feature the abrupt onset of numerous somatic symptoms such as palpitations, sweating, tremulousness, dyspnea, chest pain, nausea, dizziness, and numbness.

Bibliography

Culpepper L. Identifying and treating panic disorder in primary care. J Clin Psychiatry. 2004;65(suppl 5):19-23. [PMID: 15078114]

Item 9   Answer: B

Educational Objective: *Diagnose Mobitz type I second-degree atrioventricular block.*

This patient has evidence for Mobitz type I second-degree atrioventricular (AV) block. Second-degree heart block is characterized by intermittent nonconduction of P waves and subsequent "dropped" ventricular beats. Second-degree heart block is divided into types, Mobitz I and Mobitz II. Mobitz type I second-degree heart block is characterized by progressive prolongation of the PR interval until a dropped beat occurs. Mobitz type I block can occur in the absence of heart disease, including in athletes and older adults; in patients with underlying heart disease, including acute ischemia; and in patients who are taking drugs that block the AV node, such as β-blockers (metoprolol), calcium channel blockers, and digoxin. This type of heart block is characteristically transient and usually requires no specific treatment; however, some patients may develop excessively slow heart rates and experience symptoms related to decreased cerebral or coronary perfusion. If treatment is necessary, it begins by identifying and correcting reversible causes of slowed conduction, such as myocardial ischemia, increased vagal tone (for example, from pain or vomiting), and discontinuation of drugs that depress AV conduction.

Mobitz type II second-degree AV block is characterized by a regularly dropped beat (for example, a nonconducted P wave every second or third beat) without progressive prolongation of the PR interval. It is often associated with evidence of additional disease in the conduction system, such as bundle branch block or bifascicular or trifascicular block. Mobitz type II second-degree block suddenly and unpredictably progresses to complete heart block and is usually treated with a pacemaker.

First-degree AV block is recognized, electrocardiographically, as a prolongation of the PR interval to greater than 0.2 sec. All P waves are conducted. First-degree block requires no specific treatment.

Third-degree AV block, or complete heart block, refers to a lack of AV conduction, characterized by lack of conduction of all atrial impulses to the ventricles.

KEY POINT

Mobitz type I second-degree atrioventricular block is characterized by progressive prolongation of the PR interval until a dropped beat occurs.

Bibliography
Da Costa D, Brady WJ, Edhouse J. Bradycardias and atrioventricular conduction block. BMJ. 2002;324:535-538. [PMID: 11872557]

Item 10   Answer: D

Educational Objective: *Treat chronic stable angina with worsening symptoms with increased dosage of a β-blocker.*

The most appropriate management at this point is to increase the patient's dose of metoprolol. Medical therapy for chronic stable coronary artery disease (CAD) includes both antianginal and vascular-protective agents. Antianginal therapy includes β-blockers, calcium channel blockers, and nitrates. Vascular-protective therapy includes aspirin, angiotensin-converting enzyme (ACE) inhibitors, and statins. This patient is already on a β-blocker, aspirin, a statin, and an ACE inhibitor. Switching to a long-acting nitrate will help relieve his angina symptoms. However, his resting heart rate of 87/min and high blood pressure suggest a suboptimal dose of β-blocker, and the patient's dosage of metoprolol should be increased. The β-blocker dose should be titrated to achieve a resting heart rate of approximately 55 to 60/min and approximately 75% of the heart rate that produces angina with exertion. The patient should be reevaluated in a few weeks to assess the response to therapy.

Ranolazine is a novel antianginal agent that is approved for the treatment of chronic stable angina. It should only be used, however, in addition to baseline therapy with a β-blocker, a calcium channel blocker, and a long-acting nitrate. Given that this patient was on suboptimal doses of metoprolol and is just being started on a long-acting nitrate, the addition of ranolazine would be premature.

Coronary angiography would not be indicated at this time because the patient is not receiving maximal medical therapy. In the setting of continued angina despite maximal medical therapy, coronary angiography could be considered.

Exercise treadmill stress testing would not provide useful information in this setting. It would only confirm the high pretest probability that this patient has underlying CAD as a cause for the current symptoms.

KEY POINT

In the treatment of chronic stable angina, the β-blocker dose should be titrated to achieve a resting heart rate of approximately 55 to 60/min and approximately 75% of the heart rate that produces angina with exertion.

Bibliography
Jawad E, Arora R. Chronic stable angina pectoris. Dis Mon. 2008; 54(9):671-689. [PMID: 18725007]

Item 11   Answer: A

Educational Objective: *Diagnose pulmonary embolism with CT pulmonary angiography.*

This patient's symptoms of chest pain and dyspnea in combination with the physical findings of asymmetric leg edema, elevated central venous pressure, tachypnea, and tachycardia suggest the possibility of pulmonary embolism. The most appropriate diagnostic test to perform next is CT pulmonary angiography to look for pulmonary emboli.

A normal echocardiogram between episodes of chest pain does not rule out unstable angina because wall motion returns to normal between ischemic episodes. However, this patient had no wall motion abnormalities during her ongoing chest pain, making acute myocardial ischemia very unlikely. Because an acute coronary syndrome is highly unlikely, coronary angiography is not indicated as the next diagnostic test.

A resting radionuclide perfusion study can be helpful in the diagnosis of coronary ischemia when the electrocardiogram is nondiagnostic but does not provide additive information to that already obtained by echocardiography.

Transesophageal echocardiography is not sensitive for detection of pulmonary emboli but may be useful in acute chest pain if aortic dissection is suspected. Ascending aortic dissection is often associated with acute aortic regurgitation, myocardial ischemia, cardiac tamponade or hemopericardium, and hemothorax or exsanguination. Considerable (>20 mm Hg) variation in systolic blood pressure in the arms may be present. Descending thoracic aortic aneurysm is more commonly associated with splanchnic ischemia, renal insufficiency, lower extremity ischemia, or focal neurologic deficit due to spinal cord ischemia. This woman has no physical findings to suggest this diagnosis.

KEY POINT

Normal wall motion on echocardiography during chest pain excludes coronary ischemia or infarction.

Bibliography
Chunilal SD, Eikelboom JW, Attia J, et al. Does this patient have pulmonary embolism? JAMA. 2003;290(21):2849-2858. [PMID: 14657070]

Item 12   Answer: D

Educational Objective: *Evaluate suspected coronary artery disease using an exercise stress test.*

The most appropriate diagnostic test for this patient is an exercise stress test. This 68-year-old woman has cardiac risk factors of smoking and hypertension, with an intermediate Framingham risk score (18% likelihood of a coronary event in 10 years). (A tool to calculate the Framingham risk score can be accessed at www.acponline.org/acp_press/essentials/calculator.htm.) In addition, she has atypical chest pain, so further evaluation is appropriate. An exercise stress test is recommended in patients with intermediate probability of coronary artery disease with a normal baseline electrocardiogram (ECG) who are able to exercise because it provides information about exercise tolerance and hemodynamic response to exercise.

An adenosine nuclear perfusion stress test is contraindicated in patients with significant bronchospastic disease and hence is not the correct choice for a patient with asthma. Furthermore, exercise stress testing is preferred over pharmacologic stress testing because of the additional physiologic information on exercise tolerance and the blood pressure and heart rate response to exercise.

Coronary angiography would only be appropriate if the patient were presenting with an acute coronary syndrome or after an abnormal stress test to determine if there is an indication for revascularization.

Dobutamine stress echocardiography is an appropriate choice in patients who are unable to exercise and are not hypertensive at rest. This patient is able to exercise, so treadmill testing is the more appropriate choice.

KEY POINT

Exercise electrocardiographic stress testing is the primary approach to the diagnosis of coronary artery disease in patients who can exercise and have a normal resting electrocardiogram.

Bibliography

Wilson JM. Diagnosis and treatment of acquired coronary artery disease in adults. Postgrad Med J. 2009;85(1005):364-365. [PMID: 19581247]

Item 13   Answer: B
Educational Objective: *Diagnose atrial flutter.*

The most likely diagnosis for this patient is atrial flutter. The presence on the electrocardiogram of multiple P waves in a "sawtooth" pattern, typically with 2:1 ventricular conduction, characterizes atrial flutter and eliminates atrial fibrillation as a diagnostic consideration. Electrocardiographically, atrial fibrillation is characterized by an absence of discernible P waves, which are replaced by fibrillatory waves that vary in amplitude, shape, and timing. The ventricular response is grossly irregular and often rapid, except when there is concomitant atrioventricular block.

Sinoatrial node dysfunction (sick sinus syndrome) is a frequent cause of pacemaker implantation. It consists of symptomatic sinus bradycardia and the tachycardia-bradycardia syndrome (alternating atrial tachyarrhythmias and bradycardia). In patients with "tachy-brady" syndrome, bradycardia usually occurs after termination of the tachycardia; atrial fibrillation is the most common tachyarrhythmia observed in this group of patients. The patient does not fulfill the diagnostic criteria for sinus node dysfunction.

Ventricular tachycardia is characterized by wide-complex QRS morphology (QRS >0.12 sec) and a ventricular rate that is greater than 100/min. In ventricular tachycardia, the ventricular rate typically ranges from 140/min to 250/min. The patient does not have a wide-complex tachycardia and, therefore, does not have ventricular tachycardia.

KEY POINT

Atrial flutter is typically a narrow-complex tachycardia characterized by multiple regular atrial contractions (flutter waves) creating a "sawtooth" baseline pattern prior to the QRS complex.

Bibliography

Sawhney NS, Anousheh R, Chen WC, Feld GK. Diagnosis and management of typical atrial flutter. Cardiol Clin. 2009;27(1):55-67, viii. [PMID: 19111764]

Item 14   Answer: D
Educational Objective: *Treat chronic stable angina with appropriate medical therapy.*

The most appropriate treatment of this patient would be to continue his current medical management. Medical therapy for chronic coronary artery disease (CAD) can be classified as antianginal or vascular protective. Antianginal medications include β-blockers, calcium channel blockers, nitrates, and ranolazine. β-Blockers reduce mortality by approximately 20%. Patients with chronic stable angina can be treated with calcium channel blockers if they are unable to tolerate β-blockers, or calcium channel blockers can be added to β-blocker therapy for difficult-to-control symptoms. All patients with chronic stable angina should carry either a sublingual or a spray form of nitroglycerin for emergency use. Ranolazine should only be considered in patients who remain symptomatic despite optimal doses of β-blockers, calcium channel blockers, and nitrates.

Vascular-protective medications include aspirin, clopidogrel, angiotensin-converting enzyme (ACE) inhibitors, and statins. Aspirin reduces the risk of stroke, myocardial infarction, sudden death, and vascular death by 33%. Although clopidogrel is beneficial in patients with acute coronary syndromes, it has small clinical benefit in patients with chronic stable angina and is associated with an increased risk of bleeding. ACE inhibitors reduce cardiovascular mortality by 17% to 23%. Statins reduce future cardiovascular events by approximately 25% to 30%. Current guidelines specify an LDL cholesterol target level of less than 100 mg/dL (2.6 mmol/L) for patients with coronary artery disease. This patient is receiving standard therapy for chronic stable angina with aspirin, β-blocker (carvedilol), ACE inhibitor (lisinopril), a statin (simvastatin), and nitroglycerin. His blood pressure is well controlled, pulse rate is appropriately reduced, and the lipid profile is at target. His symptoms are infrequent and stable; no change in his medical therapy is needed.

Coronary angiography is reserved for patients with acute coronary symptoms, angina increasing in severity, markedly abnormal stress tests, sudden cardiac death, or diagnostic difficulties and is not indicated in this clinically stable patient. Because this patient's symptoms are well controlled with the current therapy, it is not necessary to add ranolazine.

KEY POINT

Most patients with chronic stable angina are treated with aspirin, a β-blocker, an ACE inhibitor, nitroglycerin, and a statin.

Bibliography

Pfisterer ME, Zellweger MJ, Gersh BJ. Management of stable coronary artery disease. Lancet. 2010;375(9716):763-72. [PMID: 20189028]

Item 15   Answer: A

Educational Objective: *Diagnose atrial fibrillation.*

The electrocardiogram is characteristic for atrial fibrillation, showing a rapid, irregularly irregular rhythm with no discernible P waves and atrial fibrillatory waves at a rate between 350 and 600 beats/min. The fibrillatory waves vary in amplitude, morphology, and intervals, creating a rough, irregular baseline between the QRS complexes. The patient's evaluation should minimally include a transthoracic echocardiogram to exclude occult valve or other structural heart disease and also to assess the size of the left atrial appendage; in addition, thyroid studies should be performed to exclude hyperthyroidism.

Atrial flutter is recognized by its saw-tooth pattern of flutter waves, most noticeable in the inferior leads II, III, and aVF; flutter waves are distinctly different from the small, chaotic fibrillation waves that are characteristic of atrial fibrillation.

Sinus tachycardia is a regular rhythm associated with P waves prior to each QRS complex. In each lead, the P-wave morphology and PR interval remain constant in shape and duration. The absence of well-defined P waves in this electrocardiogram rules out sinus tachycardia.

Ventricular tachycardia is characterized by wide-complex QRS morphology (QRS >0.12 sec) and a ventricular rate ranging from 140-250/min. This patient's QRS complexes are narrow, excluding ventricular tachycardia as a diagnosis.

KEY POINT

Atrial fibrillation is characterized electrocardiographically by an irregularly irregular rhythm with no discernible P waves and atrial fibrillation waves creating an irregular baseline.

Bibliography

Zimetbaum P. Atrial fibrillation. Ann Intern Med. 2010;153(11):ITC61. [PMID: 21135291]

Item 16   Answer: E

Educational Objective: *Avoid screening for asymptomatic coronary artery disease.*

No additional testing for coronary artery disease (CAD) is the best management option for this patient. He is at low risk for CAD, and he is asymptomatic. In addition, he only has a 4% probability of a major coronary event over the next 10 years (www.acponline.org/acp_press/essentials/calculator.htm). The American College of Cardiology/American Heart Association, American College of Physicians, and U.S. Preventive Services Task Force all agree that there is little evidence to support routine testing for CAD in adults who are low risk and asymptomatic. Screening for CAD in adults who are asymptomatic is not recommended because the probability of a false-positive test is much greater than the probability of a true positive test. For patients with an intermediate probability of CAD, noninvasive stress testing with an exercise stress test provides the most useful information.

Coronary angiography should be reserved for patients with chronic CAD who have lifestyle-limiting angina despite medical therapy, markedly positive results on noninvasive stress testing, successful resuscitation from sudden cardiac death, or documented ventricular tachycardia. Coronary angiography can also be considered in patients with nonspecific chest pain to completely exclude CAD as a cause for the current symptoms if they have had recurrent hospitalizations. Coronary calcium testing may be considered in asymptomatic persons with a 10% to 20% Framingham 10-year risk category (intermediate risk) and in young persons with a strong family history of premature cardiovascular disease. The diagnostic accuracy of CT angiography to detect obstructive CAD is approximately 90%. Because CT angiography provides no functional information (that is, the extent of ischemia), a markedly abnormal study is followed by referral to coronary angiography or stress testing to determine the ischemic burden. Recent consensus guidelines suggest that the benefits of CT angiography are greatest in symptomatic patients with an intermediate pretest probability of CAD.

KEY POINT

There is little evidence to support routine testing for coronary artery disease in adults who are low risk and asymptomatic.

Bibliography

Snow V, Barry P, Fihn SD, Gibbons RJ, Owens DK, Williams SV, Weiss KB, Mottur-Pilson C; ACP; ACC Chronic Stable Angina Panel. Evaluation of primary care patients with chronic stable angina: guidelines from the American College of Physicians. Ann Intern Med. 2004;141 (1):57-64. [PMID: 15238371]

Item 17   Answer: C

Educational Objective: *Diagnose atrioventricular reentrant tachycardia (Wolff-Parkinson-White syndrome).*

The most likely diagnosis is atrioventricular reentrant tachycardia. The patient presents with a history of tachycardia and recent syncope. The electrocardiogram shows a short PR interval and the presence of a delta wave, which signifies preexcitation. These features, together with tachycardia, make the diagnosis of Wolff-Parkinson-White syndrome, a type of atrioventricular reentrant tachycardia.

There are no clinical features to suggest idioventricular tachycardia or slow ventricular tachycardia, which is demonstrated electrocardiographically as a wide QRS complex and a heart rate between 60/min and 100/min. Atrial flutter is recognized by the characteristic negative sawtooth deflections in

ECG leads II, III, and aVF, with a positive deflection in V_1, findings that are not present in this patient's electrocardiogram. Multifocal atrial tachycardia characteristically occurs in the setting of chronic lung disease and is manifested by three or more P-wave configurations on the electrocardiogram with associated tachycardia.

KEY POINT

The combination of a short PR interval and a delta wave plus tachycardia confirms the diagnosis of Wolff-Parkinson-White syndrome, a type of atrioventricular tachycardia.

Bibliography

Lee KW, Badhwar N, Scheinman MM. Supraventricular tachycardia–part I. Curr Probl Cardiol. 2008;33(9):467-546. [PMID: 18707990]

Item 18   Answer: A
Educational Objective: *Evaluate progressive chronic angina pectoris with coronary angiography.*

Coronary angiography is the most appropriate option in this patient with continued anginal symptoms despite optimal medical therapy. Compared with optimal medical therapy, a strategy of coronary angiography and revascularization provides no benefit in patients with chronic stable angina. This patient, however, remains highly symptomatic despite optimal medical therapy, and therefore may benefit from coronary angiography and revascularization. Coronary revascularization is beneficial in patients with chronic stable angina and the following conditions: angina pectoris refractory to medical therapy; a large area of ischemic myocardium and high-risk criteria on stress testing; high-risk coronary anatomy, including left main coronary artery stenosis or three-vessel disease; and significant coronary artery disease with reduced left ventricular systolic function. In appropriately selected patients, revascularization, either a percutaneous coronary intervention or coronary artery bypass grafting surgery, has been shown to reduce angina, increase longevity, and improve left ventricular performance.

Exercise treadmill stress testing would not be useful for this patient's management as it would only confirm the known diagnosis of coronary artery disease. Results of an exercise stress test would not influence therapeutic decisions.

β-Blockers, such as metoprolol, reduce myocardial oxygen demand by reducing heart rate and contractility, thereby reducing myocardial oxygen consumption. However, this patient's heart rate is already reduced to 48/min and his blood pressure is under excellent control. Increasing the dose of metoprolol in these circumstances is unlikely to produce further benefit and may not be tolerated because of unacceptably low pulse rate and blood pressure.

For patients with unstable angina, admission to the coronary care unit and intravenous heparin and nitroglycerin would be beneficial. This patient has chronic stable angina, character-ized by progressive exertional angina for 2 months without episodes of pain while at rest or prolonged episodes of pain.

KEY POINT

Coronary angiography is indicated in patients with chronic stable angina who experience lifestyle-limiting angina despite optimal medical therapy.

Bibliography

Jawad E, Arora R. Chronic stable angina pectoris. Dis Mon. 2008;54 (9):671-689. [PMID: 18725007]

Item 19   Answer: D
Educational Objective: *Diagnose ventricular tachycardia.*

The most likely diagnosis is ventricular tachycardia. The electrocardiogram demonstrates sinus rhythm that is suddenly interrupted by the onset of ventricular tachycardia. Ventricular tachyarrhythmias consist of ventricular tachycardia, ventricular fibrillation, and torsades de pointes (a special subset of polymorphic ventricular tachycardia). Ventricular tachyarrhythmias are characterized by wide QRS complex morphology (QRS >0.12 sec) and ventricular rates greater than 100/min. In ventricular tachycardia, the ventricular rate typically ranges from 140 to 250/min; in torsades de pointes, the ventricular rate ranges from 200 to 300/min; and in ventricular fibrillation, the rate is typically above 300/min.

Atrial fibrillation is characterized by an irregularly irregular rhythm, an irregular baseline (atrial fibrillatory waves), and the absence of P waves, which is inconsistent with this patient's electrocardiographic findings.

Supraventricular tachycardia with a wide QRS complex, usually due to coexisting bundle branch block or preexcitation (Wolff-Parkinson-White syndrome), can mimic ventricular tachycardia. Differentiating ventricular tachycardia from supraventricular tachycardia with aberrant conduction is important because the treatment differs markedly. Ventricular tachycardia is more common than supraventricular tachycardia with aberrancy, particularly in patients with structural heart disease. A key point is that any wide QRS tachycardia should be considered to be ventricular tachycardia until proven otherwise. The most important differentiating point is the history of ischemic heart disease. In the presence of known structural heart disease, especially a prior myocardial infarction, the diagnosis of ventricular tachycardia is almost certain. The presence of cannon waves (large *a* waves) in the jugular venous pulsations and varying intensity of the first heart sound support the diagnosis of atrioventricular dissociation caused by either ventricular tachyarrhythmias or heart block.

KEY POINT

A wide QRS tachycardia in the presence of known structural heart disease, especially a prior myocardial infarction, is almost certainly ventricular tachycardia.

Bibliography

Srivathsan K, Ng DW, Mookadam F. Ventricular tachycardia and ventricular fibrillation. Expert Rev Cardiovasc Ther. 2009;7(7):801-809. [PMID: 19589116]

Item 20   Answer: B

Educational Objective: *Treat non–ST-elevation myocardial infarction with a β-blocker.*

The most appropriate additional treatment for this patient is metoprolol. This patient's elevated troponin I level and ST-segment depression and T-wave inversions on electrocardiogram are indicative of a non–ST-elevation myocardial infarction (NSTEMI). Early intravenous β-blocker therapy reduces infarct size, decreases the frequency of recurrent myocardial ischemia, and improves short- and long-term survival. β-Blockers diminish myocardial oxygen demand by reducing heart rate, systemic arterial pressure, and myocardial contractility; in addition, prolongation of diastole augments perfusion to the injured myocardium. β-Blocker therapy can be used in left ventricular dysfunction if heart failure status is stable.

An intra-aortic balloon pump is indicated for an acute coronary syndrome with cardiogenic shock that is unresponsive to medical therapy, acute mitral regurgitation secondary to papillary muscle dysfunction, ventricular septal rupture, or refractory angina. The intra-aortic balloon pump reduces afterload during ventricular systole and increases coronary perfusion during diastole. Patients with refractory cardiogenic shock who are treated with an intra-aortic balloon pump have a lower in-hospital mortality rate than patients who are not treated. This patient has no indication for an intra-aortic balloon pump.

Calcium channel blockers, such as verapamil, are also effective antianginal medications, but data are conflicting as to whether calcium channel blockers reduce mortality in patients with NSTEMI. Therefore, β-blockers are first-line therapy for unstable angina and NSTEMI unless contraindications are present. With ongoing ischemia despite β-blocker therapy, a calcium channel blocker can be added. However, there is no indication for starting verapamil rather than metoprolol at this time.

There is no role for the routine use of warfarin in the treatment of acute coronary syndrome, including NSTEMI. Warfarin is not associated with improved patient outcome as compared to treatment without warfarin. Warfarin may be considered in patients at increased risk for thromboembolism, such as those with atrial fibrillation.

KEY POINT

In patients with myocardial infarction, early intravenous β-blocker therapy reduces infarct size, decreases the frequency of recurrent myocardial ischemia, and improves short- and long-term survival.

Bibliography

Hillis LD, Lange RA. Optimal management of acute coronary syndromes. N Engl J Med. 2009;360(21):2237-2240. [PMID: 19458369]

Item 21   Answer: A

Educational Objective: *Diagnose acute severe mitral regurgitation due to papillary muscle rupture.*

The most likely diagnosis is acute mitral valve regurgitation due to papillary muscle rupture. The clinical history of chest pain and dyspnea a week ago and the electrocardiographic findings of Q waves in leads II, III, and aVF strongly suggest an acute inferior wall myocardial infarction. The presence of a new systolic murmur and respiratory distress several days after an acute myocardial infarction indicates the possibility of either a ventricular septal rupture or mitral regurgitation. Papillary muscle rupture generally presents several days after the infarct event. Severe mitral regurgitation complicating an acute myocardial infarct is more common with inferior versus anterior infarcts and should be suspected in patients with pulmonary edema and respiratory distress in that setting. The murmur of mitral regurgitation may not be prominent because of the acutely elevated left atrial pressure and relatively lower transmitral systolic pressure gradient. Echocardiography is diagnostic, and early clinical recognition with aggressive support (intra-aortic balloon pump, afterload reduction if blood pressure allows) is essential, providing a bridge to surgical repair.

A left ventricular aneurysm may result in late-appearing complications of acute myocardial infarction. A ventricular aneurysm may be associated with intractable ventricular tachyarrhythmias, systemic emboli, or heart failure. It is not associated with a new holosystolic murmur.

Pulmonary embolism can complicate acute myocardial infarction and should be considered in any patient with new-onset pleuritic chest pain, dyspnea, and hypotension. However, pulmonary embolism is not associated with a new holosystolic murmur.

Ventricular free wall rupture typically leads to pericardial tamponade manifesting as sudden hypotension and death. Ventricular free wall rupture typically occurs 1 to 4 days after acute myocardial infarction. Patients usually present with cardiovascular collapse, tamponade, or pulseless electrical activity.

KEY POINT

The presence of a new systolic murmur and respiratory distress several days after an acute myocardial infarction indicates the possibility of either a ventricular septal rupture or mitral regurgitation.

Bibliography

Topalian S, Ginsberg F, Parrillo JE. Cardiogenic shock. Crit Care Med. 2008;36:S66-S74. [PMID: 18158480]

Item 22   Answer: B

Educational Objective: *Treat ST-elevation myocardial infarction with thrombolytic therapy.*

The best management option for this patient is immediate thrombolytic therapy. The patient is experiencing an acute inferior wall ST-elevation myocardial infarction (STEMI). The diagnosis is established by the presence of chest pain and ST-segment elevations in leads II, III, and aVF. The treatment for an acute STEMI is either revascularization or thrombolytic therapy. The patient has no contraindications for thrombolytic therapy. She is currently hemodynamically stable without cardiogenic shock. The treatment of choice is percutaneous coronary intervention (PCI) provided that it can be done immediately or in less than 60 minutes if transfer to another hospital is necessary. Since the nearest hospital with PCI capability is 3 hours away, immediate thrombolytic therapy is the most appropriate treatment for this patient.

Thrombolytic agents are an alternative to primary PCI in suitable candidates with STEMI. By lysing the clot that is limiting blood flow to the myocardium, thrombolytics restore perfusion to the ischemic area, reduce infarct size, and improve survival. Thrombolytics should be administered within 12 hours after the onset of chest pain; the earlier the administration, the better the outcome.

Aggressive medical therapy would not be the correct option for this patient given the electrocardiographic findings, her relatively young age, and the ability to treat her with a thrombolytic agent.

Transfer for coronary artery bypass graft surgery would not be the correct option given that the patient's coronary anatomy has not yet been defined and there would be an unacceptable delay if she were transferred for coronary angiography. Most patients presenting with a STEMI can be treated effectively with percutaneous coronary intervention or thrombolytic therapy. Bypass surgery in the setting of an acute infarction is therefore rarely performed. Bypass surgery may be preferred in patients who have a large amount of myocardium at ischemic risk owing to proximal left main disease or multivessel disease, especially if the left ventricular ejection fraction is reduced. However, this is predicated by first performing coronary angiography and knowing the coronary anatomy.

KEY POINT

Thrombolytic agents are an alternative to primary percutaneous coronary intervention in suitable candidates with ST-elevation myocardial infarction and should be administered within 12 hours after the onset of chest pain.

Bibliography

Hillis LD, Lange RA. Optimal management of acute coronary syndromes. N Engl J Med. 2009;360(21):2237-2240. [PMID: 19458369]

Item 23   Answer: A

Educational Objective: *Diagnose first-degree atrioventricular block.*

This electrocardiogram shows first-degree atrioventricular block and is otherwise unremarkable. First degree atrioventricular block is diagnosed when the PR interval is greater than 0.20 sec. It is often associated with a soft S_1. The presence of first-degree heart block suggests atrioventricular nodal disease but rarely requires therapy. First-degree atrioventricular block is also associated with acute reversible conditions, including inferior myocardial infarction, rheumatic fever, and digitalis intoxication. Additionally, any medication that slows conduction through the atrioventricular node (for example, diltiazem) can potentially produce a first-degree atrioventricular block.

Second-degree atrioventricular block is established when not all beats are conducted from the atria to the ventricles ("dropped beats"). It is recognized in the tracing by the presence of isolated P waves that are not followed by a QRS complex.

Third-degree (complete) atrioventricular heart block is characterized by complete absence of conduction from the atria to the ventricles; the P waves and the QRS complexes are completely independent of each other. Careful analysis will show that the P wave rate and the QRS rate are different and that the PR interval is different for every QRS complex.

The electrocardiographic diagnosis of ventricular preexcitation is based on a short PR interval (<0.11 sec), prolonged QRS duration, and slurred onset of the QRS (delta wave) complex. None of these findings are present.

KEY POINT

First-degree atrioventricular block is diagnosed when the PR interval is greater than 0.20 sec.

Bibliography

Ufberg JW, Clark JS. Bradydysrhythmias and atrioventricular conduction blocks. Emerg Med Clin North Am. 2006;24(1):1-9, v. [PMID: 16308110]

Item 24   Answer: C

Educational Objective: *Diagnose right ventricular infarction complicating an inferior wall ST-elevation myocardial infarction.*

The most likely cause of hypotension in this patient is right ventricular infarction. Right ventricular infarction occurs in approximately 20% of patients with an inferior wall ST-elevation myocardial infarction (STEMI). This diagnosis should be considered in patients with the clinical triad of hypotension, clear lung fields, and jugular venous distention. The diagnosis can be made using a right-sided electrocardiogram, on which ST-segment elevation in leads V_3R and V_4R will be seen. Treatment for right ventricular infarction consists of rapid restoration of blood flow to the right ventricle with either thrombolytic therapy or primary percutaneous coronary intervention, aggressive volume loading with intravenous normal saline to increase filling of the right ventricle, and dopamine or dobutamine if hypotension persists.

Increased vagal tone can cause bradycardia and decreased right ventricular preload, resulting in hypotension early in the course of a myocardial infarction. Although increased vagal tone is commonly associated with inferior wall myocardial infarction, the patient's tachycardia suggests an alternative diagnosis.

Pericardial tamponade from rupture of the left ventricular free wall usually leads to sudden hypotension and death. Free wall rupture is second only to heart failure as the most common cause of death for patients who die in hospitals after myocardial infarction. Ventricular free wall rupture typically occurs 1 to 4 days after acute myocardial infarction. It would be unlikely for pericardial tamponade to be present upon initial presentation unless the patient had chest pain for several days prior to the hospitalization.

A ventricular septal defect manifests as a new systolic murmur, hypotension, and respiratory distress 1 to 3 days following the onset of a myocardial infarction. It would be exceedingly uncommon for a patient to present initially with a ventricular septal defect unless symptoms of chest pain were present for several days.

KEY POINT

In the setting of an inferior wall ST-elevation myocardial infarction, the clinical triad of hypotension, clear lung fields, and jugular venous distention suggests a right ventricular infarction.

Bibliography
Reynolds HR, Hochman JS. Cardiogenic shock: current concepts and improving outcomes. Circulation. 2008;117(5):686-697. [PMID: 18250279]

Item 25   Answer: D
Educational Objective: *Diagnose ventricular septal defect following ST-elevation myocardial infarction.*

The most likely diagnosis is a ventricular septal defect. Mechanical complications occur in roughly 0.1% of patients with ST-elevation myocardial infarction (STEMI) and usually occur 2 to 7 days after infarction. Late complications following STEMI include cardiogenic shock, ventricular septal defect, mitral regurgitation, free wall rupture, and left ventricular thrombus. This patient's progressive hypotension, respiratory distress, and new systolic murmur and thrill suggest either ischemic mitral regurgitation or a ventricular septal defect. Following echocardiography to confirm the diagnosis, this patient should undergo emergent surgery to repair the defect or valve.

Patients with aortic dissection typically present with severe, sharp, tearing chest pain. The pain may radiate widely and be associated with syncope, systemic ischemia (related to impaired blood flow to an organ or limb), or heart failure (aortic valve

disruption, tamponade). Ascending aortic dissection is often associated with acute aortic regurgitation (diastolic murmur at the base of the heart), myocardial ischemia, cardiac tamponade or hemopericardium, and hemothorax or exsanguination. A new systolic murmur and thrill are not compatible with aortic dissection.

Pericardial tamponade may occur following an STEMI from hemorrhagic pericarditis or free wall rupture. Pericardial tamponade from rupture of the left ventricular free wall usually leads to sudden hypotension and death. Ventricular free wall rupture typically occurs 1 to 4 days after acute myocardial infarction. Patients usually present with cardiovascular collapse, tamponade, or pulseless electrical activity. It is not associated with a new, loud systolic murmur or palpable thrill.

A massive pulmonary embolism may produce cardiovascular collapse and hypoxemia but cannot explain the new systolic murmur or left-sided heart failure.

KEY POINT

A ventricular septal defect following an ST-elevation myocardial infarction results in respiratory distress, hypotension, a new systolic murmur, and a palpable thrill.

Bibliography
Poulsen SH, Praestholm M, Munk K, Wierup P, Egeblad H, Nielsen-Kudsk JE. Ventricular septal rupture complicating acute myocardial infarction: clinical characteristics and contemporary outcome. Ann Thorac Surg. 2008;85(5):1591-1596. [PMID:18442545]

Item 26   Answer: D
Educational Objective: *Diagnose sinoatrial node dysfunction.*

This patient has symptomatic sinoatrial node dysfunction (also called sick sinus syndrome). Sinoatrial node dysfunction comprises a collection of pathologic findings that result in bradycardia. These include sinus arrest, sinus exit block, and sinus bradycardia. This patient has sinus bradycardia and sinus arrest. Approximately 50% of patients with sinoatrial node dysfunction also have associated supraventricular tachycardia, most often atrial fibrillation or atrial flutter. The tachycardia-bradycardia syndrome is characterized by rapid ventricular conduction during episodes of atrial fibrillation, but resting bradycardia between episodes. Symptomatic sinus node dysfunction is an indication for pacemaker placement, even if the bradycardia occurs as a consequence of drug therapy, if there is no acceptable alternative.

Atrioventricular nodal block is classified as first, second, or third degree. First-degree block is defined by prolongation of the PR interval to greater than 0.2 sec and usually is not associated with alterations in heart rate. There are two types of second-degree block, both recognized electrocardiographically by the presence of a P wave that is not followed by a ventricular complex. Mobitz type I block (Wenckebach block) manifests as progressive prolongation of the PR interval until there is a dropped beat, whereas Mobitz type II block manifests as a dropped beat without progressive PR-interval prolongation. Mobitz type I block usually does not progress to complete heart block, but Mobitz type II block, which is usually associated with a bundle branch block, typically progresses to third-degree block. Second-degree block may be associated with bradycardia, depending upon the frequency of blocked atrial impulses. Third-degree block is the complete absence of conduction of atrial impulses to the ventricle and is the most common cause of marked bradycardia; ventricular rates are usually 30-50/min. This patient has no evidence of atrioventricular block.

KEY POINT

Sinoatrial node dysfunction comprises a collection of pathologic findings (sinus arrest, sinus exit block, and sinus bradycardia) that result in bradycardia.

Bibliography

Ufberg JW, Clark JS. Bradydysrhythmias and atrioventricular conduction blocks. Emerg Med Clin North Am. 2006;24(1):1-9, v. [PMID: 16308110]

Item 27   Answer: A

Educational Objective: *Diagnose heart block due to donepezil.*

The medication most likely responsible for the patient's heart block is donepezil. Donepezil inhibits acetylcholinesterase. Its activity occurs preferentially in the central nervous system, but mild peripheral cholinergic side effects are common. These effects include increased vagal tone, bradycardia, and, occasionally, atrioventricular block. In this patient, this side effect became manifest when the dosage of donepezil was increased. In patients with preexisting heart block, cholinesterase inhibitors should be used with caution.

Memantine inhibits the glutamatergic *N*-methyl-D-aspartate receptor on central neurons. The side effects of memantine include hallucinations, confusion, restlessness, anxiety, dizziness, headache, fatigue, and constipation.

Trazodone does not commonly cause slowing of cardiac conduction, although it may be associated with palpitations and ventricular ectopy. Vitamin E at a high dose can cause loose stools and may inhibit vitamin K carboxylase, but it is not associated with cardiac side effects.

KEY POINT

Donepezil, an acetylcholinesterase inhibitor, may cause mild peripheral cholinergic side effects, including increased vagal tone, bradycardia, and atrioventricular block.

Bibliography

Feldman H, Gauthier S, Hecker J, et al. A 24-week, randomized, double-blind study of donepezil in moderate to severe Alzheimer's disease. Neurology. 2001;57:613-620. [PMID: 11524468]

Item 28   Answer: D

Educational Objective: *Treat an unstable patient with a cardiac arrhythmia with electrical cardioversion.*

Electrical cardioversion is indicated for an unstable patient with any arrhythmia, other than sinus tachycardia, including atrial fibrillation with a rapid ventricular rate. This patient has persistent tachycardia, worsening mental status, hypoxia, and hypotension consistent with significant hemodynamic instability. Immediate cardioversion is often the safest choice even in hemodynamically stable patients, particularly in those with wide complex tachycardia. After termination of the arrhythmia, the electrocardiogram can provide clues regarding the presence of previous myocardial infarction, left ventricular hypertrophy, or long QT syndrome, and an echocardiogram provides evaluation for structural heart disease and assessment of left ventricular function. Exercise testing can screen for significant coronary artery disease and provoke exercise-associated tachycardias. In newly diagnosed cardiomyopathy, cardiac catheterization is often necessary to evaluate for coronary artery disease as the cause of myocardial dysfunction. CT pulmonary angiography can evaluate the patient for pulmonary emboli; however, none of these studies are indicated until the patient's cardiac rhythm is stabilized with immediate cardioversion.

KEY POINT

Electrical cardioversion is indicated in hemodynamically unstable patients with an arrhythmia.

Bibliography

Zimetbaum P. Atrial fibrillation. Ann Intern Med. 2010;153(11):ITC61. [PMID: 21135291]

Item 29   Answer: B

Educational Objective: *Identify hyperthyroidism as the cause of sinus tachycardia.*

Measuring the TSH level is an appropriate first step to determine the underlying cause of the sinus tachycardia. Sinus tachycardia originates from the sinoatrial node and is defined as a rate of greater than 100/min. Common causes of sinus tachycardia include normal response to exercise and situations associated with increased catecholamine release (fear, pain, anxiety, alcohol withdrawal) as well as fever, hypovolemia, sepsis, heart failure, pulmonary embolism, and hypoxia. Hyperthyroidism is a relatively common cause of sinus tachycardia. Other clues suggesting hyperthyroidism in this patient include difficulty sleeping and unexplained weight loss. In patients with hyperthyroidism, treatment with a β-blocker may provide some symptomatic relief until the underlying thyroid disease is treated.

Adenosine bolus injection is highly effective at terminating atrioventricular (AV) nodal reentrant tachycardia and providing diagnostic information in unclear cases such as revealing flutter waves during adenosine-induced AV block or revealing an underlying atrial tachycardia. Adenosine has no role in managing patients with sinus tachycardia.

An exercise stress test is used to diagnose coronary artery disease. This patient is asymptomatic, has good exercise tolerance, and has no other signs or symptoms of coronary artery disease. Therefore, an exercise stress test is not warranted.

Sinoatrial ablation is indicated for patients with atrial tachycardia that uses part of the sinoatrial node as a reentry circuit. Sinoatrial node ablation is rarely used to treat inappropriate sinus tachycardia. This is a condition characterized by an elevated resting sinus rate in the absence of a recognized cause and an exaggerated rate response to exercise. Most patients with inappropriate sinus tachycardia respond to β-blockers or nondihydropyridine calcium channel blockers, but some refractory cases are treated with sinoatrial node ablation.

KEY POINT

Determining the underlying cause of sinus tachycardia is necessary to guide appropriate treatment.

Bibliography
DeVoe JE, Judkins DZ, Woods L. Clinical inquiries. What is the best approach to the evaluation of resting tachycardia in an adult? J Fam Pract. 2007;56(1):59-61. [PMID: 1721790]

Item 30   Answer: D
Educational Objective: *Treat atrial fibrillation with metoprolol and warfarin.*

This patient is best treated with metoprolol and warfarin. There are two strategies in the treatment of persistent or paroxysmal atrial fibrillation: controlling the ventricular response rate to atrial fibrillation (rate control) and using antiarrhythmic drugs to maintain sinus rhythm (rhythm control). There is no survival advantage associated with either of these strategies, but for older patients (age >70 years), rate control is associated with improved quality-of-life scores. More hospitalizations and adverse drug reactions occur in patients receiving rhythm control compared with rate control. This elderly patient would be at significant risk of drug side effects from antiarrhythmic therapy. Therefore, this patient should receive medication to control the ventricular rate, such as metoprolol, and not an antiarrhythmic agent, such as amiodarone. The use of anticoagulation for stroke prevention is not affected by choice of approach.

In patients with nonvalvular atrial fibrillation, warfarin with a target INR of 2.0 to 3.0 has been shown to decrease stroke risk by an average of 62%, compared with a 19% decrease with aspirin therapy. To determine whether the risk of stroke is high enough to warrant chronic anticoagulation, risk stratification scores have been developed. The CHADS$_2$ risk score for assessing the risk of stroke associated with atrial fibrillation has been validated in a large population. Points are scored for the presence of the following specific risk factors for stroke: *C*ongestive heart failure, *H*ypertension, *A*ge >75 years, *D*iabetes,

and *S*troke or transient ischemic attack (TIA). Patients are given 2 points for a history of stroke or TIA (the strongest risk factor) and 1 point for all other risk factors. The risk of stroke is lowest in patients with a CHADS$_2$ score of 0 (1.2%). The risk is 18% for a CHADS$_2$ score of 6 (maximum score). Patients with a CHADS$_2$ score of 3 or greater and patients with a history of TIA or stroke are at high risk and should be considered for chronic anticoagulation with warfarin. This patient's 10-minute episode of arm weakness is very suggestive of TIA, placing him in the highest risk category for stroke. Patients with a CHADS$_2$ score of 1 or 2 should be assessed on an individual basis for aspirin versus warfarin therapy.

Not all patients with newly diagnosed atrial fibrillation require acute anticoagulation with heparin. Asymptomatic patients with good rate control who require long-term anticoagulation with aspirin or warfarin can have this therapy initiated as an outpatient.

KEY POINT

Most patients with atrial fibrillation are treated with a combination of rate control and long-term anticoagulation.

Bibliography
Zimetbaum P. Atrial fibrillation. Ann Intern Med. 2010;153(11):ITC61. [PMID: 21135291]

Item 31   Answer: D
Educational Objective: *Manage benign premature ventricular contractions.*

The most appropriate management for this patient is no additional investigation or therapy. He is very active and has no symptoms associated with the premature ventricular contractions (PVCs). Physical examination is normal and no findings suggest structural heart disease. Finally, the family history includes no worrisome features to suggest premature or sudden cardiac death syndromes. PVCs often are not associated with symptoms, although they can cause palpitations or a sensation that the heart has stopped, owing to the post-PVC compensatory pause. PVCs at rest in the setting of a structurally normal heart appear to be associated with little to no increased risk of cardiovascular events, particularly in patients younger than 30 years. Repetitive or complex ectopy in the setting of heart disease is associated with increased mortality risk, although the risk is due to the underlying pathophysiologic substrate, and suppression of ambient ventricular arrhythmias does not reduce mortality. Some patients have bothersome symptoms associated with PVCs. If symptoms can be clearly correlated with PVCs, treatment may be appropriate, although many patients respond well to simple reassurance. First-line therapy is almost always a β-blocker such as metoprolol or a calcium channel blocker such as verapamil. However, antiarrhythmic drug therapy is associated with side-effects, so treatment cannot be undertaken without a discussion of its risks and benefits. Additional investigation in this asymptomatic young and healthy patient is unlikely to change his management. Therefore, echocardiography, arrhythmia monitoring, and exercise stress testing is not indicated.

KEY POINT

Premature ventricular contractions at rest in the setting of a structurally normal heart appear to be associated with little to no increased risk of cardiovascular events, particularly in patients younger than 30 years.

Bibliography

Ng GA. Treating patients with ventricular ectopic beats. Heart. 2006;92 (11):1707-12. [PMID: 17041126]

Item 32   Answer: D

Educational Objective: *Treat patients at risk for sudden death with an implantable cardioverter-defibrillator.*

The most appropriate treatment for this patient is an ICD. Sustained ventricular tachycardia (VT) occurs most commonly in patients with previous myocardial infarction, and it is the scar formed by the infarction that provides the anatomic substrate for reentry. Areas of fibrosis interspersed with viable myocardial tissue are present in the border zone of dense scar tissue and impart the required conduction delay critical to the establishment of reentry circuits. Symptoms depend on the underlying state of the patient, and some patients can be asymptomatic, particularly if the VT rate is slow. In general, medical therapy (amiodarone, procainamide, flecainide) does not improve survival in patients with VT and structural heart disease; thus, most patients are candidates for ICD placement. Large clinical trials have demonstrated ICD therapy improves survival rates in patients with hemodynamically unstable VT after cardiac arrest who have ischemic or nonischemic cardiomyopathy and ejection fractions less than 35%. In patients with left ventricular dysfunction in the absence of VT, ICD implantation has also been shown to improve survival. The primary eligibility criterion for ICD implantation for primary prevention of sudden cardiac death in the setting of heart failure is left ventricular ejection fraction less than 35%, regardless of the presence or absence of coronary disease or the occurrence of arrhythmia.

KEY POINT

The primary eligibility criterion for implantable cardioverter-defibrillator implantation for primary prevention of sudden cardiac death in the setting of heart failure is left ventricular ejection fraction less than 35%.

Bibliography

Cevik C, Nugent K, Perez-Verdia A, Fish RD. Prophylactic implantation of cardioverter defibrillators in idiopathic nonischemic cardiomyopathy for the primary prevention of death: a narrative review. Clin Cardiol. 2010;33(5):254-60. [PMID: 20513063]

Item 33   Answer: B

Educational Objective: *Manage a patient with ventricular fibrillation arrest in the setting of acute myocardial infarction.*

The best option for the patient at this time is to continue medical management. Ventricular tachyarrhythmias are common in the setting of acute myocardial infarction, occurring in up to 20% of patients. Despite a sixfold increase in in-hospital mortality, the overall mortality at 1 year is not increased in patients with ventricular fibrillation that occurs early in this setting. Therefore, unlike sudden cardiac death occurring in other settings, cardiac arrest occurring within the first 48 hours of transmural acute myocardial infarction does not require defibrillator placement.

Primary ventricular fibrillation should be distinguished from ventricular fibrillation that occurs later in the course, usually as a result of heart failure. Before the advent of the implantable cardioverter-defibrillator, ventricular fibrillation occurring late in the hospital course was associated with an 85% 1-year mortality rate. All patients, even those who have not suffered arrhythmia during myocardial infarction, should be reevaluated after myocardial infarction by transthoracic echocardiogram to further stratify risk. If the ejection fraction is found to be reduced (<35%), the patient may be a candidate for defibrillator placement.

Amiodarone has not been shown to improve overall mortality following myocardial infarction. In the general population of cardiac arrest survivors, amiodarone does not improve mortality.

Implantable cardioverter-defibrillator placement is not indicated for patients who experience ventricular arrhythmias less than 48 hours after an acute ST-elevation myocardial infarction. Implantable cardioverter-defibrillators have demonstrated a mortality benefit for essentially all other groups of cardiac arrest survivors.

The typical indications for a pacemaker include symptomatic sinoatrial node dysfunction (sinus bradycardia, intra-atrial block, exit block) and symptomatic bradycardia due to advanced second- or third-degree heart block. This asymptomatic man with no evidence of bradycardia or advanced heart block on his electrocardiogram has no indication for a pacemaker. Pacemaker placement does not prevent sudden death due to ventricular tachyarrhythmias.

KEY POINT

Cardiac arrest occurring within the first 48 hours of an acute, transmural myocardial infarction does not require secondary prevention therapy other than standard post–myocardial infarction care.

Bibliography

Kusumoto F. A comprehensive approach to management of ventricular arrhythmias. Cardiol Clin. 2008;26(3):481-496, vii. [PMID: 18538192]

Item 34 Answer: C
Educational Objective: *Diagnose familial long QT syndrome.*

This patient most likely has long QT syndrome (LQTS). Cardiac events in patients with LQTS include syncope and cardiac arrest due to torsade de pointes ventricular tachycardia. LQTS may be either congenital or acquired. This patient probably has congenital LQTS, suggested by recurrent syncope triggered by activity and a family history of early sudden death (cousin drowning). Her mother is probably affected as well. Risk factors for acquired LQTS include female sex, hypokalemia, hypomagnesemia, structural heart disease, previous QT-interval prolongation, and a history of drug-induced arrhythmia. (An extensive list of offending agents can be found at www.azcert.org/medical-pros/drug-lists/drug-lists.cfm.) Other cardiac causes of syncope and sudden death in young patients include hypertrophic cardiomyopathy and arrhythmogenic right ventricular dysplasia.

Left bundle branch block (LBBB) and right bundle branch block (RBBB) are electrocardiographic patterns that increase in frequency with age. LBBB most often occurs in patients with underlying heart disease. In older patients, LBBB is associated with increased mortality. In younger patients, however, LBBB is not associated with syncope or sudden death and the prognosis is generally excellent. RBBB is similarly associated with increased mortality in older patients with underlying heart disease. When RBBB is not associated with underlying cardiac disease, patient outcomes are generally excellent, and RBBB is an unlikely cause of this patient's symptoms.

First-degree atrioventricular block is characterized by prolongation of the PR interval to longer than 0.2 sec; it usually is not associated with alterations in heart rate and has no association with syncope or sudden death.

KEY POINT

Cardiac events in patients with long QT syndrome include syncope and cardiac arrest due to torsade de pointes ventricular tachycardia.

Bibliography
Goldenberg I, Zareba W, Moss AJ. Long QT syndrome. Curr Probl Cardiol. 2008;33(11):629-694. [PMID: 18835466]

Item 35 Answer: A
Educational Objective: *Treat New York Heart Association class IV heart failure with digoxin.*

Digoxin is the most appropriate therapy to initiate in this patient. The role of digoxin in treating heart failure patients in sinus rhythm is primarily for symptom control rather than improving survival. Treatment with digoxin has not been shown to affect mortality but has been shown to reduce hospitalizations. Digoxin can be added to other therapy in patients with New York Heart Association class III or IV heart failure for symptom control. Maintaining lower serum concentrations of digoxin is as effective as maintaining higher concen-

trations, and potential toxicities are avoided. Higher digoxin levels (≥1.2 ng/mL [1.5 nmol/L] versus 0.5-0.8 ng/mL [0.6-1.0 nmol/L]) appear to be associated with higher mortality in patients with systolic heart failure. The primary reason to use an angiotensin receptor blocer (ARB) instead of an angiotensin-converting enzyme (ACE) inhibitor, such as lisinopril, is to avoid the side effect of cough. Combined treatment with an ACE inhibitor and an ARB is generally not recommended, because concurrent therapy is significantly associated with increased risk of medication nonadherence and adverse effects, including worsening renal function and symptomatic hypotension, whereas the additional benefit of using these two medications together is not well established. ACE inhibitors are currently preferred over ARBs for most patients, because there is more clinical experience with these agents.

There is no role for the routine anticoagulation of heart failure patients with warfarin (or aspirin) because there is no apparent benefit and an increased risk of bleeding. Major guidelines generally agree that warfarin should be considered in a patient with a heart failure and a previous thrombotic event (for example, stroke or pulmonary embolism) and in patients with an underlying atrial fibrillation heart rhythm.

KEY POINT

Digoxin alleviates symptoms and decreases hospitalizations, but it provides no survival benefit in patients with heart failure.

Bibliography
Goldberg LR. Heart failure. Ann Intern Med. 2010;152(11):ITC61-16; quiz ITC616. [PMID: 20513825]

Item 36 Answer: D
Educational Objective: *Diagnose heart failure due to peripartum cardiomyopathy.*

This patient most likely has heart failure due to peripartum cardiomyopathy. Peripartum cardiomyopathy is defined as heart failure with a left ventricular ejection fraction less than 45% that is diagnosed between 3 months before and 6 months after delivery in the absence of an identifiable cause. It is usually diagnosed during the first month postpartum. This patient has clinical features consistent with heart failure (progressive dyspnea), evidence of left ventricular dysfunction (tachycardia, elevated central venous pressure, S_3 and S_4, displaced and diffuse apical impulse, mitral regurgitant murmur, pulmonary crackles), and confirmatory chest radiography (pleural effusions and interstitial infiltrates).

Acute myocardial infarction may occur during pregnancy and in the postpartum period. It may be related to atherosclerotic coronary artery disease or coronary artery dissection and vasculitis and carries a high risk of maternal mortality and morbidity. This patient's presentation, however, does not suggest an acute coronary syndrome, given the absence of chest pain or electrocardiographic changes.

Aortic dissection may occur in the peripartum or postpartum period and is a particular concern in patients with aortopathy related to Marfan syndrome, familial thoracic aortic aneurysmal disease, or bicuspid aortic valve–related aortopathy. However, the current presentation does not suggest aortic dissection given the absence of chest pain, the presence of equal and normal blood pressures in the upper extremities, and the presence of normal lower extremity pulses. Additionally, aortic dissection is usually associated with an abnormal chest radiograph (widened mediastinum, abnormal aortic contour), and the absence of these findings argues strongly against the diagnosis. Aortic dissection cannot explain the patient's findings of a dilated left ventricle and signs of heart failure.

Coarctation of the aorta may rarely present initially as hypertension during pregnancy. However, the patient's current physical examination findings of easily palpable lower extremity pulses without delay and the absence of hypertension argue against coarctation. In addition, rib notching is not reported on the chest radiograph.

KEY POINT

The presence of elevated central venous pressure, pulmonary crackles, ventricular gallops (S$_3$ or S$_4$), any cardiac murmur, and lower extremity edema all increase the likelihood of heart failure.

Bibliography
Goldberg LR. Heart failure. Ann Intern Med. 2010;152(11):ITC61-15; quiz ITC616. [PMID: 20513825]

Item 37   Answer: A
Educational Objective: *Evaluate a patient with new-onset heart failure with cardiac angiography.*

The most appropriate diagnostic test for this patient is a cardiac angiography. This patient has typical angina (substernal chest pain precipitated by exertion and relieved by rest) and new-onset heart failure, as evidenced by symptoms (exertional dyspnea and orthopnea), examination findings (elevated jugular venous pressure, pulmonary crackles, and an S$_3$ and S$_4$), and echocardiogram with a subnormal ejection fraction. Definitive testing for coronary artery disease (CAD) by cardiac catheterization is warranted. The primary aim of an evaluation for CAD is to identify possible targets for revascularization (percutaneous or surgical) with the goals of reducing angina, improving systolic function, reducing the risk of heart failure progression, and improving survival.

For patients with an intermediate likelihood of CAD who have no features of unstable angina, stress testing is the preferred approach when assessing for CAD. An exercise stress test is recommended in a patient with an intermediate probability of disease and a normal resting electrocardiogram (ECG). A nuclear medicine stress test is helpful if the resting ECG is abnormal. In this patient, however, the pretest probability for CAD is high based on his age, sex, and the presence of typical anginal symptoms. Because a negative result on stress test-

ing in a patient with a high pretest probability of CAD would have a high likelihood of being a false negative, catheterization would still be needed for a definitive diagnosis, as well as for planning therapy.

A radionuclide ventriculogram can be useful in confirming the ejection fraction if clarification is needed. In this patient, however, the ejection fraction value is provided by the echocardiogram. Furthermore, a radionuclide ventriculogram would not assist in determining the cause of the new-onset heart failure.

KEY POINT

Patients with new-onset heart failure and angina should be evaluated with cardiac catheterization and angiography if they are possible candidates for revascularization.

Bibliography
Goldberg LR. Heart failure. Ann Intern Med. 2010;152(11):ITC61-15; quiz ITC616. [PMID: 20513825]

Item 38   Answer: B
Educational Objective: *Evaluate new-onset heart failure with echocardiography.*

An echocardiogram should be obtained in all patients with newly diagnosed or suspected heart failure to determine whether the heart failure is systolic or diastolic and whether there are any structural or functional abnormalities that may be causing the heart failure (such as regional wall abnormalities, pericardial disease, or valvular abnormality). All of these issues may have a significant impact on management and prognosis.

B-type natriuretic peptide (BNP) is a hormone synthesized by the cardiac ventricles in response to increased wall stress due to pressure or volume overload. BNP assays have become a useful tool in the diagnosis of acute heart failure and differentiating it from noncardiac causes of dyspnea. A patient with a BNP concentration below 100 pg/mL is unlikely to have acute heart failure, whereas a patient with a concentration higher than 500 pg/mL has a high likelihood of having heart failure. BNP level will likely be elevated in this patient, confirming the presence of volume overload. The physical examination, history, and chest radiograph concordantly suggest volume overload and heart failure, and a BNP level confirming this would not be helpful.

A radionuclide ventriculogram would accurately assess ventricular ejection fraction but would not provide other cardiac structural or functional information that may impact management. A radionuclide ventriculogram, therefore, is not the most appropriate next test.

Ischemia is a major cause of left ventricular dysfunction. Given the potential significant benefits of revascularization in appropriate candidates, including improved ventricular function and reduced morbidity and mortality, diligent evaluation for coronary artery disease should be undertaken for most patients with heart failure. A stress test would be appropriate in this patient if there were a higher clinical suspicion for coronary disease or ischemia causing new-onset heart failure. However, given the lack of anginal symptoms, the patient's relatively young age, and lack of risk factors, clinical suspicion at this point is low. Finally, and importantly, an exercise stress test is contraindicated in a patient with decompensated heart failure, such as this patient.

KEY POINT

An echocardiogram should be obtained in all patients with newly diagnosed or suspected heart failure.

Bibliography
Abraham J, Abraham TP. The role of echocardiography in hemodynamic assessment in heart failure. Heart Fail Clin. 2009;5(2):191-208. [PMID: 19249688]

Item 39   Answer: B

Educational Objective: *Treat New York Heart Association class I or II systolic heart failure with a β-blocker.*

Treatment with an angiotensin-converting enzyme (ACE) inhibitor (such as lisinopril) and a β-blocker (such as carvedilol) is indicated for all patients with systolic heart failure regardless of symptoms or functional status, including asymptomatic or very functional patients. The combination of these two classes of medications has additive benefits with regard to morbidity and mortality in systolic heart failure. This patient is already taking an ACE inhibitor, so a β-blocker such as carvedilol should be added. β-Blockers should not be initiated or increased during decompensated states, such as volume overload or hypotension, because the transient decline in cardiac output may worsen a decompensated state.

Amlodipine is the only calcium channel blocker demonstrated to have a neutral (rather than detrimental) effect on morbidity and mortality in heart failure. Thus, it is an acceptable agent to use for angina or hypertension that is not adequately controlled with ACE inhibitors or β-blockers. However, this patient has neither angina nor uncontrolled hypertension, and amlodipine is not indicated.

Digoxin is indicated for patients with moderately to severely symptomatic heart failure (New York Heart Association [NYHA] class III-IV) or for rate control in patients with atrial fibrillation. Digoxin improves symptoms and reduces hospitalizations, but it does not affect survival. Spironolactone is indicated only for treatment of NYHA class III or IV heart failure; in this setting, its use is associated with a 30% reduction in mortality. This patient, however, is only minimally symptomatic (NYHA class II); treatment with either digoxin or spironolactone is not indicated.

There are currently no robust data to support addition of an angiotensin receptor blocker (ARB), such as losartan, to ACE inhibitor therapy for treatment of systolic heart failure. No definitive improvement in survival has been demonstrated using the combination of these two agents. ARBs are currently recommended only for patients who are intolerant of ACE inhibitors, primarily owing to ACE inhibitor–induced cough.

KEY POINT

Treatment with an angiotensin-converting enzyme inhibitor and a β-blocker is indicated for all patients with systolic heart failure regardless of symptoms or functional status, including asymptomatic or very functional patients.

Bibliography
Goldberg LR. Heart failure. Ann Intern Med. 2010;152(11):ITC61-15; quiz ITC616. [PMID: 20513825]

Item 40   Answer: D

Educational Objective: *Treat a patient with heart failure with a β-blocker and an angiotensin-converting enzyme inhibitor.*

This patient should be started on lisinopril in addition to metoprolol. Angiotensin-converting enzyme (ACE) inhibitors, such as lisinopril, are indicated for treatment of all New York Heart Association (NYHA) functional classes of systolic heart failure, including asymptomatic (NYHA class I) patients. ACE inhibitors reduce mortality and morbidity in asymptomatic and symptomatic patients and delay the onset of clinical heart failure in patients with asymptomatic left ventricular dysfunction. Overall, ACE inhibitor therapy reduces mortality by about 20%, risk for myocardial infarction by about 20%, and hospitalization for heart failure by 30% to 40%.

For patients intolerant of ACE inhibitors owing to hyperkalemia or renal insufficiency, the combination of hydralazine and a nitrate is a suitable alternative, with hemodynamic effects of vasodilation and afterload reduction. Treatment with this combination is also associated with a reduction in mortality, although to a lesser degree than is seen with ACE inhibitors, and this combination does not have the same positive impact on quality of life as an ACE inhibitor.

The role of digoxin in treating heart failure patients in sinus rhythm is primarily for symptom control rather than improving survival. Treatment with digoxin has not been shown to affect mortality but has been shown to reduce hospitalizations. Digoxin can be added to other therapy in patients with NYHA class III or IV heart failure for symptom control. Maintaining lower serum concentrations of digoxin is as effective as maintaining higher concentrations, and potential toxicities are avoided.

Eplerenone is a selective aldosterone blocker that is currently approved for treatment of hypertension and for left ventricular dysfunction after myocardial infarction. Eplerenone is a suitable alternative to spironolactone in treatment of severe heart failure (NYHA class III or IV) if gynecomastia develops as a side effect of spironolactone treatment.

This patient has NYHA class II heart failure (symptoms with moderate exertion) and does not meet the criteria for treatment with digoxin or an aldosterone agonist.

KEY POINT

Angiotensin-converting enzyme inhibitors are indicated for treatment of all New York Heart Association (NYHA) functional classes of systolic heart failure, including asymptomatic (NYHA class I) patients.

Bibliography

Goldberg LR. Heart failure. Ann Intern Med. 2010;152(11):ITC61-15; quiz, ITC616. [PMID: 20513825]

Item 41   Answer: D

Educational Objective: *Treat a patient with New York Heart Association functional class III or IV heart failure with spironolactone.*

The most appropriate addition to this patient's treatment is spironolactone. She has symptoms consistent with New York Heart Association (NYHA) class III functional status (symptoms develop with mild activity), and she does not appear volume-overloaded on examination (normal central venous pressure and no S_3, pulmonary crackles, or edema). Spironolactone is indicated for treatment of severe (NYHA functional class III or IV) systolic heart failure in addition to standard therapy with an angiotensin-converting enzyme (ACE) inhibitor, β-blocker, and diuretic as needed. Spironolactone further blocks the actions of aldosterone, which is not completely suppressed by chronic ACE inhibitor therapy; aldosterone has adverse effects of sodium retention, potassium wasting, and myocardial fibrosis. The addition of spironolactone is associated with a 30% relative reduction in mortality.

Serum creatinine and potassium levels should be serially monitored in patients taking spironolactone. Contraindications to spironolactone therapy include a serum creatinine level greater than 2.5 mg/dL (221 µmol/L) in men or 2.0 mg/dL (176.8 µmol/L) in women or a potassium level greater than 5 meq/L (5 mmol/L).

It is generally not recommended to add angiotensin receptor blocker therapy, such as losartan, to ACE inhibitor therapy because the risk of adverse side effects, such as hyperkalemia and hypotension, is increased.

The addition of metolazone to loop diuretic therapy can be useful to increase diuretic effectiveness. However, this patient appears euvolemic on her current diuretic regimen, so enhanced diuresis is not needed.

First-generation calcium channel blockers (such as nifedipine) have been shown to increase the risk of heart failure decompensation and hospitalization. Amlodipine and felodipine are the only calcium channel blockers with demonstrated neutral effects on mortality in patients with heart failure. These agents can be used in patients with heart failure for the management of hypertension or angina not adequately controlled with other agents such as ACE inhibitors or β-blockers.

KEY POINT

Angiotensin-converting enzyme inhibitors, β-blockers, and spironolactone reduce mortality in patients with New York Heart Association class III or IV heart failure.

Bibliography

Goldberg LR. Heart failure. Ann Intern Med. 2010;152(11):ITC61-15; quiz ITC616. [PMID: 20513825]

Item 42   Answer: A

Educational Objective: *Diagnose atrial fibrillation as the cause of clinical deterioration in a patient with aortic stenosis.*

New-onset atrial fibrillation is the most likely cause of the patient's new symptoms. Aortic valve sclerosis, or valve thickening without outflow obstruction, is present in more than 25% of persons older than 65 years. Patients are often diagnosed when an asymptomatic murmur is auscultated or following an incidental echocardiographic finding. The progression from aortic sclerosis to stenosis is slow, and fewer than 20% of patients develop valve obstruction over the next 10 years. When mild stenosis is present, however, progressive valve stenosis proceeds more rapidly. Classic manifestations of aortic stenosis are angina, syncope, and heart failure. In early stages, aortic stenosis may present subtly with dyspnea or a decrease in exercise tolerance. Atrial fibrillation can be associated with rapid and severe clinical deterioration due to the more rapid rate and loss of atrial contribution to left ventricular filling. Angina occurs in more than 50% of patients with severe stenosis, due in part to maldistribution of coronary flow in the hypertrophied myocardium. Patients with aortic stenosis have increased sensitivity to ischemic injury, and subsequently have higher mortality. Frank syncope associated with aortic stenosis is rare, with prospective studies documenting sudden cardiac death rates less than 1% annually.

Endocarditis should be suspected if an abnormal murmur is heard on examination, particularly in patients with a compelling history or concurrent fever. Incidence is higher in patients with underlying valve abnormalities and prosthetic valves. Because of the absence of fever and the presence of atrial fibrillation as a more likely cause of clinical deterioration, infective endocarditis is unlikely.

Patients with a history of rheumatic fever may have involvement of multiple heart valves, but this is not the case in patients with degenerative aortic sclerosis. Furthermore, the physical examination findings of chronic mitral regurgitation include a holosystolic murmur, heard best at the apex, with radiation laterally or posteriorly. The auscultatory findings for mitral stenosis include an opening snap with a low-pitched middiastolic murmur that accentuates presystole. These findings are not present, making mitral stenosis or regurgitation unlikely.

In patients with aortic stenosis, atrial fibrillation can be associated with rapid and severe clinical deterioration due to the more rapid rate and loss of atrial contribution to left ventricular filling.

Bibliography

Kappetein AP, van Geldorp M, Takkenberg JJ, Bogers AJ. Optimum management of elderly patients with calcified aortic stenosis. Expert Rev Cardiovasc Ther. 2008;6(4):491-501. [PMID: 18402539]

Item 43   Answer: A
Educational Objective: *Diagnose failure of a prosthetic aortic heart valve.*

Failure of a prosthetic aortic valve often leads to aortic insufficiency. Bioprosthetic valves are less durable than mechanical valves because of the progressive degenerative calcification of the biologic material. In the first generation of bioprosthetic valves, only about 50% of aortic and 30% of mitral prostheses were still working after 15 years. Although newer valves are more durable and have larger valve areas and improved hemodynamics, they are still prone to progressive calcific degeneration. Physical examination in patients with chronic aortic regurgitation shows a widened pulse pressure with bounding peripheral and carotid pulses. Auscultatory findings include an early to holodiastolic murmur along the left upper sternal border, which is high pitched and may be better heard when the patient is at end-expiration, leaning forward.

The characteristic physical examination findings in atrial septal defect are fixed splitting of the S_2 and a right ventricular heave. A pulmonary midsystolic flow murmur and a tricuspid diastolic flow rumble caused by increased flow through the right-sided valves from a large left-to-right shunt may be heard.

Aortic coarctation is usually diagnosed in childhood by the association of a systolic murmur with systemic hypertension and reduced femoral pulse amplitude. More than 50% of patients with aortic coarctation also have a bicuspid aortic valve. When coarctation is severe, the murmur may be continuous and a murmur from collateral intercostal vessels may also be audible and palpable. An ejection click and aortic systolic murmur suggest the presence of a bicuspid aortic valve. An S_4 is common.

The auscultatory findings for rheumatic mitral stenosis include an opening snap with a low-pitched middiastolic murmur that accentuates presystole and is best heard over the mitral valve area. The S_1 may be intensified owing to higher left atrial pressures.

New-onset ventricular septal defect in adults usually occurs 5 to 7 days following a myocardial infarction. It is characterized by the development of cardiogenic shock and a new systolic murmur. A thrill along the left sternal border may also be present. This patient does not have a history consistent with myocardial infarction and does not have the typical findings.

Failure of a prosthetic aortic valve often leads to aortic insufficiency.

Bibliography

Choudhry NK, Etchells EE. The rational clinical examination. Does this patient have aortic regurgitation? JAMA. 1999;281(23):2231-8. [PMID: 10376577]

Item 44   Answer: D
Educational Objective: *Manage an asymptomatic benign murmur.*

This patient has a benign midsystolic murmur that is grade 2/6 in intensity and requires no further evaluation or intervention. Midsystolic murmurs grade 2/6 or less are considered innocent murmurs, especially when they are short in duration, associated with a physiologically split (normal) S_2, and are not accompanied by any other abnormal cardiac sounds or murmurs. The most common etiology of this type of murmur in persons older than 65 years is minor valvular abnormalities due to aortic sclerosis. Aortic sclerosis is characterized by focal areas of valve thickening leading to mild valvular turbulence, producing the auscultated murmur. A hyperdynamic circulation (for example, from severe anemia, thyrotoxicosis, or pregnancy) also may produce an innocent midsystolic pulmonary or aortic flow murmur. A physiologically split S_2 (apparent during inspiration, absent during exhalation) excludes severe aortic stenosis.

Endocarditis prophylaxis is not indicated. The only patients who should receive endocarditis prophylaxis are those with prosthetic cardiac valves, those with a known history of prior infective endocarditis, those with unrepaired cyanotic congenital heart disease, those with complex congenital heart disease with residual abnormalities, and cardiac transplant recipients with valve abnormalities.

Transthoracic echocardiography is indicated when a grade 3/6 or greater systolic murmur is heard on examination, in the presence of any diastolic or continuous murmur, or if a new murmur is diagnosed in the interval since a normal prior physical examination; none of these criteria are met by this patient.

A screening cardiac stress test is not warranted because she has no symptoms indicative of angina or risk factors for coronary artery disease. In a patient with a low pretest probability of coronary artery disease, an exercise stress test would carry a high false-positive rate.

Short, soft, midsystolic murmurs in the elderly are usually benign and caused by minor, age-related changes of the aortic valve (aortic sclerosis).

Bibliography

Etchells E, Bell C, Robb K. Does this patient have an abnormal systolic murmur? JAMA. 1997;277(7):564-571. [PMID: 9032164]

Item 45   Answer: C

Educational Objective: *Diagnose mitral stenosis.*

This patient's clinical history and physical examination findings are consistent with rheumatic mitral valve stenosis. Cardiac auscultation reveals the typical findings of mitral stenosis, including an accentuation of P_2 (evidence of elevated pulmonary arterial pressure), an opening snap (a high-pitched apical sound best heard with the diaphragm of the stethoscope), and a low-pitched, rumbling diastolic murmur.

Mitral stenosis is usually caused by rheumatic valve disease. In the United States, clinical presentation tends to be 20 to 30 years after the initial episode of rheumatic fever, and most cases occur in women. Patients with mitral stenosis may be asymptomatic for some time, but become symptomatic with additional hemodynamic stress, such as the increased volume load of pregnancy. This hemodynamic stress may precipitate an arrhythmia, such as atrial fibrillation, that can further exacerbate heart failure symptoms.

The diagnosis of acute aortic regurgitation is suggested in patients with rapid onset of dyspnea, exercise intolerance, or chest pain (aortic dissection). Physical findings include tachycardia, hypotension, a soft S_1 (due to premature closure of the mitral valve), an S_3 and/or S_4 gallop, an accentuated pulmonic closure sound, and pulmonary crackles. The typical murmur of aortic regurgitation may not be prominent in acute disease as aortic and left ventricular diastolic pressures equilibrate quickly, resulting in a short and soft (sometimes inaudible) diastolic murmur at the base of the heart.

The characteristic physical examination finding in atrial septal defect is fixed splitting of the S_2. A pulmonic midsystolic murmur at the base of the heart and a tricuspid diastolic flow rumble may be heard at the lower left sternal border owing to increased flow through the valves from the left-to-right shunt.

The murmur of tricuspid regurgitation is a systolic murmur that is best heard at the lower left sternal border and characteristically increases in intensity with inspiration. Tricuspid regurgitation usually occurs as a secondary consequence of pulmonary hypertension, right ventricular chamber enlargement with annular dilatation, or endocarditis.

KEY POINT

Typical findings of mitral stenosis include an opening snap and a low-pitched, rumbling diastolic murmur.

Bibliography

Chizner MA. The diagnosis of heart disease by clinical assessment alone. Dis Mon. 2002;48(1):7-98. [PMID: 11807426]

Item 46   Answer: C

Educational Objective: *Diagnose hypertrophic cardiomyopathy.*

In this patient, the physical examination is most consistent with hypertrophic cardiomyopathy. The systolic murmur of hypertrophic cardiomyopathy is caused by obstruction in the left ventricular outflow tract from the thickened interventricular septum. In severe cases, systolic anterior motion of the mitral valve apparatus into the left ventricular outflow tract contributes to the systolic murmur. If mitral valve leaflet coaptation is affected, there may be concurrent mitral regurgitation. The stand-to-squat maneuver and passive leg lift transiently increase venous return (preload), which increases left ventricular chamber size and volume. As a consequence, there is less relative obstruction and turbulence in the left ventricular outflow tract, decreasing murmur intensity. Handgrip exercise also diminishes murmur intensity, by increasing afterload and decreasing the relative pressure gradient across the left ventricular outflow tract. The Valsalva maneuver and the squat-to-stand maneuver transiently decrease venous return, with the septum and anterior mitral leaflet brought closer together. Turbulent flow—and the murmur—are increased. Transthoracic echocardiography can confirm a diagnosis of hypertrophic cardiomyopathy.

Aortic coarctation in an adult is characterized by hypertension and a continuous or late systolic murmur that may be heard over the back. Because pulses distal to the aortic obstruction are decreased, aortic coarctation is also associated with abnormal differences in upper and lower extremity blood pressures. The carotid upstroke is normal in coarctation.

A congenital bicuspid aortic valve is a common cause of calcific aortic stenosis. The murmur of aortic stenosis is an early systolic murmur that often radiates toward the carotid arteries. Hypertrophic cardiomyopathy is associated with rapid upstrokes of the carotid arteries, helping to distinguish it from aortic stenosis, which is associated with a carotid artery pulsation that has a slow up-rise and is diminished in volume. In addition, the murmur of aortic stenosis decreases with the Valsalva maneuver. Finally, although the presence of a bicuspid aortic valve accelerates the process of aortic calcification, patients typically develop stenosis in their thirties or forties, not in the late teens or early twenties.

The murmur associated with a ventricular septal defect is a harsh systolic murmur located parasternally that radiates to the right sternal edge and may be associated with a palpable thrill but no change in the carotid artery pulsation. Maneuvers that increase afterload, such as isometric handgrip exercise, increase the left-sided murmurs of mitral regurgitation and ventricular septal defect.

KEY POINT

The Valsalva maneuver and the squat-to-stand maneuver increase the murmur of hypertrophic cardiomyopathy.

Bibliography
Etchells E, Bell C, Robb K. Does this patient have an abnormal systolic murmur? JAMA. 1997;277(7):564-571. [PMID:9032164]

Item 47   Answer: A
Educational Objective: *Diagnose aortic valve regurgitation.*

This patient most likely has aortic regurgitation. Physical findings of chronic aortic regurgitation may include cardiomegaly, tachycardia, a widened pulse pressure, a thrill at the base of the heart, a soft S_1 and a sometimes absent aortic closure sound, and an S_3 gallop. The characteristic high-pitched diastolic murmur begins immediately after S_2 and is heard best at the second right or third left intercostal space with the patient leaning forward, and in end-expiration. Manifestations of the widened pulse pressure may include the Traube sign (pistol-shot sounds over the peripheral arteries), the de Musset sign (head bobs with each heartbeat), the Duroziez sign (systolic and diastolic murmur heard over the femoral artery), and the Quincke sign (systolic plethora and diastolic blanching in the nail bed with nail compression).

Mitral stenosis is associated with accentuation of P_2 (evidence of elevated pulmonary arterial pressure), an opening snap (a high-pitched apical diastolic sound best heard with the diaphragm of the stethoscope) followed by a low-pitched, rumbling diastolic murmur best heard with the bell of the stethoscope at the apex with the patient in the left lateral decubitus position. Presystolic accentuation of the murmur may be present. As the severity of the stenosis worsens, the opening snap moves closer to S_2 as a result of increased left atrial pressure, and the murmur increases in duration.

A small patent ductus arteriosus in an adult produces a continuous murmur that envelopes the S_2 and is characteristically heard beneath the left clavicle. Patients with a moderate-sized patent ductus arteriosus may present with symptoms of heart failure, a continuous "machinery-type" murmur best heard at the left infraclavicular area, and bounding pulses with a wide pulse pressure.

Tricuspid valve regurgitation usually occurs as a secondary consequence of pulmonary hypertension, right ventricular chamber enlargement with annular dilatation, or endocarditis. The murmur of tricuspid regurgitation occurs during systole and is loudest at the lower left sternal border and becomes louder with inspiration.

KEY POINT

The characteristic high-pitched diastolic murmur of chronic aortic regurgitation begins immediately after S_2 and is heard best with the patient leaning forward, and in end-expiration at the second right or third left intercostal space.

Bibliography
Choudhry NK, Etchells EE. The rational clinical examination. Does this patient have aortic regurgitation? JAMA. 1999;281(23):2231-2238. [PMID: 10376577]

Item 48   Answer: D
Educational Objective: *Diagnose mitral valve prolapse.*

Mitral valve prolapse is the most common cause of mitral regurgitation. The prevalence in the United States is 2% to 3% with equal sex distribution. The classic auscultatory findings are a midsystolic click followed by a late apical systolic murmur. A squat-to-stand maneuver transiently decreases preload on the heart. This decreases left ventricular chamber size and increases systolic buckling of the redundant mitral valve into the left atrium, moving the midsystolic click earlier in systole and increasing mitral regurgitation.

Most patients with mitral valve prolapse have either minimal or no mitral regurgitation, and the prognosis is benign, with annual mortality below 1%. Serious complications, which are rare, include significant mitral regurgitation, infective endocarditis, and arrhythmia.

The murmur of aortic stenosis is an early systolic murmur that is heard best at the right second intercostal space but can be heard anywhere from the cardiac base to the apex. The murmur often radiates toward the carotid arteries. The murmur of aortic stenosis decreases with the Valsalva maneuver.

Aortic coarctation in an adult is characterized by hypertension and a continuous or late systolic murmur that may be heard over the back. Because pulses distal to the aortic obstruction are decreased, aortic coarctation is also associated with abnormal differences in upper and lower extremity blood pressures.

The murmur of hypertrophic cardiomyopathy is a harsh systolic murmur heard best near the lower left sternal border between the sternum and apex. The Valsalva maneuver and the squat-to-stand maneuver transiently increase the intensity of the murmur. Handgrip exercise increases afterload and decreases the relative pressure gradient across the left ventricular outflow tract, so murmur intensity for hypertrophic cardiomyopathy is decreased. Carotid upstrokes are brisk. There is no midsystolic click.

KEY POINT

The classic auscultatory findings of mitral valve prolapse are a midsystolic click followed by a late apical systolic murmur.

Bibliography
Foster E. Clinical practice. Mitral regurgitation due to degenerative mitral-valve disease. N Engl J Med. 2010;363(2):156-65. [PMID: 20647211]

Item 49   Answer: D

Educational Objective: *Follow a patient with an asymptomatic bicuspid aortic valve and preserved left ventricular function.*

The most appropriate management for this patient is clinical follow-up in 1 year. This patient has a bicuspid aortic valve with moderate aortic regurgitation. Echocardiography demonstrates normal left ventricular size and systolic function. Pulmonary pressures are in the normal range, and there is no evidence of adverse hemodynamic effects of valve regurgitation on the ventricle (ventricular size and function are normal). No specific treatment is needed at this time. However, because worsening of aortic regurgitation can be insidious, routine clinical follow-up is indicated in at least yearly intervals, typically with repeat transthoracic echocardiography to monitor for disease progression. The presence of a bicuspid aortic valve is associated with ascending aorta dilatation, and transthoracic echocardiography can also monitor for aortic enlargement. Most patients with bicuspid valves will eventually develop aortic stenosis, regurgitation, or aortic root dilatation or dissection that will require surgery.

Antibiotic endocarditis prophylaxis is now recommended only in patients with prosthetic cardiac valves, those with a known history of prior infective endocarditis, cardiac transplant recipients with valve abnormalities, those with unrepaired cyanotic congenital heart disease, and those with complex congenital heart disease with residual abnormalities. This patient, therefore, should not receive antibiotic endocarditis prophylaxis.

Aortic valve replacement surgery is recommended in patients with severe aortic regurgitation and cardiopulmonary symptoms. In asymptomatic patients with severe regurgitation, surgery is recommended once there are signs of left ventricular enlargement or adverse hemodynamic effects on the left ventricle, or if the ejection fraction falls below 50% to 55%. This patient is asymptomatic, and his left ventricular size and function are normal.

A β-blocker (such as metoprolol) is indicated for all stages of systolic heart failure, even asymptomatic patients with left ventricular ejection fractions less than 50%. This patient has no evidence of systolic heart failure either by symptoms or echocardiographic evidence. There is no evidence that treatment with a β-blocker delays the time to aortic valve replacement; therefore, metoprolol is not indicated.

KEY POINT

Asymptomatic patients with chronic aortic regurgitation and normal left ventricular size and function have an excellent prognosis and do not require prophylactic surgery.

Bibliography

Maurer G. Aortic regurgitation. Heart. 2006;92(7):994-1000. [PMID: 16775114]

Section 2

Endocrinology and Metabolism
Questions

Item 1 [Basic]

A 48-year-old man comes to the office for a routine physical examination. The patient is asymptomatic but overweight. Although he has no pertinent personal medical history, he has a strong family history of diabetes mellitus. He currently takes no medications.

Results of physical examination are normal, except for a BMI of 29.

Results of routine laboratory studies show a fasting plasma glucose level of 158 mg/dL (8.8 mmol/L). These results are confirmed 2 days later.

Which of the following terms best describes his current glycemic status?

(A) Impaired fasting glucose
(B) Impaired glucose tolerance
(C) Metabolic syndrome
(D) Type 2 diabetes mellitus

Item 2 [Basic]

A 68-year-old woman is re-evaluated after laboratory studies show a fasting plasma glucose level of 113 mg/dL (6.3 mmol/L). She has a family history of type 2 diabetes mellitus.

On physical examination, blood pressure is 142/88 mm Hg and BMI is 29. Other vital signs and examination findings are normal.

She undergoes an oral glucose tolerance test, during which her 2-hour plasma glucose level increases to 135 mg/dL (7.5 mmol/L).

Which of the following is the most appropriate treatment recommendation?

(A) Acarbose
(B) Metformin
(C) Ramipril
(D) Rosiglitazone
(E) Diet and exercise

Item 3 [Advanced]

A 51-year-old man is evaluated for a 9-month history of chronic abdominal pain. He has a long-standing history of alcoholism and has been admitted to the hospital several times in the past 8 years for acute pancreatitis. He reports a 5.5-kg (12.1-lb) weight loss over the past year. He currently takes no medications.

Vital signs are normal; BMI is 23. Physical examination reveals a scaphoid-appearing abdomen with normal bowel sounds and diffuse abdominal tenderness to palpation without guarding.

A fasting plasma glucose level is 175 mg/dL (9.7 mmol/L), and a repeat fasting plasma glucose level is 182 mg/dL (10.1 mmol/L). Urine ketones are negative.

A CT scan of the abdomen reveals diffuse pancreatic calcifications.

Which of the following is the best categorization of this patient's diabetes mellitus?

(A) Late-onset autoimmune diabetes of adulthood
(B) Secondary diabetes
(C) Type 1 diabetes
(D) Type 2 diabetes

Item 4 [Basic]

An obese 44-year-old woman is evaluated for persistent hyperglycemia. For the past 3 months, she has followed a strict regimen of diet and exercise in an attempt to control her hyperglycemia. Home blood glucose monitoring has shown preprandial levels between 120 and 160 mg/dL (6.7 and 8.9 mmol/L) and occasional postprandial levels exceeding 200 mg/dL (11.1 mmol/L). She takes no medications.

Vital signs and physical examination findings are normal, except for a BMI of 30.

Laboratory studies show a serum creatinine level of 0.8 mg/dL (70.7 µmol/L); the urine is negative for microalbuminuria.

Which of the following is the most appropriate treatment?

(A) Begin exenatide
(B) Begin glimepiride
(C) Begin metformin
(D) Begin pioglitazone
(E) Continue the diet and exercise for an additional 3 months

Item 5 [Advanced]

A 78-year-old man is evaluated in the hospital for poor glycemic control before undergoing femoral-popliteal bypass surgery. He has been on the vascular surgery ward for 3 weeks with a nonhealing foot ulcer. The patient has an extensive history of arteriosclerotic cardiovascular disease, including peripheral vascular disease, and a 20-year-history of type 2 diabetes mellitus. His most recent hemoglobin A_{1c} value, obtained on admission, was 8.9%. His diabetes regimen consists of glipizide. While in the hospital, his plasma glucose levels have generally been in the 200 to 250 mg/dL (11.1 to 13.9 mmol/L) range. He is eating well.

In addition to stopping glipizide, which of the following is most appropriate treatment for this patient?

(A) Basal insulin and rapid-acting insulin before meals
(B) Continuous insulin infusion
(C) Neutral protamine Hagedorn (NPH) insulin twice daily
(D) Sliding scale regular insulin

Item 6 [Advanced]

A 48-year-old man is evaluated for mild blurring of his central vision bilaterally. He has had type 1 diabetes mellitus for 24 years. The patient is referred for an immediate retinal examination, which reveals macular edema and new neovascularization.

Which of the following is the most appropriate next management step?

(A) Addition of aspirin
(B) Addition of atorvastatin
(C) Decrease in the insulin dosage
(D) Retinal photocoagulation

Item 7 [Basic]

A 67-year-old woman is seen for a follow-up visit. She has had several hypoglycemic episodes that have become increasingly frequent over the past 6 months. Her current medications are neutral protamine Hagedorn (NPH) insulin, 20 units, and regular insulin, 5 units, both injected before breakfast and supper. A review of her glucose log shows blood glucose readings ranging between 70 and 150 mg/dL (3.9 and 8.3 mmol/L) when fasting and 50 and 250 mg/dL (2.8 and 13.9 mmol/L) during the day. Her last measured hemoglobin A_{1c} value was 7.8%.

Which of the following changes is most appropriate?

(A) Change to insulin glargine and insulin lispro
(B) Change to oral metformin and sitagliptin
(C) Decrease the dosages of NPH and regular insulin by 10%
(D) Increase her caloric intake

Item 8 [Basic]

A 20-year-old woman is brought to the emergency department by her college roommate. The patient is lethargic with rapid respirations. Her roommate reports that the patient has had a cough, fever, and chills for the 3 days. She has a 12-year history of type 1 diabetes mellitus. During the previous 24 hours, the patient has had poor oral intake and has not taken her insulin. Today she developed abdominal pain, nausea, and vomiting.

On physical examination, the patient is lethargic but arousable. Temperature is 35.5°C (96.0°F), blood pressure is 90/68 mm Hg, pulse rate is 120/min, and respiration rate is 28/min and deep. The cardiopulmonary examination is normal. Bowel sounds are diminished but present. Palpation elicits generalized tenderness, but no peritoneal signs are present. Other than lethargy, the neurologic examination is normal.

Which the following tests will establish the diagnosis?

(A) Serum glucose and electrolytes and urine ketones
(B) Serum glucose and potassium, complete blood count, and urinalysis
(C) Serum glucose, electrolytes, and ketones and arterial blood gases
(D) Serum glucose, phosphate, and potassium and arterial blood gases
(E) Serum ketones and carbon dioxide, complete blood count, and urine ketones

Item 9 [Advanced]

An 83-year-old obtunded woman is evaluated in the emergency department. She has a history of type 2 diabetes mellitus treated with insulin glargine. The patient developed nausea, vomiting, and diarrhea 2 days ago. Her oral intake was limited, and she did not receive her insulin. Today, the patient was found minimally responsive.

On physical examination, the patient responds only to noxious stimuli with groaning. Temperature is 35.9°C (96.7°F), blood pressure is 90/50 mm Hg, pulse rate is 120/min, and respiration rate is 14/min. She has dry mucous membranes, and her skin demonstrates prolonged tenting. Other than obtundation, the neurologic examination is normal.

Glucose	976 mg/dL (54.2 mmol/L)
Blood urea nitrogen	46 mg/dL (16.4 mmol/L)
Creatinine	2.1 mg/dL (185.6 mmol/L)
Electrolytes	
Sodium	132 meq/L (132 mmol/L)
Potassium	4.8 meq/L (4.8 mmol/L)
Chloride	98 meq/L (98 mmol/L)
Carbon dioxide	22 meq/L (22 mmol/L)
Osmolality	335 mosm/kg H_2O
Serum ketones	Negative
Arterial pH	7.33

Which of the following is the best next management step for this patient?

(A) Administer broad-spectrum antibiotics
(B) Bicarbonate replacement
(C) Insulin administration
(D) Intravenous fluid administration
(E) Potassium replacement

Item 10 [Basic]

A 23-year-old woman with type 1 diabetes mellitus is admitted to the hospital with a diagnosis of community-acquired pneumonia and lethargy. Before admission, her insulin pump therapy was discontinued because of confused mentation.

On physical examination, temperature is 37.5°C (99.5°F), blood pressure is 108/70 mm Hg, pulse rate is 100/min, and respiration rate is 24 min. There are decreased breath sounds in the posterior right lower lung. Neurologic examination reveals altered consciousness.

Blood urea nitrogen	38 mg/dL (13.6 mmol/L)
Creatinine	1.4 mg/dL (123.8 µmol/L)
Electrolytes	
Sodium	130 meq/L (130 mmol/L)
Potassium	5.0 meq/L (5.0 mmol/L)
Chloride	100 meq/L (100 mmol/L)
Bicarbonate	14 meq/L (14 mmol/L)
Glucose	262 mg/dL (14.5 mmol/L)
Urine ketones	Positive

Rapid infusion of normal saline is initiated.

Which of the following is the most appropriate next management step?

(A) Add insulin glargine
(B) Add neutral protamine Hagedorn (NPH) insulin
(C) Implement a sliding scale for regular insulin
(D) Start an insulin drip

Item 11 [Basic]

A 50-year-old man is evaluated during a routine physical examination. He is asymptomatic, has no medical problems, and takes no medications. He is a nonsmoker and drinks two alcoholic beverages daily. His father, uncle, and a brother had myocardial infarctions between the ages of 55 and 60 years.

On physical examination, vital signs are normal. BMI is 28. On the skin examination, he has soft, nontender, yellow plaques measuring between 0.5 and 1 cm on his upper eyelids. The remainder of the physical examination results are normal.

Which of the diagnostic studies should be done next?

(A) Aminotransferase and alkaline phosphatase
(B) Serum ferritin
(C) Serum glucose and hemoglobin A_{1c}
(D) Serum lipids
(E) Thyroid-stimulating hormone

Item 12 [Basic]

A 41-year-old man is evaluated for follow-up of a lipid profile obtained a month ago. He is a smoker with a 15 pack-year history. He works in an office and does not regularly exercise. He does not have hypertension and does not have a family history of premature coronary heart disease.

On physical examination, vital signs are normal. BMI is 38. His waist circumference is 94 cm (43 in). The remainder of his physical examination results are normal.

Serum glucose (fasting)	98 mg/dL (5.4 mmol/L)
Total cholesterol	188 mg/dL (4.8 mmol/L)
HDL cholesterol	31 mg/dL (0.8 mmol/L)
LDL cholesterol	128 mg/dL (3.3 mmol/L)
Triglycerides	145 mg/dL (1.6 mmol/L)

Which of the following is the most appropriate next management step?

(A) Initiate fibrate therapy
(B) Initiate lifestyle modifications
(C) Initiate statin therapy
(D) Ultrasonography to measure carotid artery intimal thickness

Item 13 [Basic]

A 38-year-old man is evaluated during a follow-up visit. A fasting lipid panel was performed 3 weeks ago. The patient does not use tobacco and has no history of heart disease, stroke, transient ischemic attack, diabetes mellitus, or renal, liver, or thyroid disease. His father has hypertension. He takes no medications and has no allergies.

Vital signs are normal; BMI is 32. Physical examination is unremarkable. Fasting lipid levels are as follows: total cholesterol, 234 mg/dL (6.1 mmol/L); HDL-cholesterol, 48 mg/dL (1.2 mmol/L); LDL-cholesterol, 158 mg/dL (4.1 mmol/L); triglycerides: 142 mg/dL (1.6 mmol/L). All other laboratory findings are within normal limits.

Which of the following is the most appropriate management option for this patient?

(A) Begin therapy with a fibrate
(B) Begin therapy with a statin
(C) Obtain lipoprotein(a) level
(D) Repeat lipid screening in 1 to 2 years

Item 14 [Basic]

A 60-year-old man with type 2 diabetes mellitus and hypertension visits the office to establish medical care. His daily medications are metformin, lisinopril, amlodipine, and aspirin.

On physical examination, blood pressure is 128/65 mm Hg and pulse is 76/min; BMI is 26. The remaining physical examination findings are normal.

Cholesterol	
Total	215 mg/dL (5.6 mmol/L)
HDL	39 mg/dL (1.0 mmol/L)
LDL	145 mg/dL (3.8 mmol/L)
Triglycerides	185 mg/dL (2.1 mmol/L)
Hemoglobin A_{1c}	6.5%

Which of the following drugs should be initiated?

(A) Colestipol
(B) Ezetimibe
(C) Niacin
(D) Simvastatin

Item 15 [Basic]

A 63-year-old man is evaluated during a follow-up appointment. One month ago, he had a transient ischemic attack. A carotid ultrasound revealed a 60% left internal carotid artery stenosis, and a transthoracic echocardiogram revealed left ventricular hypertrophy. He is currently asymptomatic. He has hypertension and quit smoking 10 years ago. He has no history of coronary artery disease and no family history of premature coronary artery disease. Current medications are hydrochlorothiazide and aspirin. An LDL-cholesterol level 6 months ago was 138 mg/dL (3.6 mmol/L), and he has been compliant with recommended lifestyle modifications.

On physical examination, blood pressure is 122/78 mm Hg. There are no focal neurologic abnormalities. Fasting lipid levels are as follows: total cholesterol, 206 mg/dL (5.3 mmol/L); HDL-cholesterol, 50 mg/dL (1.3 mmol/L); LDL-cholesterol, 128 mg/dL (3.3 mmol/L); triglycerides, 144 mg/dL (1.6 mmol/L).

Which of the following is the most appropriate management option to reduce the risk of stroke and coronary artery events in this patient?

(A) Add atorvastatin
(B) Add nicotinic acid
(C) Change hydrochlorothiazide to amlodipine
(D) Change hydrochlorothiazide to carvedilol

Item 16 [Advanced]

A 55-year-old woman is evaluated for a 7-month history of worsening fatigue. She also reports that her hair is thinning and she has an unexplained weight gain of 4.1 kg (9 lb) despite trying to limit food intake. She has no other medical problems and takes no medications.

On physical examination, temperature is 36.7°C (98.0°F), blood pressure is 120/70 mm Hg, pulse rate is 60/min, and respiration rate is 12/min. BMI is 27. The thyroid is twice its normal size. Her voice is normal, and deep tendon reflexes are 2+ throughout. The remainder of the physical examination is normal.

Laboratory evaluation reveals a serum thyroid-stimulating hormone (TSH) level of 14.1 μU/mL (14.1 mU/L) and a free thyroxine level of 0.9 ng/dL (12 pmol/L).

Which of the following tests are necessary before initiating therapy?

(A) Measurement of thyroid peroxidase (TPO) antibody
(B) Radionuclide uptake scanning
(C) Measurement of thyroglobulin level
(D) No additional tests

Item 17 [Advanced]

A 42-year-old woman is evaluated for an asymmetric enlargement of her thyroid. She is otherwise asymptomatic, and she has no risk factors for thyroid cancer.

On physical examination, a possible thyroid nodule is palpated on the left side. A complete blood count, routine serum chemistry tests, and thyroid-stimulating hormone level (TSH) are normal. Ultrasound examination reveals a 2.2-cm left-sided solid nodule.

What is the appropriate next step in the evaluation of this patient?

(A) Fine-needle aspiration of the thyroid nodule
(B) Measurement of serum free thyroxine (T$_4$)
(C) Measurement of thyroglobulin level
(D) Thyroid scan and radioactive iodine uptake test
(E) Thyroidectomy

Item 18 [Advanced]

A 23-year-old woman comes to the office for follow-up. She has a 5-year history of hypothyroidism and has been on a stable dose of levothyroxine for the past 3 years. She is now 4 weeks pregnant with her first child.

Physical examination findings are noncontributory.

Results of laboratory studies 2 months ago showed a serum thyroid-stimulating hormone (TSH) level of 2.9 μU/mL (2.9 mU/L) and a free thyroxine level of 1.4 ng/dL (18.1 pmol/L).

Which of the following is the most appropriate management?

(A) Add iodine therapy
(B) Measure her free triiodothyronine (T$_3$) level
(C) Recheck her serum TSH level
(D) Continue current management

Item 19 [Advanced]

An 18-year-old woman is evaluated for tachycardia, nervousness, decreased exercise tolerance, and weight loss of 6 months' duration. She has otherwise been healthy. Her sister has Graves disease. She takes no medications.

On physical examination, blood pressure is 128/78 mm Hg, pulse rate is 124/min, respiration rate is 16/min, and BMI is 19. There is no proptosis. An examination of the neck reveals a smooth thyroid gland that is greater than 1.5 times the normal size. Cardiac examination reveals regular tachycardia. Her lungs are clear to auscultation.

Human chorionic gonadotropin	Negative
Thyroid-stimulating hormone	<0.01 μU/mL (0.01 mU/L)
Thyroxine (T$_4$), free	5.5 ng/dL (71.0 pmol/L)
Triiodothyronine (T$_3$), free	9.1 ng/L (14.0 pmol/L)

Which of the following is the most appropriate treatment for this patient?

(A) Atenolol
(B) Atenolol and methimazole
(C) Methimazole
(D) Radioactive iodine and methimazole

Item 20 [Advanced]

A 26-year-old woman is evaluated for a 2-week history of constipation, fatigue, and weight gain. Three months ago, she began experiencing nervousness, heat intolerance, and weight loss but says these symptoms abated after 6 weeks. The patient delivered a healthy infant 14 weeks ago. After thyroid function tests performed 8 weeks postpartum revealed a thyroid-stimulating hormone (TSH) level of 0.02 µU/mL (0.02 mU/L) and a free thyroxine (T$_4$) level of 3.5 ng/dL (45.2 pmol/L), she was placed on atenolol, 25 mg/d.

On physical examination, blood pressure is 115/70 mm Hg, pulse rate is 50/min, respiration rate is 14/min, and BMI is 23.3. No proptosis or inflammatory changes are noted on ocular examination. Examination of the neck reveals no tenderness or bruits; the thyroid gland cannot be palpated.

Which of the following is the best next step in management?

(A) Methimazole
(B) Repeat measurement of TSH and free T$_4$ levels
(C) Thyroid scan and 24-hour radioactive iodine uptake test
(D) Thyroid ultrasonography

Item 21 [Advanced]

A 75-year-old man is admitted to the intensive care unit with sepsis associated with pneumonia, hypoxemic respiratory failure requiring ventilator support, and hypotension. He is treated appropriately with volume resuscitation, vasopressors, and antibiotic therapy and is extubated 5 days later.

On physical examination, blood pressure is 110/75 mm Hg, pulse rate is 88/min, and respiration rate is 16/min. Examination of the neck reveals a thyroid gland of normal size and without nodules. There are no tremors in the extremities.

Because results of admission laboratory studies showed mild hyponatremia, additional blood tests are performed to evaluate the hyponatremia.

Cortisol (8 AM)	30 µg/dL (828 nmol/L) (normal range, 5-25 µg/dL [138-690 nmol/L])
Thyroid-stimulating hormone	0.23 µU/mL (0.23 mU/L)
Thyroxine (T$_4$), free	0.9 ng/dL (11.6 pmol/L)
Triiodothyronine (T$_3$), free	0.4 ng/L (0.6 pmol/L)

Which of the following is the most appropriate next management step?

(A) Brain MRI
(B) Levothyroxine administration
(C) Repeat thyroid function tests in 6 weeks
(D) Ultrasonography of the thyroid gland

Item 22 [Advanced]

A 51-year-old woman is evaluated in the office following an emergency department visit for abdominal pain. The pain spontaneously resolved. A CT scan in the emergency department revealed an incidentally discovered 1.4-cm left adrenal nodule with smooth borders and low attenuation and vascularity. She is otherwise healthy and takes no medications.

On physical examination, temperature is 36.5°C (97.7°F), blood pressure is 120/80 mm Hg, pulse rate is 60/min, and respiration rate is 14/min. The remainder of the physical examination is normal.

A comprehensive metabolic profile, including electrolytes, is normal.

Which of the following diagnostic tests should be done next?

(A) Aldosterone and renin levels and overnight suppression test
(B) Aldosterone and renin levels and dehydroepiandrosterone sulfate (DHEA-S) and testosterone levels
(C) Plasma metanephrine levels and overnight dexamethasone suppression test
(D) Plasma metanephrine levels, DHEA-S, and testosterone levels
(E) No additional tests

Item 23 [Advanced]

A 43-year-old man is evaluated for drug-resistant hypertension. Hypertension was diagnosed 1 year ago and has been difficult to control despite maximum dosages of lisinopril, metoprolol, and nifedipine. The patient reports feeling well.

On physical examination, temperature is 36.5°C (97.7°F), blood pressure is 146/92 mm Hg, pulse rate is 88/min, respiration rate is 17/min, and BMI is 27. Results of the general physical examination and funduscopic examination are unremarkable.

Electrolytes	
Sodium	143 meq/L (143 mmol/L)
Potassium	3.3 meq/L (3.3 mmol/L)
Chloride	101 meq/L (101 mmol/L)
Bicarbonate	33 meq/L (33 mmol/L)
Creatinine	1.0 mg/dL (88.4 µmol/L)
Spot urine potassium	Inappropriately high
Urinalysis	Normal

Which of the following is the most appropriate next diagnostic test?

(A) CT of the adrenal glands
(B) Determination of serum aldosterone to plasma renin activity ratio
(C) Digital subtraction renal angiography
(D) Measurement of plasma metanephrine and normetanephrine levels

Item 24 [Advanced]

A 34-year-old woman is seen for follow-up after results of laboratory studies confirm hypercortisolism.

Adrenocorticotropic hormone	Elevated
Urine free cortisol	Elevated
Cortisol (8 AM)	
After 1 mg of dexamethasone the night before	Elevated
After 8 mg of dexamethasone the night before	Partial suppression

Which of the following is the most appropriate next diagnostic test?

(A) Adrenal CT
(B) Adrenal MRI
(C) Cosyntropin stimulation test
(D) Pituitary MRI

Item 25 [Basic]

A 55-year-old woman is evaluated for a 6-month history of recurrent episodes of palpitations, sweating, and headaches. Medical history is otherwise unremarkable. She takes no medications.

On physical examination, the patient appears anxious. Temperature is 36.9°C (98.4°F), blood pressure is 158/96 mm Hg, pulse rate is 88/min, respiration rate is 18/min, and BMI is 30. Findings from a general physical examination, including examination of the thyroid gland, are otherwise unremarkable.

Laboratory studies show elevated plasma epinephrine and norepinephrine levels.

Which of the following is the most appropriate next management step?

(A) Abdominal CT scan
(B) Adrenalectomy
(C) Bilateral adrenal vein sampling
(D) Metaiodobenzylguanidine (MIBG) scan

Item 26 [Advanced]

A 65-year-old woman is evaluated for a 3-week history of fatigue, nausea, and poor appetite. In the week before symptom onset, she had acute bronchitis with productive cough and fever. The patient has a 2-year history of osteoarthritis of the knees that requires intra-articular corticosteroid injections every 3 to 4 months; her last injection was 3 months ago. Her only other medication is acetaminophen.

On physical examination, the patient looks tired. Temperature is 37.5°C (99.5°F), blood pressure is 112/58 mm Hg, pulse rate is 92/min, respiration rate is 17/min, and BMI is 32. The patient has cushingoid features and central obesity. There are multiple ecchymoses on the upper and lower extremities. Decreased axillary and pubic hair is noted. There is bony hypertrophy and small effusions of the knees bilaterally but no evidence of warmth or erythema.

Adrenocorticotropic hormone (AM)	Low normal
Cortisol (8 AM)	
Initial measurement	Low
After cosyntropin stimulation	Low normal

Which of the following is the most likely cause of this patient's recent symptoms?

(A) Adrenal adenoma
(B) Exogenous corticosteroids
(C) Pituitary microadenoma
(D) Primary adrenal insufficiency

Item 27 [Basic]

A 47-year-old woman is hospitalized for pyelonephritis. The patient has a 6-year history of primary adrenal insufficiency and has been doing well on therapy with oral hydrocortisone and fludrocortisone. She reports missing two doses of the hydrocortisone today because of nausea. She is started on rapid intravenous infusion of normal saline and ceftriaxone.

On physical examination, temperature is 38.9°C (102.0°F), blood pressure is 92/58 mm Hg supine and 76/50 mm Hg sitting, pulse rate is 98/min supine and 112/min sitting, and respiration rate is 19/min.

Results of laboratory studies reveal a serum sodium level of 125 meq/L (125 mmol/L) and a serum potassium level of 5.5 meq/L (5.5 mmol/L).

Which of the following should be administered next?

(A) Infusion of 3% saline
(B) Stress dosage of intravenous hydrocortisone
(C) Usual dosage of fludrocortisone alone
(D) Usual dosage of oral hydrocortisone alone

Item 28 [Basic]

A 66-year-old woman is found to have a T-score of -2.7 at her hip following a routine screening dual energy x-ray absorptiometry (DEXA) scan. The patient is otherwise healthy, has no obvious risk factors for osteoporosis, and takes no medicines.

Calcium	9.8 mg/dL (2.5 mmol/L)
Phosphorus	3.8 mg/dL (1.2 mmol/L)
25-Hydroxy vitamin D	22 ng/mL (54.9 nmol/L)
Alkaline phosphatase	90 U/L
Parathyroid hormone	20 pg/mL (20 ng/L)

In addition to starting oral bisphosphonate therapy, which of the following should be done next?

(A) Add estrogen replacement therapy
(B) Order a parathyroid scan
(C) Recommend increased sun exposure
(D) Start vitamin D and calcium supplementation

Item 29 [Advanced]

A 62-year-old woman is evaluated during a follow-up visit for hypertension. She has no symptoms and is monogamous with her husband of 35 years. Her only medication is hydrochlorothiazide. She received an influenza vaccination 3 months ago and a herpes zoster vaccination 1 year ago. Her last Pap smear was 14 months ago and results were normal, as were results of the previous three annual Pap smears.

On physical examination, blood pressure is 136/72 mm Hg and weight is 62 kg (136 lb). Other general physical examination findings are normal.

The total cholesterol level is 188 mg/dL (4.9 mmol/L) and the HDL-cholesterol level is 54 mg/dL (1.4 mmol/L).

Which of the following is the most appropriate health maintenance intervention for this patient?

(A) Abdominal ultrasonography
(B) Dual-energy x-ray absorptiometry
(C) Pap smear
(D) Pneumococcal vaccine

Item 30 [Basic]

A 69-year-old woman is evaluated for a loss of 2 inches in height over the past 5 years. She is currently taking adequate dosages of supplemental calcium and vitamin D. Results of dual-energy x-ray absorptiometry show a T score of –2.5. An evaluation for secondary causes of osteoporosis is unrevealing.

Which of the following agents should be initiated in this patient?

(A) Alendronate
(B) Calcitonin
(C) Estrogen
(D) Raloxifene
(E) Teriparatide

Item 31 [Advanced]

A 70-year-old woman is evaluated for worsening gastro-esophageal reflux disease with heartburn. She first noticed this symptom 1 month ago when she began taking alendronate, 70 mg orally once weekly, for osteoporosis. Current medications are alendronate, calcium, and ergocalciferol.

The alendronate is discontinued.

Which of the following is now the most appropriate treatment for this patient's osteoporosis?

(A) Calcitonin
(B) Intravenous zoledronate
(C) Raloxifene
(D) Teriparatide

Item 32 [Basic]

A 72-year-old woman is evaluated for mid and low back pain. Her pain has been present for several months, but last week she experienced sharp and intense pain after picking up a basket of wet laundry. Her medical history is unremarkable, and she takes no medications. She does not smoke cigarettes and does not drink alcohol.

On physical examination, BMI is 18. She has tenderness over the middle and lower thoracic regions. Spine radiographs show compression fractures at T10, L1, and L2.

Calcium	9.8 mg/dL (2.5 mmol/L)
Phosphorus	3.9 mg/dL (1.3 mmol/L)
Alkaline phosphatase	88 U/L
Bone mineral density	Spine T-score : –2.6
	Total hip T-score: –1.9

Which of the following is the most likely diagnosis?

(A) Normal bone density
(B) Osteopenia
(C) Osteoporosis
(D) Secondary osteoporosis

Section 2

Endocrinology and Metabolism
Answers and Critiques

Item 1   **Answer: D**

Educational Objective: *Diagnose type 2 diabetes mellitus.*

This patient has type 2 diabetes mellitus. The diagnosis of diabetes mellitus can be established by a fasting plasma glucose level of at least 126 mg/dL (7.0 mmol/L), a random plasma glucose level of at least 200 mg/dL (11.1 mmol/L) and symptoms of hyperglycemia (for example, polyuria, polydipsia, or blurred vision), or a 2-hour oral glucose tolerance test (OGTT) result of at least 200 mg/dL (11.1 mmol/L). In 2010, the American Diabetes Association endorsed a hemoglobin A_{1c} value of 6.5% of greater as diagnostic of diabetes.

Impaired fasting glucose, impaired glucose tolerance, or both mark the transition from normal glucose tolerance to type 2 diabetes mellitus. Impaired fasting glucose is diagnosed when the fasting plasma glucose level is in the range of 100 to 125 mg/dL (5.6 to 6.9 mmol/L), and impaired glucose tolerance—an analogous prediabetic state—is diagnosed when the plasma glucose level at the 2-hour mark of an OGTT is 140 to 199 mg/dL (7.8 to 11.0 mmol/L).

For a diagnosis of the metabolic syndrome to be made, information about the patient's blood pressure (≥130/85 mm Hg), lipid levels (triglyceride level ≥150 mg/dL [1.7 mmol/L]; HDL-cholesterol <40 mg/dL in men [1.0 mmol/L]), fasting plasma glucose level (≥110 mg/dL [6.1 mmol/L]), and waist circumference (>40 in [>102 cm] in men) is necessary. Insufficient data have been provided for this diagnosis.

KEY POINT

Type 2 diabetes mellitus is diagnosed when the fasting plasma glucose level is 126 mg/dL (7.0 mmol/L) or greater, the random plasma glucose level is 200 mg/dL (11.1 mmol/L) or greater, the plasma glucose level is 200 mg/dL (11.1 mmol/L) or greater after a 2-hour oral glucose tolerance test, or the venous hemoglobin A_{1c} value is 6.5% or greater.

Bibliography

American Diabetes Association. Standards of medical care in diabetes—2010. Diabetes Care. 2010;33 Suppl 1:S11-61. [PMID: 20042772]

Item 2   **Answer: E**

Educational Objective: *Treat prediabetes with diet and exercise.*

The most appropriate treatment for this patient is diet and exercise. She has impaired fasting glucose (IFG), defined as a fasting plasma glucose level in the range of 100 to 125 mg/dL (5.6 to 6.9 mmol/L), and should begin a program of intensive lifestyle change, including 30 minutes of exercise most days of the week and a calorie-restricted diet, to achieve weight reduction on the order of 7% of body weight.

Diet and exercise is the recommended approach for patients with either IFG or impaired glucose tolerance (IGT), the prediabetic states. The relative risk reduction (RRR) in the incidence of diabetes in patients with IGT associated with intensive lifestyle change is 58%.

Pharmacologic therapy with glucose-lowering drugs is not indicated for this patient with isolated IFG. In pharmacologic studies of diabetes prevention, acarbose therapy resulted in only a 25% RRR, which is inferior to that obtained with diet and exercise.

Metformin therapy is associated with an RRR of 31%, which is also inferior to the 58% RRR obtained with diet and exercise. Metformin therapy may be considered in patients with both IFG and IGT, who constitute a higher risk group. This patient does not have IGT (fasting plasma glucose level of 140 to 199 mg/dL [7.7 to 11.0 mmol/L] at the 2-hour mark of an oral glucose tolerance test) and so should not receive metformin.

Modulators of the renin-angiotensin axis, such as ramipril and other angiotensin-converting enzyme inhibitors, do not contribute to diabetes prevention.

Rosiglitazone and pioglitazone have been associated with 62% and 81% RRRs, respectively, in the incidence of diabetes. These agents, however, are not endorsed for routine pharmacologic use in patients with prediabetes because of their costs and adverse effects, including edema, increased fracture risk in women, and possible increased cardiovascular morbidity.

KEY POINT

Patients with prediabetes should be advised to adopt a program of lifestyle change to prevent progression to type 2 diabetes mellitus.

Bibliography

Vijan S. Type 2 diabetes. Ann Intern Med. 2010;152(5):ITC31-15. [PMID: 20194231]

Item 3   Answer: B

Educational Objective: *Diagnose secondary diabetes related to chronic pancreatitis.*

This patient has secondary diabetes related to chronic pancreatitis. Diabetes mellitus is generally categorized as type 1, type 2, gestational, and secondary diabetes. This patient's diabetes is the last type, which consists of a group of unrelated conditions that are associated with hyperglycemia through effects on either insulin availability or insulin sensitivity. These include various endocrine disorders, such as Cushing syndrome and acromegaly; several pancreatic conditions, such as acute and chronic pancreatitis and pancreatic cancer; drug-induced hyperglycemia; and several genetic syndromes. This patient has a history of alcohol abuse, a history of recurrent pancreatitis, and pancreatic calcifications on an abdominal CT scan, which collectively confirm the diagnosis of chronic pancreatitis.

Some older patients previously diagnosed with type 2 diabetes mellitus have autoimmune beta-cell destruction, albeit of a more gradually progressive nature (termed latent autoimmune diabetes of adulthood). Such patients develop absolute insulin deficiency over time. Late-onset autoimmune diabetes of adulthood is a possibility in this patient, given his age (51 years), his lean body habitus, and the insidious onset of diabetes. However, it would be much less common than secondary diabetes in this man with confirmed chronic pancreatitis.

This patient's clinical presentation is atypical for type 1 diabetes, which usually has an acute or subacute onset and is characterized by polyuria, polydipsia, polyphagia, ketonemia or ketonuria, and weight loss.

Most patients with type 2 diabetes are obese or at least have abdominal obesity (high waist-to-hip ratio). This patient is of normal body weight, and his scaphoid-appearing abdomen makes type 2 diabetes even less likely.

KEY POINT

Secondary causes of diabetes mellitus may result from diseases of the exocrine pancreas, endocrinopathies, genetic syndromes, and drugs or chemicals.

Bibliography

Vijan S. Type 2 diabetes. Ann Intern Med. 2010;152(5):ITC31-15. [PMID: 20194231]

Item 4   Answer: C

Educational Objective: *Treat type 2 diabetes mellitus with metformin.*

The most appropriate treatment for this patient is to begin metformin. Various oral and injectable agents are available for the initial management of type 2 diabetes, most of which reduce hyperglycemia to a similar degree. Because of its low cost, effectiveness, good tolerability, relative safety, favorable effects on body weight, and absence of hypoglycemia as a side effect, metformin remains the best first-line agent available. Metformin is contraindicated in patients with renal insufficiency (serum creatinine level >1.4 mg/dL [123.8 µmol/L] for women and >1.5 mg/dL [132.6 µmol/L] for men). For this patient, ongoing attempts at lifestyle change are unlikely to reduce her blood glucose level further. Therefore, initiation of metformin therapy is most likely to improve her glycemic control.

Exenatide, an injectable agent, is only approved for use in combination regimens with oral agents and is inappropriate in most circumstances as monotherapy. Glimepiride could be used but is associated with weight gain and the risk of hypoglycemia. Overall, it remains a less attractive choice than metformin in most patients, including this one. Pioglitazone is also available for monotherapy, but its side effects of weight gain, edema, increased peripheral bone fracture rates in women, and high cost make it less attractive than metformin as a first-line therapy.

KEY POINT

Metformin is recommended as the initial pharmacologic therapy for most patients with type 2 diabetes mellitus.

Bibliography

Nathan DM, Buse JB, Davidson MB, et al. Medical management of hyperglycemia in type 2 diabetes: a consensus algorithm for the initiation and adjustment of therapy: a consensus statement of the American Diabetes Association and the European Association for the Study of Diabetes. Diabetes Care. 2009;32(1):193-203. [PMID: 18945920]

Item 5   Answer: A

Educational Objective: *Manage hyperglycemia in a hospitalized patient with basal and preprandial insulins.*

The most appropriate treatment for this patient is basal and preprandial insulin administration. He has uncontrolled diabetes mellitus during hospitalization. Recent guidelines recommend attempting to improve glycemic control in all hospitalized patients (140 to 200 mg/dL [7.8 to 11.1 mmol/L). Thus, a basal-bolus insulin regimen consisting of a long-acting insulin and a rapid-acting insulin analogue before meals is recommended for this hospitalized patient. Such an approach allows for a more easily titratable regimen and can conveniently be held during diagnostic testing or procedures when nutritional intake is interrupted.

Continuous insulin infusions are difficult to administer outside the intensive care unit in most hospitals. Therefore, initiating one is not the best treatment for this patient and may not even be necessary to obtain good glycemic control.

A regimen of neutral protamine Hagedorn (NPH) insulin twice daily will likely improve glycemic control but is not as easily titratable as a basal-bolus correction and does not prevent postprandial glucose spikes.

Sliding scale regular insulin has been associated with increased hyperglycemic and hypoglycemic excursions and has been found to result in inferior glycemic control compared with a basal-bolus correction regimen in hospitalized patients. Initiating this approach is therefore inappropriate.

KEY POINT

A basal-bolus insulin regimen consisting of a long-acting insulin and a rapid-acting insulin analogue before meals is recommended for hospitalized patients with uncontrolled diabetes.

Bibliography

Umpierrez GE, Smiley D, Zisman A, et al. Randomized study of basal-bolus insulin therapy in the inpatient management of patients with type 2 diabetes (RABBIT 2 trial). Diabetes Care. 2007;30(9):2181-2186. [PMID:17513708]

Item 6   Answer: D

Educational Objective: *Manage diabetic retinopathy and macular edema with panretinal photocoagulation.*

Panretinal photocoagulation is the most appropriate next step in management. Diabetic retinopathy is a well-recognized microvascular complication of type 1 diabetes mellitus and is one of the leading causes of visual loss in adults in the United States. Diabetic retinopathy is classified as nonproliferative (with hard exudates, microaneurysms, and minor hemorrhages), which is not associated with visual decline, and proliferative (with "cotton-wool spots" and neovascularization), which is associated with loss of vision. Changes in retinal blood flow occur after several years of diabetes. These changes cause retinal ischemia, which in turn promotes growth factors that stimulate proliferation of new blood vessels. This process leads to scarring and fibrosis. Fibrous tissue can put traction on the retina, which can cause retinal detachment with resultant vision loss. New vessels can also become more permeable and leak serum, which causes macular edema. Tight glycemic control has been shown to decrease the incidence and progression of retinopathy. Blood pressure reduction appears to exert as great a beneficial effect on retinopathy as glycemic control. Once proliferative retinopathy or macular edema is established, vision can be preserved by appropriately timed laser photocoagulation.

Randomized clinical trials have detected no beneficial effect of aspirin on the incidence or progression of proliferative retinopathy or visual loss. At the same time, other studies have not demonstrated harm to the optic system of patients who must take aspirin for cardiovascular protection.

Although lipid-lowering drugs, such as atorvastatin, have been associated in some studies with reduced rates of retinopathy, they cannot alter the course of established retinopathy and are not indicated in this patient.

Abrupt rapid improvement in glycemic control has been associated with modest worsening of diabetic retinopathy in early studies, but there is no evidence that allowing control to deteriorate by reducing the intake of insulin will improve retinopathy. This patient's glycemic control has been stable, so his insulin regimen should not be changed.

KEY POINT

Laser photocoagulation of the retina can help preserve vision in patients with proliferative diabetic retinopathy and/or macular edema.

Bibliography

Fante RJ, Durairaj VD, Oliver SC. Diabetic retinopathy: an update on treatment. Am J Med. 2010;123(3):213-216. [PMID: 20193825]

Item 7   Answer: A

Educational Objective: *Improve glucose control with the addition of basal and preprandial insulins.*

The most appropriate therapeutic change is to substitute insulin glargine and insulin lispro for her current diabetes medications. Basal and rapid-acting insulin analogues, when dosed properly, reduce the risk of hypoglycemia. Current choices of long- or intermediate-acting basal insulins include insulin glargine, insulin detemir, and neutral protamine Hagedorn (NPH) insulin. The optimal basal insulin should be peakless and have a 24-hour duration of action. Both insulin glargine and, to a lesser extent, insulin detemir meet these requirements. NPH insulin, on the other hand, does not and is usually administered twice daily because its duration of action typically extends only 12 to 18 hours with a peak of activity at 4 to 8 hours after administration, which can precipitate hypoglycemic episodes at other times. In one study, the risk of hypoglycemia was significantly higher during the overnight hours in patients taking NPH insulin versus insulin glargine at bedtime. An ideal prandial insulin has a brisk peak and a short overall duration of action to properly cover postprandial glucose excursions. Such pharmacokinetics are found with the rapid-acting insulin analogues lispro, aspart, and glulisine. In contrast, regular insulin has a duration of action of 6 to 8 hours and so is not an optimal preprandial product.

She should be encouraged to switch to a regimen of four injections of insulin per day, with a once daily injection of a basal insulin, such as insulin glargine, and mealtime injections of a rapid-acting analogue, such as insulin lispro.

Patients with advanced type 2 diabetes mellitus who are on insulin should not be transferred to oral agents because the need for insulin suggests an already significant insulin deficiency that oral agents are unlikely to overcome. Glycemic control would inevitably deteriorate.

Decreasing the dosage of NPH and regular insulin may diminish her overnight hypoglycemic episodes but would also result in higher blood glucose levels. Therefore, this change in the patient's diabetes regimen is not appropriate.

Increasing caloric intake to combat hypoglycemia is rarely indicated. Ideally, the insulin regimen should be adjusted on the basis of the patient's nutritional intake, not vice-versa.

The combination of basal and rapid-acting insulin analogues, when dosed properly, reduces the risk of hypoglycemia.

Bibliography

Vijan S. Type 2 diabetes. Ann Intern Med. 2010;152(5):ITC31-15. [PMID: 20194231]

Item 8   Answer: C

Educational Objective: *Diagnose diabetic ketoacidosis.*

This patient has diabetic ketoacidosis (DKA), and the tests to establish the diagnosis are serum glucose, electrolytes, and ketones and arterial blood gases. The most life-threatening acute complication of diabetes is DKA, which mostly affects patients with type 1 diabetes and is sometimes its presenting manifestation. At presentation, patients with DKA usually report a several-day history of polyuria, polydipsia, and blurred vision, culminating in nausea, vomiting, abdominal pain, dyspnea, and altered mental status. Physical examination typically reveals deep, labored breathing (Kussmaul respirations), a fruity odor to the breath (from acetone), poor skin turgor, tachycardia, and hypotension. This complication can occur as a result of precipitating acute stresses such as infections (influenza, pneumonia, or gastroenteritis) or acute myocardial infarction; in patients with insulin pumps, when a technical interruption of insulin infusion occurs; and in patients who are nonadherent to their medication regimen. In almost all instances, DKA is entirely preventable if patients practice regular glucose monitoring and understand the need for increased insulin doses during acute stress events. The diagnosis of DKA is based on a blood glucose level less than 250 mg/dL (13.9 mmol/L), anion gap metabolic acidosis (arterial pH <7.30), a serum carbon dioxide level less than 15 meq/L (15 mmol/L), and positive serum or urine ketone concentrations.

The diagnosis of diabetic ketoacidosis is based on a blood glucose level less than 250 mg/dL (13.9 mmol/L), anion gap metabolic acidosis (arterial pH <7.30), a serum carbon dioxide level less than 15 meq/L (15 mmol/L), and positive serum or urine ketone concentrations.

Bibliography

Wilson JF. In the clinic. Diabetic ketoacidosis. Ann Intern Med. 2010;152(1):ITC1-1-ITC1-15. [PMID: 20048266]

Item 9   Answer: D

Educational Objective: *Treat hyperglycemic hyperosmolar syndrome with intravenous fluids.*

The next management step for this patient is rapid infusion of intravenous fluids. This patient has hyperglycemic hyperosmolar syndrome. Diagnostic criteria include plasma glucose level greater than 600 mg/dL (33.3 mmol/L), arterial pH greater than 7.30, serum bicarbonate greater than 15 mg/dL (15 mmol/L), serum osmolality greater than 320 mosm/kg H_2O, and absent urine or serum ketones. Patients with this disorder usually have a precipitating factor, such as severe infection, myocardial infarction, or new kidney insufficiency. Management of hyperglycemic hyperosmolar syndrome mainly involves identifying the underlying precipitating illness and restoring a markedly contracted plasma volume. Normal saline, which is already comparatively hypotonic in such patients, is usually chosen first to replenish the extracellular space. If the patient has hypotension, fluids should be administered as rapidly as tolerated to restore plasma (intravascular) volume. When blood pressure is restored and urine output is established, administration rates should be slowed and hypotonic solutions should be administered. The total body water deficit can be calculated by using standard formulas, with the goal of replacing one-half the deficit during the first 24 hours and the remainder during the next 2 to 3 days.

Insulin reduces glucose levels but should be administered only after expansion of the intravascular space has begun. If given earlier, movement of glucose into cells theoretically can reduce circulating volume further, which threatens cerebral, kidney, and coronary perfusion.

Electrolytes should be monitored, especially potassium, because the potassium level may fall as urine output is restored and kidney function improves with intravenous fluid therapy; in addition, potassium is shifted intracellularly by the administration of insulin therapy. Potassium should not be administered until urine output is verified, because these patients are prone to acute kidney injury. Mild metabolic acidosis does not require bicarbonate therapy, because normalization of circulating volume will quickly correct this defect. Antibiotics are not required unless a bacterial infection is identified.

Management of hyperglycemic hyperosmolar syndrome involves identifying the underlying precipitating illness and restoring plasma volume with intravenous fluids.

Bibliography

Kitabchi AE, Nyenwe EA. Hyperglycemic crises in diabetes mellitus: diabetic ketoacidosis and hyperglycemic hyperosmolar state. Endocrinol Metab Clin North Am. 2006;35(4):725-51. [PMID: 17127143]

Item 10   Answer: D

Educational Objective: *Treat diabetic ketoacidosis with an insulin drip.*

This patient should be started on an insulin drip. Discontinuation of insulin pump therapy resulted in inadequate insulin coverage; as a result, the patient developed diabetic ketoacidosis, as evidenced by the plasma glucose level of 262 mg/dL (14.5 mmol/L), the positive urine ketones, and an anion gap. It is imperative to recognize that patients with insulin-deficient diabetes mellitus can develop ketoacidosis with only moderate glucose elevations. This patient should now be started on an insulin drip in a monitored setting. Intravenous insulin infusion is usually the preferred method of insulin delivery in an emergency because dehydration may be severe (which decreases subcutaneous absorption) and rapid titration of insulin may be required. Her plasma glucose level should be measured every 1 to 2 hours and adjustments made to the insulin infusion, as required, to gradually normalize her glucose level and reverse the ketoacidosis. After the metabolic abnormalities have been corrected and the patient is ready to be transferred to subcutaneous administration of insulin (usually when the patient starts eating), intravenous and subcutaneous insulin administration need to be overlapped to avoid rebound ketoacidosis. Short-acting or rapid-acting insulins should be given for 1 to 2 hours or intermediate or long-acting insulins for 2 to 3 hours before terminating the insulin infusion to ensure adequate overlap.

Insulin glargine and neutral protamine Hagedorn (NPH) insulin are long-acting preparations that do not provide the flexibility needed to aggressively treat diabetic ketoacidosis.

The use of sliding scale insulin will not allow for adequate insulin coverage, and the ketoacidosis can be expected to progress.

KEY POINT

Ketoacidosis can develop in insulin-deficient patients with only moderate plasma glucose elevations; an insulin drip is the most effective treatment of diabetic ketoacidosis.

Bibliography

Wilson JF. In the clinic. Diabetic ketoacidosis. Ann Intern Med. 2010; 152(1):ITC1-15. [PMID: 20048266]

Item 11   Answer: D
Educational Objective: *Diagnose xanthelasma.*

The patient's skin lesions are xanthelasmas, which are the most common type of xanthomas. Xanthomas are the characteristic skin conditions associated with primary (due to genetic defects) or secondary hyperlipidemias. Xanthomas are yellow, orange, reddish, or yellow-brown papules, plaques, or nodules. If the infiltration is deep, the xanthoma may be nodular and have normal-appearing overlying skin. The type of xanthoma closely correlates with the type of lipoprotein that is elevated. Xanthelasma is a type of xanthoma characterized by soft, nontender, nonpruritic plaques localized to the eyelids. Xanthelasma can occur without hyperlipidemia, but is often associated with familial dyslipidemias.

Other types of xanthomas include eruptive xanthomas, which present as clusters of erythematous papules typically on the extensor surfaces. They are most often associated with extremely high (greater than 3000 mg/dL [33.9 mmol/L]) serum triglyceride levels. Eruptive xanthomas regress with treatment of hypertriglyceridemia. Plane xanthomas are yellow-to-red plaques found in skin folds of the neck and trunk. They can be associated with familial dyslipidemias and a variety of hematologic malignancies. Tendon xanthomas are subcutaneous nodules occurring on the extensor tendons. They are associated with familial hypercholesterolemia.

Hypothyroidism is associated with elevated lipid levels and can be a cause of secondary hyperlipidemias. However, hypothyroidism is not directly associated with the formation of xanthomas and usually does not result in lipid levels high enough to cause xanthomas. An elevated serum ferritin suggests the diagnosis of hemochromatosis, but hemochromatosis is not associated with xanthomas. Although liver chemistry tests may be abnormal in patients with extremely elevated lipid levels and are important to monitor during lipid therapy with statins, they are not associated with xanthoma formation. Type 2 diabetes is often seen in association with dyslipidemias, but abnormal glucose levels are not directly related to xanthoma formation.

KEY POINT

Xanthelasma is characterized by soft, nontender, nonpruritic plaques localized to the eyelids and may be associated with familial dyslipidemias.

Bibliography

Pitambe HV, Schulz EJ. Life-threatening dermatoses due to metabolic and endocrine disorders. Clin Dermatol. 2005;23(3):258-266. [PMID: 15896541]

Item 12   Answer: B
Educational Objective: *Manage isolated low HDL cholesterol with therapeutic lifestyle changes.*

The most appropriate next management step is to recommend lifestyle modifications. In evaluating and managing low HDL cholesterol, it is important to remember the primary target of therapy is LDL cholesterol. After LDL cholesterol has been evaluated and managed, non-HDL cholesterol is evaluated as a secondary target in patients with elevated triglycerides. This patient has isolated low HDL cholesterol. Because of insufficient evidence of risk reduction from controlled trials, ATP III has not set a specific goal for raising HDL cholesterol. In patients in whom the HDL cholesterol remains low despite use of statins or fibrates to treat high LDL or non-HDL cholesterol, or in patients with isolated low HDL cholesterol such as this patient, the first management step is institution of lifestyle interventions, including exercise, tobacco cessation, and weight management, because these interventions are capable of increasing the HDL cholesterol level.

The patient does not meet criteria for statin therapy because his LDL cholesterol goal is 130 mg/dL (3.4 mmol/L) and his measured LDL cholesterol is 128 mg/dL (3.3 mmol/L). His LDL cholesterol goal is based on the presence of two cardiovascular risk factors: smoking and low HDL cholesterol. Fibrate therapy is not indicated to treat his triglycerides because his non-HDL cholesterol, measured as total cholesterol-HDL cholesterol, is 157 mg/dL (4.0 mmol/L) and is below his target of 160 mg/dL (4.1 mmol/L). The non-HDL cholesterol goal is calculated as 30 mg/dL (0.8 mmol/L) above the patient's LDL cholesterol goal. Fibrate therapy would be indicated if the patient had a coronary heart disease equivalent such as diabetes or peripheral vascular disease, because fibrate therapy in this setting results in reduced mortality. Ultrasonography is not needed to determine carotid intimal thickness, because such information will not modify therapeutic decisions.

KEY POINT

In patients with isolated low HDL cholesterol, the first management step is institution of lifestyle interventions, including exercise, tobacco cessation, and weight management.

Bibliography

Kopin L, Lowenstein C. In the clinic. Dyslipidemia. Ann Intern Med. 2010;153(3):ITC21. [PMID: 20679557]

Item 13   Answer: D
Educational Objective: *Manage hyperlipidemia in a low-risk patient.*

The best management for this patient is to repeat a fasting lipid level in the future. This patient has hyperlipidemia, defined by a total cholesterol level above 200 mg/dL (5.2 mmol/L). The LDL-cholesterol goal varies depending on the presence or absence of five major cardiovascular risk factors: cigarette smoking, hypertension, older age (men ≥45 years; women ≥55 years), low HDL-cholesterol level (<40 mg/dL [1.0 mmol/L]), and a family history of coronary artery disease (first degree male relative <55 years; female relative <65 years).

In patients with zero or one risk factor, the LDL cholesterol goal is below 160 mg/dL (4.1 mmol/L). This patient has no major risk factors. Because his current LDL-cholesterol level is below 160 mg/dL (4.1 mmol/L), no therapy is indicated. The U.S. Preventive Services Task Force (USPSTF) concluded that the optimal interval for repeat screening is uncertain. It would be reasonable to repeat screening every 5 years, as recommended by the National Cholesterol Education Program, or select a shorter interval if the lipid levels are close to the threshold for treatment, as in this patient.

Fibrate therapy would be indicated for hypertriglyceridemia (>200 mg/dL [2.3 mmol/L]) in the setting of elevated non–HDL-cholesterol levels, which is not present in this patient.

Statin therapy would be appropriate for this patient with no risk factors if his LDL-cholesterol level were above 190 mg/dL (5.0 mmol/L) and would be optional if the level were between 160 mg/dL and 190 mg/dL (4.1 and 5.0 mmol/L).

Lipoprotein(a) [Lp(a)] level determination is not recommended for routine practice. Lp(a) is associated with increased risk for CAD but does not appear to be an independent predictor of risk of CAD.

KEY POINT

In patients with zero or one cardiovascular risk factor, the LDL cholesterol goal is below 160 mg/dL (4.1 mmol/L).

Bibliography

Kopin L, Lowenstein C. In the clinic. Dyslipidemia. Ann Intern Med. 2010;153(3):ITC21. [PMID: 20679557]

Item 14   Answer: D
Educational Objective: *Treat elevated LDL-cholesterol in a patient with diabetes mellitus.*

The most appropriate therapy is initiation of a statin, such as simvastatin. This patient has multiple risk factors for coronary artery disease, including diabetes mellitus, hypertension, and hypercholesterolemia. Diabetes is a coronary artery disease equivalent risk factor, and patients with diabetes have the same LDL-cholesterol goal as patients who have had a myocardial infarction, namely, below 100 mg/dL (2.6 mmol/L). A statin is the first-line treatment for cholesterol reduction. A 40-mg daily dose of simvastatin would likely reduce the LDL-cholesterol level by 30% and achieve the target goal.

Colestipol interrupts bile acid reabsorption and reduces LDL-cholesterol levels by 10% to 15%. It is often used as a second-line drug with statins because it acts synergistically to induce LDL receptors. However, colestipol can interfere with the absorption of this patient's other medications and, for this reason, is not the best initial management of his hyperlipidemia.

Although ezetimibe reduces LDL-cholesterol levels by reducing cholesterol absorption from the intestine, there are presently no clinical trial results showing that this medication reduces cardiovascular disease events, in contrast to statins. Therefore, ezetimibe should be reserved as an adjunct to other cholesterol-lowering medications if goal level is not achieved or for patients intolerant or allergic to other proven medications.

Niacin is an effective medication for modestly lowering LDL-cholesterol levels and increasing HDL-cholesterol levels but is often not tolerated because of its adverse effects (nausea and flushing), particularly at the dosage needed to achieve adequate reduction of the LDL-cholesterol level. Niacin would be a poor choice for this patient because it can cause glucose intolerance, potentially worsening his glucose control.

KEY POINT

The indication to initiate cholesterol-lowering medication and the goal level for treatment are dependent on the absolute level of LDL-cholesterol and the estimated risk for a coronary artery disease event.

Bibliography

Kopin L, Lowenstein C. In the clinic. Dyslipidemia. Ann Intern Med. 2010;153(3):ITC21. [PMID: 20679557]

Item 15   Answer: A

Educational Objective: *Treat hyperlipidemia in a patient with a history of transient ischemic attack.*

The most appropriate treatment is to begin atorvastatin. This patient with carotid artery disease and a transient ischemic attack (TIA) is considered by the Adult Treatment Panel III to have coronary artery–equivalent disease. In such patients, the LDL-cholesterol goal is lower than 100 mg/dL (2.6 mmol/L) to reduce the risk for future coronary events. Additionally, the American Heart Association/American Stroke Association and the National Stroke Association recommend aggressive risk factor reduction for the secondary prevention of stroke following an ischemic stroke or TIA. There is also accumulating evidence that reduction of blood pressure and treatment with a statin may prevent recurrent stroke even in patients with no evidence of hypertension or hyperlipidemia based upon current thresholds for treatment.

Changing antihypertensive medication to a β-blocker or calcium channel blocker in this patient is not indicated. The 2006 American Heart Association/American Stroke Association guidelines support the use of diuretics and an angiotensin-converting enzyme inhibitor.

Nicotinic acid is a lipid-lowering agent that, in addition to reducing LDL-cholesterol level, reduces triglyceride level and increases HDL-cholesterol level. However, statins are first-line therapy for lowering the LDL-cholesterol level in the absence of contraindications, and this patient has normal levels of triglycerides and HDL-cholesterol.

KEY POINT

In patients who have had a stroke or transient ischemic attack, the LDL-cholesterol goal is less than 100 mg/dL (2.6 mmol/L).

Bibliography

O'Regan C, Wu P, Arora D, Perri D, Mills EJ. Statin therapy in stroke prevention: a meta-analysis involving 121,000 patients. Am J Med. 2008;121(1):24-33. [PMID: 18187070]

Item 16   Answer: D

Educational Objective: *Diagnose hypothyroidism.*

This patient requires no additional testing before levothyroxine therapy is initiated for her hypothyroidism. Hashimoto disease is the most common cause of hypothyroidism, and confirmation of this diagnosis with measurement of TPO antibody is not necessary. Measurement of TPO antibody levels may be helpful in patients with subclinical hypothyroidism (elevated thyroid-stimulating hormone [TSH] level but normal free thyroxine [T_4]). In these patients, increased titers of TPO antibody confer an increased risk of hypothyroidism (~4% per year), which escalates as TSH levels rise above the reference range.

The radioactive iodine uptake (RAIU) test measures thyroid gland iodine uptake over a timed period, usually 24 hours.

Patients with thyrotoxicosis typically have an above-normal or high-normal RAIU, which is inappropriate in the context of a suppressed TSH level. In patients with thyroiditis or exposure to exogenous thyroid hormone, the RAIU will be below normal (<5% at 24 hours). Radionuclide uptake scanning has no role in the evaluation of hypothyroidism.

Thyroglobulin, a glycoprotein integral in follicular storage of thyroid hormone, can be detected in serum. Thyroglobulin levels can be elevated in hyperthyroidism and destructive thyroiditis. Intake of exogenous thyroid hormone generally suppresses thyroglobulin levels, which makes its measurement useful in patients with thyrotoxicosis due to surreptitious use of thyroid hormone. Thyroglobulin is also an effective tumor marker in patients with papillary or follicular thyroid cancer after thyroidectomy and radioactive iodine ablation therapy, because normal thyroid release of thyroglobulin should no longer be present. Measurement of thyroglobulin levels has no role in the evaluation of hypothyroidism.

KEY POINT

Hashimoto disease is the most common cause of hypothyroidism, and confirmation of this diagnosis with measurement of TPO antibody is not necessary.

Bibliography

McDermott MT. In the clinic. Hypothyroidism. Ann Intern Med. 2009;151(11):ITC61. [PMID: 19949140]

Item 17   Answer: A

Educational Objective: *Evaluate a thyroid nodule.*

The appropriate next step in the evaluation of this patient is a fine-needle aspiration of the thyroid nodule. The prevalence of palpable thyroid nodules is 4% to 7%. The cancer risk for a thyroid nodule is 5% to 10%. Factors associated with increased cancer risk include extremes of age (<20 or >60 years), male sex, a history of head or neck irradiation, a family history of thyroid cancer (especially medullary thyroid cancer), nodule size larger than 1 cm, rapid nodule growth, and hoarseness. Fine-needle aspiration is a simple method of determining the presence of malignancy. Sensitivity is approximately 90% to 95%, with a false-negative rate of 1% to 11%. Guidelines recommend biopsy of any nodule greater than 1 cm in diameter, and biopsy of smaller nodules should be considered in patients with cancer risk factors.

Limited laboratory testing is typically required in the evaluation of a thyroid nodule. Beyond a routine complete blood count and serum chemistry panel, the serum thyroid-stimulating hormone (TSH) level should be measured, because the result will help guide the evaluation (autonomously functioning nodules and multinodular goiters that suppress TSH levels are rarely malignant). Concomitant measurement of the serum free thyroxine (T_4) level is also reasonable if patients have thyroid-related symptoms but unnecessary in an asymptomatic patient with a normal TSH level such as this patient.

Thyroglobulin, a glycoprotein integral in follicular storage of thyroid hormone, can be detected in serum of normal patients. Thyroglobulin levels can be elevated in hyperthyroidism and destructive thyroiditis and is an excellent thyroid cancer marker in patients who have undergone thyroidectomy or radioactive iodine ablation. In this patient with an intact thyroid gland, a thyroglobulin level measurement will not be helpful.

A thyroid scan and radioactive iodine uptake test are appropriate in the context of a suppressed serum TSH level because a toxic nodule or multinodular goiter may be present. Because such hyperfunctional nodules rarely harbor cancer (<1%), their evaluation and management are far different. This patient does not have a suppressed TSH, and a thyroid scan and radioactive iodine uptake test is not indicated.

Although surgery is sometimes considered for nodules larger than 4 cm in diameter, surgery has no role in this asymptomatic patient with a smaller nodule.

KEY POINT

Guidelines recommend biopsy of any nodule greater than 1 cm in diameter, and biopsy of smaller nodules should be considered in patients with cancer risk factors.

Bibliography

Miller MC. The patient with a thyroid nodule. Med Clin North Am. 2010;94(5):1003-15. [PMID: 20736109]

Item 18   Answer: C

Educational Objective: *Manage hypothyroidism during pregnancy by monitoring TSH level.*

The most appropriate next step is to recheck this patient's serum thyroid-stimulating hormone (TSH) level. Because a fetus depends on maternal thyroid hormone for the first 10 to 12 weeks of gestation, the thyroid levels of pregnant women with hypothyroidism should be carefully monitored. Recent guidelines recommend that TSH and total thyroxine (T_4) levels be monitored throughout pregnancy because standard free T_4 levels are not as accurate in pregnant patients. The total T_4 level should be kept stable at approximately 1.5 times the normal range, and the TSH level should be kept in the lower range of normal. This may require an increase in their levothyroxine dosage of approximately 35% to 50% as early as the first trimester. Because of estrogen elevation during pregnancy, thyroid-binding globulin (TBG) levels increase. However, without an increase in the dosage of levothyroxine, free T_4 levels may decrease as more T_4 becomes bound by TBG. After delivery, TBG levels decrease, as do thyroid hormone requirements.

Although maternal iodine replacement has been successfully used in countries with prevalent iodine deficiency, its use in patients who are iodine sufficient can be associated with catastrophic results, such as a fetal goiter (pharmacologic amounts of iodine blocks release of thyroid hormone). Because significant iodine deficiency in the United States is rare, iodine therapy in pregnant U.S. women is not indicated.

Measurement of the free triiodothyronine (T_3) level is not useful in the evaluation of hypothyroidism because T_3 levels typically remain within the reference range until the point of severe hypothyroidism. This pattern is unaltered by pregnancy.

Continuing the current management is inappropriate because undertreatment of maternal hypothyroidism can have a potentially negative effect on fetal neurocognitive development.

KEY POINT

Levothyroxine requirements may increase 30% to 50% during the first trimester of pregnancy.

Bibliography

McDermott MT. In the clinic. Hypothyroidism. Ann Intern Med. 2009;151(11):ITC61. [PMID: 19949140]

Item 19   Answer: B

Educational Objective: *Treat Graves disease with atenolol and methimazole.*

The most appropriate medical regimen for this patient with Graves disease is atenolol and methimazole. Graves disease can present with either subclinical or overt thyrotoxicosis. Physical examination may reveal tachycardia; an elevated systolic blood pressure with a widened pulse pressure; a palpable goiter, which is classically smooth; a thyrotoxic stare due to lid retraction; proptosis; and, infrequently, an infiltrative dermopathy. To control her tachycardia, a β-blocker, such as atenolol, is indicated. Given the clinical and laboratory findings, this patient is also moderately hyperthyroid. To treat her hyperthyroidism, either methimazole or propylthiouracil can be used. Methimazole, which generally has fewer side effects and results in quicker achievement of the euthyroid state than propylthiouracil, is preferred in most patients. Because of a presumed immunomodulatory effect, antithyroidal drugs result in drug-free remission rates of between 30% and 50% in patients with Graves disease who are treated for 1 year.

Atenolol alone would only address this patient's adrenergic symptoms and not reduce her thyroid hormone levels, and methimazole alone would not immediately address her tachycardia.

Radioactive iodine therapy preceded or followed by adjunctive therapy with an antithyroidal drug is occasionally used to treat Graves disease. The drug is given in an attempt to decrease the risk of a transient worsening of the thyrotoxicosis after thyroid ablation. Because antithyroidal drugs render the thyroid radioresistant, they must be stopped for several days before and after giving the radioactive iodine. Although an occasional patient becomes euthyroid after radioactive iodine administration, the expected outcome is hypothyroidism, which typically occurs within 2 to 3 months of therapy, at which time thyroid hormone replacement therapy is begun.

KEY POINT

Methimazole has fewer side effects and results in quicker achievement of the euthyroid state than does propylthiouracil in patients with hyperthyroidism.

Bibliography

Nakamura H, Noh JY, Itoh K, Fukata S, Miyauchi A, Hamada N. Comparison of methimazole and propylthiouracil in patients with hyperthyroidism caused by Graves' disease. J Clin Endocrinol Metab. 2007;92(6):2157-2162. [PMID: 17389704]

Item 20   Answer: B

Educational Objective: *Diagnose the hypothyroid stage of postpartum thyroiditis.*

The best next management step is repeat measurement of the thyroid-stimulating hormone (TSH) and free thyroxine (T_4) levels. Postpartum thyroiditis, which occurs in approximately 5% of women in the United States within a few months of delivery, is a variant of painless thyroiditis. At presentation, patients may have transient thyrotoxicosis alone, transient hypothyroidism alone, or thyrotoxicosis that is followed by hypothyroidism and then by recovery. This patient most likely has postpartum thyroiditis that is now in the hypothyroid phase after a period of transient thyrotoxicosis. The hypothyroidism can be confirmed by remeasuring her TSH and free T_4 levels.

In this patient, the absence of a goiter and eye disease points away from Graves disease, as does the recent development of symptoms associated with hypothyroidism.

Methimazole therapy is inappropriate for this patient because she most likely has hypothyroidism, not hyperthyroidism. If transient hypothyroidism is confirmed by a high TSH level and low free T_4 level, thyroid hormone replacement, not methimazole, can be considered for bothersome symptoms.

With postpartum thyroiditis, results of thyroid scans and radioactive iodine uptake tests will be low during the thyrotoxic phase and then become elevated during the hypothyroid phase as the thyroid gland recovers and becomes very avid for iodine as stores are repleted. Before such testing can be advised, however, the results of current thyroid function tests are required to assess the patient's thyroid hormone status and determine if scan results suggest Graves disease or, what is more likely, recovery thyroiditis.

Ultrasound of the thyroid gland can be used to distinguish the high vascular flow of Graves disease from the low-flow pattern of autoimmune thyroiditis. A more direct test of this patient's thyroid function, however, is measurement of the TSH and free T_4 levels, which can quantify thyroid function and provide a baseline with which to compare future thyroid function test results.

KEY POINT

Postpartum thyroiditis can cause postpartum thyrotoxicosis, hypothyroidism, or a period of both.

Bibliography

McDermott MT. In the clinic. Hypothyroidism. Ann Intern Med. 2009;151(11):ITC61. [PMID: 19949140]

Item 21   Answer: C

Educational Objective: *Diagnose euthyroid sick syndrome.*

This patient should have repeat thyroid function tests in 6 to 8 weeks. With his history of a recent severe illness, the results of his thyroid function tests (low thyroid-stimulating hormone [TSH] and free triiodothyronine [T_3] levels and a low-normal free thyroxine [T_4] level) are most consistent with changes from a nonthyroidal illness (collectively known as euthyroid sick syndrome). The classic pattern consists of low TSH and free T_3 levels with a free T_4 level in the normal to low-normal range (or even frankly low with a prolonged illness). Reverse T_3 levels are elevated (if measured), but because results of this measurement typically take several weeks to obtain, reverse T_3 level results are seldom used clinically. The best next step is to allow the patient to recover for 4 to 8 weeks and then repeat the thyroid function tests. If results of these tests are not normal after recovery, further workup can commence.

Brain MRI is not appropriate for this patient because no clinical finding suggests pituitary dysfunction. Furthermore, if evaluation of the pituitary gland were required, MRI of the sella turcica would be most appropriate.

There are no data showing that T_4 replacement therapy is beneficial for nonthyroidal illness. Therefore, initiation of levothyroxine is not appropriate.

Thyroid ultrasonography does not help determine changes in thyroid function and thus is not useful for this patient.

KEY POINT

Severe illness can cause euthyroid sick syndrome, which is associated with abnormal results on thyroid function tests that often normalize after recovery.

Bibliography

Adler SM, Wartofsky L. The nonthyroidal illness syndrome. Endocrinol Metab Clin North Am. 2007;36(3):657-672, vi. [PMID: 17673123]

Item 22   Answer: C

Educational Objective: *Evaluate an incidentally discovered adrenal adenoma.*

Plasma-free metanephrine levels and overnight dexamethasone suppression test should be done next. The increasing use of imaging studies has revealed many previously unrecognized, often asymptomatic adrenal masses (adrenal incidentalomas). Initial assessment should include a careful history and physical examination to find any suggestion of malignant disease or clinical evidence of hormone hypersecretion. Most patients with metastatic cancer of the adrenal glands have clinical evidence of disease elsewhere. Imaging characteristics of the mass (size, CT attenuation, vascularity) can provide important clues. The risk of primary or metastatic cancer is nearly 2% for tumors less than 4 cm in diameter but increases to 25% for tumors 6 cm or larger. Metastatic lesions to the adrenal glands tend to have a high CT attenuation (>20 Hounsfield units) and are often bilateral. Primary adrenocortical carcinoma tends to be large with irregular borders and may include areas of necrosis. Pheochromocytoma, adrenal carcinoma, and metastatic disease to the adrenal glands are often vascular, whereas benign adrenal adenomas are not highly vascular.

Because overt clinical manifestations are typically scant, screening tests are often necessary to identify potentially functioning adrenal incidentalomas secreting cortisol, aldosterone, or catecholamines. Subclinical Cushing syndrome is the most common abnormality associated with adrenal incidentalomas. Because these patients have no symptoms or physical findings of Cushing syndrome, the possibility of autonomous hypersecretion of glucocorticoids should be evaluated with an overnight dexamethasone suppression test. Additionally, measurements of plasma catecholamines are reasonable screening tests to rule out pheochromocytoma, which can be asymptomatic or associated with intermittent symptoms.

Adrenal incidentalomas are unlikely to secrete aldosterone, but patients should be screened for that possibility if they have hypertension or hypokalemia, both of which are absent in this patient. Similarly, excess adrenal androgen production is rare, except when the mass represents adrenal cancer, and screening is not routinely performed in the absence of clinical signs or symptoms of feminization in men or hyperandrogenism in women, which is also absent in this patient.

KEY POINT

Hypersecretion of glucocorticoids and catecholamines should be evaluated in all patients, including asymptomatic patients, with incidentally discovered adrenal adenoma.

Bibliography
Nieman LK. Approach to the patient with an adrenal incidentaloma. J Clin Endocrinol Metab. 2010;95(9):4106-13. [PMID: 20823463]

Item 23   Answer: B
Educational Objective: *Diagnose hyperaldosteronism with measurement of the serum aldosterone to plasma renin activity ratio.*

The most appropriate next diagnostic test is determination of the serum aldosterone to plasma renin activity ratio. This patient has drug-resistant hypertension (uncontrolled hypertension on three drugs, including a diuretic), unprovoked hypokalemia, and probable metabolic alkalosis; he also has an inappropriately high urine potassium level. In this setting, primary hyperaldosteronism is a very likely cause of his hypertension and hypokalemia, especially given his age. The best screening test for primary hyperaldosteronism is a determination of the ratio of serum aldosterone (in ng/dL) to plasma

renin activity (in ng/mL/min). A ratio greater than 20, particularly when the serum aldosterone level is greater than 15 ng/dL (414 pmol/L), is consistent with the diagnosis of primary hyperaldosteronism.

After biochemical confirmation of hyperaldosteronism, localization procedures are appropriate to differentiate aldosterone-producing adenomas, which are amenable to surgical resection, from bilateral hyperplasia, which is medically treated. Given the high incidence of incidental adrenal lesions, however, imaging studies, such as CT of the adrenal glands, should not be performed before biochemical testing that confirms the presence of hyperaldosteronism.

This patient does not fit the demographic or clinical profile of a patient with renovascular hypertension, and thus evaluating the renal arteries with digital subtraction renal angiography is not indicated. Renovascular hypertension due to fibromuscular disease of the renal arteries usually presents in patients younger than 35 years, and azotemia is rarely present. Atherosclerotic renovascular hypertension is more common in patients older than 55 years and is frequently associated with vascular disease in other vessels; azotemia is often present.

Other than sustained hypertension, this patient did not have any of other symptoms or signs suggestive of a pheochromocytoma (palpitations, headache, tremor, diaphoresis). Therefore, screening for a pheochromocytoma with measurement of the plasma metanephrine and normetanephrine levels is less likely to be helpful than is screening for hyperaldosteronism.

KEY POINT

The best screening test for primary hyperaldosteronism is a determination of the ratio of serum aldosterone to plasma renin activity.

Bibliography
Funder JW, Carey RM, Fardella C, et al; Endocrine Society. Case detection, diagnosis, and treatment of patients with primary aldosteronism: an Endocrine Society clinical practice guideline. J Clin Endocrinol Metab. 2008;93(9):3266-3281. [PMID: 18552288]

Item 24   Answer: D
Educational Objective: *Evaluate a patient with suspected Cushing disease with pituitary MRI.*

The most appropriate next diagnostic test for this patient is pituitary MRI. She has biochemical features of adrenocorticotropic hormone (ACTH)–dependent Cushing syndrome (hypercortisolism and elevated ACTH). The cause of the ACTH hypersecretion is either a pituitary adenoma or an ectopic source, such as a carcinoid tumor. In this patient, partial suppression was achieved with high-dose dexamethasone, which suggests an ACTH-secreting pituitary microadenoma. High-dose dexamethasone is usually not successful in suppressing ACTH production from an ectopic source. However, there are exceptions, so caution must be exercised in interpretation. In such instances, expert consultation is highly recommended.

Adrenal imaging is indicated if the hypercortisolism is ACTH independent (hypercortisolism and normal or low ACTH level). In patients with hypercortisolism associated with suppressed ACTH secretion, a CT scan of the adrenal glands often shows a tumor (adenoma or carcinoma). However, this patient's ACTH level was elevated and adrenal imaging is not indicated with either a CT or MRI scan.

The cosyntropin stimulation test is used to determine the adrenal reserve by measuring the response to a standard dose of synthetic adrenocorticotropic hormone. The test does not detect Cushing syndrome but, rather, adrenal insufficiency and is therefore not indicated for this patient.

KEY POINT

Adrenocorticotropic hormone (ACTH)–dependent hypercortisolism is most commonly caused by a pituitary tumor or an ectopic ACTH source, such as a carcinoid tumor.

Bibliography
Findling JW, Raff H. Cushing's syndrome: important issues in diagnosis and management. J Clin Endocrinol Metab. 2006;91(10):3746-3753. [PMID: 16868050]

Item 25   Answer: A
Educational Objective: *Diagnose pheochromocytoma with abdominal CT scan.*

The most appropriate next management step for this patient is an abdominal CT scan. She has the classic symptoms of pheochromocytoma—palpitations, sweating, headaches, and hypertension. Additionally, biochemical testing revealed increased plasma levels of catecholamines. Most pheochromocytomas are located in the adrenal medulla, although some are extra-adrenal in origin. CT has sensitivities of 93% to 100% in detecting adrenal pheochromocytoma and approximately 90% in detecting extra-adrenal catecholamine-secreting paragangliomas. MRI is as sensitive as CT in detecting adrenal pheochromocytomas and superior to CT in detecting extra-adrenal catecholamine-secreting paragangliomas.

An adrenalectomy is appropriate only when a tumor is confirmed. An adrenalectomy would not be indicated if the source of the catecholamines were confirmed to be extra-adrenal.

If an abdominal CT shows no masses, the next best localizing study would be a metaiodobenzylguanidine (MIBG) scan. MIBG scintigraphy is highly specific (99%) but less sensitive (80%) than CT techniques. MIBG scintigraphy is generally reserved for patients with equivocal CT results, extra-adrenal catecholamine-secreting tumors, or suspected malignancy.

Adrenal vein sampling is a technically difficult and hazardous procedure, especially in a patient with a pheochromocytoma. The availability of the highly specific and sensitive MIBG scan should take precedence over this more hazardous procedure.

KEY POINT

CT has sensitivities of 93% to 100% in detecting adrenal pheochromocytoma, and approximately 90% in detecting extra-adrenal catecholamine-secreting paragangliomas.

Bibliography
Young WF Jr. Adrenal causes of hypertension: pheochromocytoma and primary aldosteronism. Rev Endocr Metab Disord. 2007;8(4):309-320. [PMID: 17914676]

Item 26   Answer: B
Educational Objective: *Diagnose chronic corticosteroid therapy as the cause of adrenal insufficiency.*

This patient has central adrenal insufficiency secondary to exogenous corticosteroid use. Systemic corticosteroids are the most common cause of central adrenal insufficiency, with supraphysiologic dosages of exogenous corticosteroids causing disruption of hypothalamic/pituitary adrenocorticotropic hormone (ACTH) production. Consequently, the adrenal cortex atrophies. When subsequently challenged by stress, the hypothalamus and pituitary gland are unable to stimulate adequate adrenal production of cortisol. This central effect of exogenous corticosteroids can occur after only 3 weeks of suppressive therapy. The patient appears to have developed Cushing syndrome as a result of chronic systemic exposure to the intra-articular injections of corticosteroids. Despite her cushingoid features, however, she has clinical and biochemical evidence of adrenal insufficiency. Her low-normal serum ACTH level and her partial response to cosyntropin stimulation indicate that she has central (secondary) adrenal insufficiency. Patients with adrenal insufficiency often decompensate during concurrent illnesses.

An adrenal adenoma could cause a suppressed ACTH level, cushingoid features, and central obesity, but her symptoms also suggest glucocorticoid deficiency. Furthermore, an adrenal adenoma would cause an elevated, not suppressed, cortisol level.

A functioning pituitary adenoma might produce excessive ACTH, but in that case both the ACTH and cortisol levels would be elevated, not suppressed as they are in this patient. A nonfunctioning pituitary adenoma might cause suppressed levels of ACTH and cortisol but there would be no signs of hypercortisolism, as seen in this patient.

Primary adrenal insufficiency (Addison disease) is typically associated with low cortisol production and elevated ACTH levels.

KEY POINT

Secondary adrenal insufficiency due to exogenous corticosteroids may be associated with suppression of both adrenocorticotropic hormone and cortisol levels and with clinical findings of excess glucocorticoids.

Bibliography
Chakera AJ, Vaidya B. Addison disease in adults: diagnosis and management. Am J Med. 2010;123(5):409-413. [PMID: 20399314]

Item 27   Answer: B

Educational Objective: *Treat adrenal insufficiency during stress with intravenous stress doses of hydrocortisone.*

Given her fever and hypotension, this patient with known primary adrenal insufficiency should receive a stress dosage of intravenous hydrocortisone. Patients with adrenal insufficiency are educated to increase their corticosteroid dosage during stressful events, such as an infection or surgery. When they do not, symptoms of adrenal insufficiency occur. Some patients, such as this one, develop nausea and vomiting that limit the use of orally administered corticosteroids. In such patients, corticosteroids should be administered parenterally. Cortisol replacement with corticosteroids and restoration of intravascular volume with normal saline are vital to treatment of acute adrenal insufficiency. Stress-level dosages of corticosteroids are considered to be 10-times the normal daily replacement dosage. For most patients, this is equivalent to 100 mg of hydrocortisone daily, administered intravenously in divided dosages three to four times per day. Once the dosage of hydrocortisone is over 60 mg per day, fludrocortisone is unnecessary because that dose of hydrocortisone has adequate mineralocorticoid activity.

Hyponatremia is a common feature of adrenal insufficiency and is easily corrected with hydrocortisone and normal saline to restore plasma volume. Administering 3% saline to correct the low sodium level is therefore inappropriate.

Fludrocortisone is a mineralocorticoid that is required in patients with primary adrenal insufficiency. Treatment with fludrocortisone is usually not necessary in a hospitalized patient receiving normal saline and high dosages of hydrocortisone, which has mineralocorticoid activity. This therapy will maintain vascular volume and suppress vasopressin, which is responsible for the hyponatremia. Fludrocortisone therapy alone is insufficient for a patient with primary adrenal insufficiency who is experiencing physiologic stress.

Although this patient requires close observation, making no changes to her therapeutic regimen (maintaining baseline dosages) would be inappropriate, given the need for a higher dosage of the corticosteroid during this stressful event.

KEY POINT

Stress-level dosages of corticosteroids are administered to patients with adrenal insufficiency during times of increased physiological stress.

Bibliography
Chakera AJ, Vaidya B. Addison disease in adults: diagnosis and management. Am J Med. 2010;123(5):409-413. [PMID: 20399314]

Item 28   Answer: D

Educational Objective: *Treat osteoporosis with bisphosphonate therapy and vitamin D and calcium.*

Vitamin D supplementation is an important part of treatment for osteoporosis. Vitamin D levels are best measured by looking at stores of 25-Hydroxy vitamin D. A wide range of "optimal" levels are reported (15-80 ng/mL [37-200 nmol/L]). Generally, levels lower than 30 ng/mL (74.8 nmol/L) are defined as insufficient, and levels lower than 20 ng/mL (49.9 nmol/L) are defined as deficient. Vitamin D is obtained through ultraviolet (sunlight) radiation and natural foods, fortified foods, and vitamin supplements. Many variables such as latitude, season, sunscreen use, and clothing prevent sunlight from being an effective method to maintain adequate vitamin D stores. Because the vitamin D content of most foods is relatively low, most patients will need vitamin D supplementation. A common supplementation strategy includes a loading dose followed by maintenance dosing. A loading dose of 50,000 IU of vitamin D is given orally once a week for 10 weeks and is then followed by a daily dose of 2000 IU. Vitamin D deficiency contributes to bone loss from decreased vitamin D-dependent intestinal calcium absorption and secondary hyperparathyroidism. Vitamin D supplements can also improve muscle strength, which can lead to fewer falls in the osteoporotic patient.

The United States Preventive Services Task Force advises against using estrogen or estrogen plus progestin for the prevention of chronic diseases, including osteoporosis, after menopause, citing data from the Women's Health Initiative that showed at least a trend toward an increased risk of breast cancer, coronary heart disease, stroke, venous thromboembolism, dementia and cognitive decline, and urinary incontinence with such use.

In patients with hyperparathyroidism, localization of abnormal parathyroid glands preoperatively by means of ultrasonography, technetium Tc 99m sestamibi scintigraphy, or MRI offers the possibility of a less invasive surgical approach. However, the accuracy of these radiologic modalities is variable. This patient's serum calcium and parathyroid hormone levels are normal, excluding hyperparathyroidism as the cause of this patient's osteoporosis.

KEY POINT

The prevention and treatment of osteoporosis includes vitamin D and calcium supplementation.

Bibliography
Kennel KA, Drake MT, Hurley DL. Vitamin D deficiency in adults: when to test and how to treat. Mayo Clin Proc. 2010;85(8):752-7. [PMID: 20675513]

Item 29   Answer: B

Educational Objective: *Screen for osteoporosis with dual-energy x-ray absorptiometry.*

Dual-energy x-ray absorptiometry is an appropriate screening test for this patient. Guidelines recommend that screening for osteoporosis begin at age 65 years for women. Women aged 60 to 64 years should be screened if they are at higher than average risk for osteoporosis. The most predictive risk factor for osteoporosis is weight below 70 kg (154 lb), as with this patient.

The U.S. Preventive Services Task Force (USPSTF) recommends against screening for abdominal aortic aneurysm in women because of the low prevalence of abdominal aortic aneurysm in this group. Abdominal ultrasonography, therefore, is not indicated.

After three consecutive negative annual cytology smears, the risk of cervical cancer is reduced to approximately 1/100,000 person-years. In this monogamous patient with three consecutive normal Pap smears whose last Pap smear was 14 months ago, it would be reasonable to increase the screening interval to every 2 to 3 years, with consideration of stopping screening at age 65 years if her Pap smears continue to be normal.

Pneumococcal vaccine is indicated for persons age 65 years and older or for those younger than 65 years who live in long-term care facilities, or who have chronic illnesses, or who are Alaskan natives or American Indians. This patient has no indication for pneumococcal vaccination at this time.

KEY POINT

Screening for osteoporosis is recommended for women age 65 years and older and in women 60 to 64 years old who are at increased risk for osteoporosis.

Bibliography

Davison KS, Kendler DL, Ammann P, et al. Assessing fracture risk and effects of osteoporosis drugs: bone mineral density and beyond. Am J Med. 2009;122(11):992-997. [PMID: 19854322]

Item 30   Answer: A

Educational Objective: *Treat osteoporosis with a bisphosphonate.*

This patient should be started on a bisphosphonate, such as alendronate. These drugs are pyrophosphate derivatives that bind to the bone surface and inhibit osteoclastic bone resorption. They are poorly absorbed and must be taken in the fasting state to optimize absorption. Alendronate is effective in lowering fracture risk in patients with osteoporosis. Zoledronate is one of several newer bisphosphonates that can be administered intravenously and is associated with a long duration of action. A single injected dose of zoledronate suppresses bone turnover markers for a full year and induces significant gains in bone mineral density over the same period. Zoledronate also reduces fracture risk.

Calcitonin nasal spray increases bone mass in the spine and decreases vertebral fractures but does not affect the incidence of hip fractures. This drug is indicated for women who are more than 5 years postmenopausal. It is a second-line drug to the bisphosphonates.

Hormone replacement therapy is no longer regarded as the mainstay of therapy for osteoporosis. In the Women's Health Initiative, the use of conjugated estrogens and medroxyprogesterone in postmenopausal women increased bone mass but also increased the risk of cardiovascular disease, breast cancer, stroke, deep venous thrombosis, and pulmonary embolism.

Raloxifene is a selective estrogen receptor modulator that has estrogen-like effects on bone but inhibits the effects of estrogen in the breast and uterus. Raloxifene increases bone mass and decreases the risk of vertebral fractures in postmenopausal women but does not affect the incidence of hip fractures. Raloxifene is not associated with adverse cardiovascular events and decreases the risk of breast cancer in high-risk women. Side effects include hot flushes and an increase in the risk of thromboembolism. It is a second-line drug to the bisphosphonates.

Teriparatide (recombinant human PTH [1-34]) is the only anabolic agent listed, whereas all the other medications are antiresorptive. When given intermittently, teriparatide stimulates osteoblastic bone formation. Given as a subcutaneous injection, teriparatide should not be used for more than 2 years. The drug significantly increases bone mass and can decrease the incidence of both vertebral and nonvertebral fractures. Animal studies have shown an increased risk of osteosarcoma; therefore, this agent should be avoided in patients with Paget disease of bone, unexplained elevation of alkaline phosphatase level, previous radiation involving the skeleton, and a history of skeletal cancer. Teriparatide should be considered in patients who are intolerant of other medications and in those with the greatest fracture risk (T-score <−3.5 or <−3.0 with a fragility fracture).

KEY POINT

Bisphosphonates are a class of drugs that can lower the fracture rate in patients with osteoporosis.

Bibliography

Bilezikian JP. Efficacy of bisphosphonates in reducing fracture risk in postmenopausal osteoporosis. Am J Med. 2009;122(2 Suppl):S14-21. [PMID: 19187808]

Item 31   Answer: B

Educational Objective: *Treat postmenopausal osteoporosis with intravenous zoledronate.*

This patient should stop taking alendronate and instead receive intravenous zoledronate. Bisphosphonates are first-line drugs for treating postmenopausal women with osteoporosis. Alendronate and risedronate reduce the risk of both vertebral and nonvertebral fractures. Some patients with osteoporosis, however, may be intolerant of oral bisphosphonates because of aggravation of underlying gastroesophageal reflux disease. For these patients, once yearly intravenous infusion of zoledronate is a potent and effective alternative. An injectable bisphosphonate, such as zoledronate, should also be considered when oral bisphosphonates are unsuccessful, contraindicated (as in esophageal stricture or achalasia), or likely to be poorly absorbed (as in uncontrolled celiac disease and inflammatory bowel disease) and when a patient is unable to remain upright for 30 to 60 minutes after dosing. An alternative to annual intravenous alendronate is intravenous ibandronate every 3 months.

Calcitonin is not a first-line drug for postmenopausal osteoporosis treatment. Its efficacy against fractures is not strong, and its effects on bone mineral density are less than those of other agents.

Although raloxifene, a selective estrogen receptor modulator, can prevent bone loss and reduces the risk of vertebral fractures, its effectiveness in reducing other fractures is uncertain. Extraskeletal risks (including risk of thromboembolism and fatal stroke) and benefits must be considered before starting postmenopausal women on raloxifene therapy. For this patient, the safer alternative of intravenous zoledronate or ibandronate is available and is recommended as first-line therapy.

Teriparatide (recombinant human parathyroid hormone [1-34]) is reserved for treating patients at high risk of fracture, including those with very low bone mineral density (T-score below −3.0) with a previous vertebral fracture and contraindications to bisphosphonate use. This therapy improves bone mineral density, stimulates new bone formation, and reduces the risk of new vertebral and nonvertebral fractures. Dosage requirements, such as daily subcutaneous injections, may limit its use. Teriparatide is an anabolic agent, whereas the other osteoporosis drugs are antiresorptive agents. Since this patient does not have a previous fracture and is probably able to tolerate once yearly intravenous zoledronate, teriparatide is not indicated.

KEY POINT

Once yearly intravenous infusion of zoledronate is a potent therapy for treating postmenopausal osteoporosis of the spine and hip.

Bibliography

Davison KS, Kendler DL, Ammann P, et al. Assessing fracture risk and effects of osteoporosis drugs: bone mineral density and beyond. Am J Med. 2009;122(11):992-927. [PMID: 19854322]

Item 32   **Answer: C**

Educational Objective: *Diagnose osteoporosis.*

This patient has osteoporosis. She had recent vertebral compression fractures in response to minimal trauma (fragility fracture). Osteoporosis is diagnosed by the presence of fragility fractures (fracture secondary to minor trauma, such as falling from a standing position), or by a bone mineral density (BMD) T-score less than −2.5 in patients who have not experienced a fragility fracture. Bone density scan results are reported in terms of T-scores (the standard deviation from the mean BMD of a young healthy population) and Z-scores (the standard deviation from the BMD of an age- and sex-matched group). At the spine, a T-score of −1 represents approximately 10% bone loss. The T-score is used to diagnose osteoporosis.

Osteopenia is defined as a BMD T-score that is between −1 and −2.5. In all patients, the presence of a fragility fracture takes priority over BMD results in diagnosing osteoporosis. This patient has also had an evaluation for causes of secondary bone loss. The normal serum calcium, phosphorus, and alkaline phosphatase levels and normal urine calcium level are consistent with osteoporosis and exclude secondary osteoporosis.

KEY POINT

Osteoporosis is diagnosed by the presence of fragility fractures or by a bone mineral density T-score less than −2.5 in patients who have not experienced a fragility fracture.

Bibliography

Davison KS, Kendler DL, Ammann P, et al. Assessing fracture risk and effects of osteoporosis drugs: bone mineral density and beyond. Am J Med. 2009;122(11):992-997. [PMID: 19854322]

Section 3

Gastroenterology and Hepatology
Questions

Item 1 [Basic]

A 42-year-old man is evaluated in the clinic for 1 day of acute onset, left-sided colicky flank pain. The pain radiates from his left upper quadrant to the left lower quadrant and upper thigh. With the onset of the pain, he has developed nausea but no vomiting. He has no other medical problems and takes no medications.

On physical examination, temperature is 37.4°C (99.3°F), blood pressure is 154/78 mm Hg, heart rate 85/min, and respiration rate is 18/min. He reports no tenderness to abdominal or costovertebral angle palpation. The remainder of the physical examination is normal.

Urinalysis shows many erythrocytes, but no leukocytes or bacteria.

Which of the following tests should be done next?

(A) Abdominal x-ray
(B) Intravenous pyelography
(C) Kidney ultrasound
(D) Noncontrast helical abdominal CT scan

Item 2 [Basic]

A 67-year-old woman is evaluated in the hospital for acute abdominal pain. She was admitted for community-acquired pneumonia, and her condition was improving on therapy with antibiotics and fluids. However, on day 3 she developed acute abdominal pain associated with nausea. Her medical history includes a 7-year history of peripheral arterial disease, type 2 diabetes mellitus, hyperlipidemia, and an episode of diverticulitis 2 years ago. Her medications are pravastatin, aspirin, dipyridamole, and metformin.

On physical examination, she is in distress; temperature is 38.3°C (101.0°F), blood pressure is 170/100 mm Hg, pulse rate is 120/min, and respiration rate is 25/min. She rates her pain as 10 out of 10. She has diffuse abdominal tenderness, more pronounced in the left lower quadrant with rebound tenderness.

Which of the following is the most appropriate next diagnostic test?

(A) Colonoscopy
(B) CT scan of the abdomen
(C) Left pelvic ultrasonography
(D) Supine and upright abdominal radiographs

Item 3 [Advanced]

A 70-year-old man is evaluated in the emergency department for severe lower abdominal and back pain that began suddenly 12 hours ago and was associated with a syncopal episode. Since that time, he has had vague lower abdominal and back discomfort. There has been no change in bowel or urinary habits and no fever or chills. The patient has a 40 pack-year history of smoking cigarettes. He also has hypertension and hyperlipidemia. His medications are atorvastatin, aspirin, lisinopril, and hydrochlorothiazide.

On physical examination, temperature is 37.7°C (99.8°F), blood pressure is 90/60 mm Hg, pulse rate is 110/min and regular, and respiration rate is 18/min. Results of the cardiac and neurologic examinations are normal. There is moderate tenderness to palpation in the infra-umbilical and suprapubic regions but no guarding or rebound tenderness. The remainder of the abdominal examination is normal.

Laboratory results include a hematocrit of 29% and a leukocyte count of 12,000/µL (12.0 × 10⁹/L). Results of liver chemistry studies and urinalysis are normal. A stool sample tests negative for occult blood. Electrocardiogram shows normal sinus rhythm and left ventricular hypertrophy. A plain abdominal radiograph shows no free air or air-fluid levels.

Which of the following is the most likely diagnosis?

(A) Acute myocardial infarction
(B) Diverticulitis
(C) Nephrolithiasis (renal colic)
(D) Ruptured abdominal aortic aneurysm

Item 4 [Advanced]

A 25-year-old woman is evaluated for a 2-year history of almost daily bloating and lower abdominal cramping; the symptoms are associated with constipation, relieved with bowel movements, and seem worse when she is under stress. She has one or two small bowel movements a week and often has a feeling of incomplete evacuation. She never has diarrhea and has not had blood in the stool, nocturnal awakening with pain or for bowel movements, or weight loss. She has taken a fiber supplement without relief. The patient is otherwise healthy, and her only medication is an oral contraceptive pill that she has been taking for 1 year.

On physical examination, vital signs are normal; there is mild lower abdominal tenderness with no rebound, guarding, or palpable abdominal masses. Hemoglobin level and serum biochemistry tests, including thyroid-stimulating hormone, are all normal.

Which of the following is the most appropriate next step in the management of this patient?

(A) Colonoscopy
(B) CT scan of the abdomen and pelvis
(C) Discontinue the oral contraceptive
(D) Reassurance and polyethylene glycol

Item 5 [Advanced]

A 75-year-old woman is evaluated in the emergency department for the acute onset of passage of bright red blood per rectum. This morning she had crampy abdominal pain and had two episodes of diarrhea after which she passed bright red blood. The patient has a history of hypertension and coronary artery disease. Medications are aspirin, ramipril, metoprolol, and simvastatin. She had a colonoscopy 6 months ago, which was normal.

On physical examination, the patient is not in acute distress; temperature is 36.8°C (98.2°F), blood pressure is 130/80 mm Hg, pulse rate is 70/min, and respiration rate is 14/min. The heart and lungs are normal. The abdomen is soft with tenderness in the left lower quadrant without rebound or guarding. Rectal examination shows the presence of bright red blood. Laboratory studies reveal a hemoglobin level of 11.9 g/dL (119 g/L), a leukocyte count of 8400/µL (8.4 × 10⁹/L), and platelet count 246,000/µL (246 × 10⁹/L). Serum electrolytes, glucose, creatinine, and urea nitrogen are normal. CT scan of the abdomen and pelvis shows segmental thickening in the sigmoid colon.

Which of the following is the most likely diagnosis?

(A) Crohn disease
(B) Irritable bowel syndrome
(C) Ischemic colitis
(D) Peptic ulcer disease

Item 6 [Basic]

A 63-year-old man is evaluated for a 2-day history of left lower quadrant abdominal pain. The pain is constant and is not relieved by a bowel movement or by positional changes. The patient is slightly nauseated and has no appetite but is not vomiting. He has never had a similar episode. The patient is otherwise healthy.

On physical examination, temperature is 38.0°C (100.4°F), blood pressure is 125/85 mm Hg, pulse rate is 95/min, and respiration rate is 14/min. There is fullness and tenderness of the left lower quadrant with no rebound or guarding; bowel sounds are decreased. Rectal examination is normal; examination of stool for occult blood is negative. Leukocyte count is 14,000/µL (14 × 10⁹/L); all other laboratory results are normal. A plain abdominal radiograph is unremarkable, and a chest radiograph shows no free air beneath the diaphragms.

Which of the following is the most appropriate next step in the evaluation of this patient?

(A) Barium enema
(B) Colonoscopy
(C) Contrast-enhanced CT scan of the abdomen and pelvis
(D) Small-bowel radiographic series

Item 7 [Advanced]

A 42-year-old man is evaluated in the hospital for a 1-year history of postprandial abdominal pain that radiates to the back, is worse after eating, and is associated with bloating and nausea. He has not lost weight. The patient has had at least five alcohol-containing drinks a day for 20 years.

On physical examination, vital signs are normal; BMI is 21. There is mild epigastric tenderness with no guarding or rebound and normal bowel sounds.

Laboratory studies reveal a normal complete blood count and normal glucose and liver chemistry tests; amylase is 221 U/L and lipase is 472 U/L. A plain film of the abdomen is shown.

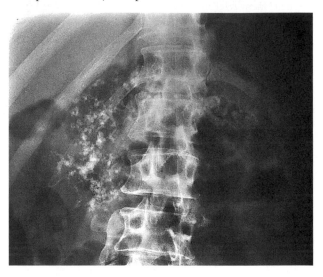

Which of the following is the most likely diagnosis?

(A) Acute cholangitis
(B) Chronic pancreatitis
(C) Diverticulitis
(D) Peptic ulcer disease

Item 8 [Advanced]

A 14-year-old boy is evaluated for a 1-week history of fever, abdominal pain, and bloody diarrhea. He reports no recent travel or medication use but did go to a barbeque 1 week ago and ate hamburgers. His medical history is otherwise unremarkable.

On physical examination, temperature is 38.4°C (101.2°F), blood pressure is 150/96 mm Hg, pulse rate is 100/min, and respiration rate is 14/min. He has petechiae on his legs. The abdomen is diffusely tender. The remainder of the examination is normal.

Hemoglobin	7.6 g/dL (76 g/L)
Leukocyte count	15,000/µL (15 × 10⁹/L)
Platelet count	46,000/µL (24 × 10⁹/L)
Blood urea nitrogen	36 mg/dL (12.8 mmol/L)
Creatinine	2.8 mg/dL (247.5 mmol/L)

Urinalysis is positive for many erythrocytes per high-power field.

Which of the following is the most appropriate next management step for this patient?

(A) Empiric antibiotics
(B) Peripheral blood smear
(C) Platelet transfusion
(D) Routine stool culture (shigella, salmonella, campylobacter)
(E) Stool for fecal leukocytes

Item 9 [Advanced]

A 64-year-old woman is evaluated for 2 weeks of nonbloody diarrhea. She was recently diagnosed with stage IV rectal cancer and underwent treatment with chemotherapy and radiation therapy 4 weeks ago. She has 10 small, loose bowel movements daily associated with tenesmus. She has no nausea, vomiting, abdominal pain, fever, or weight loss.

On physical examination, vital signs are normal. The abdomen is soft, and no evidence of rectal fissures or fistulas is seen.

Which is the following is the most appropriate diagnostic test?

(A) Abdominal/pelvic CT scan
(B) Flexible sigmoidoscopy
(C) Stool culture
(D) Stool osmolality

Item 10 [Advanced]

A 41-year-old man is evaluated for an 8-month history of midepigastric pain that is worse after eating and six to eight oily bowel movements a day usually occurring after a meal. He has lost 6.8 kg (15 lb) over the past 6 months. The patient drinks six to eight cans of beer a day, and he has been admitted to the hospital twice with acute pancreatitis. He takes no medications.

On physical examination, BMI is 21. He has normal bowel sounds and mid-epigastric tenderness but no evidence of hepatosplenomegaly or masses. Rectal examination reveals brown stool that is negative for occult blood. The remainder of the examination is normal. Plain radiograph of the abdomen shows a normal bowel gas pattern and is otherwise normal.

Fasting plasma glucose	124 mg/dL (6.9 mmol/L)
Aspartate aminotransferase	191 U/L
Alanine aminotransferase	82 U/L
Amylase	132U/L
Lipase	289 U/L

Which of the following tests is most likely to establish the diagnosis in this patient?

(A) Colonoscopy
(B) CT scan of the abdomen
(C) Measurement of serum antiendomysial antibodies
(D) Stool for leukocytes, culture, ova, and parasites

Item 11 [Basic]

A 30-year-old woman is evaluated for a 9-month history of cramping midepigastric discomfort that is relieved by defecation; the discomfort is sometimes accompanied by bloating. The stool is often watery. She has not had fever, chills, or weight loss. The patient is otherwise healthy and takes no medications; there is no family history of gastrointestinal disease.

On physical examination, the patient is afebrile; blood pressure is 105/70 mm Hg, pulse rate is 72/min, and respiration rate is 14/min; BMI is 23. The abdomen is soft and not tender or distended; the stool is brown and negative for occult blood. Complete blood count and serum biochemistry studies, including liver studies, vitamin B_{12}, vitamin D, and thyroid-stimulating hormone, are normal. A flexible sigmoidoscopy is normal.

Which of the following is the most appropriate management for this patient?

(A) Colonoscopy
(B) CT enteroscopy
(C) Gluten-free diet
(D) Symptomatic management

Item 12 [Basic]

A 74-year-old woman is evaluated in the emergency department with a 2-day history of diarrhea characterized by ten bowel movements daily, with worsening abdominal pain and fever. Five weeks ago, the patient was hospitalized with necrotizing fasciitis of the right thigh for which she underwent debridement, received nafcillin and clindamycin therapy, and was discharged after 2 weeks. On discharge, she was prescribed a 2-week course of nafcillin, which she completed 1 week ago.

On physical examination, temperature is 38.6°C (101.5°F), blood pressure is 90/55 mm Hg, pulse rate is 122/min, and respiration rate is 24/min. The abdomen is distended and tender to palpation, and bowel sounds are absent.

Laboratory studies indicate a leukocyte count of 32,500/μL (32.5×10^9/L). Stool, blood, and urine samples are obtained for culture.

Which of the following is the most likely diagnosis?

(A) *Clostridium difficile* infection
(B) Crohn disease
(C) Diverticulitis
(D) Diverticulosis
(E) Ischemic colitis

Item 13 [Advanced]

A 30-year-old man is evaluated for a 3-day history of fever and diarrhea. He has not recently traveled and he is otherwise healthy.

On physical examination, he appears fatigued but not severely ill. Temperature is 38.7°C (101.7°F); other vital signs are normal. There is mild diffuse abdominal tenderness to deep palpation. A stool specimen is submitted for diagnostic testing and is found to be positive for *Salmonella* species.

Which of the following is the most appropriate next step in management?

(A) Administer loperamide
(B) Begin oral ciprofloxacin
(C) Begin oral metronidazole
(D) Reassure and set up follow-up phone call

Item 14 [Basic]

A 24-year-old man is evaluated for a 6-day history of malaise, fatigue, and jaundice following a camping trip in rural Mexico 3 weeks ago. His alcohol consumption is approximately 6 beers per week, never exceeding more than 2 beers per occasion. Two weeks ago he participated in a marathon race and finished the race without incident. His sister was recently diagnosed with primary biliary cirrhosis. The remainder of his history is unremarkable.

On examination, temperature is 37.8°C (100.0°F), blood pressure is 132/72 mm Hg, pulse rate is 104/min, and the respiration rate is 16/min. BMI is 21. Examination shows sclera icterus and hepatomegaly. The remainder of the examination findings are normal.

Bilirubin (total)	4.6 mg/dL (78.7 µmol/L)
Bilirubin (direct)	3.5 mg/dL (59.9 µmol/L)
Aspartate aminotransferase	1123 U/L
Alanine aminotransferase	1350 U/L
Alkaline phosphatase	185 U/L

Which of the following patterns of hepatic injury is present?

(A) Cholestatic injury
(B) Hepatocellular injury
(C) Mixed hepatocellular and cholestatic injury
(D) Nonhepatic injury pattern (muscle injury)

Item 15 [Advanced]

A 30-year-old woman is evaluated because of an abnormal serum total bilirubin level detected when she had a life insurance examination. Medical history is unremarkable. Her only medication is an oral contraceptive agent. Physical examination is normal.

Hemoglobin	13.9 g/dL (139 g/L)
Mean corpuscular volume	88 fL
Red cell distribution width	10.8%
Serum total bilirubin	2.4 mg/dL (41.0 µmol/L)
Serum direct bilirubin	0.2 mg/dL (3.4 µmol/L)
Serum aspartate aminotransferase	23 U/L
Serum alanine aminotransferase	22 U/L
Serum alkaline phosphatase	82 U/L

Which of the following is the most appropriate management at this time?

(A) Discontinue the oral contraceptive agent
(B) No further intervention required
(C) Obtain a reticulocyte count and haptoglobin level
(D) Repeat the liver chemistry tests in 3 months
(E) Schedule abdominal ultrasonography

Item 16 [Basic]

A 62-year-old man is evaluated in the hospital following an episode of acute cholecystitis 3 days ago. He had symptoms of right upper quadrant abdomin several times over the past few months, but they resolved spontaneously. At the time of hospital admission, ultrasonography showed an enlarged gallbladder with a thickened wall and evidence of stones in the gallbladder. He was treated with antibiotics and analgesics and his symptoms resolved. He currently feels well. He has no significant medical history.

On physical examination, temperature is normal, blood pressure is 112/64 mm Hg, pulse rate is 68/min, and respiration rate is 12/min. BMI is 28. He is not jaundiced. On abdominal examination, normal bowel sounds are present without tenderness. Murphy sign is absent.

Which of the following is the most appropriate next step in the management of this patient?

(A) Cholecystectomy
(B) Endoscopic retrograde cholangiopancreatography (ERCP) with sphincterotomy
(C) Low-fat diet and weight loss
(D) Ursodeoxycholic acid

Item 17 [Advanced]

A 42-year-old man is evaluated for a 1-month history of progressive jaundice, pruritus, and dark urine. The patient has a 15-year history of ulcerative colitis. He is treated with mesalamine and occasionally requires corticosteroid therapy. He takes no other medications.

On physical examination, vital signs are normal. There is jaundice and hepatomegaly but no splenomegaly, ascites, or abdominal tenderness. There is no asterixis.

Hemoglobin	14 g/dL (140 g/L)
Aspartate aminotransferase	150 U/L
Alanine aminotransferase	180 U/L
Bilirubin (total)	4.2 mg/dL (71.8 µmol/L)
Alkaline phosphatase	450 U/L

Which of the following is the most likely diagnosis?

(A) Gilbert syndrome
(B) Hepatitis A
(C) Hepatitis C
(D) Primary sclerosing cholangitis

Item 18 [Basic]

A 64-year-old woman is evaluated in the emergency department for a 3-week history of postprandial right upper quadrant abdominal pain that has become increasingly intense. The pain is now constant, radiates to her right shoulder, and is accompanied by fever, nausea, and vomiting.

On physical examination, temperature is 38.3°C (101.0°F), blood pressure is 110/65 mm Hg, pulse rate is 110/min, and respiration rate is 20/min. There is pain on palpation in the right upper quadrant of the abdomen with a Murphy sign. There is no rebound, tenderness, or jaundice.

Bilirubin (total) 2.0 mg/dL (34.2 µmol/L)
Aspartate aminotransferase 40 U/L
Alanine aminotransferase 120 U/L
Amylase 58 U/L
Lipase 36 U/L

Ultrasonography shows pericholecystic fluid with stones in the gallbladder. The wall of the gallbladder is thickened (6 mm), and there is no dilatation of the bile ducts.

Which of the following is the most likely diagnosis?

(A) Acute cholangitis
(B) Acute cholecystitis
(C) Acute pancreatitis
(D) Gallbladder dyskinesia

Item 19 [Advanced]

A 63-year-old man comes to the emergency department because of significant epigastric pain, nausea, and fever of 24 hours' duration. On physical examination, the patient is jaundiced. Temperature is 38.5°C (101.3°F), blood pressure is 100/68 mm Hg, and pulse rate is 100/min. Abdominal examination discloses significant right upper quadrant tenderness.

Leukocyte count 12,100/µL (12.1 × 10⁹/L)
Serum alkaline phosphatase 315 U/L
Serum aspartate aminotransferase 103 U/L
Serum alanine aminotransferase 117 U/L
Serum lipase 240 U/L
Serum total bilirubin 2.9 mg/dL (49.6 µmol/L)

Abdominal ultrasonography shows a dilated 11-mm common bile duct and a gallbladder containing multiple stones.

Which of the following is the most likely diagnosis accounting for all the patient's findings?

(A) Acute cholangitis
(B) Acute cholecystitis
(C) Acute pancreatitis
(D) Cholelithiasis

Item 20 [Advanced]

A 59-year-old woman is evaluated in the emergency department for a 9-hour history of epigastric pain, nausea, and vomiting. She had been previously healthy.

On physical examination, the patient appears ill. Temperature is 36.5°C (97.8°F), blood pressure is 148/84 mm Hg, pulse rate is 112/min, and respiration rate is 14/min. BMI is 30. Abdominal examination reveals diffuse tenderness.

Leukocyte count 28,200/µL (28.2 × 10⁹/L)
Total bilirubin 3.4 mg/dL (58.1 µmol/L)
Alkaline phosphatase 164 U/L
Alanine aminotransferase 224 U/L
Aspartate aminotransferase 142 U/L
Amylase 410 IU/L
Lipase 360 IU/L

Ultrasonography shows cholelithiasis and a dilated common bile duct.

Which of the following is the most appropriate next step in the management of this patient?

(A) Emergency laparoscopic cholecystectomy
(B) Endoscopic retrograde cholangiopancreatography (ERCP)
(C) Jejunal enteral feedings
(D) Magnetic resonance cholangiopancreatography (MRCP)

Item 21 [Basic]

A 55-year-old woman is evaluated in the hospital for a 2-day history of severe epigastric abdominal pain, nausea and vomiting, and anorexia. The patient has no significant medical history, takes no medications, and does not drink alcohol.

On physical examination, temperature is 38.0°C (100.4°F), blood pressure is 124/76 mm Hg, pulse rate is 99/min, and respiration rate is 16/min. There is scleral icterus and jaundice. There is mid-epigastric and right upper quadrant tenderness.

Aspartate aminotransferase 656 U/L
Alanine aminotransferase 567 U/L
Bilirubin (total) 5.6 mg/dL (95.8 µmol/L)
Amylase 1284 U/L
Lipase 6742 U/L
Triglycerides 250 mg/dL (2.8 mmol/L)

Abdominal ultrasonography shows a biliary tree with a dilated common bile duct of 12 mm and cholelithiasis but no choledocholithiasis.

Which of the following is the most likely diagnosis?

(A) Alcoholic pancreatitis
(B) Autoimmune pancreatitis
(C) Gallstone pancreatitis
(D) Hypertriglyceridemic pancreatitis

Item 22 [Advanced]

A 34-year-old woman is evaluated for continued severe mid-epigastric pain that radiates to the back, nausea, and vomiting 5 days after being hospitalized for alcohol-related pancreatitis. She has not been able eat or drink since being admitted.

On physical examination, temperature is 38.2°C (100.8°F), blood pressure is 132/84 mm Hg, pulse rate is 101/min, and respiration rate is 20/min. There is no scleral icterus or jaundice. The abdomen is distended and diffusely tender with hypoactive bowel sounds but no peritoneal signs.

Aspartate aminotransferase 189 U/L
Alanine aminotransferase 151 U/L
Bilirubin (total) 1.1 mg/dL (18.8 µmol/L)
Amylase 388 U/L
Lipase 924 U/L

CT scan of the abdomen shows a diffusely edematous pancreas with multiple peripancreatic fluid collections and no evidence of pancreatic necrosis.

Which of the following is the most appropriate next step in the management of this patient?

(A) Begin prednisone
(B) Enteral nutrition with nasojejunal feeding tube
(C) Intravenous imipenem
(D) Pancreatic débridement

Item 23 [Basic]

A 68-year-old man is evaluated for a 15-year history of acid reflux symptoms and a 6-month history of worsening midsternal burning chest discomfort. The pain is nonexertional and exacerbated by lying down or bending over. He also notes occasional difficulty swallowing solids described as a sensation of food "sticking" at about the level of the lower sternum. The pain is partially alleviated by over-the-counter antacids, but they have no effect on the dysphagia. He does not smoke or drink, he has no other medical problems, and he takes no prescription medications.

On physical examination, vital signs are normal. BMI is 27. Cardiopulmonary and abdominal examinations are unremarkable.

Which of the following is the most appropriate initial diagnostic test for this patient?

(A) Ambulatory esophageal pH monitoring
(B) Empiric treatment with omeprazole
(C) *Helicobacter pylori* testing
(D) Upper endoscopy

Item 24 [Advanced]

A 30-year-old woman is evaluated in the emergency department for abdominal pain and hematemesis. She undergoes upper endoscopy, which demonstrates a 1-cm duodenal ulcer with a clean base. *Helicobacter pylori* is seen on biopsy, and the patient is discharged home with appropriate therapy for *H. pylori*. She is adherent to her therapy and her symptoms rapidly resolve.

The patient returns to the office 3 months later with 3 weeks of midepigastric abdominal discomfort; regurgitation; and burning chest discomfort that worsens with bending over, lying down, or after eating large meals. Repeat endoscopy demonstrates complete healing of her duodenal ulcer; erosive esophagitis is present.

Which of the following is the most appropriate treatment for this patient?

(A) Metoclopramide
(B) Omeprazole
(C) Ranitidine
(D) Sucralfate

Item 25 [Advanced]

A 61-year-old man is evaluated for a 3-week history of abdominal discomfort and early satiety. During this time, he has experienced a 1.4-kg (3-lb) weight loss. For the past 10 days he has treated these symptoms with an over-the-counter proton pump inhibitor with partial relief of symptoms. He takes no other medications.

On physical examination, temperature is 37°C (98.6°F), blood pressure is 132/76 mm Hg, pulse rate is 68/min, and respiration rate is 12/min. His abdominal examination reveals a rounded, soft abdomen with active bowel sounds. No masses are palpable. Deep epigastric palpation results in mild tenderness.

Upper endoscopy reveals a 9-mm ulcer in the gastric antrum proximal to the pylorus.

Which of the following is the most appropriate management for this patient's ulcer?

(A) Biopsy
(B) Omeprazole, amoxicillin, and clarithromycin
(C) Rapid urease test
(D) Urea breath test

Item 26 [Basic]

A 65-year-old woman is evaluated 1 week after undergoing an esophagogastroduodenoscopy for persistent abdominal pain. The procedure showed a 1-cm, clean-based ulcer in the duodenal bulb and scattered antral erosions. Biopsy specimens from the stomach showed nonspecific gastritis but no evidence of *Helicobacter pylori* infection. Serum antibody testing for *H. pylori* was also negative. Proton pump inhibitor therapy was started, and the patient's symptoms were alleviated. The patient has a history of mild osteoarthritis and osteoporosis. Medications are over-the-counter ibuprofen for arthritis and a calcium supplement, vitamin D, and alendronate.

On physical examination, vital signs are normal. The abdominal examination reveals no tenderness, hepatomegaly, or palpable masses. Complete blood count is normal.

Which of the following is the most appropriate next step in the management of this patient?

(A) Measure serum gastrin
(B) Perform fecal antigen test for *Helicobacter pylori*
(C) Repeat endoscopy and ulcer biopsy
(D) Stop the alendronate
(E) Stop the ibuprofen

Item 27 [Basic]

A 46-year-old man is evaluated for a 5-month history of intermittent midabdominal discomfort that occurs after eating. Each episode lasts between 30 minutes and 1 hour. The discomfort is described as fullness; he reports no symptoms characteristic of esophageal reflux or biliary colic. He has no vomiting, dysphagia, or changes in bowel habits. He has gained approximately 4.5 kg (10 lb) during the past 5 months. Medical history includes low back pain for which he takes ibuprofen. He has no family history of malignancy.

On physical examination, vital signs are normal. BMI is 28. The remainder of the physical examination is normal.

A metabolic panel and complete blood count are normal.

What is the most appropriate next management step for this patient?

(A) Start metoclopramide
(B) Stop ibuprofen
(C) Obtain an upper endoscopy
(D) Test for *Helicobacter pylori* infection

Item 28 [Basic]

A 58-year-old woman is evaluated for a 3-month history of burning midepigastric pain after eating and early satiety. The pain feels the same as a gastric ulcer she had 10 years ago. She reports no associated sour taste, belching, bloating, or worsening symptoms with recumbency or at night. She has no nausea, vomiting, painful swallowing, changes in bowel habits, or weight loss. She is otherwise in good health and has no symptoms of anxiety or depression.

On physical examination, vital signs are normal. Mild midepigastric tenderness is present, but her physical examination is otherwise normal.

A thyroid-stimulating hormone level, complete blood count, and metabolic panel are normal. An upper endoscopy is performed and it is normal. Testing for *H. pylori* is negative.

Which of the following is the most appropriate management for this patient?

(A) Ambulatory esophageal pH monitoring
(B) Psychiatric evaluation
(C) Surgical evaluation
(D) Trial of a proton pump inhibitor (PPI)

Item 29 [Advanced]

A 57-year-old woman is evaluated for recurrent gastrointestinal bleeding. She has a history of heartburn without dysphagia but no other medical problems. She has no obvious source of bleeding. She reports no menstrual blood loss, hematochezia, hematemesis, easy bruising, or bleeding. She takes no medications other than therapeutic doses of ferrous sulfate with which she is adherent. Three months ago, an upper endoscopy was normal except for a hiatal hernia. A colonoscopy was normal.

Her stool continues to test positive for fecal occult blood. Hemoglobin is 10.2 g/dL (102 g/L). Serum iron studies are compatible with iron deficiency.

Which of the following is the most appropriate next step in the management of this patient?

(A) Barium swallow
(B) Double balloon enteroscopy
(C) Repeat colonoscopy
(D) Repeat upper endoscopy

Item 30 [Advanced]

A 78-year-old man hospitalized 3 days ago for heart failure is evaluated for 1 day of cramping left lower abdominal pain and the explosive passage of two bloody stools. His medical history is remarkable for hypertension and type 2 diabetes. Medications are lisinopril, metoprolol, furosemide, digoxin, insulin glargine, and premeal insulin lispro.

On physical examination, the patient is slightly uncomfortable. Temperature is 37.2°C (99.0°F), blood pressure is 130/68 mm Hg, pulse rate is 60/min, and respiration rate is 12/min. Bowel sounds are present. An S_3 is present and lung auscultation reveals clear lungs fields. The abdomen is tender in the left lower quadrant without rebound or guarding. No masses or tenderness is found on rectal examination.

Hemoglobin is 11.1 g/dL (111 g/L). *Clostridium difficile* toxin assay is negative.

Colonoscopy shows petechial hemorrhages interspersed with areas of pale, edematous mucosa in the sigmoid region.

Which of the following is the most likely diagnosis?

(A) Acute mesenteric ischemia
(B) Diverticulitis
(C) Diverticulosis
(D) Ischemic colitis

Item 31 [Basic]

A 68-year-old man is evaluated in the emergency department for a 6-hour history of nausea and vomiting with some bright-red emesis. For the past 2 hours he has felt lightheaded and weak.

On physical examination, temperature is 37.0°C (98.6°F), blood pressure is 88/51 mm Hg, pulse rate is 114/min, and respiration rate is 18/min. Nasogastric aspiration shows a mixture of coffee grounds and dark blood. The abdomen is not tender, and bowel sounds are normal. Laboratory studies reveal a hemoglobin level of 9.4 g/dL (94 g/L); all other tests are normal. Intravenous omeprazole therapy is begun, and the patient is stabilized with infusion of normal saline and transfusion of two units of packed erythrocytes.

Which of the following is the best management option for this patient?

(A) Esophagogastroduodenoscopy
(B) Immediate surgical intervention
(C) Observation
(D) Octreotide infusion
(E) Ranitidine infusion

Item 32 [Basic]

A 60-year-old man hospitalized for advanced cirrhosis complicated by ascites and encephalopathy is evaluated for massive hematemesis and hypotension. The patient's medications are spironolactone, propranolol, furosemide, and lactulose.

On physical examination, temperature is 35.6°C (96.1°F), blood pressure is 80/50 mm Hg, pulse rate is 146/min, and respiration rate is 20/min. The patient has just vomited red blood. Laboratory studies show a hemoglobin level of 9 g/dL

(90 g/L), a platelet count of 60,000/µL (60×10^9/L), and an INR of 3.

Which of the following is the most appropriate initial management of this patient?

(A) Arteriography
(B) Esophagogastroduodenoscopy
(C) Intravenous nadolol
(D) Rapid volume replacement

Item 33 [Basic]

A 76-year-old man is evaluated in the emergency department after having suddenly passed a large amount of red and maroon blood per rectum. He has not had abdominal pain, nausea, vomiting, fever, or weight loss. He had a colonoscopy 1 year ago that showed a benign polyp and diverticulosis. He is otherwise healthy and takes no medications.

On physical examination, the patient is pale; blood pressure is 105/65 mm Hg and pulse rate is 100/min. Abdominal examination is normal; there is dried blood in the perianal area, and rectal examination reveals fresh blood on the examination glove.

Laboratory studies reveal a hemoglobin level of 10.1 g/dL (101 g/L) and normal biochemical studies, including blood urea nitrogen. Leukocyte count is 5600/µL (5.6×10^9/L) and platelet count is 348,000/µL (348×10^9/L); prothrombin time and activated partial thromboplastin time are normal.

Intravenous access is obtained and volume resuscitation with normal saline is begun. A nasogastric tube aspirate is positive for bile but negative for blood.

Which of the following is the most likely cause of the gastrointestinal bleeding?

(A) Colon cancer
(B) Colonic ischemia
(C) Diverticulosis or vascular ectasia
(D) Inflammatory bowel disease

Item 34 [Basic]

A 51-year-old woman has a 3-month history of intermittent rectal bleeding and pain on defecation. Bloody streaks cover the stool, and the toilet paper is also bloody. She is otherwise well and takes no medications.

One month before the bleeding developed, she underwent an elective orthopedic surgical procedure and required narcotic drugs for several weeks postoperatively. The narcotics caused significant constipation. The patient had her first screening colonoscopy less than 1 year ago, and results were normal. At that time, a retroflexed view of the rectum revealed small internal hemorrhoids.

Visual inspection of the anal opening reveals small external hemorrhoids and several anal skin tags. Hemoglobin is 13.9 g/dL (139 g/L).

Which of the following is most likely causing this patient's rectal bleeding and pain?

(A) Anal fissure
(B) Colon cancer
(C) Colonic diverticula
(D) Rectal cancer

Item 35 [Advanced]

A 45-year-old woman is evaluated during a routine office visit. She was diagnosed with chronic active hepatitis B infection 10 years ago. She has no symptoms and no other medical problems. A liver biopsy performed 3 years ago revealed changes consistent with chronic active inflammation with no cirrhosis. She is taking interferon alfa.

On physical examination, vital signs are normal. No evidence of telangiectasias or other stigmata of chronic liver disease is present. The abdomen is unremarkable without evidence of hepatomegaly, liver tenderness, or ascites. The remainder of the examination findings are normal.

Serum aspartate aminotransferase is 200 U/L and alanine aminotransferase is 100 U/L. (unchanged from 6 months ago). Prothrombin time and activated partial thromboplastin time are normal. Hepatitis C antibody is negative.

Which of the following is the most appropriate screening strategy for hepatocellular carcinoma in this patient?

(A) α-Fetoprotein
(B) Abdominal ultrasonography
(C) CT of the liver with contrast
(D) Screening is not indicated

Item 36 [Basic]

A 22-year-old college student has recently returned from a 3-month anthropology course in Thailand where she lived with a local village family. She has a 2-week history of fatigue and nausea with occasional vomiting and a 2-day history of jaundice. She was previously well, takes no medications, and has no history of liver disease, injection drug use, blood transfusions, sexual exposures, or known exposure to anyone with hepatitis. She took malarial prophylaxis and her hepatitis B vaccination status is current. She does not recall vaccination for hepatitis A.

Physical examination is significant only for jaundice and a slightly enlarged, nontender liver. There are no spider angiomata or signs of encephalopathy.

Aspartate aminotransferase	1586 U/L
Alanine aminotransferase	1897 U/L
Total bilirubin	6.2 mg/dL (106.0 µmol/L)

Which of the following is the most likely diagnosis?

(A) Hepatitis A
(B) Hepatitis B
(C) Hepatitis C
(D) Hepatitis D

Item 37 [Basic]

A 55-year-old man is hospitalized for a 2-week history of jaundice and altered mental status. The patient has a 10-year history of alcohol dependence. His family reports that he had been drinking heavily every day until about 3 weeks ago.

On physical examination, the patient is confused and lethargic; temperature is 38.0°C (100.4°F), blood pressure is 90/60 mm Hg, pulse rate is 120/min, and respiration rate is 30/min. Examination reveals scleral icterus. There is no guarding on palpation of the abdomen. The liver edge is tender and palpable. There is no ascites, edema, or evidence of bleeding.

INR	4.0
Bilirubin (total)	37.0 mg/dL (632.7 µmol/L)
Aspartate aminotransferase	175 U/L
Alanine aminotransferase	73 U/L
Hepatitis B surface antigen	Negative
Hepatitis B surface antigen antibody	Positive
Hepatitis C antibody	Negative
Hepatitis A antibody (IgM)	Negative
Hepatitis A antibody (IgG)	Positive
Antinuclear antibody titer	Negative

Ultrasonography shows an enlarged, fatty liver with no nodules, ascites, pericholecystic fluid, or bile duct dilatation.

Which of the following is the most likely diagnosis?

(A) Alcoholic hepatitis
(B) Autoimmune hepatitis
(C) Hepatitis A
(D) Hepatitis B
(E) Hepatitis C

Item 38 [Basic]

A 38-year-old woman is evaluated for abnormal liver chemistry tests detected in an evaluation for new-onset fatigue, joint pains, and jaundice. She has a history of autoimmune hypothyroidism, and her only medications are levothyroxine and a multivitamin. She has never used illicit drugs and does not drink alcohol. Her mother has systemic lupus erythematosus.

On physical examination, the patient is afebrile. Blood pressure is 130/75 mm Hg, pulse rate is 80/min, and respiration rate is 14/min. There is scleral icterus; the rest of the examination is normal.

Bilirubin (total)	6.0 mg/dL (102.6 µmol/L)
Bilirubin (direct)	3.6 mg/dL (61.6 µmol/L)
Aspartate aminotransferase	890 U/L
Alanine aminotransferase	765 U/L
Alkaline phosphatase	100 U/L
Antinuclear antibody	Titer 1:40
Anti–smooth muscle antibody	Titer 1:640
Antimitochondrial antibody	Negative

Viral serologic tests are negative.

Which of the following is the most likely diagnosis?

(A) Acute cholecystitis
(B) Autoimmune hepatitis
(C) Drug-induced liver injury
(D) Primary biliary cirrhosis

Item 39 [Basic]

A 32-year-old man is evaluated for a 2-week history of nausea, malaise, low-grade fever, vomiting, and jaundice. Other than having multiple sex partners, he has no other significant medical history and takes only ibuprofen for headache and fever.

On physical examination, temperature is 37.6°C (99.7°F), blood pressure is 110/75 mm Hg, pulse rate is 90/min, and respiration rate is 22/min. Examination reveals scleral icterus, jaundice, hepatomegaly, asterixis, and somnolence. There are no stigmata of chronic liver disease.

Bilirubin (total)	17.5 mg/dL (299.2 µmol/L)
Aspartate aminotransferase	8790 U/L
Alanine aminotransferase	7650 U/L
INR	2.3
Hepatitis B surface antigen	Positive
Hepatitis B core antigen (IgM)	Positive
Hepatitis C virus RNA	Negative
Hepatitis A IgM antibody	Negative
Hepatitis A IgG antibody	Positive

Ultrasonography shows hepatomegaly and increased echogenicity, a normal spleen, and perihepatic ascites. There is no ductal dilatation.

Which of the following is the most likely diagnosis?

(A) Acute hepatitis A
(B) Acute hepatitis B
(C) Chronic hepatitis B
(D) Hepatitis C

Item 40 [Basic]

A 55-year-old woman recently had elevated liver chemistry tests detected on examination for life insurance. She has no symptoms of liver disease and no history of jaundice, ascites, lower extremity edema, or encephalopathy. While in college she received 3 units of blood following a major motor vehicle accident that resulted in a ruptured spleen. She has no other significant medical history and takes no medications. She has had only one sex partner in her lifetime.

On physical examination, vital signs are normal. There are spider angiomata on the upper body, and a nodular liver edge is noted.

Bilirubin (total)	1.1 mg/dL (18.8 µmol/L)
Aspartate aminotransferase	48 U/L
Alanine aminotransferase	96 U/L
Hepatitis C antibody	Positive
Hepatitis B surface antigen	Negative
Hepatitis A antibody (IgM)	Negative
Hepatitis A antibody (IgG)	Positive

Abdominal CT scan shows changes in the liver consistent with cirrhosis.

Which of the following is the most likely diagnosis?

(A) Hepatitis A
(B) Hepatitis B
(C) Hepatitis C
(D) Hepatitis D

Item 41 [Advanced]

A 60-year-old woman is evaluated for a 2-week history of jaundice, weight gain, and increased abdominal girth. She has no fever or abdominal pain. Her medical history is significant for type 2 diabetes, hyperlipidemia, and obesity. She drinks 2 twelve-ounce bottles of beer per week and has never exceeded this amount. She was an intravenous drug abuser for 10 years beginning at the age of 20 years but has not used any illicit drugs since then. Her medications are metformin, glyburide, pravastatin, and aspirin.

On physical examination, vital signs are normal. BMI is 32. She is jaundiced. Spider angiomata are present over the upper chest. Her abdomen is protuberant and nontender with shifting dullness. The liver and spleen are not palpable. The ankles show pitting edema.

Serum aspartate aminotransferase	165 U/L
Serum alanine aminotransferase	160 U/L
Serum alkaline phosphatase	123 U/L
Total bilirubin	5.6 mg/dL (95.8 µmol/L)
Anti-hepatitis C antibody	Negative
Hepatitis B surface antigen	Negative
Antibody to hepatitis B surface antigen	Positive

Which of the following is the most likely cause of the patient's liver disease?

(A) Alcohol
(B) Chronic hepatitis B infection
(C) Chronic hepatitis C infection
(D) Nonalcoholic steatohepatitis
(E) Primary biliary cirrhosis

Item 42 [Advanced]

A 40-year-man is evaluated for fatigue, yellow eyes, and increasingly severe pruritus over the past 8 weeks. He reports no fever, abdominal pain, recent travel, or risk factors for hepatitis. He was diagnosed with ulcerative colitis at age 32 years, and the disease has been well controlled with sulfasalazine. He does not drink alcohol, and he takes no other medications.

On examination, vital signs are normal. Scleral icterus is present. Spider angiomata are present over the upper chest, and gynecomastia is present. The abdomen is nontender, and the liver and spleen are not palpable. No ascites are present.

Serum aspartate aminotransferase	125 U/L
Serum alanine aminotransferase	130 U/L
Serum alkaline phosphatase	550 U/L
Total bilirubin	3.6 mg/dL (61.6 µmol/L)
Hepatitis A IgG antibody	Positive
Hepatitis A IgM antibody	Negative
Antimitochondrial antibody	Negative

Which of the following is the most likely cause of the patient's liver disease?

(A) Autoimmune hepatitis
(B) Hepatitis A
(C) Primary biliary cirrhosis
(D) Primary sclerosing cholangitis

Item 43 [Basic]

A 43-year-old woman has a 3-month history of gradually increasing abdominal distention and jaundice. She has no other symptoms, and her medical history is noncontributory.

On physical examination, the patient has jaundice, palmar erythema, and spider angiomata. Abdominal examination discloses hepatosplenomegaly and moderate ascites.

Aspartate aminotransferase	53 U/L
Alanine aminotransferase	47 U/L
Alkaline phosphatase	123 U/L
Total bilirubin	3.2 mg/dL (54.7 µmol/L)
Albumin	2.9 g/dL (29 g/L)

Abdominal ultrasonography shows hepatomegaly, a coarse echotexture of the liver, patent portal and hepatic veins, mild splenomegaly, moderate ascites, and no bile duct dilatation. Paracentesis is performed. The ascitic fluid leukocyte count is 80/µL, and albumin is 0.7 g/dL (7 g/L). Gram stain and culture are pending.

Which of the following is the most likely cause of the ascites?

(A) Cirrhosis
(B) Nephrotic syndrome
(C) Ovarian cancer
(D) Tuberculosis

Item 44 [Advanced]

A 45-year-old man is evaluated in the emergency department for lethargy and disorientation. The patient has a history of alcoholic cirrhosis complicated by esophageal variceal bleeding, ascites, and edema. His medications are furosemide, spironolactone, propranolol, and lactulose. He has been sober for 1 year.

On physical examination, the patient is somnolent but arousable. He is afebrile; blood pressure is 100/78 mm Hg, pulse rate is 65/min, and respiration rate is 12/min. There are no focal neurologic deficits; the pupils are equal and reactive to light. There is shifting abdominal dullness and 2+ lower extremity edema. The stool is negative for occult blood.

Leukocyte count	5600/μL (5.6×10^9/L)
Glucose (random)	112 mg/dL (6.2 mmol/L)
Creatinine	1.8 mg/dL (159.1 μmol/L)
Sodium	135 meq/L (135 mmol/L)
Potassium	3.5 meq/L (3.5 mmol/L)
Chloride	100 meq/L (100 mmol/L)
Bicarbonate	28 meq/L (28 mmol/L)
Bilirubin (total)	4.0 mg/dL (68.4 μmol/L)
Aspartate aminotransferase	78 U/L
Alanine aminotransferase	45 U/L
Albumin	2.7 g/dL (27 g/L)
Ammonia	230 μg/dL (135 μmol/L)

Urinalysis is positive for leukocytes. Urine dipstick is positive for 3+ leukocyte esterase and nitrites. CT scan of the head is normal. A diagnostic peritoneal fluid tap excludes spontaneous bacterial peritonitis. Diuretics are discontinued and empiric antibiotic therapy is started.

Which of the following is the most appropriate management for this patient?

(A) Corticosteroids
(B) Hemodialysis
(C) Increase lactulose therapy
(D) Transjugular intrahepatic portosystemic shunt

Item 45 [Advanced]

A 45-year-old man with alcoholic cirrhosis is admitted to the hospital for worsening ascites and abdominal pain. His medications are propranolol, lactulose, spironolactone, and furosemide.

On physical examination, temperature is 37.2°C (99.0°F), blood pressure is 110/60 mm Hg, pulse rate is 56/min, and respiration rate is 16/min. Tense ascites is present, and the abdomen is tender to palpation. The remainder of the examination is noncontributory.

Admission serum creatinine is 0.8 mg/dL (70.7 μmol/L). A diagnostic paracentesis reveals 350 leukocytes/μL. Cefotaxime and albumin infusions are begun.

On hospital day 3 the patient is oliguric. Laboratory studies reveal a blood urea nitrogen level of 15 mg/dL (5.4 mmol/L) and a serum creatinine level of 2.0 mg/dL (176.8 μmol/L). Urinalysis reveals a spot urine sodium of 10 meq/L (10 mmol/L). Furosemide and spironolactone are discontinued and infusions of normal saline and albumin are initiated, but he remains oliguric.

Kidney ultrasound shows normal kidney size, and there is no hydronephrosis.

Which of the following is the most likely cause of his acute kidney injury?

(A) Hepatorenal syndrome
(B) Obstructive nephropathy
(C) Prerenal azotemia
(D) Renal artery stenosis

Item 46 [Basic]

A 24-year-old woman with a 1-year history of Crohn disease is evaluated for tender bumps on her shins. She has been experiencing more abdominal pain and increased bowel movements for the past 3 months. Starting 2 weeks ago, she developed low-grade fever, increased fatigue, and arthralgia. Her only medication is sulfasalazine.

On physical examination, vital signs are normal. On abdominal examination, bowel sounds are present and palpation produces slight tenderness in the right lower quadrant. A typical skin lesion found on the lower extremity is shown (Plate 1).

Which of the following is the most likely diagnosis for the skin finding?

(A) Dermatitis herpetiformis
(B) Erythema nodosum
(C) Pyoderma gangrenosum
(D) Rheumatoid nodule

Item 47 [Basic]

A 55-year-old man is evaluated for a 4-month history of frequent and urgent defecation with loose and bloody stool, mild abdominal cramping, and fatigue. He has up to eight bowel movements a day and often wakes at night with symptoms. He does not have fever, nausea, or vomiting, but he has lost 3 kg (7 lb). He has mild joint pain in his knees and ankles that also began 4 months ago, is worse in the morning, and resolves somewhat during the day. The patient is a former cigarette smoker but quit smoking 2 years ago. He has no other medical problems.

On physical examination, vital signs are normal. There is mild lower abdominal tenderness without rebound or guarding; there are no palpable abdominal masses. Examination of the rectum shows gross blood.

Laboratory studies reveal a hemoglobin level of 12.3 g/dL (123 g/L) with a mean corpuscular volume of 76 fL. Fecal leukocytes are present, but stool culture is negative. Colonoscopy shows continuous erythema, friability, and loss of vascular pattern from the rectum to the splenic flexure; the rest of the colon and terminal ileum is normal. Histology shows cryptitis, crypt abscesses, and crypt architecture distortion.

Which of the following is the most likely diagnosis?

(A) Crohn colitis
(B) Infectious colitis
(C) Ischemic colitis
(D) Microscopic colitis
(E) Ulcerative colitis

Item 48 [Advanced]

A 52-year-old man is evaluated for a 5-month history of three to four loose, bloody stools a day with mild urgency, abdominal cramping, and fatigue. He has not lost weight during this episode. He is otherwise healthy.

On physical examination, vital signs are normal. There is mild lower abdominal tenderness without rebound or guarding; there are no palpable abdominal masses. Examination of the rectum shows gross blood. Colonoscopy shows continuous mild erythema and loss of vascular pattern from the rectum to the transverse sigmoid colon; the rest of the colon and terminal ileum are normal. Biopsy specimens from the abnormal mucosa show cryptitis, crypt abscesses, and distortion of crypt architecture.

Which of the following is the most appropriate therapy for this patient?

(A) Azathioprine
(B) Ciprofloxacin
(C) Infliximab
(D) Mesalamine
(E) Metronidazole

Item 49 [Advanced]

A 65-year-old woman is evaluated for a 6-month history of watery, nonbloody diarrhea; she has from 3 to 20 bowel movements a day. She also has abdominal cramps and bloating and has lost 2.2 kg (5 lb) since the beginning of the episode. She had been previously healthy. She has not traveled recently, been hospitalized, or used antibiotics.

On physical examination, the vital signs are normal. The heart rate is regular and the chest is clear. The abdomen is soft with slight distention.

Colonoscopy is grossly normal. Multiple biopsy specimens are obtained.

Which of the following is the most likely diagnosis?

(A) *Clostridium difficile* colitis
(B) Crohn disease
(C) Microscopic colitis
(D) Tropical sprue
(E) Ulcerative colitis

Gastroenterology and Hepatology
Answers and Critiques

Item 1　　**Answer: D**

Educational Objective: *Diagnose nephrolithiasis with helical CT scan.*

A noncontrast helical abdominal CT scan should be the next diagnostic test. Acute renal colic is characterized by the sudden onset of unilateral flank pain. Acute renal colic also may cause nausea and vomiting, and patients with stones located in the ureters or urethra may have irritative symptoms such as urinary urgency and frequency. Nearly 90% of patients with nephrolithiasis have either gross or microscopic hematuria. Noncontrast helical abdominal CT has replaced intravenous pyelography as the gold standard for diagnosing kidney stones. This test reveals urinary tract obstruction with hydronephrosis, detects stones as small as 1 mm in diameter, and helps evaluate other potential causes of abdominal pain and hematuria. However, noncontrast helical abdominal CT is expensive and has a higher radiation exposure than other imaging studies.

Most kidney stones are radiopaque and are easily visualized on plain radiographs of the abdomen, which are inexpensive, noninvasive, and widely available. However, false-negative results may occur in patients with small stones or radiolucent stones composed of uric acid or related to use of indinavir, and with interference of the overlying bowel. Similarly, vascular calcification and phleboliths may cause false-positive results for kidney stones. As such, plain abdominal radiography has a low sensitivity and specificity for the diagnosis of this condition.

Intravenous pyelography has a high sensitivity and specificity in the diagnosis of kidney stones. However, this study requires bowel preparation and the use of intravenous iodinated contrast agents, which are contraindicated in patients with acute kidney injury and chronic kidney disease.

Kidney ultrasonography has a low sensitivity for kidney stones but a higher specificity than plain abdominal radiography. This study is relatively inexpensive, widely available, and provides a functional assessment of the severity of the stone disease. Kidney ultrasonography also can detect urinary tract obstruction with associated hydronephrosis but may not reveal small stones or stones in the ureters and urethra.

KEY POINT

Noncontrast helical abdominal CT scan is the imaging modality of choice for the diagnosis of nephrolithiasis.

Bibliography

Goldfarb DS. In the clinic. Nephrolithiasis. Ann Intern Med. 2009;151(3):ITC2. [PMID: 19652185]

Item 2　　**Answer: D**

Educational Objective: *Evaluate acute abdominal pain with supine and upright abdominal radiographs.*

The most appropriate next diagnostic tests are supine and upright abdominal radiographs. The term *acute abdomen* refers to sudden and severe abdominal pain less than 24 hours in duration. Rebound tenderness and severe diffuse abdominal pain are suggestive of an acute abdomen with peritonitis. Pain that is acute in onset generally points to acute inflammatory, infectious, or ischemic causes. Upper abdominal pain is usually of gastric, hepatobiliary, or pancreatic origin, whereas pain in the lower abdomen originates from the hindgut and genitourinary organs. All patients with abdominal pain should have measurements of serum amylase and lipase to evaluate for acute pancreatitis.

Chest radiograph and supine and upright abdominal radiographs should be obtained in every patient with significant acute abdominal pain to exclude bowel obstruction or perforation or intrathoracic processes (for example, pneumonia, pneumothorax, or aortic dissection) that can present as abdominal pain. This patient's history of diverticulitis suggests possible diverticular rupture.

Colonoscopy is not indicated in a patient with acute peritoneal signs and has the potential to worsen the situation by causing a perforation of inflamed bowel wall.

Although an abdominal CT scan is usually necessary for a definitive diagnosis of acute abdominal pain, initial screening with supine and upright abdominal radiographs should be done first to look for air-fluid levels, suggestive of a bowel obstruction, and free peritoneal air, suggestive of a perforated viscus.

Based on its relatively low cost, convenience, and noninvasive nature, ultrasonography has been utilized as a diagnostic tool for acute diverticulitis. However, the examination remains operator-dependent and, in the absence of well-designed prospective comparative studies, it remains a second-line diagnostic tool.

KEY POINT

In patients with acute abdominal pain, initial screening should include supine and upright abdominal radiographs to look for air-fluid levels, suggestive of a bowel obstruction, and free peritoneal air, suggestive of a perforated viscus.

Bibliography

Cartwright SL, Knudson MP. Evaluation of acute abdominal pain in adults. Am Fam Physician. 2008;77(7):971-978. [PMID: 18441863]

Item 3   Answer: D

Educational Objective: *Diagnose ruptured abdominal aortic aneurysm.*

The patient's clinical presentation—severe abdominal or back pain with syncope followed by abdominal discomfort—is typical for a ruptured abdominal aortic aneurysm (AAA) that has been locally contained, preventing his immediate death. The sentinel event of severe sudden abdominal and back pain associated with loss of consciousness marks the occurrence of rupture. Leukocytosis and anemia are common. A CT scan should be performed for diagnosis, and the aneurysm should be repaired emergently.

Contained rupture of AAA, when misdiagnosed, is most often mistaken for renal colic, acute myocardial infarction, or diverticulitis. Renal colic may produce severe pain in the lower back, flank, or groin. Typically, the pain waxes and wanes. It is unlikely that renal colic would present with syncope, and the normal urinalysis also makes this diagnosis unlikely.

Acute myocardial infarction can be associated with syncope, and the electrocardiogram is not always diagnostic, particularly if there are findings such as left ventricular hypertrophy, which may obscure subtle abnormalities. However, the presence of abdominal and lower back pain rather than chest pain makes this diagnosis less likely.

Diverticulitis would present with fever and crampy abdominal pain, most commonly in the left lower quadrant and often associated with a change in bowel habits. Leukocytosis may be present. Syncope associated with the onset of pain would be a very unusual presentation for this entity.

KEY POINT

Abdominal pain, back pain, and syncope often herald an abdominal aortic aneurysm rupture.

Bibliography

Lederle FA. In the clinic. Abdominal aortic aneurysm. Ann Intern Med. 2009;150(9):ITC5-1-15; quiz ITC5-16. [PMID: 19414835]

Item 4   Answer: D

Educational Objective: *Diagnose and treat constipation-predominant irritable bowel syndrome.*

The most appropriate next step in the management of this patient is reassurance and polyethylene glycol. This patient has irritable bowel syndrome. As a young woman, she fits the demographic profile, and she meets the Rome III criteria, with abdominal pain relieved by defecation and a change in bowel habits. The most recent diagnostic criteria require the presence of at least two of three symptoms occurring for 3 months (not necessarily consecutive) during a 12-month period. These symptoms include pain relieved with defecation, onset associated with change in stool frequency, or onset associated with change in the consistency of the stool. In clinical practice, these criteria have a positive predictive value of 98%. Importantly, she has no alarm indicators, including older age, male sex, nocturnal awakening, rectal bleeding, weight loss, or family history of colon cancer. In the absence of alarm symptoms, additional tests have a diagnostic yield of 2% or less. Furthermore, laboratory studies indicate no anemia or thyroid deficiency. Irritable bowel syndrome is a clinical diag-

nosis, and there are no laboratory, radiographic, or endoscopic findings that aid in diagnosis. Additional evaluation is not only unnecessary and expensive but also potentially harmful, especially when invasive procedures are ordered. The patient should be reassured that although this problem is annoying and inconvenient, it is not life-threatening. Because fiber supplementation has not been helpful, a nonabsorbed osmotic laxative such as polyethylene glycol will likely provide her significant relief.

There is no indication for the patient to undergo a CT scan or colonoscopy. Oral contraceptives are not typically associated with the syndrome, and she began taking the medication after the onset of her symptoms.

KEY POINT

Irritable bowel syndrome is a clinical diagnosis that can be made confidently when patients meet the Rome III criteria and do not have alarm indicators.

Bibliography

Wilson JF. In the clinic. Irritable bowel syndrome. Ann Intern Med. 2007;147(1):ITC7-1-ITC7-16. [PMID: 17606954]

Item 5   Answer: C

Educational Objective: *Diagnose ischemic colitis.*

This patient likely has ischemic colitis, the most frequent form of ischemia of the gastrointestinal tract. This type of ischemia usually affects the elderly with atherosclerotic disease, and in most cases is transient and resolves with conservative management. Patients with acute colonic ischemia usually present with rapid onset of abdominal pain and tenderness over the affected bowel. Rectal bleeding or bloody diarrhea usually develops within 24 hours of the onset of abdominal pain. The typical finding on CT scan is thickening of the bowel wall in a segmental pattern, which is not specific for ischemia and can be seen in infectious colitis and Crohn disease. The finding of patchy segmental ulcerations on colonoscopy in a patient with a compatible history establishes the diagnosis. Colonic strictures are a rare complication.

The patient's acute onset of symptoms with bloody diarrhea is not consistent with Crohn disease. Patients with Crohn disease commonly present with a chronic history of abdominal pain, diarrhea, and weight loss. Peptic ulcer disease could present with bright red rectal bleeding but only in the setting of a large and rapid bleed and could not explain the findings on the CT scan. Irritable bowel syndrome is a diagnosis of exclusion and does not present with rectal bleeding and the changes noted on the CT scan.

KEY POINT

Ischemic colitis presents most commonly in elderly patients with atherosclerotic vascular disease with crampy abdominal pain and bloody stool; in most cases it is self-limited.

Bibliography

Sreenarasimhaiah J. Diagnosis and management of ischemic colitis. Curr Gastroenterol Rep. 2005;7(5):421-426. [PMID: 16168242]

Item 6   Answer: C

Educational Objective: *Evaluate diverticulitis with CT scan.*

The most appropriate next step in the evaluation of this patient is a contrast-enhanced CT scan of the abdomen and pelvis. This patient's left lower quadrant pain, fever, and elevated leukocyte count are classic symptoms and signs of diverticulitis. The most sensitive imaging modality to confirm this diagnosis as well as evaluate for any complications such as perforation, abscess, obstruction, and fistula is a contrast-enhanced CT scan of the abdomen and pelvis. A number of prospective investigations have reported a sensitivity of 69% to 95% and specificity of 75% to 100% for CT scan in acute diverticulitis. The presence of severe disease found on CT scan was prognostically very useful by accurately predicting failure of medical treatment and risk of secondary complications.

Colonoscopy is generally avoided during an episode of acute diverticulitis for concern of increased risk of perforation with air insufflation; furthermore, colonoscopy would miss the extraluminal complications such as abscess formation. A small-bowel series evaluates the small intestine, which is not affected in diverticulitis. Before the availability of CT scanning, barium enema was used to diagnose diverticulitis but, like colonoscopy, presents a risk for perforation and is not sensitive to the presence of extraluminal complications.

KEY POINT

The best imaging modality to confirm suspected diverticulitis and evaluate for extraluminal complications is a contrast-enhanced CT scan.

Bibliography
Sheth AA, Longo W, Floch MH. Diverticular disease and diverticulitis. Am J Gastroenterol. 2008;103(6):1550-1556. [PMID: 18479497]

Item 7   Answer: B

Educational Objective: *Diagnose chronic pancreatitis confirmed by pancreatic calcification.*

The diagnosis of chronic pancreatitis should be strongly considered in the appropriate clinical setting, such as a patient with a history of alcoholism who presents with chronic upper abdominal pain radiating to the back, diabetes, and steatorrhea. Such patients may not need additional testing. However, most patients have only nonspecific abdominal pain and elevated pancreatic enzyme levels and require diagnostic radiographic imaging studies. The presence of pancreatic calcifications on plain films or CT scan confirms the diagnosis. Plain films of the abdomen will show pancreatic calcifications in some patients, as it did in this patient. Most patients, however, require abdominal CT scans to detect the calcifications and to exclude other causes of pain.

Acute cholangitis is associated with biliary obstruction and is characterized by the triad of pain, fever, and jaundice, which are absent in this patient. If biliary obstruction involves the pancreatic duct as well, pancreatic enzymes may be elevated. Acute cholangitis is not compatible with an illness lasting 1 year.

Diverticulitis is another acute illness characterized by left lower quadrant pain, fever, and localized abdominal tenderness. Nei-

ther acute cholangitis nor diverticulitis is associated with pancreatic calcifications. Acute diverticulitis is not associated with pancreatic enzyme elevations.

Pain associated with peptic ulcer disease is likely to be epigastric, is usually described as burning or gnawing, and tends to occur during fasting or at night. It is not associated with elevated pancreatic enzyme levels or pancreatic calcifications.

KEY POINT

The diagnosis of chronic pancreatitis should be strongly considered in patients with a history of alcoholism presenting with chronic upper abdominal pain radiating to the back, diabetes, steatorrhea, and pancreatic calcifications on abdominal radiographs.

Bibliography
Conwell DL, Banks PA. Chronic pancreatitis. Curr Opin Gastroenterol. 2008;24(5):586-590. [PMID: 19122499]

Item 8   Answer: B

Educational Objective: *Diagnose hemolytic uremic syndrome.*

The most appropriate next management step is a peripheral blood smear. This patient likely has hemolytic uremic syndrome (HUS), which is characterized by thrombocytopenia and thrombotic microangiopathy. Thrombotic microangiopathy is a clinical syndrome that affects multiple organ systems but is always characterized by thrombocytopenia and microangiopathic hemolytic anemia (schistocytes on the peripheral blood smear, elevated reticulocyte count, and elevated lactate dehydrogenase level). Thrombotic microangiopathy may manifest as thrombotic thrombocytopenic purpura or HUS. HUS is usually caused by infection with Shiga toxin–producing *Escherichia coli* (O157:H7), often related to ingestion of contaminated, under-cooked beef, or by complement dysregulation caused by genetic mutations. Additional manifestations of HUS may include acute kidney injury and neurologic findings (for example, headache, confusion) but the only diagnostic criteria are thrombocytopenia and microangiopathic hemolytic anemia in the absence of any other potential cause.

Antibiotics are not recommended in the treatment of HUS. Studies in children have shown either no benefit or increased complications when antibiotics are used. The mainstay of treatment is supportive, with adequate fluids and close monitoring of electrolytes and blood counts; dialysis may be required for acute renal failure. Transfusion of packed red blood cells may be indicated if anemia worsens, but platelet transfusion is controversial, because it may worsen the thrombotic process and is typically used only when bleeding is significant.

Routine stool cultures only test for salmonella, shigella, and campylobacter. Therefore, in patients with bloody diarrhea, stool should also be sent specifically for *E. coli* O157:H7 testing. Fecal leukocyte testing has poor sensitivity and specificity in the diagnosis of infectious diarrhea, will not specifically diagnose HUS, and will not add useful diagnostic information.

Hemolytic uremic syndrome diagnosis is based on the presence of microangiopathic hemolytic anemia and thrombocytopenia.

Bibliography

Razzaq S. Hemolytic uremic syndrome: an emerging health risk Am Fam Physician. 2006;74(6):991-6. [PMID: 17002034]

Item 9   Answer: B

Educational Objective: *Diagnose radiation proctitis.*

Flexible sigmoidoscopy is the most appropriate next diagnostic test. The most likely cause of diarrhea in this patient is radiation proctitis, which occurs commonly in patients receiving pelvic radiation. Acute radiation proctitis usually manifests within 6 weeks of therapy with symptoms of diarrhea and tenesmus. The proctitis is due to direct radiation injury to the rectal mucosal and usually resolves soon after radiation is discontinued. Chronic proctitis can occur months to years after treatment and is associated with a worse prognosis. Diagnosis is established by endoscopic findings of mucosal telangiectasia, with biopsy showing submucosal fibrosis and arteriole endarteritis.

The temporal relationship between the patient's radiation therapy and onset of her diarrheal symptoms within 6 weeks most strongly suggests radiation proctitis. Evaluation for an infectious cause of diarrhea is unlikely to establish a diagnosis, because the pretest probability of an infectious cause of diarrhea is low. Abdominal/pelvic CT scan will not be helpful, because no specific radiologic features define radiation proctitis; the diagnosis is established by direct visualization of the affected mucosa.

Measuring stool osmolality may occasionally be helpful in distinguishing osmotic diarrhea from secretory diarrhea and in those few patients suspected of having factitious diarrhea (low stool osmolality). This test will not be helpful in a patient with a history compatible with radiation proctitis.

Acute radiation proctitis can cause diarrhea and tenesmus within 6 weeks of therapy.

Bibliography

Leiper K, Morris AI. Treatment of radiation proctitis. Clin Oncol (R Coll Radiol). 2007;19(9):724-9. [PMID: 17728120]

Item 10   Answer: B

Educational Objective: *Diagnose chronic pancreatitis with abdominal CT scan.*

The test most likely to establish the diagnosis is CT scan of the abdomen. This patient has chronic pancreatitis secondary to alcohol abuse, which has resulted in malabsorption. The three classic findings in chronic pancreatitis are abdominal pain that is usually mid-epigastric, postprandial diarrhea, and diabetes mellitus secondary to pancreatic endocrine insufficiency. Malabsorption occurs in patients with chronic pancreatitis when approximately 80% of the pancreas is destroyed. Malabsorption presents with diarrhea and steatorrhea, weight loss, and deficiencies of fat-soluble vitamins because the dam-

aged pancreatic gland is no longer producing the pancreatic exocrine enzymes to absorb food. Additional clues to the diagnosis include elevated pancreatic enzyme levels and liver chemistry tests. Patients with a typical presentation may not need additional testing. However, most patients with chronic pancreatitis have only nonspecific abdominal pain (and normal pancreatic enzyme concentrations) and require diagnostic radiographic imaging studies. The presence of pancreatic calcifications on radiographs confirms the diagnosis. Plain films of the abdomen will show pancreatic calcifications in approximately 30% of patients. Most patients, however, require abdominal CT scans, which are able to detect pancreatic calcification in up to 90% of patients. CT scanning can also exclude other causes of pain.

Antiendomysial antibodies are a marker for celiac disease, which is unlikely in this patient with an evident history of pancreatic malabsorption. Although colonoscopy is indicated as a screening tool for average risk asymptomatic patients beginning at the age of 50 years and for patients with a change in bowel habits and weight loss, this patient's history suggests pancreatic malabsorption, and colonoscopy is less likely than abdominal CT scan to confirm the diagnosis. Stool studies are appropriate for determining the cause of an acute infectious diarrhea, but this patient has had diarrhea for 8 months, and infectious diarrhea is not usually associated with such a degree of weight loss or elevation of pancreatic enzymes.

Patients with chronic pancreatitis present with abdominal pain and, in more severe cases, malabsorption and endocrine insufficiency.

Bibliography

Witt H, Apte MV, Keim V, Wilson JS. Chronic pancreatitis: challenges and advances in pathogenesis, genetics, diagnosis, and therapy. Gastroenterology. 2007;132(4):1557-1573. [PMID:17466744]

Item 11   Answer: D

Educational Objective: *Diagnose and treat diarrhea-predominant irritable bowel syndrome.*

The most appropriate management for this patient is symptom control. Irritable bowel syndrome (IBS) is the most common gastrointestinal condition diagnosed in the United States. This patient presents with symptoms that meet the Rome III criteria for IBS. The Rome criteria were developed to establish consensus guidelines for diagnosis of functional bowel disorders. Criteria for IBS are symptoms of recurrent abdominal pain or discomfort and a marked change in bowel habit for at least 6 months, with symptoms experienced on at least 3 days a month for at least 3 months. Two or more of the following must also apply: (1) pain is relieved by a bowel movement; (2) onset of pain is related to a change in frequency of stool; and/or (3) onset of pain is related to a change in the appearance of stool. In this otherwise healthy young woman, reassurance that she has a chronic but not a life-threatening disease with recommendation of a high-fiber diet should be the initial therapy.

CT enteroscopy or colonoscopy would be premature at this point given the absence of alarm symptoms: fever, weight loss, blood in stool, abnormal physical examination, family history of inflammatory bowel disease or colon cancer, or pain or diarrhea that awakens/interferes with sleep.

This patient does not have evidence of malabsorption, anemia, or weight loss to suggest a diagnosis of celiac disease; therefore, an empiric gluten-free diet would be inappropriate. An empiric gluten-free diet is never appropriate without first establishing the histological diagnosis of celiac disease with a small-bowel biopsy.

KEY POINT

Irritable bowel syndrome is a clinical diagnosis of exclusion and, in the absence of alarm symptoms, invasive workup is not necessary.

Bibliography
Wilson JF. In the clinic. Irritable bowel syndrome. Ann Intern Med. 2007;147(1):ITC7-1-ITC7-16. [PMID: 17606954]

Item 12 Answer: A
Educational Objective: *Diagnose a patient with severe* Clostridium difficile *infection.*

This patient most likely has severe *Clostridium difficile* infection (CDI). CDI typically presents with watery diarrhea, although the range of symptoms span an asymptomatic carrier state to severe fulminant colitis with toxic megacolon. Patients with CDI and associated colitis typically have diarrhea up to 10 or 15 times daily, lower abdominal pain, cramping, fever, and leukocytosis that often exceeds 15,000/µL (15 x 10^9/L). CDI with colitis is most commonly associated with prior antibiotic administration. The colitis is produced by two toxins, A and B. These have different mechanisms of action, but both are highly potent and cause cytotoxicity at extremely low concentrations. The toxins can be detected in the clinical laboratory and the presence of either toxin confirms the diagnosis. Treatment of severe CDI with colitis consists of oral vancomycin and intravenous metronidazole.

The typical presentation of Crohn disease is abdominal pain, diarrhea, and weight loss that occurs over a period of months, if not years. This patient's severe and rapidly progressive course is not consistent with Crohn disease.

Patients with uncomplicated diverticulitis present with abdominal pain and fever. Physical examination discloses left lower quadrant abdominal tenderness. Leukocytosis is present, and urinalysis may show sterile pyuria due to inflammation close to the bladder. The patient's 2 day history of severe diarrhea is not consistent with diverticulitis. Diverticulosis consists of the presence of diverticula in the colon. Diverticulosis is common in aging Western populations and is not associated with pain or diarrhea.

Ischemic colitis symptoms include left lower quadrant abdominal pain and bloody diarrhea, which are often self-limited. Treatment is supportive and includes intravenous fluids and bowel rest. Most symptoms resolve within 48 hours. This patient's progressive symptoms are not consistent with a diagnosis of ischemic colitis.

KEY POINT

Patients with previous exposure to antibiotics may develop *Clostridium difficile* infection and associated colitis, which is characterized by diarrhea up to 10 or 15 times daily, lower abdominal pain, cramping, fever, and leukocytosis.

Bibliography
Bartlett JG, Gerding DN. Clinical recognition and diagnosis of Clostridium difficile infection. Clin Infect Dis. 2008;46:S12-S18. [PMID: 18177217]

Item 13 Answer: D
Educational Objective: *Manage* Salmonella *gastroenteritis.*

This patient has *Salmonella* gastroenteritis, but he does not require treatment at this time. Because *Salmonella* gastroenteritis is usually self-limited, antibiotic treatment is generally not required for most healthy persons. If the diarrhea worsens to the point that he cannot replace lost fluids or if he shows evidence of toxicity (persistent high fever, declining mentation, end-organ dysfunction) or likely bacteremia, he will need more aggressive intervention.

Treatment is recommended only for (1) immunocompetent patients younger than 2 years or older than 50 years to avoid the increased incidence of complications in these age groups; (2) immunocompetent patients with severe illness requiring hospitalization; (3) immunocompetent patients with known or suspected atherosclerotic plaques or endovascular or bone prostheses because of seeding of salmonellae to these areas during a bloodstream infection; and (4) immunocompromised patients, such as patients with uncontrolled HIV infection or those requiring corticosteroids and other immunosuppressive agents.

There is a great temptation to treat patients with documented or suspected bacterial diarrhea. Although there is evidence that antibacterial treatment of *Shigella* or travelers' diarrhea (caused by certain toxin-producing strains of *Escherichia coli*) might hasten recovery, the benefits of early treatment are modest and diminish with time. The treatment of presumed or documented *Salmonella* diarrhea is even more problematic. For most patients with salmonellosis, recovery occurs equally fast with or without antibiotics. In addition, there may be a delay in clearing the salmonellae from the stool of antibiotic-treated patients, and the effects of the antibiotics can independently contribute to toxicity, including *Clostridium difficile* toxin–mediated diarrhea.

Of the antibiotics that might be useful in treating salmonellosis, ciprofloxacin would be reasonably likely to be effective in vitro, although resistance to the fluoroquinolones is increasing in many parts of the world.

Metronidazole would not have any benefit for *Salmonella* or any other bacterial diarrhea. The use of antidiarrheal agents such as loperamide is probably safe for individuals with travelers' diarrhea but is not recommended for potentially invasive pathogens such as *Salmonella*. In addition, patients with fever, bloody stools, or signs of systemic toxicity should not be given bowel paralytics because these agents can worsen the acute disease course.

KEY POINT

Because *Salmonella* gastroenteritis is usually self-limited, antibiotic treatment is generally not required for most healthy persons.

Bibliography
Pawlowski SW, Warren CA, Guerrant R. Diagnosis and treatment of acute or persistent diarrhea. Gastroenterology. 2009;136(6):1874-1886. [PMID: 19457416]

Item 14   Answer: B

Educational Objective: *Diagnose hepatocellular injury pattern on laboratory testing.*

This patient has acute hepatocellular damage associated with mild hyperbilirubinemia that could be caused by acute hepatitis. Hepatocellular injury most often results in an elevation of serum alanine aminotransferase (ALT) and aspartate aminotransferase (AST) concentrations, which reflect release of intracellular enzymes from injured hepatocytes. AST is also released from other tissues, such as the heart and skeletal muscle. Therefore, elevations of ALT, which is minimally produced in nonhepatic tissues, are more specific for diagnosing liver disease. Hepatocyte dysfunction is often associated with conjugated hyperbilirubinemia, in which the direct bilirubin fraction is greater than 50%.

Cholestatic injury (cholestasis), which consists of a lack of or an abnormality in the flow of bile, is indicated primarily by an elevation of serum alkaline phosphatase and relatively minimal elevations of AST and ALT. Cholestasis may occur without jaundice because of the capacity of the liver to continue to secrete bile sufficiently until the injury to the bile ducts is significant. Profound disruption of the bile secretory mechanisms is likely to result in conjugated hyperbilirubinemia with elevation of the direct fraction of serum bilirubin. The first evaluative step in a patient with a cholestatic pattern of injury is to obtain an ultrasound study to determine if intrahepatic or extrahepatic biliary obstruction is present.

Liver disorders can also present with a mixed pattern of liver injury that is characterized by moderate to severe elevations of aminotransferase, alkaline phosphatase, and bilirubin levels. Hepatitis B and C are examples of conditions that can occasionally present with a mixed liver injury pattern.

This patient's predominantly elevated aminotransferase levels with mildly elevated alkaline phosphatase concentration and direct bilirubin fraction clearly points to a hepatocellular injury pattern. A nonhepatic injury pattern, such as muscle injury, would be associated with striking elevations of AST, lesser elevations of ALT, and would not be associated with elevations of conjugated bilirubin.

KEY POINT

Hepatocellular injury most often results in an elevation of serum alanine aminotransferase (ALT) and aspartate aminotransferase (AST) concentrations and often is associated with direct hyperbilirubinemia.

Bibliography

Burke MD. Liver function: test selection and interpretation of results. Clin Lab Med. 2002;22(2):377-90. [PMID: 12134466]

Item 15   Answer: B

Educational Objective: *Diagnose Gilbert syndrome.*

This patient has indirect (unconjugated) hyperbilirubinemia, which in an asymptomatic patient with a normal hemoglobin level and otherwise normal liver tests is suggestive of Gilbert syndrome. Bilirubin is measured as conjugated (direct) and unconjugated (indirect) fractions. In patients with cholestatic diseases leading to jaundice, approximately half of the bilirubin is measured as the conjugated fraction. Predomi-nance of the unconjugated fraction indicates either the overproduction of bilirubin (as occurs in hemolysis) or impairment of bilirubin conjugation. The latter is relatively common, given the 5% prevalence of Gilbert syndrome in the general population. This benign syndrome, also known as constitutional hepatic dysfunction and familial nonhemolytic jaundice, is characterized by total bilirubin concentrations up to 3.0 mg/dL (51.3 mmol/L) resulting from a reduced expression of the enzyme that conjugates bilirubin. Gilbert syndrome is the most common inherited disorder of bilirubin metabolism. In adults, it is a benign disorder, and no additional diagnostic studies or therapy is required at this time.

Cholestasis due to an oral contraceptive agent will cause conjugated (direct) hyperbilirubinemia and an elevated serum alkaline phosphatase level, neither of which this patient has. Patients with hemolysis significant enough to cause unconjugated hyperbilirubinemia generally have a low hemoglobin level and abnormal values for mean corpuscular volume (low) and red cell distribution width (high). Abdominal ultrasonography may be a helpful study for patients with direct hyperbilirubinemia, which is usually associated with liver disease, but is not indicated in this patient who has indirect hyperbilirubinemia and no evidence of liver disease.

KEY POINT

The incidental finding of indirect (unconjugated) hyperbilirubinemia in an asymptomatic patient with a normal hemoglobin level and otherwise normal liver tests is indicative of Gilbert syndrome.

Bibliography

Krier M, Ahmed A. The asymptomatic outpatient with abnormal liver function tests. Clin Liver Dis. 2009;13(2):167-177. [PMID: 19442912]

Item 16   Answer: A

Educational Objective: *Manage symptomatic gallstone disease.*

The best management for this patient is elective cholecystectomy before hospital discharge. Most patients with asymptomatic stones are managed conservatively. About 70% of patients with gallstones and single or infrequent episodes of pain have a rate of biliary complications of 1% to 2% per year. Patients with an episode of complicated biliary disease (acute cholecystitis or gallstone pancreatitis) have a 30% chance of having a recurrence of complicated disease within 3 months. This patient has had recurrent episodes of biliary colic and cholecystitis and is at risk for complicated gallbladder disease. In uncomplicated gallbladder disease, laparoscopic cholecystectomy is preferred to open laparotomy, because it results in shorter hospital stays, less pain, and a more rapid recovery.

ERCP with sphincterotomy is indicated for patients with biliary obstruction due to choledocholithiasis. It has no role in removing nonobstructing stones from the gallbladder.

Although ursodeoxycholic acid may decrease the risk for future stone formation in some patients, it is less effective than cholecystectomy in patients with existing stones, and its use is limited to patients who are unable to undergo surgery. Dietary changes and weight loss may be useful for preventing development of gallstones, but do not treat stones that are already present.

Cholecystectomy provides definitive therapy for patients with symptomatic gallstone disease.

Bibliography

Sanders G, Kingsnorth AN. Gallstones. BMJ. 2007;335(7614):295-9. [PMID: 17690370]

Item 17   Answer: D

Educational Objective: *Diagnose primary sclerosing cholangitis.*

This patient likely has primary sclerosing cholangitis, a chronic cholestatic liver disease associated with inflammatory bowel disease and characterized by fibrosis, inflammation, and stricturing of the biliary tree. Up to 85% of affected patients have underlying inflammatory bowel disease, but less than 5% of patients with inflammatory bowel disease have primary sclerosing cholangitis. Cholestatic liver diseases primarily cause elevation of serum alkaline phosphatase values and minor elevations of the aminotransferase levels. The disorder is more common in patients with ulcerative colitis than with Crohn disease. Most patients are diagnosed while asymptomatic with abnormal results on liver biochemistry tests, but jaundice and pruritus can occur in patients with advanced disease. The diagnosis is usually made by endoscopic retrograde cholangiopancreatography, which is especially useful in advanced disease where histologic samples can be taken to rule out cholangiocarcinoma and stents can be placed if there is a dominant stricture. Magnetic resonance cholangiopancreatography can also be used.

Gilbert syndrome is a common disorder associated with indirect hyperbilirubinemia. Patients with this syndrome generally have a serum total bilirubin level of less than 3.0 mg/dL (51.3 μmol/L), whereas the serum direct bilirubin level is less than or equal to 0.3 mg/dL (5.1 μmol/L). A presumptive diagnosis of Gilbert syndrome can be made in an otherwise healthy patient who has indirect hyperbilirubinemia, normal liver enzyme values, and a normal hemoglobin concentration (which excludes hemolysis). This patient does not fulfill the criteria for Gilbert syndrome.

Patients with acute hepatitis C are usually asymptomatic and therefore rarely present clinically, but 60% to 85% of persons who acquire acute hepatitis C develop chronic infection. The cholestatic picture in the absence of other signs of advanced liver disease is inconsistent with chronic hepatitis C. Patients with acute hepatitis A often have fatigue, nausea, mild upper abdominal pain, and jaundice. Serum aspartate aminotransferase and alanine aminotransferase values are usually greater than 500 U/L. Hepatitis A does not present with a cholestatic biochemical profile as seen in this patient.

Patients with acute hepatitis have a marked elevation of aminotransferases, whereas patients with primary sclerosing cholangitis have a cholestatic pattern (primary elevation of bilirubin and alkaline phosphatase levels).

Bibliography

Broomé U, Bergquist A. Primary sclerosing cholangitis, inflammatory bowel disease, and colon cancer. Semin Liver Dis. 2006;26(1):31-41. [PMID:16496231]

Item 18   Answer: B

Educational Objective: *Diagnose acute cholecystitis.*

The patient likely has acute cholecystitis; she has a history of biliary colic, including pain that radiates to the right shoulder, a Murphy sign elicited on examination, fever, leukocytosis, mild bilirubin and aminotransferase elevation, gallstones and pericholecystic fluid, and thickening of the gallbladder wall on ultrasonography. When ultrasonography reveals gallstones and a positive ultrasonographic Murphy sign, the positive predictive value for acute cholecystitis is 92%. Murphy sign is interruption of deep inspiration when pressure is applied beneath the right costal arch. When the patient has the additional findings of gallstones and gallbladder wall thickening (>3 mm), the positive predictive value is 95% for acute cholecystitis. Surgical cholecystectomy is advisable once gallstones lead to such complications as acute cholecystitis.

Acute cholangitis is associated with biliary obstruction and the subsequent development of a suppurative infection within the biliary tree. Obstruction is most often due to gallstones. Charcot triad (pain, fever, and jaundice) occurs in most patients with cholangitis. The absence of biliary tract obstruction on ultrasonography rules out acute cholangitis.

Although the presentation of pancreatitis varies, the most common signs and symptoms are the sudden onset of constant, severe upper abdominal pain associated with nausea and vomiting. The hallmark of diagnosis is the presence of markedly increased levels of circulating pancreatic enzymes, which are not found in this patient.

Gallbladder dyskinesia, characterized by a reduced rate of gallbladder emptying, is controversial as a cause of right upper quadrant pain. Some patients have features that overlap with those of functional bowel disease. It is not associated with fever, a positive Murphy sign, hyperbilirubinemia, or gallstones.

The classic findings of acute cholecystitis are biliary colic, a Murphy sign, fever, leukocytosis, mild bilirubin and aminotransferase elevation, gallstones, pericholecystic fluid, and thickening of the gallbladder wall on ultrasonography.

Bibliography

Trowbridge RL, Rutkowski NK, Shojania KG. Does this patient have acute cholecystitis? [erratum in JAMA. 2009;302(7):739]. JAMA. 2003;289(1):80-86. [PMID: 12503981]

Item 19   Answer: A

Educational Objective: *Diagnose acute cholangitis.*

This patient has classic acute cholangitis. The clinical diagnosis is based upon the presence of Charcot triad (fever, jaundice, and right upper quadrant abdominal pain). In this setting, bile duct dilation, with stones in the gallbladder, suggests acute cholangitis due to choledocholithiasis. Broad-spectrum antibiotics to cover aerobic and anaerobic gram-negative bacilli and enterococci should be started immediately. Endoscopic retrograde cholangiopancreatography with sphincterotomy should then be performed to remove impacted stones.

Patients with acute cholecystitis may have right upper quadrant pain and gallstones, but the bilirubin level is usually not greater than 2 mg/dL (34.2 μmol/L), and aminotransferase levels are normal. Uncomplicated cholecystitis is not associated with common bile duct obstruction. Patients with simple cholelithiasis are generally asymptomatic. This patient may have pancreatitis that is related to obstruction of the common bile duct and is supported by the finding of elevated lipase level. However, pancreatitis alone cannot explain all of this patient's symptoms and in particular cannot account for the right upper quadrant pain or dilated common bile duct.

KEY POINT

The clinical diagnosis of acute cholangitis is based upon the presence of fever, jaundice, and right upper quadrant abdominal pain and the finding of common bile duct obstruction.

Bibliography

Attasaranya S, Fogel EL, Lehman GA. Choledocholithiasis, ascending cholangitis, and gallstone pancreatitis. Med Clin North Am. 2008; 92:925-960, x. [PMID: 18570948]

Item 20   Answer: B

Educational Objective: *Manage gallstone pancreatitis with ERCP.*

The most appropriate next step in management is ERCP. Patients with acute pancreatitis usually have the sudden onset of epigastric pain, often radiating to the back. These symptoms are often accompanied by nausea, vomiting, fever, and tachycardia. The physical examination shows epigastric tenderness, abdominal distension, hypoactive bowel sounds, and occasional guarding. The diagnosis is confirmed by laboratory results showing serum concentrations of amylase and lipase at least three times the upper limit of normal. Abdominal ultrasonography should be used to detect cholelithiasis in patients with suspected gallstone pancreatitis. ERCP is recommended in patients with evidence of gallstone pancreatitis and suspected biliary obstruction. Biliary obstruction is suspected if cholelithiasis or choledocholithiasis is present, bile ducts are dilated, and liver enzymes are elevated. Aminotransferase concentrations rise initially in gallstone pancreatitis, with subsequent rise of alkaline phosphatase and bilirubin if obstruction persists. ERCP with sphincterotomy has been shown to lower morbidity and mortality in these patients, significantly reducing rates of cholangitis and biliary sepsis.

Although elective cholecystectomy will be required in the future, ERCP is the preferred immediate intervention for removing obstructing stones in acute pancreatitis. MRCP may be used to evaluate biliary obstruction if ultrasonography is nondiagnostic. In a patient with choledocholithiasis identified by ultrasonography, MRCP is unlikely to provide additional diagnostic information and cannot be used therapeutically to remove the obstructing stone. Finally, definitive treatment should not be delayed to obtain further imaging studies. Jejunal enteral feedings are indicated in patients with severe pancreatitis when it is anticipated the patient will not be able to eat for a prolonged period of time. In this case, it is likely the patient will be able to resume oral intake after the obstructing stone is removed.

KEY POINT

ERCP with sphincterotomy and stone extraction is the initial treatment of choice for gallstone pancreatitis.

Bibliography

Gupta K, Wu B. In the clinic. Acute pancreatitis. Ann Intern Med. 2010; 153(9):ITC51-5. [PMID: 21041574]

Item 21   Answer: C

Educational Objective: *Diagnose gallstone pancreatitis.*

The most likely diagnosis is gallstone pancreatitis. This patient has a classic presentation of acute pancreatitis with the acute onset of epigastric abdominal pain, nausea, and vomiting associated with markedly elevated pancreatic enzymes. About 80% of all cases of acute pancreatitis are due to gallstones and alcohol abuse. About 10% of cases are classified as idiopathic; obstruction, drugs, and metabolic, genetic, infectious, and vascular disorders cause the remaining 10% of cases. The presence of stones in the gallbladder, a dilated bile duct, and elevated aminotransferase levels highly suggest gallstones as the cause of pancreatitis. The scleral icterus, jaundice, and elevated bilirubin level suggest continuing bile duct obstruction. Abdominal ultrasonography has a sensitivity of only 50% to 75% for choledocholithiasis, and a common duct stone should be suspected in the correct clinical situation even when ultrasonography does not show a stone. Endoscopic retrograde cholangiopancreatography (ERCP) with sphincterotomy and stone removal is the most appropriate procedure in patients with acute gallstone pancreatitis.

The absence of alcohol consumption excludes alcoholic pancreatitis. Patients whose serum triglyceride level exceeds 1000 mg/dL (11.3 mmol/L) may develop hypertriglyceridemic pancreatitis, but this patient's triglyceride level is only high normal. Autoimmune pancreatitis is a type of chronic pancreatitis. Findings include hypergammaglobulinemia, diffuse pancreatic enlargement, a mass lesion in the pancreas, an irregular main pancreatic duct, and the presence of autoantibodies such as antinuclear antibody. Patients are usually asymptomatic or have only mild symptoms. This patient's acute onset of pain and evidence of gallstone disease is not compatible with the diagnosis of autoimmune pancreatitis.

KEY POINT

The presence of stones in the gallbladder, a dilated bile duct, and elevated aminotransferase levels highly suggest gallstones as the cause of acute pancreatitis.

Bibliography

Wang GJ, Gao CF, Wei D, Wang C, Ding SQ. Acute pancreatitis: etiology and common pathogenesis. World J Gastroenterol. 2009;15(12):1427-1430. [PMID: 19322914]

Item 22   Answer: B

Educational Objective: *Manage severe acute pancreatitis with enteral nutrition.*

The most appropriate management step is enteral nutrition with nasojejunal tube feeding. This patient has moderate to severe acute pancreatitis and after 5 days remains febrile, continues to be in pain, and cannot take in any oral nutrition. The patient will likely have an extended period before being able to take in oral nutrition. Two routes are available for providing nutrition in patients with severe acute pancreatitis: enteral nutrition and parenteral nutrition. Enteral nutrition is provided through a feeding tube, ideally placed past the ligament of Treitz so as not to stimulate the pancreas. Parenteral nutrition is provided through a large peripheral or central intravenous line. Enteral nutrition is preferred over parenteral nutrition because of its lower complication rate. Enteral nutrition is associated with a significantly lower incidence of infections, reduced surgical interventions to control complications of pancreatitis, and a reduced length of hospital stay.

Imipenem therapy is only helpful in acute pancreatitis when there is evidence of pancreatic necrosis. Pancreatic necrosis is diagnosed by a contrast-enhanced CT scan that shows nonenhancing pancreatic tissue. In patients with noninfected pancreatic necrosis, antibiotics may decrease the incidence of sepsis, systemic complications (for example, respiratory failure), and local complications (for example, infected pancreatic necrosis or pancreatic abscess). There is no benefit from antibiotic use in acute pancreatitis without pancreatic necrosis, and such treatment may lead to development of nosocomial infections with resistant pathogens. Similarly, pancreatic débridement is recommended only in patients with pancreatitis and infected pancreatic necrosis. There is no role for corticosteroid therapy in patients with acute pancreatitis of any etiology. Corticosteroid use may increase the risk for nosocomial related infections and metabolic complications such as hyperglycemia.

KEY POINT

Enteral feeding is the preferred route for providing nutrition in patients with severe acute pancreatitis.

Bibliography

Petrov MS, van Santvoort HC, Besselink MG, van der Heijden GJ, Windsor JA, Gooszen HG. Enteral nutrition and the risk of mortality and infectious complications in patients with severe acute pancreatitis: a meta-analysis of randomized trials. Arch Surg. 2008;143(11):1111-1117. [PMID: 19015471]

Item 23　　Answer: D

Educational Objective: *Evaluate gastroesophageal reflux disease (GERD) alarm symptoms with upper endoscopy.*

The initial diagnostic test for this patient is upper endoscopy. His presentation is typical for GERD: burning pain relieved by antacids and worsened by lying down and bending forward. Response to empiric treatment with a proton pump inhibitor such as omeprazole would be sufficiently sensitive and specific to diagnose GERD; however, this patient also has the alarm symptom of dysphagia. Upper endoscopy should be performed next to evaluate for acid-induced esophageal stricture and esophageal carcinoma.

Testing for *H. pylori* is not indicated for patients with GERD, because the presence or absence of *H. pylori* does not correlate with the presence or absence of GERD or guide therapy. Ambulatory esophageal pH monitoring is the gold standard for diagnosing GERD and is typically used in patients in whom the diagnosis is uncertain or who are unresponsive to

empiric therapy. In this patient who presents with symptoms typical for GERD with alarm symptoms, the primary goal of testing is to establish the presence of a GERD complication such as acid stricture or esophageal carcinoma.

KEY POINT

In patients with gastroesophageal reflux disease, endoscopy is indicated for patients with alarm symptoms.

Bibliography

Wilson JF. In the clinic. Gastroesophageal reflux disease. Ann Intern Med. 2008;149(3):ITC2-1-15; quiz ITC2-16. [PMID: 18678841]

Item 24　　Answer: B

Educational Objective: *Treat erosive esophagitis with a proton pump inhibitor.*

The standard of care for the medical management of gastroesophageal reflux disease (GERD), including patients with erosive esophagitis, is proton pump inhibitor (PPI) therapy. Although histamine₂ receptor antagonist therapy relieves symptoms and heals esophagitis in 50% to 60% of patients, PPI therapy provides results in the 80% range. Five PPIs are available in the United States: omeprazole, esomeprazole, lansoprazole, pantoprazole, and rabeprazole; they all have similar efficacy.

A promotility agent such as metoclopramide can theoretically be beneficial in the treatment of patients with GERD by increasing lower esophageal sphincter pressure, enhancing gastric emptying, or improving peristalsis. However, promotility agents have significant side effects and the FDA has imposed a black box warning on metoclopramide, and specialty guidelines recommend against the use of metoclopramide because of questionable efficacy and numerous side effects.

Sucralfate (aluminum sucrose sulfate) is a topical therapy for peptic ulcer disease and GERD. Sucralfate adheres to the mucosal surface and promotes healing by an unknown mechanism. Sucralfate is approximately as effective as a histamine₂ receptor antagonist for the treatment of GERD and nonerosive esophagitis but substantially less effective than a PPI and has no role in the treatment of erosive esophatitis.

KEY POINT

Proton pump inhibitor therapy is the treatment of choice for erosive or severe esophagitis.

Bibliography

Wang WH, Huang JQ, Zheng GF, Xia HH, Wong WM, Lam SK, Wong BC. Head-to-head comparison of H2-receptor antagonists and proton pump inhibitors in the treatment of erosive esophagitis: a meta-analysis. World J Gastroenterol. 2005;11(26):4067-77. [PMID: 15996033]

Item 25　　Answer: A

Educational Objective: *Biopsy a gastric ulcer.*

The most appropriate management for this patient's gastric ulcer is biopsy. Biopsies of all gastric ulcers should be performed, because even small, benign-appearing gastric ulcers may harbor malignancy. In benign ulcers, biopsies can also provide evidence for the presence of *Helicobacter pylori* infection and guide appropriate therapy.

Testing for *H. pylori* is indicated in patients with active peptic ulcer disease (duodenal or gastric) and in patients with a history of peptic ulcer disease who have not been previously treated for *H. pylori* infection. The most commonly used endoscopic tests include biopsy and histologic assessment and the rapid urease test. The sensitivity of the rapid urease test can be reduced by as much as 25% in patients who have taken a proton pump inhibitor (PPI), such as omeprazole, within 2 weeks or bismuth or antibiotic therapy within 4 weeks of the endoscopy; therefore, biopsy followed by histologic evaluation for evidence of *H. pylori* infection is the endoscopic test of choice for this patient. The sensitivity of urea breath testing, like that of the rapid urease test, is reduced by medications that affect urease production such as a PPI.

Treatment for peptic ulcer disease is guided by the biopsy and presence of *H. pylori* infection. In the presence of documented infection, triple therapy consisting of a PPI, amoxicillin, and clarithromycin is the most commonly used initial treatment. Triple therapy is not indicated in the absence of documented infection. In this patient, triple therapy should be withheld pending documentation of infection.

KEY POINT

Biopsies of all gastric ulcers should be performed, because even small, benign-appearing gastric ulcers may harbor malignancy.

Bibliography

McColl KE. Clinical practice. Helicobacter pylori infection. N Engl J Med. 2010:29;362(17):1597-604. [PMID: 20427808]

Item 26   Answer: E
Educational Objective: *Treat peptic ulcer disease by stopping an NSAID.*

The most appropriate next step in the management of this patient is to stop the ibuprofen. The two most common causes of peptic ulcer disease are NSAIDs and *Helicobacter pylori* infection, which account for more than 90% of cases. This patient has a history of arthritis for which she takes over-the-counter ibuprofen; many patients who take such non-prescription medications are unaware that they are taking an NSAID that can cause ulcer disease.

H. pylori infection has been ruled out in this patient by the negative histology for the organism as well as negative serum antibody testing; therefore, no further testing for *H. pylori* is needed.

Measuring serum gastrin should be considered in a patient in whom there is a suspicion of an acid hypersecretion state, such as a gastrinoma (Zollinger-Ellison syndrome), clinical features of which include multiple peptic ulcers, ulcers in unusual locations, severe esophagitis, or fat malabsorption, none of which this patient has.

Malignancy always needs to be considered in a patient with a gastric ulcer; therefore, biopsies of the ulcer and follow-up endoscopy to ensure ulcer healing would be recommended. However, this patient has a duodenal ulcer, which is much less likely to represent a malignancy, and biopsy of the ulcer or follow-up endoscopy to assess for healing is not needed.

Alendronate therapy for osteoporosis has been associated with esophagitis and rare cases of gastric or duodenal ulcers; however, stopping alendronate without considering the more common causes of peptic ulcer disease would not be appropriate at this time.

KEY POINT

The two most common causes of peptic ulcer disease are NSAIDs and *Helicobacter pylori* infection, which account for more than 90% of cases.

Bibliography

Jones R, Rubin G, Berenbaum F, Scheiman J. Gastrointestinal and cardiovascular risks of nonsteroidal anti-inflammatory drugs. Am J Med. 2008;121(6):464-474. [PMID: 18501223]

Item 27   Answer: B
Educational Objective: *Diagnose NSAID use as a cause of dyspepsia.*

For a patient with dyspepsia who is taking nonsteroidal anti-inflammatory drugs (NSAIDs) and has no concerning alarm features, stopping the NSAID is the most appropriate next step. NSAIDs are the drugs most frequently associated with dyspepsia. If stopping or changing the NSAID is not a viable option, initiation of a proton pump inhibitor is warranted.

Metoclopramide is a treatment that may have efficacy in patients with dysmotility-like dyspepsia. However, this diagnosis is based on patient symptoms (early satiety, nausea), a normal upper endoscopy, and absence of other more common causes of dyspepsia such as NSAID use.

NSAID use is a much more common cause of dyspepsia than *Helicobacter pylori* infection. Testing for *H. pylori* before stopping the ibuprofen may lead to unnecessary treatment or misdiagnosis in this patient. Simply stopping or changing the NSAID may obviate the need for further testing for *H. pylori* and unnecessary treatment if the patient's dyspepsia improves. If symptoms continue after stopping the NSAID, testing for *H. pylori* is warranted.

Alarm features such as unexplained iron deficiency anemia, unintentional weight loss, dysphagia, odynophagia, palpable abdominal masses, or jaundice would necessitate an urgent upper endoscopy. Because the incidence of malignancy is significantly greater in patients older than 55 years, upper endoscopy is indicated in any patient older than 55 years with new-onset dyspepsia even without alarm features. This patient has no indication for upper endoscopy.

KEY POINT

NSAIDs are potential causes of dyspepsia and should be stopped or changed in patients with dyspeptic symptoms.

Bibliography

Talley NJ, Vakil NB, Moayyedi P. American Gastroenterological Association technical review on the evaluation of dyspepsia. Gastroenterology. 2005;129(5):1756-80. [PMID: 16285971]

Item 28   Answer: D
Educational Objective: *Empirically treat functional dyspepsia with a proton pump inhibitor.*

The most appropriate management for this patient is an empiric trial with a proton pump inhibitor (PPI). Functional dyspepsia is defined as chronic or recurrent discomfort in the epigastrium with no organic cause determined. Upper endoscopy is necessary to rule out organic causes, and only after this is performed can the diagnosis of functional dyspepsia be distinguished from organic dyspepsia (e.g., dyspepsia caused by peptic ulcer disease, reflux esophagitis, malignancy). Because this patient's functional dyspepsia symptoms are ulcer-like, an empiric trial of a PPI is the recommended treatment.

Ambulatory esophageal pH monitoring, which consists of inserting a pH monitor in the distal esophagus and recording the results over a period of 24 hours, is the most accurate means to confirm the diagnosis of gastroesophageal reflux disease (GERD). The technique also allows determination of an association between symptoms and the amount and pattern of esophageal acid exposure. This procedure may be helpful when the diagnosis of GERD is in doubt or appropriate GERD therapy is nonsuccessful. This patient's symptoms are not compatible with GERD and ambulatory pH monitoring is not indicated.

Functional dyspepsia does not have an apparent organic cause that requires surgery. Therefore, surgical consultation is not indicated. With no other signs or symptoms to suggest a psychiatric illness, psychiatric consultation is not warranted.

KEY POINT

An empiric trial of a proton pump inhibitor is indicated for ulcer-like functional dyspepsia.

Bibliography
Tack J, Lee KJ. Pathophysiology and treatment of functional dyspepsia. J Clin Gastroentrol. 2005:39(5 suppl 3):S211-S216. [PMID: 15798487]

Item 29   Answer: D
Educational Objective: *Diagnose gastrointestinal bleeding of obscure cause.*

The next step in the management of this patient is to repeat the upper endoscopy. Initial endoscopy may miss lesions that are difficult to see or bleed intermittently. Between one third and two thirds of sources of gastrointestinal bleeding of obscure etiology are found within the reach of upper endoscopy, which is typically the next procedure performed following nondiagnostic upper and lower endoscopy. Repeat upper endoscopy is particularly appealing in this patient with a hiatal hernia because of the possibility of Cameron lesions. Cameron lesions are linear gastric ulcers or erosions in the hiatal hernia sac. Cameron lesions are usually an incidental finding and are seen in 5% of patients with hiatal hernias who undergo endoscopic examination, but they can cause chronic or, less often, acute blood loss.

If repeat upper endoscopy is negative, consideration can be given to repeat colonoscopy or capsule endoscopy. In wireless capsule endoscopy, a patient swallows a video capsule that, by intestinal motility, passes through the stomach and into the small intestine. The video capsule transmits images to a recording device worn by the patient. This procedure has been shown to detect sources of bleeding in 70% of patients and is considered the test of choice following upper and lower endoscopy studies.

Barium swallow has a low sensitivity and specificity in the diagnosis of gastrointestinal bleeding compared with upper endoscopy and can interfere with subsequent endoscopic studies. The double balloon endoscope is a system that uses two latex balloons, one mounted on the endoscope and a second balloon on the overtube, which are successively inflated and deflated to pleat the bowel over the endoscope and achieve deep intubation of the small intestine. Double balloon endoscopy may be performed through an oral or a transanal route and has replaced intraoperative enteroscopy in many cases. The role for double balloon endoscopy is to evaluate or treat findings seen on capsule endoscopy, for evaluation of ongoing bleeding when bleeding is brisk enough that the need for endoscopic hemostasis is expected, and as a complementary test when a small-bowel source of bleeding remains a concern despite a nondiagnostic capsule endoscopy.

KEY POINT

In gastrointestinal bleeding of obscure origin, repeat upper endoscopy will identify a bleeding source in a significant proportion of patients.

Bibliography
Concha R, Amaro R, Barkin JS. Obscure gastrointestinal bleeding: diagnostic and therapeutic approach. J Clin Gastroenterol. 2007;41(3):242-51. [PMID: 17426461]

Item 30   Answer: D
Educational Objective: *Diagnose ischemic colitis.*

The most likely diagnosis is ischemic colitis. Although an underlying cause is often not identified, colonic ischemia can occur in association with colonic hypoperfusion in the setting of aortic or cardiac bypass surgery, prolonged physical exertion (for example, long-distance running), and any cardiovascular event accompanied by hypotension. Medications such as oral contraceptives, drugs such as cocaine, vasculitides, and hypercoagulable states have also been identified as risk factors. Most patients with colonic ischemia are older than 60 years and usually present with left lower quadrant pain, urgent defecation, and red or maroon rectal bleeding that does not require transfusion. Patients may have mild tenderness over the involved segment of colon; hypovolemia and peritonitis are rare. Colonoscopic findings are generally segmental and include hemorrhagic nodules, linear and circumferential ulceration, and gangrene. Therapy includes intravenous fluids and antibiotics to cover anaerobes and gram-negative bacteria, although data to support this latter practice are weak.

Most patients with acute mesenteric ischemia are older than 50 years. Severe abdominal pain is almost invariably present, but early physical examination findings are minimal, illustrating the classic teaching of "pain out of proportion to examination." Although occult blood–positive stool is common, overt bleeding is rare. Late signs and symptoms include nausea, vomiting, fever, hematemesis, obstruction, back pain, and shock.

Diverticular disease encompasses both diverticular hemorrhage and diverticulitis. Diverticulosis is an important cause of massive painless lower gastrointestinal bleeding in older patients. Diverticulitis results from obstruction at the diverticulum neck by fecal matter, leading to mucus and bacterial overgrowth. Because 85% of diverticulitis occurs in the sigmoid or left colon, left lower quadrant pain is the most common clinical manifestation, often accompanied by fever and leukocytosis; overt rectal bleeding is typically not seen. In patients with suspected diverticulitis, colonoscopy is not performed because of the risk of colonic perforation.

KEY POINT

Most patients with colonic ischemia are older than 60 years and usually present with left lower quadrant pain, urgent defecation, and red or maroon rectal bleeding that does not require transfusion.

Bibliography

Feuerstadt P, Brandt LJ. Colon ischemia: recent insights and advances. Curr Gastroenterol Rep. 2010;12(5):383-90. [PMID: 20690005]

Item 31   Answer: A

Educational Objective: *Recognize risks of rebleeding in a patient with upper gastrointestinal bleeding.*

Upper endoscopy should be performed at the time of an upper gastrointestinal bleed after appropriate volume resuscitation to provide a diagnosis as to the cause of bleeding, provide a prognosis, and perform endoscopic guided therapy if required. For example, an ulcer with a visible vessel has an approximately 50% risk of rebleeding if not treated endoscopically. These ulcers can be effectively treated with injection therapy, thermal coagulation via endoscopic probes, or mechanical modalities such as endoclips. Clean-based ulcers rebleed in less than 5% of cases and do not require endoscopic therapy.

There is a 5% to 10% rebleeding rate for endoscopic hemostasis. In these patients, endoscopic therapy may be repeated if the patient remains hemodynamically stable. If repeat endoscopy is unsuccessful or the bleeding vessel is inaccessible or too large, surgical consultation should be obtained. However, endoscopic intervention is the first management choice for upper gastrointestinal bleeding.

Intravenous omeprazole has been shown to reduce the risk of recurrent upper gastrointestinal bleeding in peptic ulcers after endoscopic hemostasis. Oral omeprazole also may decrease rebleeding. A meta-analysis showed that adjuvant high-dose proton pump inhibitor therapy following endoscopic hemostasis for ulcers at high risk of rebleeding reduces rebleeding, surgery, and mortality. Octreotide may have a marginal benefit by decreasing the rate of nonvariceal bleeding but is inferior to intravenous proton pump inhibitors. Ranitidine, a histamine H_2 blocker, is inferior to proton pump inhibitors as an adjunct to endoscopic therapy, and there is no benefit of adding a histamine H_2 blocker to proton pump inhibitor therapy.

KEY POINT

Upper endoscopy should be performed at the time of an upper gastrointestinal bleed after appropriate volume resuscitation to provide a diagnosis as to the cause of bleeding, provide a prognosis, and perform endoscopic guided therapy if required.

Bibliography

Cappell MS, Friedel D. Initial management of acute upper gastrointestinal bleeding: from initial evaluation up to gastrointestinal endoscopy. Med Clin North Am. 2008;92(3):491-509, xi. [PMID: 18387374]

Item 32   Answer: D

Educational Objective: *Manage upper gastrointestinal bleeding with restoration of the intravascular volume.*

The first step in the management of acute variceal hemorrhage is the restoration of the intravascular volume using a large bore peripheral intravenous line or a central line. Packed erythrocytes are used as needed to replace blood loss and clotting factors are replaced as needed. Platelet transfusions may be indicated if values fall below $50,000/\mu L$ ($50 \times 10^9/L$).

Following restoration of the intravascular volume, this patient should undergo urgent esophagogastroduodenoscopy and band ligation of esophageal varices. Band ligation has been shown to be as effective as sclerotherapy for preventing early rebleeding. Therapy should also be started with intravenous octreotide, which reduces portal venous blood inflow through inhibition of the release of vasodilatory hormones and is more effective for controlling bleeding than placebo; however, its ultimate effect on survival is unknown.

Arteriography is not first-line therapy in patients with a variceal bleed from venous portal hypertension, and no intervention should take precedence over restoration of the intravascular volume. Arteriography is reserved for patients with a presumed arterial source of bleeding as can be seen in peptic ulcer disease or tumors anywhere along the gastrointestinal tract. In such cases, arteriography can be used to identify and embolize the specific vessel involved. This method is usually reserved for cases in which the patient is actively bleeding and either endoscopic therapy has failed to stop the bleeding or the presence of active bleeding interferes with identification of the bleeding site and the patient is unstable.

Intravenous nadolol is not appropriate because this patient is hypotensive and needs volume replacement and endoscopic intervention rather than medical therapy. A nonselective β-blocker is useful in the primary and secondary prevention of variceal bleeding but not as acute therapy.

KEY POINT

Volume restoration is a priority management intervention for gastrointestinal bleeding in hemodynamically unstable patients.

Bibliography

Cappell MS, Friedel D. Initial management of acute upper gastrointestinal bleeding: from initial evaluation up to gastrointestinal endoscopy. Med Clin North Am. 2008;92(3):491-509, xi. [PMID: 18387374]

Item 33   Answer: C

Educational Objective: *Diagnose diverticulosis or vascular ectasia as the most likely cause of painless lower gastrointestinal bleeding.*

The most likely sources of painless lower gastrointestinal bleeding are diverticulosis and vascular ectasia. After hemodynamic stabilization, the next step is to distinguish upper from lower gastrointestinal bleeding. The presence of blood or coffee-ground–like material on gastric lavage indicates ongoing or recent upper gastrointestinal bleeding and the need for upper endoscopy. Negative nasogastric tube lavage is reliable in ruling out upper gastrointestinal bleeding only if the aspirate contains bile (a yellow or green fluid that tests positive for bile with a urine dipstick), indicating passage of the tube beyond the pylorus into the duodenum.

The most common causes of acute, severe lower gastrointestinal bleeding are colonic diverticula, angiectasia (also known as angiodysplasia), colitis (for example, inflammatory bowel disease, infection, ischemia, or radiation), and colonic neoplasia. Bleeding from a colonic diverticulum and vascular ectasia is typically acute and painless. Ischemic colitis typically occurs in older individuals with significant cardiac and peripheral vascular disease who present with abdominal pain and only a small amount of bleeding. Patients with inflammatory bowel disease and bleeding usually have an established history of inflammatory bowel disease and abdominal pain. The patient's recent colonoscopy and large-volume bleeding make a neoplasm unlikely.

KEY POINT

The most likely sources of painless lower gastrointestinal bleeding are diverticulosis and vascular ectasia.

Bibliography
Zuccaro G. Epidemiology of lower gastrointestinal bleeding. Best Pract Res Clin Gastroenterol. 2008;22(2):225-232. [PMID: 18346680]

Item 34   Answer: A

Educational Objective: *Diagnose anal fissure as a cause of painful hematochezia.*

This patient most likely has an anal fissure that is causing rectal outlet bleeding and pain with defecation and that is probably due to her recent constipation. An anal fissure is a tear in the lining of the anal canal. Careful rectal examination by gently spreading the buttocks apart may reveal the fissure, but this finding may not always be present. The patient may have too much pain to allow digital rectal examination or anoscopy. Chronic fissures are often accompanied by external skin tags, as seen in this patient. Recurrent or nonhealing fissures should raise concern for underlying diseases, particularly Crohn disease.

Rectal cancer and colon cancer must always be considered in someone with new-onset rectal outlet bleeding. However, this patient underwent colonoscopy less than 1 year ago, and results were normal. Even if this patient had colonic diverticula, the fact that her bleeding occurs with painful defecation and has been present over a 3-month period is not typical of diverticular bleeding, which tends to cause significant acute painless hematochezia that often stops spontaneously.

KEY POINT

Anal fissures generally cause rectal outlet bleeding and pain with defecation.

Bibliography
Chong PS, Bartolo DC. Hemorrhoids and fissure in ano. Gastroenterol Clin North Am. 2008;37(3):627-644, ix. [PMID: 18794000]

Item 35   Answer: B

Educational Objective: *Screen for hepatocellular carcinoma in a patient with hepatitis B.*

The most appropriate screening strategy for hepatocellular carcinoma in this patient is liver ultrasonography. Hepatocellular carcinoma is the most common primary intrahepatic tumor and the fastest growing cause of cancer-related death in men in the United States. The cancer usually develops in patients with cirrhosis. The most common causes of cirrhosis leading to hepatocellular carcinoma are chronic hepatitis B and hepatitis C viral infections and alcoholic liver disease; however, patients with chronic hepatitis B infection in the absence of cirrhosis may develop hepatocellular carcinoma. Patients with a compatible ultrasound imaging study and a subsequent serum α-fetoprotein level greater than 500 ng/mL (500 µg/L) can be diagnosed with hepatocellular carcinoma without a biopsy. The optimal time to initiate a screening program and its ideal frequency are unknown.

Combined use of α-fetoprotein measurement and ultrasonography increases the sensitivity of detection but at the expense of increased false-positive results. α-Fetoprotein is not specific for hepatocellular carcinoma and should not be used alone as a screening test unless ultrasound is not available. Liver CT scanning exposes the patient to unnecessary radiation, particularly if screening is performed frequently.

KEY POINT

Patients with chronic hepatitis B infection In the absence of cirrhosis may develop hepatocellular carcinoma and should undergo periodic screening.

Bibliography
Lim SG, Mohammed R, Yuen MF, Kao JH. Prevention of hepatocellular carcinoma in hepatitis B virus infection. J Gastroenterol Hepatol. 2009;24(8):1352-7. [PMID: 19702903]

Item 36   Answer: A

Educational Objective: *Diagnose hepatitis A.*

This patient most likely has acute hepatitis A. The patient has clinical symptoms and laboratory findings consistent with acute hepatitis (fatigue, jaundice, aminotransferase concentrations >1000 U/L). The major routes of transmission are ingestion of contaminated food or water and contact with an infected person. Groups at particularly high risk include people living in or traveling to underdeveloped countries, children in day care centers, men who have sex with men, and perhaps people who ingest raw shellfish. Although any of the hepatitis viruses can cause symptomatic acute hepatitis, hepatitis A is the most likely infection in a traveler to an undeveloped country without other risk factors. Hepatitis A is almost always a self-limited infection, although acute hepatitis A may rarely present as fulminant hepatitis that may require liver transplantation. The clinical course may include a prolonged cholestatic phase characterized by persistence of jaundice for up to 6 months. Treatment of acute hepatitis A is supportive. Serum immune globulin should be administered to all household and intimate contacts within 2 weeks of exposure. Hepatitis A virus vaccine should be offered to travelers who go to underdeveloped countries, men who have sex with men, injection drug users, and patients with chronic liver disease.

Hepatitis B, C, and D are less likely without a history of parenteral exposure. Hepatitis D virus (HDV or delta agent) depends upon the presence of HBsAg for its replication and, therefore, cannot survive on its own. In a patient infected with hepatitis B, HDV infection may present as an acute hepatitis (in which case it is a coinfection) or an exacerbation of preexisting chronic hepatitis (in which case it is a superinfection). Patients with a history of injection drug use are at greatest risk for acquiring HDV infection. Finally, acute hepatitis C rarely causes symptoms.

KEY POINT

Patients with acute hepatitis generally have fatigue, nausea, vomiting, jaundice, and aminotransferase values greater than 1000 U/L.

Bibliography

Brundage SC, Fitzpatrick AN. Hepatitis A. Am Fam Physician. 2006;73:2162-2168. [PMID: 16848078]

Item 37　　Answer:　A
Educational Objective: *Diagnose alcoholic hepatitis.*

This patient has severe alcoholic hepatitis. Excessive alcohol intake may cause liver disease directly or may increase the risk of an unfavorable outcome in patients with preexisting liver disease. This patient with chronic alcohol abuse has many of the characteristic findings of alcoholic hepatitis: a history of recent heavy alcohol use, elevated serum aspartate aminotransferase (AST) and alanine aminotransferase (ALT) values (usually less than 500 U/L and frequently less than 300 U/L), AST to ALT ratio greater than 2 to 1, elevated alkaline phosphatase concentration, jaundice, coagulopathy, and encephalopathy. Moreover, other major causes of acute and chronic liver disease have been excluded.

The patient's serology tests confirm past infection with hepatitis B virus and current immunity (positive hepatitis B surface antigen antibody). Similarly, the serologic tests for hepatitis A are compatible with past infection and current immunity (positive IgG hepatitis A antibody). The negative hepatitis C antibody serology rules out chronic hepatitis C virus infection.

Autoimmune hepatitis is an inflammatory condition of the liver of unknown cause. It primarily develops in persons 20 to 40 years of age, but all age groups and most ethnic groups are affected. Women develop autoimmune hepatitis more often than men. Most patients present with features of chronic liver disease. Antinuclear antibody, anti–smooth-muscle antibody, or antibody to liver/kidney microsome type 1 (anti-LKM1) is present in 87% of patients and helps to support a diagnosis of autoimmune hepatitis. Finally, autoimmune hepatitis does not cause a fatty liver.

KEY POINT

Patients with alcoholic hepatitis have a history of recent heavy alcohol use, elevated serum aspartate aminotransferase (AST) and alanine aminotransferase (ALT) concentrations, an AST:ALT ratio greater than 2 to 1, and elevated alkaline phosphatase concentration.

Bibliography

Lucey MR, Mathurin P, Morgan TR. Alcoholic hepatitis. N Engl J Med. 2009;360(26):2758-2769. [PMID: 19553649]

Item 38　　Answer:　B
Educational Objective: *Diagnose autoimmune hepatitis.*

This patient has autoimmune hepatitis, a disorder that occurs most commonly in girls and young women. Like this patient with hypothyroidism, many affected patients have other autoimmune disorders and a family history of autoimmunity. These patients usually present with vague symptoms. Fatigue, which occurs in 85% of patients, is the most common presenting symptom, followed by jaundice (46%), anorexia (30%), myalgias (30%), and diarrhea. On physical examination, most patients have an enlarged liver. Patients can have aminotransferase concentrations into the thousands (but typically less than 500 IU at presentation), elevated bilirubin, often near-normal alkaline phosphatase, and hypergammaglobulinemia. Autoimmune serologic tests, specifically antinuclear antibodies, anti–smooth muscle antibodies, and antibody to liver/kidney microsome type 1 (anti-LKM1), may be positive but are not detected in up to 25% of patients.

Primary biliary cirrhosis is a chronic progressive cholestatic liver disease of unknown cause. It is an autoimmune disorder that occurs predominantly in women (80% to 90% of cases) between 40 and 60 years of age. The diagnostic triad associated with primary biliary cirrhosis includes a cholestatic liver profile, positive antimitochondrial antibody titers, and compatible histologic findings on liver biopsy. Serum alkaline phosphatase level is usually elevated 10 times or more above normal. The patient's near-normal alkaline phosphatase concentration and negative antimitochondrial antibody essentially rule out primary biliary cirrhosis.

Although drug-induced liver injury can cause similar liver test abnormalities, the patient has not taken any new medications recently, making this diagnosis unlikely, and levothyroxine would be a very unusual cause of drug-induced hepatitis. Additionally, drug-induced hepatitis is not associated with positive anti–smooth muscle antibody findings. She has no pain to suggest acute cholecystitis.

KEY POINT

Laboratory findings in patients with autoimmune hepatitis include elevated serum aminotransferase values, hypergammaglobulinemia, mild hyperbilirubinemia, mildly elevated serum alkaline phosphatase values, and the presence of autoantibodies.

Bibliography

Krawitt EL. Clinical features and management of autoimmune hepatitis. World J Gastroenterol. 2008;14(21):3301-3305. [PMID: 18528927]

Item 39　　Answer:　B
Educational Objective: *Diagnose acute hepatitis B.*

The markedly elevated aminotransferase levels, positive hepatitis B surface antigen, and IgM antibody to hepatitis B core antigen establish the diagnosis of acute hepatitis B infection. Patients at greatest risk for exposure to hepatitis B virus infection are those with a history of multiple sexual partners and injection drug users. Most adult patients will clear their infection after a few months. However, about 5% patients develop acute progressive hepatitis B with hepatic decompensation and need urgent liver transplantation, as does this patient.

These patients tend to have an elevated INR and a rising bilirubin level and may develop encephalopathy, a marker of fulminant hepatic failure.

Patients with chronic hepatitis B have positive hepatitis B surface antigen and positive IgG antibody to hepatitis B core antigen; IgM antibody to hepatitis B core antigen is negative. In addition, this patient's fulminant course is not compatible with chronic hepatitis B infection.

Acute hepatitis A is diagnosed by the presence of IgM antibody to hepatitis A virus (IgM anti-HAV), which appears at the onset of the acute phase of the illness and becomes undetectable in 3 to 6 months. IgG anti-HAV also becomes positive during the acute phase but persists for decades and is a marker of immunity to further infection. A person with a positive IgG anti-HAV titer but a negative titer for IgM anti-HAV has had hepatitis A in the remote past or has received hepatitis A vaccine.

Patients with acute hepatitis C are usually asymptomatic and therefore rarely present clinically, but 60% to 85% of persons who acquire acute hepatitis C develop chronic infection. Although determination of antibody to hepatitis C virus (HCV) is a reliable and inexpensive test for diagnosing hepatitis C, the diagnostic "gold standard" is the presence of HCV RNA in serum.

KEY POINT

Positive hepatitis B surface antigen and IgM antibody to hepatitis B core antigen establish the diagnosis of acute hepatitis B infection.

Bibliography

Liang TJ. Hepatitis B: the virus and disease. Hepatology. 2009;49(suppl 5):S13-S21. [PMID: 19399811]

Item 40   Answer: C

Educational Objective: *Diagnose chronic hepatitis C virus infection.*

This patient most likely has chronic hepatitis C infection. Hepatitis C virus (HCV) is the most common bloodborne infection in the United States. Although screening of blood products and reduced transmission among injection drug users have resulted in a decreasing number of new HCV infections, the number of deaths is increasing because of the "backlog" of chronic infections and the long duration of chronic infection before cirrhosis develops. Patients with acute hepatitis C are usually asymptomatic and therefore rarely present clinically, but 60% to 85% of persons who acquire acute hepatitis C develop chronic infection. The anti-HCV antibody test is the screening test for at-risk persons; a positive test in a person with one of the risk factors confirms exposure to the virus. The HCV RNA test is required to determine active infection rather than just exposure to the virus.

Hepatitis A does not cause chronic liver disease. The patient's serology is compatible with either a past infection with hepatitis A virus or immunization with hepatitis A vaccine.

Hepatitis B virus (HBV) causes 20% to 30% of cases of acute viral hepatitis and 15% of cases of chronic viral hepatitis in the United States. Multiple sex partners and injection drug use are the major risk factors for disease acquisition in this country.

This patient is negative for hepatitis B surface antigen and therefore does not have chronic hepatitis B infection.

Hepatitis D virus (HDV or the delta agent) is a defective virus that requires the presence of HBsAg to replicate. In the United States, injection drug users with hepatitis B are the group at highest risk for acquiring hepatitis D.

KEY POINT

The anti–hepatitis C virus antibody test is the screening test for at-risk persons; a positive test in a person with one of the risk factors confirms exposure to the virus.

Bibliography

Jou JH, Muir AJ. In the clinic. Hepatitis C. Ann Intern Med. 2008; 148(11):ITC6-1-ITC6-16. [PMID: 18519925]

Item 41   Answer: D

Educational Objective: *Diagnose nonalcoholic steatohepatitis as the cause of cirrhosis.*

The most likely cause of this patient's liver disease is nonalcoholic steatohepatitis (NASH). Ascites and elevated aminotransferase and bilirubin levels suggest portal hypertension caused by cirrhosis. Nonalcoholic fatty liver disease (NAFLD) consists of variable degrees of fat accumulation, inflammation, and fibrosis in the absence of significant alcohol intake. Fatty liver disease in the absence of inflammation is more common in women than in men and occurs in 60% of obese patients. NASH is a subcategory of NAFLD defined as the presence of inflammation occurring in about 20% of obese patients of which 2% to 3% will develop cirrhosis. NASH is most commonly seen in patients with underlying consequences of obesity, including insulin resistance, hypertension, and hyperlipidemia (metabolic syndrome). NAFLD is usually diagnosed when patients with characteristic clinical risk factors are found to have mildly to moderately elevated serum aminotransferase concentrations. Imaging with ultrasonography, CT, or MRI can confirm the presence of steatosis. Liver biopsy is sometimes necessary to establish the diagnosis of NASH.

Alcohol and chronic hepatitis C infection are the most common causes of cirrhosis in the United States; however, this patient does not have evidence of hepatitis C infection (negative anti-hepatitis C antibody) nor does she consume alcohol in sufficient quantity to cause cirrhosis (6 alcoholic drinks per day for men and 3 alcoholic drinks per day for women for 10 years). Although chronic hepatitis B infection can lead to cirrhosis, this patient's serologies indicate immunity to hepatitis B (negative hepatitis B surface antigen, positive anti-hepatitis B surface antibody), not chronic hepatitis B infection. Although primary biliary cirrhosis is more common in women than men, it is characterized by marked elevations of the alkaline phosphatase (cholestatic liver disease) not seen in this patient.

KEY POINT

Nonalcoholic steatohepatitis (NASH) is associated with obesity, type 2 diabetes, and hyperlipidemia and is a potential cause of cirrhosis.

Bibliography

Hashimoto E, Tokushige K. Prevalence, gender, ethnic variations, and prognosis of NASH. J Gastroenterol. 2011;46(suppl 1):63-9. [PMID: 20844903]

Item 42   Answer: D

Educational Objective: *Diagnose primary sclerosing cholangitis.*

This patient has cholestatic liver disease characterized by striking elevations of the alkaline phosphatase level and only modest elevations of the aminotransferase levels. The most likely diagnosis is primary sclerosing cholangitis. The most common symptoms of primary sclerosing cholangitis are pruritus and fatigue; as the disease progresses, most patients develop jaundice. Primary sclerosing cholangitis is a chronic condition that usually presents in the fourth or fifth decade of life; it is more common in men than in women and is characterized by progressive bile duct inflammation and destruction and, ultimately, fibrosis of the intrahepatic and extrahepatic bile ducts, leading to cirrhosis. The cause of the disorder is unknown, but a strong association exists with ulcerative colitis, which is present in more than 80% of patients with primary sclerosing cholangitis. However, the severity of ulcerative colitis does not correlate with the severity of primary sclerosing cholangitis, and treatment of ulcerative colitis does not significantly affect the prognosis of cholangitis.

Primary biliary cirrhosis, another cholestatic liver disease, is a slowly progressive autoimmune disease that mainly affects women older than 25 years. Pruritus usually predates the development of jaundice, and patients often have other immune disorders such as hypothyroidism, Sjögrenor sicca syndrome, and systemic sclerosis (scleroderma); antimitochondrial antibodies are found in 95% of cases.

Autoimmune hepatitis is more common in women and usually presents in adulthood. Approximately 50% of patients are asymptomatic and are diagnosed as a result of screening tests. In most cases, serum aminotransferase levels are elevated, ranging from mild increases in serum concentrations to values greater than 1000 U/L. Hyperbilirubinemia may occur with a normal or near-normal serum alkaline phosphatase level. Certain autoantibodies may be elevated, including anti-smooth-muscle antibody, antinuclear antibody, and rarely anti-liver-kidney-microsomal antibody type 1.

Many adults have IgG antibodies to hepatitis A, indicating previous exposure and immunity to the virus. Unlike hepatitis B and hepatitis C, hepatitis A does not cause chronic liver disease.

KEY POINT

Primary sclerosing cholangitis is strongly associated with ulcerative colitis and is associated with marked elevations of alkaline phosphatase.

Bibliography

Chapman R, Fevery J, Kalloo A, Nagorney DM, Boberg KM, Shneider B, Gores GJ; American Association for the Study of Liver Diseases. Diagnosis and management of primary sclerosing cholangitis. Hepatology. 2010;51(2):660-78. [PMID: 20101749]

Item 43   Answer: A

Educational Objective: *Diagnose cirrhosis as the cause of ascites.*

This patient has cirrhosis with ascites. Ascites is the most common complication of portal hypertension secondary to cirrhosis. Any patient who develops new-onset ascites should undergo diagnostic paracentesis. Initial evaluation of ascitic fluid should include measurement of albumin and cell count with differential, Gram stain, and culture. The serum-to-ascites albumin gradient (SAAG) is calculated by subtracting the ascitic fluid albumin level from the serum albumin level. A gradient greater than 1.1 g/dL (11 g/L) indicates that the patient has portal hypertension with a high degree of accuracy. In addition to cirrhosis, other causes of portal hypertension, such as constrictive pericarditis, right-sided heart failure, and the Budd-Chiari syndrome, should be considered. A gradient of less than 1.1 g/dL (11 g/L) is not associated with portal hypertension but with conditions that can cause ascites by other mechanisms, including infection, inflammation, or low serum oncotic pressure, such as the nephrotic syndrome, malignancy, or tuberculosis. Analysis of this patient's ascitic fluid shows a SAAG of 2.2 g/dL (22 g/L), which is consistent with ascites due to sinusoidal hypertension from a chronic liver disease such as cirrhosis.

KEY POINT

Ascitic fluid analysis showing a serum-to-ascites albumin gradient greater than 1.1 g/dL is consistent with ascites caused by chronic liver disease, such as cirrhosis, right-sided heart failure, and the Budd-Chiari syndrome.

Bibliography

Wong CL, Holroyd-Leduc J, Thorpe KE, Straus SE. Does this patient have bacterial peritonitis or portal hypertension? How do I perform a paracentesis and analyze the results? JAMA. 2008;299(10):1166-1178. [PMID: 18334692]

Item 44   Answer: C

Educational Objective: *Manage hepatic encephalopathy.*

The most appropriate management for this patient is to increase the lactulose therapy. This patient has severe encephalopathy manifested by worsening somnolence. Encephalopathy progresses from subtle findings, such as reversal of the sleep-wake cycle or mild mental status changes, to irritability, confusion, slurred speech, and ultimately coma if not recognized and treated. There can be multiple inciting causes of encephalopathy in patients with cirrhosis, including dehydration, infection (especially spontaneous bacterial peritonitis), diet indiscretions, gastrointestinal bleeding, and medications. This patient likely became worse with the development of the urinary tract infection.

The best course of management is to treat the infection and to discontinue the diuretics and increase the lactulose to respond to the encephalopathy. The dose of lactulose should be titrated to achieve two to three soft stools per day with a pH below 6.0. Approximately 70% to 80% of patients with hepatic encephalopathy improve on lactulose therapy, and treatment is usually well tolerated.

Corticosteroids have no role in the reversal of hepatic encephalopathy. Transjugular intrahepatic portosystemic shunt (TIPS) is not appropriate because placement of TIPS is likely to precipitate worsening hepatic encephalopathy as more blood is bypassed through the shunt rather than processed by the liver. There is no role for hemodialysis in the treatment of hepatic encephalopathy and there appear to be no other indications for dialysis (severe acidosis, hyperkalemia, renal failure with hypervolemia).

KEY POINT

First-line therapy for hepatic encephalopathy is lactulose.

Bibliography

Kalaitzakis E, Bjornsson E. Lactulose treatment for hepatic encephalopathy, gastrointestinal symptoms, and health-related quality of life. Hepatology. 2007;46(3):949-950. [PMID:17879365]

Item 45   Answer: A

Educational Objective: *Diagnose hepatorenal syndrome.*

This patient most likely has hepatorenal syndrome, which is defined as development of kidney failure in patients with portal hypertension and normal renal tubular function. Intense renal vasoconstriction leads to a syndrome of acute kidney dysfunction characterized by increased renal sodium avidity, a relatively normal urine sediment, and oliguria in some patients. This condition is diagnosed after other causes of acute kidney injury such as prerenal azotemia, renal parenchymal disease, or obstruction have been excluded. Spontaneous bacterial peritonitis, vigorous diuretic therapy, paracentesis without volume expansion, and gastrointestinal bleeding also may precipitate hepatorenal syndrome. The most effective treatment for hepatorenal syndrome is liver transplantation.

Although patients with complete obstruction have significantly decreased urine output, those with partial obstruction may have polyuria caused by loss of tubular function or excretion of excess retained solute. Kidney ultrasonography in most patients with obstruction reveals hydronephrosis and was absent in this patient.

This patient had no signs of hypovolemia such as hypotension or tachycardia, and his kidney dysfunction did not improve after discontinuation of diuretics and administration of volume replacement with normal saline albumin. This makes prerenal azotemia an unlikely diagnosis.

The diagnosis of renal artery stenosis as the cause of this acute kidney injury is unlikely considering his end-stage cirrhosis, no evidence of hypertension, and no signs of diffuse vascular disease.

KEY POINT

The hepatorenal syndrome is defined as development of kidney dysfunction in patients with portal hypertension after exclusion of prerenal azotemia, renal parenchymal disease, or obstruction.

Bibliography

Arroyo V, Fernandez J, Ginès P. Pathogenesis and treatment of hepatorenal syndrome. Semin Liver Dis 2008;28:81-95. [PMID: 18293279]

Item 46   Answer: B

Educational Objective: *Diagnose erythema nodosum associated with inflammatory bowel disease.*

The most likely diagnosis is erythema nodosum. Extraintestinal manifestations occur in approximately 10% to 20% of patients with inflammatory bowel disease at some time in the course of their disease. Erythema nodosum, which manifests as small, exquisitely tender nodules on the anterior tibial surface, is the most common cutaneous manifestation of inflammatory bowel disease and occurs more commonly in Crohn disease, whereas pyoderma gangrenosum is more common in ulcerative colitis. The typical clinical presentation of erythema nodosum is the sudden onset of one or more tender, erythematous nodules on the anterior legs that are more easily palpated than visualized. The eruption is often preceded by a prodrome of fever, malaise, and arthralgia. A residual ecchymotic appearance is common as the lesions age. In patients with inflammatory bowel disease, treating the underlying bowel disease usually results in remission of erythema nodosum.

Dermatitis herpetiformis is characterized by grouped, pruritic, erythematous papulovesicles on the extensor surfaces of the arms, legs, central back, buttocks, and scalp. A genetic predisposition is linked to the same genes associated with celiac disease. Virtually all patients with dermatitis herpetiformis have celiac disease, but gastrointestinal symptoms occur in only about 25% of patients.

Pyoderma gangrenosum occurs in approximately 10% of patients with ulcerative colitis. Pyoderma gangrenosum is an uncommon, neutrophilic, ulcerative skin disease. Lesions tend to be multiple and to appear on the lower extremities. They begin as tender papules, pustules, or vesicles that spontaneously ulcerate and progress to painful ulcers with a purulent base and undermined, ragged, violaceous borders.

Rheumatoid nodules are the most common cutaneous manifestation of rheumatoid arthritis. They may be asymptomatic or painful and interfere with function. Rheumatoid nodules are frequently found in the subcutaneous tissue just distal to the elbow on the extensor surface of the forearm. Nodules also may be found on the extensor surface of the hand and over the Achilles tendons. Rheumatoid nodules and inflammatory bowel disease are not linked.

KEY POINT

Erythema nodosum, which manifests as small, exquisitely tender nodules on the anterior tibial surface, is the most common cutaneous manifestation of inflammatory bowel disease.

Bibliography

Requena L, Yus ES. Erythema nodosum. Dermatol Clin. 2008;26(4): 425-38, v. [PMID: 18793974]

Item 47   Answer: E

Educational Objective: *Diagnose ulcerative colitis.*

This patient has mild to moderate left-sided ulcerative colitis based on his clinical presentation and endoscopic and histologic findings. His ex-smoking status, microcytic anemia, and the presence of arthritis, which is the most common extraintestinal manifestation of inflammatory bowel disease, further support the diagnosis. Ulcerative colitis typically involves the rectum and extends proximally with contiguous inflammation that is generally limited to the mucosa of the colon and rectum. Patients usually present with bloody diarrhea associated with rectal discomfort, fecal urgency, and cramps. Although most patients have bloody diarrhea, those with proctitis can present with constipation.

Although many colitides can have overlapping clinical, endoscopic, and even histologic features, there are important differences to consider. Microscopic colitis presents with nonbloody diarrhea, and colonoscopy shows normal mucosa macroscopically and histology shows either increased intraepithelial lymphocytes (lymphocytic colitis) or an increased submucosal collagen layer (collagenous colitis). Bleeding is less often a feature of Crohn colitis, and endoscopic inflammatory changes are patchy and generally spare the rectum but can extend throughout the entire gastrointestinal tract; histologic features, however, may be indistinguishable from those of ulcerative colitis. Infectious colitis usually presents with more acute symptoms, and chronic changes such as crypt architecture distortion are absent. Ischemic colitis also generally has a more acute course and spares the rectum because of the dual blood supply to this region and is often associated with other evidence of atherosclerotic vascular disease.

KEY POINT

Ulcerative colitis typically involves the rectum and extends proximally with contiguous inflammation that is generally limited to the mucosa of the colon and rectum.

Bibliography

Baumgart DC, Sandborn WJ. Inflammatory bowel disease: clinical aspects and established and evolving therapies. Lancet. 2007; 369(9573): 1641-1657. [PMID:17499606]

Item 48   Answer: D
Educational Objective: *Treat ulcerative colitis.*

The most appropriate treatment is mesalamine. This patient has mild left-sided ulcerative colitis based on his clinical presentation, endoscopic, and histologic findings. Topical therapy is appropriate for distal disease. Options include cortisone foam and mesalamine or corticosteroid suppositories for proctitis and hydrocortisone or mesalamine enemas for left-sided colitis. Oral 5-aminosalicylates, including sulfasalazine, mesalamine, balsalazide, and olsalazine, are appropriate for distal disease that does not respond to topical therapy or for mild to moderate pancolitis.

Oral prednisone is used when symptoms do not respond to 5-aminosalicylates. Because prednisone and other corticosteroids have many acute and chronic toxic effects that are dose- and duration-dependent, the lowest effective dose should be given for the shortest time. Azathioprine (AZA) or 6-mercaptopurine (6-MP) may be used for patients who have incomplete disease remission while on corticosteroids. However, because both agents have delayed onset of action, concomitant administration of either AZA or 6-MP together with a 3- to 4-month course of prednisone is often necessary.

Antibiotics, including both metronidazole and ciprofloxacin, have not been shown to be effective in ulcerative colitis.

Infliximab is a chimeric antibody against tumor necrosis factor α; in patients with severe disease or who do not respond to corticosteroid therapy for remission, infliximab may be effective, but it would not be an appropriate first-line medication for mild ulcerative colitis.

KEY POINT

First-line therapy for induction and maintenance of remission in mild to moderate ulcerative colitis is mesalamine or another 5-aminosalicylate agent.

Bibliography

Ng SC, Kamm MA. Therapeutic strategies for the management of ulcerative colitis. Inflamm Bowel Dis. 2009;15(6):935-950. [PMID: 18985710]

Item 49   Answer: C
Educational Objective: *Diagnose microscopic colitis.*

This patient most likely has microscopic colitis, which is characterized by chronic watery diarrhea without bleeding. There are two types of microscopic colitis: collagenous colitis and lymphocytic colitis. The average age of onset for collagenous colitis is in the sixth decade of life and it tends to affect more women than men. The average age of onset for lymphocytic colitis is in the seventh decade of life, and women seem to be affected slightly more often than men. The cause of microscopic colitis is unknown. One theory is that the use of NSAIDs may contribute to the development of the disorder. Another theory is that it is caused by an autoimmune response. Colonoscopy in affected patients is grossly normal; to make a diagnosis, several biopsies must be taken from the colon. In collagenous colitis, biopsy specimens show more than normal amounts of collagen beneath the lining of the colon. In lymphocytic colitis, the specimen may also show an increased number of lymphocytes. Loperamide, diphenoxylate, and bismuth subsalicylate, either alone or in combination, are effective and well tolerated when used as initial therapy.

Ulcerative colitis is characterized by bloody diarrhea associated with rectal discomfort, which this patient does not have. Fever, weight loss, tachycardia, dehydration, and significant abdominal tenderness or rebound indicates more severe disease. Endoscopic findings can be subtle in patients with mild ulcerative colitis, and examination may show only mucosal edema and erythema. Increased inflammation causes friability, ulceration, and bleeding. Patients with Crohn disease commonly present with abdominal pain, diarrhea, and weight loss. Disease involving the small intestine often causes nonbloody diarrhea, whereas hematochezia is more likely when the colon is involved. Endoscopic examination may show aphthous ulcers or large ulcers that can coalesce and cause a "cobblestone" appearance. The patient has not taken any antibiotics and does not have other established risk factors for *Clostridium difficile* colitis, including recent hospitalization, advanced age, and severe illness. Colonoscopy will show pseudomembranes appearing as raised yellow or off-white plaques scattered over the colorectal mucosa. She has not traveled out of the country recently, and therefore, is not at risk for tropical sprue.

KEY POINT

Microscopic colitis is characterized by chronic watery diarrhea without bleeding; the diagnosis must be made by histologic examination of colonoscopic biopsy specimens.

Bibliography

Tysk C, Bohr J, Nyhlin N, Wickbom A, Eriksson S. Diagnosis and management of microscopic colitis. World J Gastroenterol. 2008;14(48): 7280-7288. [PMID: 19109861]

Section 4

General Internal Medicine
Questions

Item 1 [Basic]

A new test to screen for prostate cancer has been developed and the results are compared with the results of needle biopsy of the prostate gland. A trial assessing the results of the new test against biopsy results is summarized below:

	Biopsy + Test –	Biopsy + Test +	Biopsy – Test +	Biopsy – Test –
Patients	5	20	15	60

What are the sensitivity and specificity for this new test?

(A) Sensitivity, 0.25; specificity, 0.75
(B) Sensitivity, 0.33; specificity, 0.67
(C) Sensitivity, 0.8; specificity, 0.8
(D) Sensitivity, 0.96; specificity, 0.96

Item 2 [Basic]

A new diagnostic test is developed and tested in an experimental setting. The test's sensitivity and specificity are 0.80. In the population of patients in which the test was used, the positive and negative predictive values were 0.57 and 0.92, respectively. The prevalence of disease in the test population was 0.25. The usual prevalence of this disease in the community is 0.025.

When used in the community, which of the following measures is most likely to decrease?

(A) Sensitivity
(B) Specificity
(C) Positive predictive value
(D) Negative predictive value
(E) Positive likelihood ratio

Item 3 [Advanced]

A 54-year-old woman is evaluated during an insurance examination that requires human immunodeficiency virus (HIV) testing. She has no symptoms of HIV disease. She has had a monogamous sexual relationship with her husband of 24 years, uses no recreational drugs, and has had one blood transfusion because of trauma from a motor vehicle accident in 1970. Results of the physical examination are normal.

Results from an enzyme-linked immunosorbent assay (ELISA) are positive, with a test sensitivity and specificity of 98%. The prevalence of HIV positivity in similar patients is approximately 1 in 10,000.

What is the probability that this patient has HIV infection?

(A) 98%
(B) 90%
(C) 10%
(D) 0.5%

Item 4 [Advanced]

A 19-year-old woman is evaluated in the emergency department for right lower-quadrant abdominal pain and fever of 3 hours' duration. The patient is not sexually active.

On physical examination, the abdomen is tender to palpation in the right lower quadrant but without evidence of guarding or rebound tenderness. Pelvic examination is normal without cervical motion tenderness or right adnexal pain. Following clinical examination, the probability of acute appendicitis is estimated to be 50%. An abdominal "appendiceal" CT scan is ordered. An appendiceal CT scan showing inflammation and a thickened appendiceal wall is associated with a likelihood ratio of 13.3 for the diagnosis of acute appendicitis.

If the CT scan is interpreted as positive for appendicitis, what is the posttest probability that the patient has appendicitis?

(A) 50%
(B) 65%
(C) 80%
(D) 95%

Item 5 [Advanced]

A series of 4 new tests (A, B, C, and D) are developed to diagnose hemachromatosis. The operating characteristics for a variety of different cut points for each of the four tests are plotted on a receiver operating characteristic (ROC) curve.

Receiver Operator Characteristic (ROC) Curve

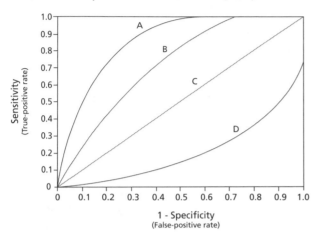

Which of the following tests has the best overall accuracy?

(A) A
(B) B
(C) C
(D) D

Item 6 [Advanced]

A 67-year-old man is evaluated during a routine physical examination. His medical history is remarkable for hypertension and hyperlipidemia. He has a 20 pack-year history of cigarette smoking but stopped smoking 18 months ago. He has no symptoms and no other medical problems. Medications are hydrochlorothiazide and simvastatin. He received his influenza vaccine this year and the pneumococcal vaccine last year. Screening colonoscopy was performed 5 years ago and was normal.

On physical examination, temperature is normal, blood pressure is 120/70 mm Hg, pulse rate is 79/min, and respiration rate is 16/min. BMI is 27. The remainder of the physical examination is normal.

Lipid panel reveals LDL and non-LDL cholesterol levels at target values.

Which of the following should be done next for this patient?

(A) Abdominal ultrasonography
(B) Dual-energy x-ray absorptiometry
(C) Pneumococcal vaccination
(D) Resting electrocardiogram

Item 7 [Advanced]

A 51-year-old man is evaluated during a routine follow-up examination in November. He was diagnosed with GOLD stage I chronic obstructive pulmonary disease 2 years ago and also has hypertension. He has a 20-pack-year history of cigarette smoking but stopped smoking 18 months ago. Current medications are inhaled albuterol as needed and hydrochlorothiazide. He had influenza and pneumococcal vaccinations 1 year ago.

Which of the following is the most appropriate immunization strategy for this patient?

(A) Pneumococcal vaccination only
(B) Trivalent intranasal live influenza and pneumococcal vaccinations
(C) Trivalent intranasal live influenza vaccination only
(D) Trivalent killed influenza and pneumococcal vaccinations
(E) Trivalent killed influenza vaccination only

Item 8 [Advanced]

A randomized clinical trial is conducted to determine if screening for lung cancer with high-resolution CT will improve patient outcomes.

Which of the following cancer screening end points is least affected by bias?

(A) Case-fatality ratio
(B) Incidence of early-stage cancer
(C) Incidence of late-stage cancer
(D) Lung cancer–specific mortality
(E) Survival of patients diagnosed with cancer

Item 9 [Advanced]

A 68-year-old woman is evaluated during a routine examination. She states that last year she had a painful rash on the right side of her back that was self-limited. She takes no medications and has no allergies.

Vital signs are normal, and the physical examination is unremarkable. Complete blood count, liver enzymes, and serum chemistry studies are all normal. She is scheduled to receive her annual influenza vaccination today.

Which of the following is the most appropriate vaccination strategy for this patient?

(A) Zoster vaccination if negative for varicella antibodies
(B) Zoster vaccination if positive for varicella antibodies
(C) Zoster vaccination now
(D) Zoster vaccination not indicated

Item 10 [Advanced]

A 30-year-old man is evaluated in the emergency department for a left foot injury that occurred 2 days ago during a camping trip. A small wood splinter became impaled in the plantar surface of his left foot. The patient removed the splinter and hiked home yesterday. He then noted mild pain and erythema surrounding the puncture site. He reports no fever or significant pain over the injury area. The patient's electronic medical record indicates that he completed the tetanus vaccination series and received a tetanus booster 8 years ago. He has never received the tetanus-diphtheria toxoid and acellular pertussis (Tdap) vaccine. He has no drug allergies.

On physical examination, vital signs are normal. There is tenderness and erythema around the wound site, and there is a small amount of purulent drainage. There is no foreign body in the wound.

The wound is cleaned, and appropriate antibiotic therapy is prescribed.

Which of the following is the most appropriate tetanus prevention strategy for the patient?

(A) Tdap vaccine
(B) Tdap vaccine and tetanus immune globulin
(C) Tetanus immune globulin
(D) No tetanus booster is required

Item 11 [Basic]

A 19-year-old asymptomatic woman is evaluated at a routine annual physical examination. The patient states she is not sexually active and has not engaged in prior sexual activity. She has a boyfriend whom she has dated for the past year. She has no pertinent family history or known drug allergies and takes no medications. She has not received a human papillomavirus vaccine.

Results of the physical examination, including a breast and pelvic examination, are normal.

Which of the following is the most appropriate option for prevention of human papillomavirus infection for this patient?

(A) Human papillomavirus (HPV) vaccine at age 21 years
(B) HPV vaccine at onset of sexual activity
(C) HPV vaccine at time of HPV seroconversion
(D) HPV vaccine now

Item 12 [Basic]

A 52-year-old man is evaluated during a routine examination that includes a discussion of health maintenance issues. After discussing screening for colorectal cancer, he refuses colonoscopy. He is willing to consider other options for screening and states that if an abnormality is found, he would be willing to undergo colonoscopy. There is no family history of colorectal cancer and no previous colonoscopy. On physical examination, vital signs and the heart, lungs, and abdomen are normal.

Which of the following is the most appropriate colorectal cancer screening strategy for this patient?

(A) Annual home fecal occult blood testing
(B) Annual office rectal examination and fecal occult blood testing
(C) Double-contrast barium enema every 10 years
(D) Flexible sigmoidoscopy every 10 years

Item 13 [Basic]

A 57-year-old woman is evaluated as a new patient. She is asymptomatic and has no significant medical history. Her father died of a myocardial infarction at age 71 years, and her 81-year-old mother is alive and healthy. There is no family history of cancer.

On physical examination, vital signs and general physical examination are normal. Laboratory results are all within normal limits.

Which of the following is an appropriate screening strategy for colon cancer in this patient?

(A) Annual digital rectal examination
(B) Colonoscopy every 10 years
(C) Double-contrast barium enema every 3 years
(D) Flexible sigmoidoscopy every 10 years

Item 14 [Basic]

A 69-year-old man is evaluated for syncope that occurred this morning while walking with his wife. Before the event, he had no palpitations, light headedness, or diaphoresis. His wife reports that he suddenly fell to the ground, striking his face, and was very pale. He regained consciousness after about 10 seconds. On regaining consciousness, he was not confused and did not experience bowel or bladder incontinence, tongue biting, chest pain, or shortness of breath. His medical history is significant for hypertension and coronary artery disease requiring percutaneous coronary intervention 1 year ago. His medications are carvedilol, simvastatin, aspirin, and lisinopril.

On physical examination, temperature is 36.6°C (97.8°F), blood pressure is 134/72 mm Hg sitting and 132/70 mm Hg after 3 minutes of standing, pulse rate is 75/min and regular, and respiration rate is 12/min. The cardiopulmonary and neurologic examinations are normal.

Electrocardiogram shows an old anterior wall myocardial infarction with evidence of new ischemic changes.

Which of the following is the most likely diagnosis?

(A) Orthostatic hypotension
(B) Seizure
(C) Situational syncope
(D) Ventricular tachycardia

Item 15 [Basic]

A 53-year-old woman is evaluated for syncope. She became dizzy after getting out of bed this morning and then briefly lost consciousness without injury. She had no diaphoresis, palpitations, or chest pain before the event. She had no incontinence, tongue biting, or postsyncopal confusion. She has recently experienced dizziness on rising too quickly from a chair. She has a 15-year history of diabetes for which she takes insulin glargine. She has a 3-year history of peripheral neuropathy and microalbuminuria. In addition to insulin, she takes lisinopril.

On physical examination, temperature is 37.1°C (98.9°F), blood pressure is 137/78 mm Hg, pulse rate is 82/min, and respiration rate is 14/min. Cardiopulmonary and vascular examinations are normal. She has significantly decreased sensation in her lower extremities bilaterally to her midshins. The remainder of the neurologic examination is normal.

Fingerstick blood glucose measurement is 140 mg/dL (7.8 mmol/L).

Which of the following diagnostic tests should be done next?

(A) 24-Hour ambulatory electrocardiography
(B) Head CT
(C) Orthostatic blood pressure measurements
(D) Ultrasound of the carotid arteries

Item 16 [Basic]

A 36-year-old woman is evaluated in the emergency department after collapsing suddenly while waiting in line at a county fair on a hot summer day. The patient states she felt nauseated and became diaphoretic and lightheaded. She sat on the ground and then lost consciousness. According to her son, she was unconscious for less than a minute, exhibited some twitching movements when she first lost consciousness, but had no incontinence, confusion, or further symptoms on regaining consciousness.

On physical examination, temperature is normal, blood pressure is 142/80 mm Hg supine and 138/78 mm Hg standing, pulse rate is 84/min supine and 92/min standing, and respiration rate is 14/min. Cardiac and neurologic examination findings are normal. An electrocardiogram is normal.

Which of the following is the most appropriate management option for this patient?

(A) Echocardiogram
(B) Electroencephalogram
(C) Exercise stress test
(D) Tilt-table testing
(E) No further testing

Item 17 [Advanced]

A 57-year-old man is evaluated in the emergency department after experiencing an episode of syncope while standing. The patient has had two other episodes of syncope in the past 6 months, both under 10 seconds in duration and occurring when sitting. There is no prodrome to the syncopal episodes. He has no palpitations and no seizure activity and denies confusion following the event. He has no cardiac history and takes no medications.

On physical examination, blood pressure is 128/75 mm Hg with no orthostatic changes, and pulse is 56/min. He has a forehead bruise. Results of the cardiac and neurologic examinations are normal.

An electrocardiogram shows left axis deviation, first-degree atrioventricular block, and right bundle branch block (trifascicular block). An echocardiogram shows normal valves, normal left ventricle size and function, and normal aortic root size.

Which of the following is the most likely diagnosis?

(A) Aortic stenosis
(B) Intermittent complete heart block
(C) Neurocardiogenic syncope
(D) Pulmonary embolism

Item 18 [Advanced]

A 76-year-old man is evaluated for a syncope event that occurred a few weeks ago. He was standing in line at the grocery store and lost consciousness without any preceding symptoms. He estimates that the duration of the episode was less than a minute, and he drove himself home. He has had two other syncopal events in the last 3 years, one while sitting, and one during a walk. He is otherwise asymptomatic with no chest pain, dyspnea, orthopnea, edema, or palpitations. He is healthy and active and he takes no medications.

On physical examination, his blood pressure is 140/85 mm Hg without orthostatic changes and his pulse rate is 82/min. Cardiopulmonary examination is normal.

The electrocardiogram and echocardiogram are both normal.

Which of the following diagnostic tests is most likely to yield useful results for this patient?

(A) Electrophysiology study
(B) Event monitoring
(C) Implantable loop recorder
(D) 24-Hour ambulatory monitoring

Item 19 [Advanced]

A 70-year-old woman is evaluated because of depressed mood, anhedonia, decreased appetite, impaired sleep, and decreased energy. Although the patient feels somewhat hopeless about the future, she adamantly states that she would never take her own life. Her judgment appears intact. Medical history is unremarkable, and she has not had previous episodes of depression. She is taking no medications. Findings on physical examination and laboratory evaluation, including thyroid function testing and vitamin B_{12} measurement, are unremarkable.

Sertraline, 50 mg/d, is begun. The patient returns for a follow-up visit 5 weeks later and reports that she is tolerating the medication well but has no significant change in symptoms, which is validated with a standardized symptom assessment tool. The sertraline is therefore increased to 100 mg/d. Six weeks later, she again reports no side effects and no improvement.

Which of the following is most appropriate at this time?

(A) Add methylphenidate
(B) Discontinue sertraline and begin citalopram
(C) Reassess in 4 weeks
(D) Refer for electroconvulsive therapy

Item 20 [Basic]

A 25-year-old woman is evaluated for a 2-month history of feeling guilty, "down", and hopeless after her fiancé ended their engagement. She is spending less time with friends, restricting previously enjoyable social activities, and having difficulty concentrating. During the past week, she has been thinking about ending her life by cutting her wrists. She lives at home with her mother and two sisters, who have expressed feelings of support and willingness to help. She has no history of previous suicide attempts. Medical history is unremarkable, and she takes no medications.

Which of the following is the most appropriate initial care for this patient?

(A) Corroborate her account by contacting her former fiancé

(B) Reassurance and careful follow-up and observation

(C) Start an antidepressant and follow up in 2 weeks

(D) Urgent mental health referral

Item 21 [Advanced]

A 72-year-old woman is evaluated for a 4-month history of insomnia with difficulty falling asleep. The patient was the major caretaker for her husband, who had advanced heart failure and died suddenly 4 months ago. She has lost 3.6 kg (8 lb) and does not have much of an appetite. The patient used to volunteer at the hospital, but she does not enjoy going there any longer. She also does not have much energy. The patient is tearful and says that nearly everything reminds her of her husband. Medical history is otherwise unremarkable. Physical examination findings are unremarkable.

Which of the following is the most appropriate management option for this patient?

(A) Begin dextroamphetamine

(B) Begin mirtazapine at bedtime

(C) Begin zolpidem at bedtime

(D) Reassure the patient

Item 22 [Basic]

A 22-year-old woman is evaluated because of decreased energy, increased sleep, weight gain, and feeling depressed. The patient always did very well academically, but since her graduation from college several months ago, she has been unable to find a job so she had to move back in with her parents. She states that her life is not working out well but denies thinking about suicide. She previously had periods of unlimited energy when she could stay up all night to do schoolwork or socialize without ever feeling tired. During some of these periods, she had several sexual partners, sometimes with men she met for the first time in a bar, and occasionally did not use condoms.

Medical history is unremarkable. She has never been treated for depression and takes no medications, including oral contraceptive agents. Findings on physical examination are unremarkable.

Which of the following is the most likely diagnosis?

(A) Attention-deficit/hyperactivity disorder

(B) Bipolar disorder

(C) Borderline personality disorder

(D) Generalized anxiety disorder

Item 23 [Basic]

A 48-year-old man is brought by his wife for evaluation. He typically drinks 1 liter of vodka daily and has done so for more than 2 years, but is now trying to quit. His last drink was almost 24 hours ago. He feels anxious and nervous and admits to having auditory hallucinations. He had a seizure previously when he stopped drinking abruptly. He has no other medical problems and takes no medications.

On physical examination, temperature is 37.2°C (99.0°F), blood pressure is 170/100 mm Hg, pulse rate is 110/min, and respiration rate is 18/min. He is tremulous and has difficulty focusing. The remainder of the examination is normal. On the Clinical Institute Withdrawal Assessment Scale for Alcohol, Revised, the patient scores 16 points. Arrangements are made to admit the patient to the hospital.

Which of the following medications should be administered now?

(A) Atenolol

(B) Clonidine

(C) Haloperidol

(D) Lorazepam

(E) Phenytoin

Item 24 [Advanced]

A 28-year-old man who is known to use cocaine is found in a parking lot, throwing himself against cars. En route to the hospital, he has a generalized tonic-clonic seizure that lasts approximately 3 minutes.

His temperature is 38.8°C (101.8°F), pulse rate is 120/min, respiration rate is 18/min, and blood pressure is 170/98 mm Hg. He is agitated, diaphoretic, and voicing paranoid thoughts. Restraints are applied, and intravenous access is obtained.

Which one of the following agents should be administered to this patient at this time?

(A) Haloperidol

(B) Lorazepam

(C) Phenytoin

(D) Propranolol

Item 25 [Advanced]

A 48-year-old man with a long history of alcohol abuse is seen for ongoing care after an inpatient stay for alcohol withdrawal. This is his third episode of acute detoxification, with the longest period of abstinence being 4 months. He does not have any current symptoms of depression and states that he is not using any illicit drugs or prescription medications. His last alcohol intake was 2 weeks before his visit to the office, and he is now enrolled in an alcohol treatment program.

Which of the following pharmacologic agents is the best adjunct to this patient's treatment?

(A) Buspirone
(B) Diazepam
(C) Disulfiram
(D) Naltrexone
(E) Paroxetine

Item 26 [Advanced]

A 46-year-old man is evaluated after being found unresponsive in a city park. Needles and syringes are found in his possession.

The patient is difficult to arouse. Temperature is 35.5°C (96.0°F), blood pressure is 130/80 mm Hg, pulse rate is 100/min, and respiration rate is 8/min. Oxygen saturation with the patient breathing ambient air is less than 80%. Fresh needle marks are found on his arms. He has decreased bibasilar breath sounds; heart sounds are normal. His pupils are dilated. Neurologic examination reveals no focal abnormalities. The patient's airway is protected.

Arterial blood gases (ambient air)
pH   7.08
P_{CO_2} 80 mm Hg (10.6 kPa)
P_{O_2} 40 mm Hg (5.3 kPa)
Bicarbonate   30 meq/L (30 mmol/L)
Calculated alveolar-
  arterial difference   Normal

Treatment is started with 100% oxygen by face mask.

Which of the following is the most appropriate intravenous antidote for this patient?

(A) Diazepam
(B) Fomepizole
(C) Naloxone
(D) Sodium thiosulfate

Item 27 [Basic]

A 58-year-old man is evaluated as a new patient. He reports that he is healthy, he drinks one martini before dinner, and has wine with dinner. There is no family history of alcohol problems. He has recently retired.

Which of the following is the best alcohol screening test for this patient?

(A) Alanine and aspartate aminotransferase concentrations
(B) CAGE questionnaire
(C) Complete blood count and mean corpuscular volume
(D) Ethanol level

Item 28 [Advanced]

A 65-year old woman is evaluated for an 8-month history of low back pain due to lumbar spinal stenosis confirmed by MRI. The patient reports daily symptoms of pain and bilateral tingling in her thighs with difficulty walking. She has no bowel or bladder incontinence. She has taken acetaminophen and ibuprofen with minimal relief of symptoms, and despite phys-

ical therapy, her symptoms have worsened. Previously she was a very active woman and her symptoms are now impairing her lifestyle. She is otherwise healthy and takes no medications.

On physical examination, vital signs are normal. Physical examination is significant for absent ankle reflexes and foot drop bilaterally. The remainder of the physical examination is normal.

Which of the following is the most appropriate next management step?

(A) Electromyography and nerve conduction study
(B) Epidural steroid injection
(C) Spinal traction
(D) Surgery

Item 29 [Advanced]

A 58-year old man is evaluated in the emergency department for severe low back pain of 3 week's duration. The patient reports no recent trauma but has felt feverish. He has no radicular symptoms and reports no bowel or bladder incontinence. He is a current smoker and active user of illicit intravenous drugs.

On physical examination, temperature is 38.9°C (102.0°F), blood pressure is 140/90 mm Hg, pulse rate is 100/min, and respiration rate is 14/min. Multiple needle marks are noted on the arms and legs. He has tenderness over the first and second lumbar vertebrae. Upper and lower extremity motor strength and sensation are normal as are the tendon reflexes. Anal sphincter tone is normal. Lower extremity and perianal sensation is intact.

Leukocyte count is 8000/µL (8×10^9/L). Erythrocyte sedimentation rate is 110 mm/h.

Which of the following is the most appropriate management?

(A) Empiric antibiotic therapy
(B) Spine CT
(C) Spine MRI
(D) Spine x-ray

Item 30 [Basic]

A 42-year-old man is evaluated for low back pain that began after he lifted a box 5 days ago. The pain is moderately severe, and almost any movement makes it worse. Lying down results in some, but not complete, relief. He reports that he has had no trouble urinating. He has no other symptoms and is otherwise healthy.

Physical examination reveals tenderness over the L4 paravertebral musculature bilaterally. His gait is slow because of the pain. Results of a straight leg raising test are normal. There is no motor weakness or sensory loss, including perineal sensation. Deep tendon reflexes are normal bilaterally.

Which of the following is the best initial management option?

(A) Acetaminophen
(B) MRI of the lumbar spine
(C) Plain radiographs of the lumbar spine
(D) Strict bed rest

Item 31 [Basic]

A 70-year-old man is evaluated because of increasing new-onset midback pain that is worse at night, interferes with his sleep, and does not improve with NSAIDs. The patient underwent radical prostatectomy for prostate cancer 2 years ago. He has had urinary incontinence since surgery, which has significantly increased over the past few weeks.

Physical examination findings include tenderness over the midthoracic vertebrae, mild flexor weakness, and hyperreflexia of the lower extremities.

Which of the following diagnostic studies should be done next?

(A) Bone scan
(B) MRI of the brain
(C) MRI of the thoracolumbar spine
(D) Plain radiographs of the thoracic spine

Item 32 [Advanced]

A 27-year-old man is evaluated for a 6-month history of cough, which is worse at night and after exposure to cold air. His cough often is brought on by his taking a deep breath or laughing. He does not have postnasal drip, wheezing, or heartburn. He has a strong family history of allergies. He received no benefit from a previous 3-month trial of gastric acid suppression therapy, intranasal corticosteroids, and an antihistamine-decongestant combination.

Physical examination findings, a chest radiograph, and spirometry results are normal.

Which of the following is most likely to provide a diagnosis of this patient's chronic cough?

(A) Bronchoscopy
(B) CT of the chest
(C) CT of the sinuses
(D) Esophageal pH monitoring over 24 hours
(E) Trial of inhaled albuterol

Item 33 [Basic]

A 52-year-old man is evaluated for a daily cough for the past 6 months. It occurs throughout the day and occasionally at night, but he does not notice any specific triggers. There is occasional production of small amounts of white sputum but no hemoptysis. He does not have any known allergies, has no new pets or exposures, and does not smoke. He does have nasal discharge. He has not noticed any wheezing and has no history of asthma. He has no symptoms of heartburn. He has had no fever, weight loss, or foreign travel, and takes no medications.

Vital signs are normal. There is a cobblestone appearance of the oropharyngeal mucosa but no mucus dripping down the oropharynx. Lungs are clear to auscultation. A chest radiograph is normal.

Which of the following is the most appropriate management for this patient?

(A) Antihistamine/decongestant combination
(B) CT scan of chest
(C) Inhaled fluticasone
(D) Proton-pump inhibitor
(E) Pulmonary function testing

Item 34 [Basic]

A 48-year-old woman is evaluated for a cough that has lasted for 3 months. She describes the cough as occurring daily, nonproductive, and without hemoptysis. She has experienced no associated dyspnea, wheezing, fever, weight loss, night sweats, or recent illness. She has not traveled recently or been exposed to anyone else who has been ill. She has never smoked. She was diagnosed with essential hypertension 6 months ago and has taken lisinopril daily since her diagnosis.

Physical examination is unremarkable. A chest radiograph is normal.

Which of the following is the most appropriate management option for this patient at this time?

(A) Discontinue the lisinopril
(B) Order a chest CT
(C) Order spirometry
(D) Start an antihistamine/decongestant combination
(E) Start a proton-pump inhibitor

Item 35 [Basic]

A 59-year-old man is evaluated because of a chronic morning cough productive of clear or yellow sputum that has been blood-tinged for the past 2 weeks. He has had no fever or weight loss. He has smoked 1.5 packs of cigarettes daily for the past 35 years.

On physical examination, blood pressure is 148/74 mm Hg, pulse rate is 88/min, and respiration rate is 20/min. Chest examination reveals decreased breath sounds throughout the thorax but no other symptoms. Other than evidence of hyperinflation, a chest radiograph is normal. The rest of the physical examination is unremarkable.

Which of the following is the most appropriate next step in management?

(A) Chest CT
(B) Cytologic evaluation and immunostaining of sputum
(C) Pulmonary function testing
(D) Follow-up in 6 months

Item 36 [Basic]

A healthy 42-year-old man has a 15-day history of a cough that was initially associated with rhinorrhea, nasal congestion, and a sore throat. All symptoms have resolved except the cough, which is productive of purulent sputum. He has not had fever, malaise, dyspnea, pleuritic chest pain, myalgia, paroxysms of coughing, or posttussive vomiting. The patient's medical history is unremarkable, he has never smoked cigarettes, and he takes no medications.

On physical examination, vital signs, including temperature, are normal. There is no pharyngeal erythema or exudate and no lymphadenopathy. The lungs are clear to auscultation.

Which of the following is the best initial management?

(A) Albuterol inhaler
(B) Azithromycin
(C) Chest radiograph
(D) Nasopharyngeal swab for influenza virus culture
(E) Symptomatic treatment

Item 37 [Basic]

A 66-year-old woman with chronic obstructive pulmonary disease is evaluated because of chronic cough and dyspnea. She currently uses a long-acting bronchodilator twice daily, an inhaled corticosteroid twice daily, ipratropium four times per day, and albuterol four to six times per day. She smokes 1 pack of cigarettes daily.

On physical examination, her vital signs are normal. Her oxygen saturation at rest and with exertion is 94%. She has diminished breath sounds, a prolonged expiratory phase, and no wheezes. Her cardiac examination is normal. Chest radiograph reveals hyperinflation, increased retrosternal airspace, and flattened hemidiaphragms bilaterally.

Which of the following should be done to manage this patient's cough and dyspnea?

(A) Help her quit smoking
(B) Increase the dosage of the inhaled corticosteroid
(C) Increase the dosage of the long-acting bronchodilator
(D) Start supplemental oxygen

Item 38 [Advanced]

A 54-year-old woman is evaluated because of a chronic cough and dyspnea on exertion of 6 years' duration. She has smoked 1.5 packs of cigarettes daily for 38 years. On physical examination, she has prolonged expiratory time and wheezes. Spirometry shows a FEV_1 of 2.2 L (66% of predicted) and an FEV_1/FVC ratio of 0.65.

If she is successful in stopping her cigarette smoking, which of the following changes in lung function can be expected?

(A) Improvement in lung function and a decrease in the rate of decline
(B) Improvement in lung function, but no decrease in the rate of decline
(C) No improvement in lung function, but a decrease in the rate of decline
(D) No improvement in lung function or decrease in the rate of decline

Item 39 [Basic]

A 49-year-old woman is evaluated for a routine physical examination. She has a sedentary lifestyle and does not exercise. She has not experienced chest pain or dyspnea. She is a current smoker with a 32-pack-year history. She takes no medications. Her father had a myocardial infarction at age 58 years.

On physical examination, her blood pressure is 132/85 mm Hg and her pulse rate is 86/min. Her BMI is 31. The remainder of the physical examination is normal.

Which of the following lifestyle modifications will have the greatest impact on reducing this patient's risk of cardiovascular disease?

(A) Aerobic exercise 30 minutes 3 or 4 days weekly
(B) Cessation of cigarette smoking
(C) Sodium-restricted diet
(D) Weight loss

Item 40 [Advanced]

A 52-year-old woman is evaluated at a routine appointment and seeks advice on smoking cessation. She smokes one and one half packs of cigarettes daily and wants help to stop. She has tried to stop smoking on three previous occasions, each time using nicotine replacement therapy, and she would like to try something different. She has a seizure disorder that is well controlled on valproate.

The patient is provided with a brief smoking cessation counseling intervention.

Which of the following is the most appropriate pharmacologic therapy?

(A) Bupropion
(B) Nortriptyline
(C) Sertraline
(D) Varenicline

Item 41 [Advanced]

A 43-year-old woman is evaluated for obesity. She has been unsuccessful at multiple attempts at weight loss, including several diets, meeting with a dietician, an exercise program, and a trial of orlistat. Medical history is remarkable for poorly controlled type 2 diabetes mellitus, hypertension, and hyperlipidemia. Medications are lisinopril, simvastatin, aspirin, metformin, and insulin glargine.

On physical examination, temperature is normal, blood pressure is 130/70 mm Hg, pulse rate is 79/min, and respiration rate is 16/min. BMI is 42. Other than changes associated with obesity, her physical examination is normal.

Hemoglobin A_{1c} is 9% and LDL cholesterol is 100 mg/dL (2.6 mmol/L).

Which of the following is the most appropriate management for her obesity?

(A) A regular walking program
(B) Bariatric surgery
(C) Low carbohydrate diet (Mediterranean style diet)
(D) Low fat diet

Item 42 [Advanced]

A 41-year-old asymptomatic man is evaluated during a routine physical examination. His only medical problem is obesity for which he has never sought treatment. Medical history is otherwise unremarkable, and he takes no medications.

On physical examination, temperature is normal, blood pressure is 127/79 mm Hg, pulse rate is 80/min, and respiration rate is 14/min. BMI is 39. Waist circumference is 112.2 cm (44 in). The remainder of the physical examination is normal.

The patient is counseled regarding his obesity.

Which of the following is the most appropriate initial evaluation for this patient?

(A) Complete blood count and serum electrolytes
(B) Electrocardiogram and chest x-ray
(C) Fasting glucose, lipid profile, and serum creatinine
(D) Sleep study and pulse oximetry

Item 43 [Advanced]

A 44-year-old woman is evaluated for obesity. She has been trying to lose weight over the past 3 years. The patient has tried several diets and has also attempted to increase her physical activity. Medical history is remarkable for type 2 diabetes mellitus, hypertension, and hyperlipidemia. Current medications are lisinopril, simvastatin, aspirin, metformin, and glipizide.

On physical examination, temperature is normal, blood pressure is 138/90 mm Hg, pulse rate is 72/min, and respiration rate is 14/min. BMI is 30. Her hemoglobin A_{1c} is 6.9%.

Which of the following is the most appropriate management option?

(A) Add orlistat
(B) Add sibutramine
(C) Discontinue glipizide, initiate insulin glargine
(D) Refer for bariatric surgery

Item 44 [Advanced]

A 41-year-old woman is evaluated for persistent nausea and vomiting after laparoscopic gastric bypass surgery 6 weeks ago for morbid obesity. The patient sometimes notices dull epigastric discomfort after the vomiting. She also has early satiety. She has lost 4.5 kg (10 lb) since her surgery. She takes naproxen for osteoarthritis.

On physical examination, vital signs are normal. BMI is 43. There is no abdominal discomfort to deep palpation.

Complete blood count, hepatic enzyme levels, and serum chemistry studies are normal.

Which of the following management options is the best choice for this patient?

(A) Omeprazole
(B) Right upper quadrant ultrasound
(C) Surgical laparotomy
(D) Upper endoscopy

Item 45 [Advanced]

A 60-year-old woman is evaluated for an unexplained weight loss during 1 year. The patient feels well and reports no fevers, night sweats, dysphagia, change in bowel habits, blood in her stool, joint pain, rash, or shortness of breath. She reports no depressed mood. She works as an accountant. She does not smoke or drink alcohol. Results of age- and sex-appropriate cancer screening tests performed 6 months ago were normal.

On physical examination, temperature is 37.0°C (98.6°F), blood pressure is 128/76 mm Hg, pulse rate is 84/min, and respiration rate is 16/min. BMI is 23. Her weight is 4.1 kg (9 lb) less than it was 12 months ago. The remainder of the physical examination is normal.

Hemoglobin	12.8 g/dL (128 g/L)
Creatinine	0.8 mg/dL (70.7 µmol/L)
Albumin	3.8 g/dL (38 g/L)
Aspartate aminotransferase	24 U/L
Alanine aminotransferase	27 U/L
C-reactive protein	0.1 mg/dL (1 mg/L)
Alkaline phosphatase	90 U/L
Lactate dehydrogenase	130 U/L
Thyroid-stimulating hormone	3 µU/mL (3 mU/L)

Chest x-ray and abdominal ultrasound examinations are normal.

Which of the following is the most appropriate management step?

(A) Begin dietary supplements
(B) Measure antinuclear antibodies
(C) Order chest CT
(D) Order upper endoscopy
(E) Re-evaluate in 6 months

Item 46 [Basic]

A 50-year-old man is evaluated for unintentional weight loss during a 1 year period. His appetite and energy level are reduced. He has lost interest in his usual activites, which he previously enjoyed. He also reports waking up several times per night. He reports no fevers, night sweats, fatigue, dysphagia, change in bowel habits, blood in his stool, joint pain, polydipsia, or shortness of breath. He works as a general contractor but has been out of work for several months. He does not smoke or drink alcohol. Results of age- and sex-appropriate cancer screening tests performed 6 months ago were normal.

On physical examination, temperature is 37.0°C (98.6°F), blood pressure is 120/74 mm Hg, pulse rate is 74/min and regular, and respiration rate is 16/min. BMI is 25.7. His weight today is 7.3 kg (16 lb) less than it was 1 year ago. The remainder of the physical examination is normal.

Hemoglobin	13.3 g/dL (133 g/L)
Fasting glucose	98 mg/dL (5.4 mmol/L)
Creatinine	1.0 mg/dL (70.7 µmol/L)
Albumin	3.7 g/dL (37 g/L)
Aspartate aminotransferase	24 U/L
Alanine aminotransferase	27 U/L
C-reactive protein	0.1 mg/dL (1 mg/L)
Alkaline phosphatase	90 U/L
Lactate dehydrogenase	130 U/L

Which of the following is the most likely cause of the patient's weight loss?

(A) Colon cancer
(B) Depression
(C) Prostate cancer
(D) Type 2 diabetes

Item 47 [Advanced]

A 65-year-old woman is seen for evaluation of unintentional weight loss. Her medical history is significant for depression that began 7 months ago and was treated with bupropion, which resulted in a rapid remission of symptoms. This was her first episode of depression. The patient now reports loss of appetite for several months but cannot precisely pinpoint when the symptom began. She has never smoked cigarettes, has no pulmonary or gastrointestinal symptoms, and has no other medical problems. Bupropion is her only medication, and she takes no supplements.

On examination, her weight has decreased by 4 kg (9 lb) from her baseline weight of 50 kg (110 lb) measured 6 months ago. No lymphadenopathy is present, and abdominal examination findings are normal.

Results of laboratory studies are normal, including a complete blood count, erythrocyte sedimentation rate determination, liver chemistry tests, and measurements of thyroid-stimulating hormone level, electrolyte levels, and serum creatinine level. A Pap test, colonoscopy, and mammography performed 1 year ago were negative for cancer.

What is the most appropriate next management step?

(A) CT of the chest, abdomen, and pelvis
(B) Discontinuation of the bupropion
(C) Initiation of an appetite stimulant, such as megestrol acetate
(D) Upper endoscopy

Item 48 [Advanced]

A 70-year-old woman is evaluated for a 6-month history of fatigue, an unintentional weight loss of 4.4 kg (10 lb), an increase in chronic cough with sputum production, and a decrease in exercise capacity. The patient has a 40-pack-year history of cigarette smoking but stopped smoking 10 years ago when chronic obstructive pulmonary disease was diagnosed. She has no other symptoms. Her medications are albuterol as needed, an inhaled corticosteroid, and salmeterol. She has been on stable dosages of these drugs for 18 months. Results of age- and sex-appropriate cancer screening tests performed 6 months ago were normal.

On physical examination, temperature is 37.5°C (99.5°F), blood pressure is 128/76 mm Hg, pulse rate is 94/min and regular, respiration rate is 16/min, and BMI is 20. A pulse oximetry reading is 60% on ambient air. Heart sounds are distant, and breath sounds are diminished bilaterally. There are no abdominal masses or organomegaly and no peripheral edema.

Hemoglobin	15 g/dL (150 g/L)
Creatinine	0.8 mg/dL (70.7 μmol/L)
Albumin	3.0 g/dL (30 g/L)
Thyroid-stimulating hormone	2.0 μU/mL (2.0 mU/L)

Spirometry shows an FEV_1 of 40% of predicted and an FEV_1 to FVC ratio of 45%. A chest radiograph shows only hyperinflation.

Which of the following is the most likely reason for this patient's weight loss?

(A) Breast cancer
(B) Cervical cancer
(C) Chronic obstructive pulmonary disease
(D) Colon cancer

Item 49 [Advanced]

A 42-year-old woman is evaluated for a 6-month history of heavy menstrual bleeding. She has been menstruating for the last 8 days and is still going through 10 pads or more a day with frequent clots. She has fatigue but no dizziness. Previous evaluation for this problem has included normal thyroid function and prolactin testing. She has no other medical problems and takes no medications. Pelvic ultrasonography has demonstrated a large posterior submucosal fibroid. A surgical treatment is planned in 2 weeks.

On examination, vital signs are normal. Her abdominal examination is benign, and the pelvic examination reveals a moderate amount of blood in the vaginal vault.

Hemoglobin level is 10.5 g/dL (105 g/L). Pregnancy test is negative.

Which of the following is the most appropriate next management step?

(A) Emergency surgery
(B) Intravenous estrogen
(C) Once daily oral contraceptives
(D) Oral medroxyprogesterone acetate
(E) Reevaluation in 1 week

Item 50 [Basic]

A 21-year-old woman is evaluated for a 7-year history of oligomenorrhea and slowly progressive hirsutism. Menses began at age 14 years and were always irregular. She has gained weight at a rate of approximately 4.5 kg (10 lb) per year. Her facial hair has become progressively thicker since age 18 years, and she now menstruates only three to four times per year. She is sexually active but does not want to become pregnant at this time. Family history is noncontributory, and she takes no medications.

On physical examination, vital signs are normal, and BMI is 28. Prominent terminal hairs are noted on the upper lip and chin, with some on the upper cheeks and chest; there is thick hair from the pubis to the umbilicus. Results of a pelvic examination and Pap smear are normal.

Dehydroepiandrosterone sulfate	4.3 µg/mL (11.6 µmol/L)
Human chorionic gonadotropin	Negative
17-Hydroxyprogesterone	105 ng/dL (3.1 nmol/L) (normal, <400 ng/dL [12.0 nmol/L])
Prolactin	11 ng/mL (11 µg/L)
Testosterone, total	84 ng/dL (2.9 nmol/L)

A progestin withdrawal challenge with medroxyprogesterone acetate results in a temporary resumption of menses.

Which of the following is the most likely diagnosis?

(A) Adrenal tumor
(B) Ovarian tumor
(C) Polycystic ovary syndrome
(D) Prolactinoma

Item 51 [Basic]

A 56-year-old woman is evaluated for hot flushes that have been interfering with her sleep and causing discomfort while at work. She wants some relief from her symptoms, which have been persistent since she experienced menopause 3 years ago. She is a nonsmoker and has no history of thromboembolic disease and no personal or family history of cancer.

Which of the following is the most appropriate treatment?

(A) Black cohosh
(B) Estrogen replacement therapy
(C) Raloxifene
(D) Red clover
(E) Soy protein

Item 52 [Advanced]

A 26-year-old woman is evaluated for a 4-month history of amenorrhea. Menses began at age 13 years. At age 18 years, the patient was placed on an oral contraceptive pill to control heavy bleeding. She discontinued the oral contraceptive pill 4 months ago because she and her husband want to become pregnant, and she has had no menses since then. There is no family history of infertility or premature menopause.

On physical examination, vital signs are normal, and BMI is 24. There is no acne, hirsutism, or galactorrhea. Examination of the thyroid gland and visual field testing yield normal findings. Pelvic examination findings are also normal. An office pregnancy test is negative.

Follicle-stimulating hormone	2 mU/mL (2 U/L)
Prolactin	17 ng/mL (17 µg/L)
Thyroid-stimulating hormone	1.1 µU/mL (1.1 mU/L)
Thyroxine (T_4), free	1.0 ng/dL (12.9 pmol/L)

Which of the following is the most appropriate next diagnostic test?

(A) Measurement of the plasma dehydroepiandrosterone sulfate level
(B) Measurement of serum estradiol level
(C) MRI of the pituitary gland
(D) Progestin withdrawal challenge

Item 53 [Advanced]

A 23-year-old woman is evaluated after having no menses for 6 months. She began menstruating at age 12 years, and menses have always been regular. The patient reports no recent weight gain, voice change, or facial hair growth; she says she may even have lost some weight recently and tends to feel warm. She is not sexually active. There is no family history of infertility or premature menopause.

On physical examination, vital signs are normal; and BMI is 22. She has no acne, hirsutism, or galactorrhea. Her thyroid gland is slightly enlarged. Visual field testing yields normal results.

Results of standard laboratory studies are normal, including thyroid-stimulating hormone and free thyroxine (T_4) levels; a human chorionic gonadotropin level is negative for pregnancy.

Which of the following is the most appropriate first step in evaluation?

(A) Brain MRI
(B) Measurement of serum follicle-stimulating hormone and prolactin levels
(C) Measurement of total serum testosterone level
(D) Pelvic ultrasonography

Item 54 [Advanced]

A 48-year-old woman presents with a history of heavy painless menstrual bleeding for the past 4 days. Her last period was 20 days ago, but before that, her periods had become more irregular over the previous 2 years, with lighter than usual bleeding.

On physical examination, the vital signs are normal. There is no evidence of hypovolemia or conjunctival pallor. The skin examination is negative for ecchymoses and petechiae. The bimanual pelvic examination reveals a nontender, normal-sized, and regular uterus. Speculum examination reveals a normal-appearing cervix with dark blood in the cervical os but no other abnormalities. A Pap smear is performed. A urine pregnancy test is negative.

Which of the following is the most appropriate next management step?

(A) Begin an oral contraceptive
(B) Begin estrogen replacement therapy
(C) Measure serum luteinizing hormone and follicle-stimulating hormone
(D) Obtain an endometrial biopsy

Item 55 [Basic]

A 56-year-old man is evaluated for a fever and a 2-day history of an expanding, well-demarcated area of warmth, swelling, tenderness, and erythema on his right foot, leg, and upper thigh. He reports feeling feverish and slightly nauseated, but has not had chills, rigors, or itching. His medical history is significant for varicose veins and chronic ankle edema. He takes no medications.

On physical examination, temperature is 37.8°C (100.0°F), blood pressure is 140/88 mm Hg, and pulse rate is 100/min.

His skin findings are shown (Plate 2). The remainder of the physical examination is normal.

Which of the following is the most likely diagnosis?

(A) Allergic contact dermatitis
(B) Atopic dermatitis
(C) Cellulitis
(D) Venous stasis dermatitis

Item 56 [Advanced]

A 65-year-old man is evaluated for a recurrent, itchy, erythematous rash that involves his eyebrows and cheeks. He has tried topical antibiotic ointment without effect. He reports no fever, photosensitivity, arthralgia, muscle weakness, flushing, or any other symptoms. He has no other medical problems and takes no medications.

On physical examination, his vital signs are normal. The rash is shown (Plate 3). The remainder of the physical examination is normal.

Which of the following is the most likely diagnosis?

(A) Dermatomyositis
(B) Rosacea
(C) Seborrheic dermatitis
(D) Systemic lupus erythematosus

Item 57 [Basic]

A 58-year-old man is evaluated because of a chronic skin rash involving the groin. The condition has been present for so long that he cannot remember when it started, but it probably has been present for a year or more. It is minimally symptomatic but does itch. He has no other medical problems and takes no medications.

The skin rash in the groin is shown (Plate 4). He also has a scaling eruption on the sides of his feet.

Which of the following is the most likely diagnosis?

(A) Cutaneous candidiasis
(B) Psoriasis
(C) Seborrheic dermatitis
(D) Tinea cruris

Item 58 [Basic]

A 28-year-old man is evaluated in the emergency department for an 8-hour history of fever, malaise, and a rash on his shoulders, lower back, arms, and palms. Ten days ago he was started on oral trimethoprim-sulfamethoxazole therapy for methicillin-resistant *Staphylococcus aureus* cellulitis. His last dose of trimethoprim-sulfamethoxazole was taken this morning. He takes no other medications and has no allergies.

On physical examination, temperature is 38.6°C (101.4°F), blood pressure is 110/70 mm Hg, pulse rate is 110/min, and respiration rate is 20/min. There are erythematous, urticarial, targetoid plaques on the shoulders that are studded with small, tense blisters. Erythematous targetoid lesions are also noted on the lower back and palms. There are small vesicles and crusts on the upper and lower lips, as well as small areas of erosion on the soft palate. His eye examination is normal. All totaled, the rash involves less than 10% of the patient's body surface area.

Which of the following is the most likely diagnosis?

(A) Allergic contact dermatitis
(B) Cellulitis
(C) "Red man syndrome"
(D) Stevens-Johnson syndrome

Item 59 [Advanced]

A 33-year-old woman is evaluated for a 3-day history of a rash on her palms. The rash first appeared on her palms as small red macules that increased in size over 24 to 48 hours, followed by the appearance of similar lesions on her arms and sores in her mouth. Three months ago she had a similar episode that resolved spontaneously. She takes no medications or supplements. She has not been exposed to anyone with similar skin lesions, but she did recently travel to North Carolina. She has a remote history of genital herpes but has had no outbreaks in several years.

On physical examination, she appears well. Temperature is 37.2°C (98.9°F), blood pressure is 118/70 mm Hg, and pulse rate is 68/min. Typical lesions are shown (Plate 5).

Which of the following is most likely diagnosis?

(A) Erythema multiforme
(B) Lyme disease
(C) Rocky Mountain spotted fever
(D) Streptococcal infection

Item 60 [Basic]

A 70-year-old man has a 1-day history of a painful rash on the left side of his chest. Three days before the rash became apparent; he developed severe pain and paresthesias in the same area.

Skin examination findings of the left side of the chest are shown (Plate 6).

The remainder of the examination findings are unremarkable.

In addition to analgesic agents, which of the following is the most appropriate treatment?

(A) Corticosteroids
(B) Intravenous acyclovir
(C) Oral famciclovir
(D) Topical penciclovir

Item 61 [Advanced]

A 45-year-old woman is evaluated in the office for a facial rash of 6 months' duration that involves the cheeks and nose. She is unsure if sun exposure worsens the rash. She does not have a rash elsewhere and does not have fatigue, ulcers, serositis, or joint pain.

Physical examination reveals a rash that is limited to the face as shown (Plate 7).

The remainder of the examination is unremarkable.

Which of the following is the most likely diagnosis?

(A) Dermatomyositis
(B) Psoriasis
(C) Rosacea
(D) Seborrheic dermatitis
(E) Systemic lupus erythematosus

Item 62 [Basic]

A 76-year-old man is seen in the office for a routine physical examination. He is healthy and has no complaints about his health, takes no medications, and does not smoke or drink alcohol. Until he retired 5 years ago, he was a farmer. On physical examination, several darkly pigmented lesions are noted on his trunk, as shown (Plate 8).

Which of the following is the most likely diagnosis?

(A) Basal cell carcinoma
(B) Malignant melanoma
(C) Seborrheic keratoses
(D) Squamous cell carcinoma

Item 63 [Advanced]

A 17-year-old male high school student is evaluated for acne. The acne has been present for 4 years but seems to be getting worse rather than better as he gets older. He has tried to control the acne by showering and scrubbing with soap and water at least twice per day. He has never been on any medications for his acne. He has no other medical problems, takes no medications, and has no allergies.

On physical examination, the acne is extensively distributed on the face, shoulders, back, and chest. The back is shown (Plate 9).

Which of the following is the best initial treatment for this patient?

(A) Oral antibiotics
(B) Oral isotretinoin
(C) Salicylic acid
(D) Topical retinoid

Item 64 [Basic]

A 34-year-old woman has a 1-week history of generalized, very pruritic, red plaques and papules that appear suddenly, last for less than 24 hours, then disappear only to reappear at a different body location. She has had these itchy bumps before, and they spontaneously resolved after 1 to 2 weeks. She has no idea what makes the rash appear or disappear. She typically treats the itching with over-the-counter antihistamines.

On physical examination, vital signs are normal. A representative skin lesion is shown (Plate 10).

What is the most likely diagnosis?

(A) Acute urticaria
(B) Angioedema
(C) Chronic urticaria
(D) Erythema multiforme

Item 65 [Basic]

A 25-year-old woman is evaluated for swollen glands located in her neck, under her arms, and in her groin. They are not tender. Two weeks ago, she had a head cold and a sore throat and felt hot and sweaty for a few days. All symptoms resolved in about a week. She has no other symptoms, and her weight has been stable. She takes no medications. She has traveled to Peru several times during the past 3 years but has never gotten ill and follows all the travel recommendations for vaccines and disease prevention. She does not smoke or use alcohol or other drugs. She has never had a sexually transmitted disease.

On physical examination, her vital signs are normal and she appears healthy. She has anterior and posterior cervical, axillary, and inguinal lymphadenopathy. The nodes are all nontender, rubbery, and mobile. Most are less than a centimeter, although the largest is 1.5 cm in the left groin.

Which of the following is the most appropriate next step in the management of this patient?

(A) Biopsy of the largest lymph node
(B) Complete blood count and chest radiograph
(C) Epstein-Barr early antigen antibody (anti-EA) test
(D) Reassurance and watchful waiting

Item 66 [Advanced]

A 42-year-old woman is evaluated for a lump under her right arm present for 1 month. It is nontender and enlarging. She has never had a mammogram. She otherwise feels well. She has no chronic medical conditions, takes no medications, and has no family history of malignancy. She does not smoke, drink alcohol, or use other drugs. She had a positive tuberculin skin test (PPD) 15 years ago that was treated with isoniazid for 9 months. HIV testing and chest radiograph were negative at the time.

On physical examination, her vital signs are normal. A 2.5-cm, firm, mobile, nontender lymph node is present in the right axilla. No dominant mass is palpated in either breast. The remainder of a complete physical examination is normal.

Which of the following is the most appropriate initial step in the management of this patient?

(A) Chest radiograph
(B) Lymph node aspirate
(C) Lymph node biopsy
(D) Repeat examination in 2 months

Item 67 [Basic]

A 66-year-old woman, who resides in a nursing home, is evaluated for urinary incontinence. Neither the nursing home staff nor family members report previous problems with incontinence. Medical history is significant for a cerebrovascular accident with severe aphasia and left hemiparesis, hypertension, and type 2 diabetes mellitus. Current medications are aspirin, dipyridamole, lisinopril, pravastatin, and glipizide.

On physical examination, temperature is 36.8°C (98.2°F), blood pressure is 164/96 mm Hg, pulse rate is 92/min, and respiration rate is 18/min. Arterial oxygen saturation is 98% on ambient air. Results of cardiopulmonary, abdominal, and rectal examinations are normal. On neurologic examination, the patient is confused. There is expressive aphasia and moderate weakness of the left arm and leg.

Complete blood count	Normal
Calcium	Normal
Creatinine	1.2 mg/dL (106.1 µmol/L)
Glucose	100 mg/dL (5.6 mmol/L)
Electrolytes	Normal
Urinalysis	2+ glucose, moderate protein, 40-50 leukocytes and 3-5 erythrocytes/hpf

Which of the following is the best management for this patient's incontinence?

(A) Begin ciprofloxacin
(B) Discontinue glipizide
(C) Insert an indwelling urinary catheter
(D) Schedule a CT scan of the head

Item 68 [Advanced]

A 78-year-old man comes for a routine annual physical examination. The patient feels well. He is accompanied by his wife, who is concerned about his hearing. The review of systems is normal, and the patient states that he does not have any difficulty hearing.

Which of the following is the best way to screen this patient for hearing impairment?

(A) Administer the Screening Hearing Handicap Inventory
(B) Perform the Weber and Rinne tests
(C) Perform the whispered-voice test
(D) Refer for audiometric testing
(E) No further evaluation is needed

Item 69 [Advanced]

An 82-year-old woman is evaluated in the office after having fallen in her home 2 days ago. She states that she "tripped." She did not have prodromal symptoms, including loss of consciousness, dizziness, lightheadedness, or imbalance. There is no history of falls. Medical history is significant for hypertension. Current medications are hydrochlorothiazide and lisinopril.

On physical examination, the patient is alert and oriented. Temperature is 36.9°C (98.5°F), blood pressure is 140/85 mm Hg without postural changes, pulse rate is 74/min, and respiration rate is 17/min. BMI is 36. Visual acuity is 20/40 in both eyes with glasses. The cardiopulmonary and neurologic examinations are normal.

Which of the following diagnostic studies should be done next?

(A) CT scan of the head
(B) "Get up and go" test
(C) 24-Hour electrocardiographic monitoring
(D) Transthoracic echocardiography

Item 70 [Advanced]

A 68-year-old man has a 6-month history of urinary incontinence that occurs two to three times each week and results in loss of about one cup of urine each time. Before most episodes, he feels the need to urinate but often is unable to get to the bathroom in time. He started wearing adult diapers 1 month ago. The patient has not had dysuria, urinary frequency or hesitancy, nocturia, or postvoid dribbling. He has recently noted some memory loss. Although his wife has taken over managing their finances, the patient continues to drive and perform all activities of daily living but has stopped playing golf because of embarrassment about his incontinence. Medical history is significant for osteoarthritis of the right knee and hyperlipidemia. Current medications are acetaminophen and pravastatin.

Vital signs are normal. Abdominal examination shows no suprapubic mass or tenderness. On rectal examination, the prostate gland is normal. His score on the Mini–Mental State Examination is 23/30 (normal is ≥24/30). The remainder of the neurologic examination is normal. Pertinent laboratory results, including serum creatinine, electrolytes, and prostate-specific antigen levels, are normal. A urinalysis is normal, and a urine culture is negative.

Which of the following medications should be prescribed?

(A) Doxazosin
(B) Imipramine
(C) Oxybutynin
(D) Phenylpropanolamine

Item 71 [Basic]

A 78-year-old asymptomatic man comes for an initial routine office visit. Medical history is significant for hypertension and hyperlipidemia, and current medications are hydrochlorothiazide, atenolol, and simvastatin. The patient has never smoked. His wife recently had a stroke, and the couple just moved from their home of many years to live in an assisted living facility. The results of a routine screening examination and laboratory tests are normal.

Which of the following screening tests should be done next?

(A) Abdominal ultrasonography
(B) Ankle-brachial index
(C) Depression screening
(D) Mini–Mental State Examination

Item 72 [Advanced]

An 89-year-old woman is evaluated for dizziness that she has had for the past year, mainly while standing and ambulating. The dizziness is described as a sense of unsteadiness. The symptoms can last for minutes to hours, and she has at least 4 to 5 episodes per day. She does not describe other motor or sensory symptoms. Medical history is remarkable for a 15-year history of type 2 diabetes mellitus, hypertension, and hyperlipidemia. Current medications are hydrochlorothiazide, ramipril, simvastatin, metformin, insulin glargine, and low-dose aspirin.

Vital signs are normal; there is no evidence of orthostasis. A cardiopulmonary examination is normal. The patient has a positive Romberg sign and is unsteady on tandem gait. Rapid alternating movements are slowed. The patient has a corrected visual acuity of 20/50 in the right eye and 20/70 in the left eye. Vibratory sense and light touch are diminished in a stocking pattern in the lower extremities. She has no motor abnormalities and no cranial nerve abnormalities. A Dix-Hallpike maneuver does not elicit vertigo or nystagmus.

A complete blood count, metabolic profile, and thyroid function studies are normal.

Which of the following management options is the best choice for this patient?

(A) Brain MRI
(B) Meclizine
(C) Physical therapy
(D) Replace aspirin with aspirin/extended-release dipyridamole

Item 73 [Basic]

A 22-year-old man comes for a routine evaluation. He feels well but has gained 6.8 kg (15 lb) during the past 4 years. He has a sedentary job as a software engineer, has a 3-pack-year history of cigarette smoking, and consumes two beers on most nights. His parents both have hypertension, and his mother has type 2 diabetes mellitus.

On physical examination, blood pressure is 140/95 mm Hg, pulse rate is 90/min, and respiration rate is 12/min; BMI is 29. There is no evidence of edema.

Laboratory studies, including a plasma fasting glucose level, fasting lipid panel, serum electrolyte level, serum creatinine level, and urinalysis results, are normal.

Which of the following is the most appropriate next management step?

(A) Atenolol
(B) Diltiazem
(C) Hydrochlorothiazide
(D) Lifestyle modifications
(E) Lisinopril

Item 74 [Advanced]

An 85-year-old woman comes for a follow-up evaluation of hypertension. She does not smoke and adheres to a Dietary Approaches to Stop Hypertension (DASH) diet. At an office visit 1 month ago, her blood pressure was 170/70 mm Hg. She was diagnosed with hypertension and chronic stable angina 7 years ago and currently takes metoprolol, sublingual nitroglycerin as needed, and aspirin.

On physical examination, blood pressure is 186/70 mm Hg, pulse rate is 60/min, and respiration rate is 12/min; BMI is 22. Cardiopulmonary examination reveals no jugular venous distention, carotid bruits, murmur, extra cardiac sounds, or pulmonary crackles. The abdomen is soft without masses or bruits. Neurologic examination findings are normal.

Electrolytes	Normal
Blood urea nitrogen	20 mg/dL (7.1 mmol/L)
Creatinine	1.2 mg/dL (106.0 μmol/L)
Urinalysis	Normal

Which of the following is the most appropriate additional therapy?

(A) Chlorthalidone
(B) Lisinopril
(C) Losartan
(D) Terazosin

Item 75 [Basic]

A 55-year-old man comes for a follow-up office visit after laboratory studies reveal a diagnosis of type 2 diabetes mellitus. He has no history of heart or kidney disease.

On physical examination, he is afebrile; blood pressure is 138/84 mm Hg, pulse rate is 78/min, and respiration rate is 16/min. BMI is 28. The remainder of the examination is normal.

Laboratory studies show normal serum electrolyte, blood urea nitrogen, and serum creatinine levels and a urine albumin-creatinine ratio of 20 mg/g.

Which of the following is the maximal allowable target blood pressure for this patient?

(A) Less than 115/75 mm Hg
(B) Less than 125/75 mm Hg
(C) Less than 130/80 mm Hg
(D) Less than 140/90 mm Hg

Item 76 [Advanced]

An asymptomatic 25-year-old man is evaluated for hypertension diagnosed during a recent pre-employment physical examination. He does not remember being told about hypertension in the past, and he has no family history of hypertension. He is not taking any medications.

On physical examination, his blood pressure is 170/60 mm Hg in both arms. The heart rate is 65/min and regular. Carotid examination is normal; estimated central venous pressure is normal. The apical impulse is displaced and sustained. An ejection click is noted at the apex and left sternal border.

There is a grade 2/6 early systolic murmur noted at the second right intercostal space. No diastolic murmur is noted over the anterior precordium. Systolic and diastolic murmurs are noted over the patient's back. There is no abdominal bruit. The lower extremity pulses are reduced and delayed.

A chest radiograph is shown.

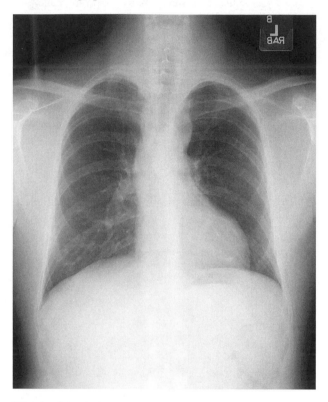

Which of the following is the most likely diagnosis in this patient?

(A) Coarctation of the aorta
(B) Essential hypertension
(C) Pheochromocytoma
(D) Renal artery stenosis

Item 77 [Advanced]

A 35-year-old man comes for a new patient evaluation. He takes no medications. His parents both have diabetes mellitus.

On physical examination, blood pressure is 165/104 mm Hg and BMI is 31. The remainder of the examination is unremarkable.

Laboratory studies, including serum electrolyte, blood urea nitrogen, and creatinine levels and urinalysis results, are normal.

Lifestyle modifications are recommended, but blood pressure findings are unchanged on a subsequent visit 2 weeks later.

Administration of which of the following is the most appropriate treatment?

(A) Hydrochlorothiazide
(B) Lisinopril and hydrochlorothiazide
(C) Metoprolol
(D) Terazosin

Item 78 [Basic]

A 50-year-old woman is evaluated during a routine office visit. She is asymptomatic and takes no medications. Her father and sister have essential hypertension.

On physical examination, vital signs are normal except for a blood pressure of 136/86 mm Hg. BMI is 24. The remainder of the physical examination, including cardiopulmonary and funduscopic examinations, is normal.

The blood pressure is confirmed on three other occasions, twice outside the office.

Which of the following is the most appropriate next step in management?

(A) Ambulatory blood pressure monitoring
(B) Hydrochlorothiazide
(C) Lifestyle modification
(D) Lisinopril

General Internal Medicine
Answers and Critiques

Item 1   Answer: C
Educational Objective: *Calculate sensitivity and specificity.*

The sensitivity and specificity of the new screening test for prostate cancer is 0.8. All tests should be compared with a gold standard, which represents the current practice standard; for prostate cancer, it is the prostate biopsy. (Figure) Sensitivity quantifies the percentage of patients with disease (in this case, patients with a positive prostate cancer biopsy) who have a positive screening test. Sensitivity is equal to a/(a + c). Specificity quantifies the percentage of normal patients (a negative biopsy for prostate cancer) with a negative screening test. Specificity is equal to d/(b + d).

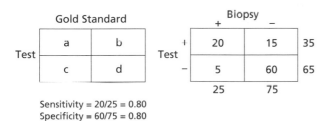

Sensitivity = 20/25 = 0.80
Specificity = 60/75 = 0.80

A highly sensitive test reduces the probability of missing the diagnosis. Because a highly sensitive screening identifies most patients with the condition, a negative screening test helps to "rule out" the diagnosis. Highly sensitive tests often have a high false-positive rate (positive test results in patients without the disease). Therefore, a positive screening test is usually followed by a highly specific (and sometimes more invasive) test, which often is the gold standard for the diagnosis. Because a highly specific test is negative in patients without the disease, a positive test helps "rule in" the diagnosis. The concepts of sensitivity and specificity can be remembered by the mnemonics "SpIN" and "SnOUT," indicating that a very specific test, when positive, rules in a disease and a highly sensitive test, when negative, rules out disease.

KEY POINT

A highly specific test, when positive, rules in a disease, and a highly sensitive test, when negative, rules out a disease.

Bibliography
Akobeng AK. Understanding diagnostic tests 1: sensitivity, specificity and predictive values. Acta Paediatr. 2007;96(3):338-41. [PMID: 17407452]

Item 2   Answer: C
Educational Objective: *Understand the effect of disease prevalence on sensitivity, specificity, likelihood ratios, and predictive values.*

The measure that is most likely to change is the positive predictive value. Sensitivity and specificity are test characteristics that do not change as populations vary. Likelihood ratios are based on sensitivity and specificity and do not change as populations vary. Predictive values address the chance of disease given a positive or negative test result and are based on the prevalence of disease in the population being tested; therefore, predictive values do change as the populations vary. As the prevalence of disease decreases (for example, the prevalence in the community compared with that in an experiment), the positive predictive value decreases and the negative predictive value increases. The opposite is true if the disease prevalence increases. The example below demonstrates these concepts.

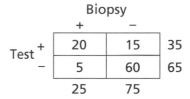

Disease prevalence 25%

Sensitivity = 20/25 = 0.80
Specificity = 60/75 = 0.80
Positive predictive value = 20/35 = 0.57
Negative predictive value = 60/65 = 0.92

Disease prevalence 2.5%

Test	Biopsy +	−	
+	20	150	170
−	5	600	605
	25	750	

Sensitivity = 20/25 = 0.80
Specificity = 600/750 = 0.80
Positive predictive value = 20/170 = 0.11
Negative predictive value = 600/605 = 0.99

Predictive values change with disease prevalence whereas sensitivity, specificity and likelihood ratios do not.

Bibliography

Akobeng AK. Understanding diagnostic tests 1: sensitivity, specificity and predictive values. Acta Paediatr. 2007;96(3):338-41. [PMID: 17407452]

Item 3   Answer: D

Educational Objective: *Calculate the positive predictive value of a diagnostic test.*

The probability that this patient has HIV disease is approximately 0.5%. The reliability of screening tests is a function of the test's sensitivity and specificity as well as the prevalence of the disease in the population under consideration. In this clinical scenario, disease prevalence of 1 in 10,000 translates to 10 patients with HIV infection in a population of 100,000 subjects. A test that is 98% sensitive will correctly identify 9.8 of these patients as having HIV infection. This is the true positive (TP) rate. This number is derived by multiplying the number of subjects with disease by the test's sensitivity (10×0.98). In this same population of 100,000 subjects, 99,990 subjects do not have disease ($100,000 - 10$). A test that is 98% specific will correctly identify 97,900 patients with a negative test result. This is the true negative (TN) rate. This number is derived by multiplying the number of subjects without disease by the test's specificity ($99,990 \times 0.98$). However, this also means that 2090 normal subjects will have a false positive (FP) test result (the difference between 99,990 subjects without HIV and 97,900 with a TN test result).

The positive predictive value (PPV) answers the question, "What is the probability that a positive test result is a true positive result?" PPV is calculated as the true positive rate divided by all positive test results. In this example, the PPV = TP/(TP + FP) = $9.8/(2090 + 9.8) = 0.0046$. This phenomenon underscores the need for specific confirmatory tests, such as Western blot analysis in this case, and the hazards of screening for disease in populations at low risk.

The positive predictive value (PPV) is calculated as the true positive rate divided by all positive test results.

Bibliography

Akobeng AK. Understanding diagnostic tests 1: sensitivity, specificity and predictive values. Acta Paediatr. 2007;96(3):338-41. [PMID: 17407452]

Item 4   Answer: D

Educational Objective: *Use a likelihood ratio to calculate posttest probability.*

The likelihood ratio (LR) of a test is the proportion of patients with the disease who test positive divided by the proportion of patients without the disease who also test positive. The numerator of this ratio is the test's sensitivity; the denomina-

tor is the false-positive rate for the test. LRs can be used to approximate the probability of disease after a test is performed, but to perform this function, three associations must be remembered: positive LRs of 2, 5, and 10 increase the probability of disease by 15%, 30%, and 45%, respectively. An appendiceal CT scan has a positive LR for appendicitis of 13.3; therefore, if the pretest probability of appendicitis was 50%, a positive scan result increases the probability for disease by roughly 45%, resulting in a posttest probability of 95% (45% added to the 50% pretest probability of disease).

Positive likelihood ratios of 2, 5, and 10 increase the probability of disease by 15%, 30%, and 45%, respectively.

Bibliography

McGee S. Simplifying likelihood ratios. J Gen Intern Med. 2002;17:646-9. [PMID: 12213147]

Item 5   Answer: A

Educational Objective: *Compare different tests using a receiver operating characteristic (ROC) curve.*

Test A has the best overall performance. Many test outcomes are continuous variables, which are arbitrarily divided at some point into normal and abnormal values by using a cut point. One way to visually compare the operating characteristics of different tests is to plot the cut points of each test on a receiver operating characteristic (ROC) curve. The ROC curve is a visual representation of the true positive rate (sensitivity) plotted as a function of the false positive rate (1.0-specificity) for different cut points. A test with the best sensitivity and specificity for each of its cut points will have a curve that "crowds" the upper left margins of the ROC curve. This concept is particularly valuable when comparing two or more tests. The test with the greatest overall accuracy will have the largest area under the ROC curve and will be located closest to the upper left corner.

In a comparison of two or more tests on a receiver operating characteristic (ROC) curve, the test with the best overall accuracy for each of its cut points will have the largest area under the ROC curve.

Bibliography

Akobeng AK. Understanding diagnostic tests 3: receiver operating characteristic curves. Acta Paediatr. 2007;96(5):644-647. Epub 2007 Mar 21. [PMID: 17376185]

Item 6   Answer: A

Educational Objective: *Screen for abdominal aortic aneurysm with abdominal ultrasonography.*

One-time screening for abdominal aortic aneurysm (AAA) with ultrasonography is recommended for all men aged 65 to 75 years who have ever smoked. Data from randomized clinical trials indicate that ultrasound identification and repair of

AAA larger than 5 cm in diameter reduces AAA-related mortality in older men. Death from abdominal aortic aneurysm rupture is rare after a single normal screening test and repeat screening in these persons is not recommended.

The U.S. Preventive Services Task Force recommends that women aged 65 years and older be screened routinely for osteoporosis and that routine screening begin at age 60 years for women at increased risk for osteoporotic fractures. The evidence is not as strong for men, but screening may be indicated for men with certain risk factors (such as long-term corticosteroid use, androgen deprivation). This man has no high-risk factors to warrant screening.

The pneumococcal vaccine is associated with substantial reductions in morbidity and mortality among the elderly and high-risk adults and is, therefore, recommended for all adults aged 65 years and older or with other risk factors (diabetes, cirrhosis, asplenia). Patients who receive their initial vaccine at older than 65 years of age should receive a second dose after 5 years. One-time revaccination is also recommended in 5 years for patients with chronic kidney disease, asplenia, or cancer or those who are immunosuppressed. This patient has no indication for revaccination.

Routine screening for coronary artery disease in asymptomatic persons without cardiovascular risk factors is not recommended. Screening electrocardiograms are not recommended because abnormalities of the resting electrocardiogram are rare, not specific for coronary artery disease, and do not predict subsequent mortality from coronary disease. Exercise testing may identify persons with coronary artery disease, but two factors limit routine testing in asymptomatic adults. First, the prevalence of significant coronary artery disease is low in this population, rendering the predictive value of a positive exercise test low (false-positive results are common). Second, abnormalities of exercise testing do not accurately predict major coronary events in asymptomatic persons.

KEY POINT

One-time screening for abdominal aortic aneurysm with ultrasonography is recommended for all men aged 65 to 75 years who have ever smoked.

Bibliography
Lederle FA. In the clinic. Abdominal aortic aneurysm. Ann Intern Med. 2009;150(9):ITC5-1-ITC5-15. [PMID: 19414835]

Item 7   Answer: E

Educational Objective: *Immunize a patient with chronic obstructive pulmonary disease against influenza with trivalent killed vaccine.*

The most appropriate immunization strategy for this patient is trivalent killed influenza vaccination. Annual influenza vaccination is recommended in patients with chronic obstructive pulmonary disease (COPD), regardless of their age. For the 2010-2011 influenza season, the Centers for Disease Control

and Prevention has recommended universal annual influenza vaccination for all persons age 6 months and older.

If this patient received influenza and pneumococcal vaccination 1 year ago, he needs only influenza vaccination. Pneumococcal vaccination is recommended for all adults older than 65 years and for younger patients who are active smokers or who have COPD, asthma, and other disorders that increase their risk for invasive pneumococcal disease. Influenza vaccination is also recommended for pregnant women whose last two trimesters coincide with the influenza season (late December through mid-March). The main vaccine used in the United States is a trivalent inactivated virus, but an intranasally administered vaccine from a trivalent live attenuated virus is also available for patients age 5 to 49 years who are not pregnant, immunosuppressed, or living with an immunosuppressed person. Because of the patient's age, the most appropriate vaccination is the trivalent killed influenza vaccination.

A single revaccination with pneumococcal vaccine is recommended in adults older than 65 years if they were vaccinated more than 5 years previously at a time when they were less then 65 years of age and in immunosuppressed patients 5 years or more after the first dose. Patients with COPD who received their first pneumococcal vaccination after age 65 years do not need revaccination.

KEY POINT

Influenza vaccination is recommended annually for all patients with chronic obstructive pulmonary disease, regardless of age.

Bibliography
Hessen MT. In the clinic. Influenza. Ann Intern Med. 2009;151(9): ICT5-1-ICT5-15. [PMID: 19894285]

Item 8   Answer: D

Educational Objective: *Recognize the relative importance of the most commonly reported end points in cancer screening studies.*

Lung cancer–specific mortality is the best end point for measuring the effect of cancer screening on patient outcomes. The case-fatality ratio (the number of deaths from a specific cancer divided by the number of patients with that cancer) is subject to serious artifacts from *length bias*, which is the preferential detection of asymptomatic, more indolent cancers by any screening test. These cancers are more likely to be detected during screening because they are detectable for a greater length of time than faster growing, more aggressive cancers. Likewise, patient survival after cancer diagnosis is artificially prolonged by screening because of length bias as well as *lead-time bias*, which is an advance in the date of cancer diagnosis without necessarily changing the patient's outcome. Although a screening test that resulted in a higher incidence of early-stage cancer would suggest an improvement in life expectancy, the relative shift in the proportion of patients diagnosed at early stages is not a good assessment of screening-test efficacy due to selection of less aggressive tumors (length bias). An absolute decrease in the incidence of late-stage (metastatic) cancer is an early indicator that a test may be effective because metastatic cancer frequently leads to death; however, lead-time bias and the resulting stage shift may still confound the absolute incidence of late-stage disease. Cause-specific mortality is least subject to the above potentially confounding effects.

KEY POINT

Cancer-specific mortality is the best end point for measuring the effect of cancer screening on patient outcomes.

Bibliography

Gates TJ. Screening for cancer: evaluating the evidence. Am Fam Physician. 2001;63:513-22. [PMID: 11272300]

Item 9 Answer: C

Educational Objective: *Immunize a patient with a previous history of herpes zoster with the zoster vaccine.*

The most appropriate strategy is zoster vaccination now. The zoster vaccine is indicated in immunocompetent patients older than 60 years for prevention of herpes zoster (shingles). Live attenuated zoster vaccine in adults 60 years or older reduces the incidence of herpes zoster by 51% and postherpetic neuralgia by 67%. The vaccine is more efficacious in preventing herpes zoster among adults 60 to 69 years of age than among those 70 years or older. On the other hand, the vaccine prevents postherpetic neuralgia to a greater extent among adults aged 70 years or more. A reported history of possible herpes zoster is not a contraindication to vaccination. While recurrence of herpes zoster is rare, there are no recognized safety concerns in giving the vaccine to a patient with a history of shingles. Excluding patients with a possible history would be a barrier to vaccination and impose a burden on physicians to assess the reliability of the prior diagnosis.

The zoster vaccine is a live vaccine and is contraindicated in people with active, untreated tuberculosis; in pregnant women; in immunocompromised patients; and in patients receiving chemotherapy, radiotherapy, or large doses of corticosteroids. Immunization should be avoided if an immunocompromised person is living in the household.

Zoster vaccine can be given concomitantly with all other live and inactivated vaccines, including influenza and pneumococcal vaccine. Zoster vaccine is given as a single subcutaneous dose. A booster dose is not recommended.

More than 99% of patients 40 years or older have serologic evidence of prior varicella infection. Therefore, routine serologic testing for varicella antibodies to determine who should be vaccinated is not cost-effective or necessary.

KEY POINT

Zoster vaccine is indicated in all patients age 60 years and older without contraindications, regardless of history of prior varicella infection.

Bibliography

Advisory Committee on Immunization Practices. Recommended adult immunization schedule: United States, 2010. Ann Intern Med. 2010;152(1):36-39. [PMID: 20048270]

Item 10 Answer: A

Educational Objective: *Provide the appropriate tetanus prevention strategy in a patient with an infected wound.*

This patient should receive tetanus-diphtheria toxoid and acellular pertussis (Tdap) vaccine. All patients evaluated for wounds should have their tetanus vaccination status reviewed. Most patients who develop tetanus are not completely vaccinated. If there is any doubt about a patient's vaccination history, the complete series should be administered. The first dose and second dose should be separated by 4 weeks, and the third dose should be given 6 to 12 months later. Because susceptibility to tetanus and diphtheria often co-exist, both tetanus and diphtheria toxoid (Td) should be administered, not just tetanus toxoid alone. It is also recommended that the Tdap vaccine be used in place of one of the Td vaccinations in adults age 19 to 64 years who have not received their single recommended booster dose of this vaccine.

Tetanus immune globulin is indicated for patients who have not completed the primary series of tetanus immunizations or in patients who have an unclear immunization history. As this patient's immunization history is clear, tetanus immune globulin is not indicated.

Tetanus booster vaccination can be omitted in patients who received a tetanus booster within the past 5 years and in patients with clean minor wounds who have received vaccination within the past 10 years. However, this patient's wound is infected, and his last booster was 8 years ago. Therefore, Tdap vaccine should be administered.

KEY POINT

Tetanus booster vaccination can be omitted in patients who received a tetanus booster within the past 5 years and in patients with clean minor wounds who have received vaccination within the past 10 years.

Bibliography

Advisory Committee on Immunization Practices. Recommended adult immunization schedule: United States, 2010. Ann Intern Med. 2010;152(1):36-39. [PMID: 20048270]

Item 11   Answer: D

Educational Objective: *Immunize against human papillomavirus.*

The most appropriate option for this patient is human papillomavirus (HPV) vaccination now. The Advisory Committee on Immunization Practices of the Centers for Disease Control and Prevention recommends HPV vaccine for cervical cancer prevention. The vaccine is recommended for all females between ages 9 and 26 years regardless of sexual activity. The vaccine has a high success rate in preventing infections with HPV strains which cause most cases of genital warts and cervical cancer.

HPV infection is predominantly spread by sexual contact. This patient states she is not sexually active. However, the vaccine should be recommended now as it is of low risk, and vaccine efficacy lasts for at least several years. The vaccine does not protect against all types of HPV, and roughly 30% of cervical cancers will not be prevented by the vaccine, so women should continue to get regular Pap smears even after completing the vaccination series.

The HPV vaccine is not effective in preventing HPV-related diseases in women who have an established infection at the time of vaccination; therefore, waiting for HPV seroconversion prior to vaccination is inappropriate.

KEY POINT

A human papillomavirus quadrivalent vaccination series should be offered to all girls and women ages 9 through 26 years, and women should continue to get regular Pap smears even after completing the vaccination series.

Bibliography

Advisory Committee on Immunization Practices. Recommended adult immunization schedule: United States, 2010. Ann Intern Med. 2010; 152(1):36-39. [PMID: 20048270]

Item 12   Answer: A

Educational Objective: *Screen for colorectal cancer with annual home fecal occult blood testing.*

The most appropriate management option for this patient is annual home fecal occult blood testing. Starting at the age of 50 years, average-risk patients should be offered several methods of screening, because personal preference and insurance coverage variations may render some methods more appropriate than others for individual patients. Even though sensitivity and specificity vary among the different screening methods, it is more important to choose and follow a screening program than it is to be concerned about which method is used. Screening methods include structural tests (such as colonoscopy and sigmoidoscopy) that can accomplish both detection and prevention (by identification and removal of precursor lesions) and stool-based tests (such as fecal occult blood testing [FOBT]), which detect existing cancers and, to a lesser degree, polyps. Annual home high-sensitivity FOBT,

sampling two to three consecutive specimens, is a method recommended by the U.S. Preventive Services Task Force (USPSTF) for screening if the patient is willing to undergo colonoscopy if results are positive. Other screening programs recommended by the USPSTF are colonoscopy every 10 years or flexible sigmoidoscopy every 5 years combined with annual high-sensitivity FOBT every 3 years.

Annual rectal examination with office FOBT is not considered adequate screening for colorectal cancer because of poor sensitivity (4.9% for advanced neoplasia and only 9% for cancer).

The American Cancer Society, U.S. Multi-Society Task Force on Colorectal Cancer, and American College of Radiology joint task force considers double-contrast barium enema an acceptable screening method; however, it should be performed every 5 years. Double contrast barium enema is not endorsed by the USPSTF. The American Cancer Society, U.S. Multi-Society Task Force on Colorectal Cancer, and American College of Radiology joint task force also differs from the USPSTF by recommending flexible sigmoidoscopy every 5 years together with an annual high-sensitivity FOBT.

KEY POINT

USPSTF endorsed colorectal cancer screening methods for average-risk patients include annual home stool testing, colonoscopy every 10 years, and flexible sigmoidoscopy every 5 years together with high-sensitivity fecal occult blood testing every 3 years.

Bibliography

Weinberg DS. In the clinic. Colorectal cancer screening. Ann Intern Med. 2008;148(3):ITC2-1-ITC2-16. [PMID: 18252680]

Item 13   Answer: B

Educational Objective: *Screen a patient at average risk for colon cancer with colonoscopy every 10 years.*

Of the listed screening strategies, colonoscopy every 10 years is the most appropriate for this patient. She is at average risk for colorectal cancer; this population includes persons with no personal or family history of colon adenoma or cancer and who do not have a condition that predisposes them to cancer, such as inflammatory bowel disease. Screening for colorectal cancer is cost effective and well tolerated; it also saves lives. Screening is feasible because the 10 to 15 years needed for a polyp to develop into cancer are sufficient time to detect and remove an adenoma. Screening in the average-risk population should be started at age 50 years; there are various effective screening strategies in average-risk patients, with surveillance intervals depending upon chosen strategy.

Annual fecal occult blood testing is a screening option but requires that two samples be collected from each of three spontaneously passed stools. Digital examination to retrieve a sample is not an acceptable substitute because it is approximately five times less sensitive compared to the technique of obtaining two samples from each of three stools. Flexible sigmoidoscopy in combination with fecal occult blood testing in 5-

year intervals is an acceptable option as well. Double-contrast barium enema is no longer considered to be a primary method of colorectal cancer screening by the U.S. Preventive Services Task Force. If double-contrast barium enema must be used for technical or anatomical reasons, the correct screening interval is 5 to 10 years.

KEY POINT

Screening for colorectal cancer in the average-risk population should be started at age 50 years.

Bibliography

Weinberg DS. In the clinic. Colorectal cancer screening. Ann Intern Med. 2008;148(3):ITC2-1-ITC2-16. [PMID: 18252680]

Item 14   Answer: D

Educational Objective: *Diagnose ventricular tachycardia as the cause of syncope.*

The most likely cause of this patient's syncope is ventricular tachycardia (VT). The patient's cardiac history, lack of presyncopal prodrome, and head laceration all suggest cardiac arrhythmia as the cause of the syncope. VT is perhaps the most feared cause of syncope because of its tendency to recur and cause sudden cardiac death. VT is most commonly seen in patients with advanced systolic heart failure and underlying ischemic heart disease. Myocardial scarring from a previous myocardial infarction can serve as the reentrant focus for ventricular arrhythmias.

Orthostatic hypotension is a frequent cause of syncope and presyncope. It is defined as a systolic blood pressure decrease of at least 20 mm Hg or a diastolic blood pressure decrease of at least 10 mm Hg within 3 minutes of standing. Orthostatic hypotension may be classified into medication-induced, neurogenic, and nonneurogenic categories. Common medications associated with orthostatic hypotension include α-adrenergic blockers, nitrates, diuretics, phosphodiesterase inhibitors, and antidepressants. Examples of diseases causing neurogenic orthostatic hypotension are diabetic or alcoholic polyneuropathy, multiple sclerosis, and multiple systems atrophy. Nonneurogenic orthostatic hypotension may be caused by disorders such as adrenal insufficiency, venous pooling, or volume depletion from an acute medical illness. This patient has no risk factors or findings suggestive of orthostatic hypotension.

The patient's syncope was witnessed by his wife who did not report any seizure activity, postictal confusion, tongue biting, or incontinence, making seizure an unlikely diagnosis.

Situational syncope is a neurocardiogenic reflex mediated in response to a particular stimulus, typically coughing, micturition, or defecation. No stimulus occurred before the syncope and no prodrome of diaphoresis, nausea, or lightheadedness was reported, making situational syncope unlikely.

KEY POINT

Ventricular tachycardia is most commonly seen in patients with advanced systolic heart failure and underlying ischemic heart disease.

Bibliography

Ouyang H, Quinn J. Diagnosis and evaluation of syncope in the emergency department. Emerg Med Clin North Am. 2010;28(3):471-85. [PMID: 20709239]

Item 15   Answer: C

Educational Objective: *Diagnose orthostatic hypotension as a cause of syncope.*

Determination of orthostatic blood pressure measurements is most likely to establish the cause of this patient's syncope. She most likely has diabetic autonomic neuropathy. Patients with autonomic neuropathy experience symptoms of dizziness due to standing-induced hypotension. Orthostatic hypotension is a frequent cause of syncope and presyncope. It is defined as a systolic blood pressure decrease of at least 20 mm Hg or a diastolic blood pressure decrease of at least 10 mm Hg within 3 minutes of standing. Orthostatic hypotension may be classified into medication-induced, neurogenic, and nonneurogenic categories. Examples of diseases causing neurogenic orthostatic hypotension are diabetic or alcoholic polyneuropathy, multiple sclerosis, and multiple systems atrophy. Patients with orthostatic hypotension should be educated to avoid rising to standing positions quickly, to wear elastic support hose, and to avoid volume depletion and large meals.

If the cause of syncope is unexplained from the initial evaluation, continuous telemetry may be useful to screen for paroxysmal arrhythmias. If symptoms are frequent, 24-hour ambulatory monitoring may be useful to exclude arrhythmia as a cause of symptoms. If symptoms are infrequent, an event monitor or loop recorder should be used. This patient's history is compatible with orthostatic hypotension, and determination of orthostatic blood pressure measurements will probably confirm the diagnosis, making further investigation unnecessary.

Neuroimaging, such as CT scanning, is of limited use in evaluating syncope. It has the highest yield in patients who are older than 65 years and have neurologic symptoms such as headache, neurologic examination abnormalities, head trauma, or are taking anticoagulants.

Bilateral carotid stenosis is a rare cause of syncope, and routine carotid duplex ultrasonography is not recommended. Typical symptoms of carotid artery stenosis include transient ischemic attack, amaurosis fugax, and stroke.

KEY POINT

Orthostatic hypotension is a frequent cause of syncope and presyncope and is defined as a systolic blood pressure decrease of at least 20 mm Hg or a diastolic blood pressure decrease of at least 10 mm Hg within 3 minutes of standing.

Bibliography

Ouyang H, Quinn J. Diagnosis and evaluation of syncope in the emergency department. Emerg Med Clin North Am. 2010;28(3):471-85. [PMID: 20709239]

Item 16   Answer: E

Educational Objective: *Diagnose vasovagal syncope by history.*

The best management option for this patient is no further testing. The patient's history is consistent with vasovagal (neurocardiogenic) syncope on the basis of the history of prolonged standing and prodromal symptoms of nausea, lightheadedness, and diaphoresis. These presyncopal warning symptoms are highly sensitive for the diagnosis of vasovagal syncope if lasting for more than 10 seconds. Brief myoclonic jerking after losing consciousness is not unusual with syncope, especially vasovagal syncope. In addition, the normal physical examination findings, the normal electrocardiogram, and the lack of orthostasis on vital sign assessment all point toward vasovagal syncope.

Advanced cardiovascular diagnostic testing, such as an echocardiogram or exercise stress test, is not needed after a first episode of syncope when symptoms are characteristic for vasovagal syncope.

An electroencephalogram might be indicated to evaluate a first, unprovoked seizure, but despite this patient's few myoclonic jerks, there is no evidence of seizure activity, such as tongue biting, incontinence, or postictal confusion.

In suspected vasovagal syncope, a tilt-table test can be useful, providing a diagnosis in up to 60% of patients when performed with pharmacologic stimulation. This test is indicated in patients with recurrent syncope and in those with one episode who are at high risk on the basis of their occupation. However, this test has poor sensitivity, specificity, and reproducibility and is not indicated in most patients with suspected vasovagal syncope.

KEY POINT

Vasovagal syncope is typically associated with a prodrome of nausea, lightheadedness, and diaphoresis.

Bibliography

Huff JS, Decker WW, Quinn JV, et al; American College of Emergency Physicians. Clinical policy: critical issues in the evaluation and management of adult patients presenting to the emergency department with syncope. Ann Emerg Med. 2007;49(4):431-444. [PMID:17371707]

Item 17   Answer: B

Educational Objective: *Diagnose intermittent complete heart block as the cause of recurrent syncope.*

This 57-year-old man has had three episodes of syncope in the past 6 months. His forehead bruise is a classic sign of syncope due to heart block, with the sudden loss of consciousness and lack of preceding symptoms resulting in the patient falling and injuring himself. Most patients with trifascicular block are asymptomatic and do not have progressive conduction system disease. Some studies suggest that only about 1% progress to complete heart block, but other studies report much higher rates.

In patients with trifascicular block, permanent pacer implantation is recommended for intermittent third-degree atrioventricular block, type II second-degree atrioventricular block, and alternating bundle branch block. A pacer is not indicated for asymptomatic trifascicular block. The first principle of diagnosis of a suspected cardiac arrhythmia is to record the abnormal rhythm. The best approach in this patient is an implantable loop recorder that continuously records the electrocardiogram and allows the patient to save the previous 30 seconds to 2 minutes (adjustable) after regaining consciousness.

Three major groups of disorders cause syncope of cardiac origin—cardiac outflow obstruction, arrhythmias, and cardiac ischemia. Causes of obstructed cardiac output leading to syncope include severe aortic stenosis, hypertrophic obstructive cardiomyopathy, and pulmonary embolism. The patient's normal examination and echocardiogram eliminates aortic stenosis and hypertrophic cardiomyopathy, and the absence of dyspnea, chest pain, and risk factors makes pulmonary embolism unlikely. Syncope associated with aortic stenosis is usually associated with exertion. The patient has no other symptoms to suggest cardiac ischemia.

Neurocardiogenic (vasovagal) syncope is one of the most common types of syncope. In neurocardiogenic syncope, triggers lead to increased parasympathetic tone, causing a drop in heart rate and blood pressure (cardioinhibitory response); decreased sympathetic tone, causing vasodilation and hypotension (vasodepressor response); or a combination of the two. The increased vagal tone seen in neurocardiogenic syncope typically causes a prodrome of nausea, diaphoresis, and pallor, which was not present in this patient.

KEY POINT

Sudden loss of consciousness irrespective of body position and lack of preceding symptoms suggest the possibility of cardiac arrhythmia.

Bibliography

Sud S, Klein GJ, Skanes AC, Gula LJ, Yee R, Krahn AD. Predicting the cause of syncope from clinical history in patients undergoing prolonged monitoring. Heart Rhythm. 2009;6(2):238-43. Epub 2008 Oct 29. [PMID: 19187918]

Item 18   Answer: C

Educational Objective: *Evaluate recurrent syncope with an implantable loop recorder.*

The test that is most likely to yield a diagnosis is the implantable loop recorder. Common causes of syncope include neurocardiogenic (vasovagal) syncope, bradyarrhythmia, tachyarrhythmia, outflow tract obstruction, and seizures. The next step in the evaluation of this patient is monitoring for an arrhythmia. The gold standard for diagnosis of an arrhythmic cause of syncope is documentation of a rhythm disturbance at the time of symptom occurrence. The choice of monitoring test should be related to the frequency of the symptoms. This patient has had recurrent, infrequent events; therefore, an implantable loop recorder would be the most likely test to result in a useful finding (either positive or negative). An implanted loop recorder records patient-activated events and automatically records bradycardic and tachycardic events; it is, therefore, significantly less prone to acquisition errors than an event monitor.

External event monitors are of two types: loop monitors, which are worn and record continuously but only save when the patient activates the monitor, and hand-held event monitors, which must be held to the chest to record. Loop monitors are useful for syncope because patient activation saves data from a short period of time (programmable and varying by company) before the monitor is activated by the patient. Hand-held event monitors are not useful for syncope, since the patient cannot activate the monitor when consciousness is lost.

This patient has had three syncopal events in 3 years. Neither a 24-hour ambulatory monitor nor an event monitor would be a good choice because of the infrequency of the patient's symptoms. He is highly unlikely to have an event during the standard 24 hours of ambulatory monitoring or the standard event monitor duration of 30 days. Event monitors are complex enough in their use that patient acquisition errors can occur, rendering the results less reliable. Since this patient has no prodromal symptoms, it is unlikely that the patient will be able to trigger the event monitor prior to the onset of syncope.

Electrophysiology study is incorrect because the diagnostic yield for syncope with an otherwise normal cardiac evaluation is extremely low.

KEY POINT

The implantable loop recorder has been shown to have the greatest diagnostic yield and cost-effectiveness for the evaluation of infrequent syncope.

Bibliography

Gould PA, Krahn AD, Klein GJ, Yee R, Skanes AC, Gula LJ. Investigating syncope: a review. Curr Opin Cardiol. 2006;21(1):34-41. [PMID: 16355027]

Item 19   Answer: B

Educational Objective: *Treat depression that does not respond to initial therapy by switching to another drug.*

The most appropriate management for this patient is switching to citalopram. The goal of depression therapy should not be simply improvement of symptoms but rather remission of depressive symptoms whenever possible. Patients with no

response to full-dose therapy within 6 weeks should receive another medication or referral for psychotherapy. The STAR*D trial found that 25% of patients with major depression who did not respond to an initial antidepressant achieved remission when another agent was substituted for the initial drug. Because this patient has not responded to an appropriate dose of sertraline after a reasonable period of time, changing to another antidepressant such as citalopram is indicated. Although both citalopram and sertraline are selective serotonin reuptake inhibitors (SSRIs), the STAR*D trial reported essentially identical responses when one SSRI was substituted for another or when an SSRI was changed to an antidepressant from a different class.

This patient has had a complete lack of response to sertraline after 3 months. Therefore, continuing this agent at the same dose for another 4 weeks is unlikely to be helpful. Similarly, augmentation with a second agent might be considered if a partial response had been achieved with sertraline, but that is not the case here. Although several case reports suggested methylphenidate might be an effective augmenter, a randomized, double-blind, placebo-controlled trial found no benefit for methylphenidate augmentation in treatment-resistant depression.

Electroconvulsive therapy is reserved for situations warranting immediate change and should be considered if profound suicidal ideation or psychotic features are present or if the patient fails to respond to multiple antidepressants. However, a trial of at least one other agent is warranted before considering electroconvulsive therapy in the absence of compelling urgency to achieve a prompt response.

KEY POINT

A patient with major depression who has not responded to one antidepressant at an appropriate dose for an adequate period should be given a different antidepressant.

Bibliography

Fancher TL, Kravitz RL. In the clinic. Depression. Ann Intern Med. 2010;152(9):ITC51-15; quiz ITC5-16. [PMID: 20439571]

Item 20   Answer: D

Educational Objective: *Manage a patient with depression with suicidal features with an urgent mental health referral.*

This patient with major depression with suicidal ideation should be urgently referred to a mental health professional. Major depression is characterized by the presence of at least five of the nine criteria for this disorder, including at least one of the two hallmark features of depressed mood and anhedonia. The nine depressive symptoms are as follows: sleep disturbance, psychomotor agitation or retardation, appetite disturbance, concentration impairment, low energy level, depressed mood, lost interest in activities, guilt or worthlessness, and suicidal ideation. This patient describes five of these symptoms (poor concentration, depressed mood, lack of interest, guilt, suicidal ideation). Urgent referral to a psychiatrist is appropriate for patients with suicidal ideation and a plan. In evaluating a patient with major depression, previous suicide attempts should be considered the best predictor of completed suicide.

Patients with suicidal ideation can be further risk stratified by assessing the level of social support. Patients with good social support can likely be safely referred to a psychiatrist for management.

Reassurance and careful follow-up is an insufficient course of action for a patient with suicidal ideation and a plan, particularly if there is no planned therapeutic intervention. Speaking with her fiancé is similarly inadequate.

Initiation of an antidepressant with follow-up in 2 weeks would be an acceptable approach for moderate depression, but not for a patient with significant suicidal or homicidal ideation or psychotic features.

KEY POINT

Patients with suicidal ideation and a plan should be either urgently referred to a psychiatrist or hospitalized for psychiatric assessment.

Bibliography
Fancher TL, Kravitz RL. In the clinic. Depression. Ann Intern Med. 2010;152(9):ITC51-15; quiz ITC5-16. [PMID: 20439571]

Item 21   Answer: B
Educational Objective: *Manage bereavement-associated depression.*

The most appropriate management option for this patient is to initiate an antidepressant, such as mirtazapine. Between 20% and 30% of spouses experience depression or complicated grief after the loss of a loved one. Most negative symptoms of bereavement peak before 6 months, and most family members are able to resume social activities and other activities of daily living by 6 months after their loved one's loss. Patients who have symptoms of major depression for at least 2 consecutive weeks 8 or more weeks after their loved one's death are candidates for pharmacologic therapy.

Major depression in the setting of bereavement cannot be diagnosed unless the symptoms persist for more than 2 months or include substantive functional impairment, morbid preoccupation with worthlessness, suicidal ideation, psychotic symptoms, or psychomotor retardation. In this patient, the symptoms have persisted for more than 2 months, and therapy is indicated. Mirtazapine would be an appropriate initial choice in this patient because it is an effective antidepressant and has a side effect of sedation. Also, weight gain sometimes occurs with mirtazapine, which may be advantageous in a depressed patient with weight loss.

Psychostimulants such as dextroamphetamine have been studied as an initial treatment of depression but with inconsistent efficacy results. Treating the insomnia with zolpidem would

not treat the underlying cause of the insomnia. Reassuring the patient does not adequately address the underlying problem, for which there is effective treatment.

KEY POINT

Patients who meet symptoms of major depression for at least 2 consecutive weeks 8 or more weeks after their loved one's death are candidates for pharmacologic therapy.

Bibliography
Fancher TL, Kravitz RL. In the clinic. Depression. Ann Intern Med. 2010;152(9):ITC51-15. [PMID: 20439571]

Item 22   Answer: B
Educational Objective: *Diagnose bipolar disorder.*

This patient most likely has bipolar disorder. Although she presents with symptoms of depression, her history includes episodes of mania or hypomania. Diagnostic criteria for mania include a distinct period of abnormally and persistently elevated, expansive, or irritable mood lasting at least 1 week. Typical symptoms include inflated self-esteem or grandiosity, decreased need for sleep, distractibility, increased goal-directed behavior, and excessive involvement in pleasurable activities that have a high potential for consequences (unrestrained buying sprees, sexual indiscretions). It is important to ask depressed patients about a personal and family history of manic symptoms in order to select an appropriate therapy.

The diagnosis of attention-deficit/hyperactivity disorder (ADHD) requires documentation of multiple symptoms of inattention or hyperactivity and impulsivity dating back to at least age 7 years. There is no history provided to indicate either these symptoms or related impairment in two or more settings, such as school and home, so ADHD appears an unlikely diagnosis.

There is also no history provided of self-harm, dysfunctional relationships, or intense anger to suggest borderline personality disorder. Although the impulsive sexual behavior could be a manifestation of borderline personality disorder, it can also be characteristic of mania or hypomania, and the overall presentation is more consistent with bipolar disorder. While there is overlap between depression and generalized anxiety disorder (GAD), with impaired concentration, sleep disturbance, and fatigue being common to both, this patient reports depression as a prominent symptom and has a history of depression as well as a history of prior manic or hypomanic periods. Thus, a diagnosis of bipolar disorder is much more apt than GAD.

KEY POINT

Diagnostic criteria for mania include a distinct period of abnormally and persistently elevated, expansive, or irritable mood lasting at least 1 week.

Bibliography
Fancher TL, Kravitz RL. In the clinic. Depression. Ann Intern Med. 2010;152(9):ITC51-15; quiz ITC5-16. [PMID: 20439571]

Item 23   Answer: D

Educational Objective: *Prevent seizures in acute alcohol withdrawal syndrome.*

Lorazepam should be administered now. Clinicians should identify the severity of alcohol withdrawal and factors that may predict the onset of serious complications. The 10-item Clinical Institute Withdrawal Assessment Scale for Alcohol, Revised, can be used to measure symptom severity and to help provide guidance in the course of treatment. Patients scoring more than 10 points usually need additional medication for withdrawal, and patients scoring more than 15 points are typically hospitalized to manage alcohol withdrawal symptoms. Benzodiazepines, such as lorazepam, are first-line therapy for patients who require pharmacologic prophylaxis or treatment for alcohol withdrawal. Patients with the alcohol withdrawal syndrome who are treated with benzodiazepines have fewer complications, including delirium tremens and alcohol-withdrawal seizures. Although shorter acting agents such as lorazepam are more commonly used, longer acting agents (chlordiazepoxide or diazepam) may be more effective in preventing seizures but can pose a risk for excess sedation in older adults and in patients with liver disease. Patients with a history of seizures should receive a prophylactic benzodiazepine on a fixed schedule, even if asymptomatic during the acute alcohol withdrawal period.

β-Blockers, such as atenolol, and clonidine can be used to control tachycardia and hypertension when needed but are adjunctive, not primary, treatments for alcohol withdrawal. Haloperidol can be used to treat agitation and hallucinosis in patients exhibiting these signs. However, β-blockers are associated with a greater incidence of delirium, and neuroleptics like haloperidol are associated with a greater incidence of seizures during withdrawal. The use of antiepileptics, such as phenytoin, is ineffective compared with benzodiazepines in preventing alcohol-related seizures.

KEY POINT

Benzodiazepines are the drug class of choice for prophylaxis of alcohol withdrawal seizures.

Bibliography

Bayard M, McIntyre J, Hill KR, Woodside J Jr. Alcohol withdrawal syndrome. Am Fam Physician. 2004;69(6):1443-50. [PMID: 15053409]

Item 24   Answer: B

Educational Objective: *Manage cocaine intoxication.*

This patient's sympathomimetic syndrome is consistent with cocaine intoxication. Clinical findings often include tachycardia, hypertension, hyperthermia, mydriasis, agitation, and psychosis. Other possible complications of cocaine abuse may be difficult to evaluate in the agitated patient. The initial treatment in this patient should include sedation with lorazepam, administered intravenously or intramuscularly. Control of agitation usually brings about a decrease in heart rate, blood pressure, and temperature.

Intravenous fluids should be administered to establish adequate urine output for possible rhabdomyolysis, and an electrocardiogram should be obtained to assess for myocardial ischemia. Laboratory studies should include measurement of serum electrolytes and serum creatine kinase and evaluation of liver function. CT scan of the brain may be indicated to rule out intracranial injury.

Haloperidol is not initially indicated for control of agitation in a patient who abuses cocaine. Haloperidol has the potential to lower the seizure threshold and would not be an initial treatment in this patient, who has already had a seizure. After agitation is controlled, haloperidol can be considered if the patient manifests psychotic features.

Drug-induced seizures, which are usually self-limited, do not respond well to phenytoin. The treatment of choice for drug-induced seizures is benzodiazepines.

Hypertension is rarely severe in cocaine abuse, and it usually responds to control of agitation. Propranolol and other β-blockers are not recommended because of the potential concern about worsening of vasoconstriction due to unopposed α-blocking effects.

KEY POINT

The initial treatment of acute cocaine intoxication is sedation with a benzodiazepine.

Bibliography

Glauser J, Queen JR. An overview of non-cardiac cocaine toxicity. J Emerg Med. 2007;32:181-6. Epub 2007 Jan 22. [PMID: 17307630]

Item 25   Answer: D

Educational Objective: *Manage alcohol dependence with naltrexone.*

This patient presents with a history of alcohol dependence. Brief interventions work for patients with at-risk alcohol use, but more aggressive therapy, potentially including pharmacotherapy, is indicated in both alcohol abuse and alcohol dependence. Naltrexone, an opioid receptor antagonist, has been shown to be effective in short-term treatment as well as in decreasing the frequency of relapse. Benzodiazepines, such as diazepam, would be used in the acute detoxification setting. Antidepressants and anxiolytics may play a role if an underlying psychiatric disorder is present but is not a primary treatment of alcohol dependence. Disulfiram has been used for years and works by leading to an accumulation of aldehyde if alcohol is consumed, resulting in vomiting, headache, and anxiety. However, studies have been inconclusive on its efficacy in enhancing abstinence.

Naltrexone, an opioid receptor antagonist, has been shown to be effective in short-term treatment of alcohol dependence as well as in decreasing the frequency of relapse.

Bibliography

In the clinic. Alcohol use. Ann Intern Med. 2009;150:ITC3-1-ITC3-15; quiz ITC3-16. Erratum in: Ann Intern Med. 2009;150:504. [PMID: 19258556]

Item 26   Answer: C

Educational Objective: *Manage hypoventilation caused by opioid overdose with naloxone.*

The most appropriate next step is intravenous administration of naloxone. The patient's acute ventilatory failure is most consistent with hypoventilation resulting from opioid intoxication. In pure hypoventilation, the alveolar-arterial difference is normal. Improved alertness after administration of naloxone confirms opioid intoxication. Naloxone has a short half-life and is typically given as a continuous intravenous infusion. If the response to naloxone is inadequate, endotracheal intubation would be appropriate.

Benzodiazepines, such as diazepam, can be used to treat cocaine toxicity. Acute cocaine toxicity is characterized by hypertension, tachycardia, hyperthermia, mydriasis, and agitation. This patient's presentation is not consistent with acute cocaine intoxication.

Intravenous fomepizole is an effective treatment for ethylene glycol and methyl alcohol poisoning. These alcohols cause an anion gap metabolic acidosis and an osmolar gap. This patient has an isolated acute respiratory acidosis that is not compatible with ethylene glycol and methyl alcohol poisoning, and thus fomepizole is not indicated.

Traditional therapy for cyanide poisoning includes inhalation of amyl nitrite followed by the administration of intravenous sodium nitrite or sodium thiosulfate. Cyanide poisoning results from inhalation of gaseous hydrogen cyanide or the ingestion of potassium or sodium cyanide. Hydrogen cyanide poisoning is also common as a result of smoke inhalation from fires. Ingestion of cyanide is most often associated with suicides and homicides. Inhalation results in seizures, coma, and cardiopulmonary arrest. Chronic exposure to low levels results in weakness and paralysis. The patient's findings are not compatible with cyanide poisoning.

KEY POINT

Continuous naloxone infusion is used to treat opioid intoxication.

Bibliography

Strang J, Kelleher M, Best D, Mayet S, Manning V. Emergency naloxone for heroin overdose. BMJ. 2006;333(7569):614-615. [PMID: 16990298]

Item 27   Answer: B

Educational Objective: *Screen a patient for alcohol problems.*

The CAGE questionnaire is the best choice to screen for alcohol problems. The CAGE questionnaire is a commonly used instrument to identify alcohol problems:

C - Have you ever felt you should cut down on your drinking?

A - Have people annoyed you by criticizing your drinking?

G - Have you ever felt bad or guilty about your drinking?

E - Eye opener: Have you ever had a drink first thing in the morning to steady your nerves or to get rid of a hangover?

With a cutoff of two positive answers, the CAGE questionnaire is 77% to 94% sensitive and 79% to 97% specific for detecting alcohol abuse or dependence in primary care settings and indicates that further assessment is warranted. Alcohol abuse may be difficult to diagnose. Patients often present with complaints that may be attributable to other medical conditions but actually are caused by alcohol consumption. These problems might include depression, insomnia, injuries, gastroesophageal reflux disease, uncontrolled hypertension, and important social problems. Other potential clues to alcohol misuse are recurrent legal or marital problems, absenteeism or loss of employment, and committing or being the victim of violence. The U.S. Preventive Services Task Force (USPSTF) recommends routine screening of adults with either directed questioning or use of a standardized tool to identify persons whose alcohol use puts them at risk. More likely to be at risk are those with prior alcohol problems, young adults, and smokers. The USPSTF found good evidence that brief behavioral counseling interventions with follow-up produce small to moderate reductions in alcohol consumption that are sustained over 6- to 12-month periods or longer.

Although the optimal interval for screening is not known, screening at the time of an initial visit is clearly important. There are multiple screening instruments; the CAGE questionnaire is one of the most widely used. Two positive responses indicate that further assessment for alcohol misuse is warranted.

The CAGE questionnaire has a reported sensitivity ranging from 43% to 94% and specificity ranging from 70% to 97%.

Laboratory tests such as an elevated mean corpuscular volume (sensitivity 63%; specificity 48%) and an elevated aspartate aminotransferase/alanine aminotransferase ratio (sensitivity 12%; specificity 91%) can be suggestive but are not diagnostic of alcohol abuse and dependence. Their relatively low sensitivities make them unsuited for screening.

Because of the short half-life of ethanol, a random ethanol level should not be used to screen for alcoholism.

Screening instruments such as the CAGE questionnaire are effective for alcohol misuse screening in the primary care setting.

Bibliography

Saitz R. Clinical practice. Unhealthy alcohol use. N Engl J Med. 2005; 352(6):596-607. [PMID:15703424]

Item 28   Answer: D

Educational Objective: *Treat lumbar spinal stenosis with surgery.*

Back pain and neurologic impairment from spinal stenosis may be treated by surgery. In considering surgical treatment for patients with back pain from radiculopathy or spinal stenosis, guidelines recommend referring patients after a minimum of 3 months to 2 years of failed nonsurgical interventions. Failure is defined as progressive neurologic deficits and severe pain that is not responsive to conservative treatment. This patient has tried conservative therapy with first-line medication treatment (NSAIDS and acetaminophen) and physical therapy, yet her symptoms have progressed. Therefore, if she is willing to consider surgical treatment, then the next appropriate step is to refer the patient for surgical consideration. Surgical treatment of spinal stenosis is usually elective.

Electromyography and nerve conduction studies are not required for the diagnosis of lumbar spinal stenosis but may be helpful in patients with atypical symptoms and when the possibility of an alternative diagnosis such as peripheral neuropathy is considered. There is currently very little evidence to support the use of corticosteroid injections in the treatment of spinal stenosis. Spinal traction is the application of constant or intermittent pulling force applied to the spine to gradually stretch the spine. Continuous or intermittent spinal traction has not been shown to be effective in patients with sciatica or spinal stenosis.

Back pain and neurologic impairment from spinal stenosis may be treated by surgery.

Bibliography

Wilson JF. In the clinic. Low back pain. Ann Intern Med. 2008;148(9): ITC5-1-ITC5-16. [PMID: 18458275]

Item 29   Answer: C

Educational Objective: *Diagnose vertebral osteomyelitis.*

The most appropriate management is urgent spine MRI. "Red flags" in this patient's presentation suggesting a systemic illness as the cause of back pain include localized pain, history of intravenous drug use, fever, and elevated erythrocyte sedimentation rate. These findings strongly suggest the possibility of vertebral osteomyelitis, infectious diskitis, or spinal epidural abscess. Most patients with vertebral osteomyelitis have back or neck pain that gradually worsens over weeks or months; fever is present in only 50% of patients and leukocytosis is typically absent, but the erythrocyte sedimentation rate is often greater that 100 mm/h. Tenderness to palpation over the involved portion of the spine is common. Vertebral osteomyelitis is most often disseminated hematogenously. Segmental arteries supply blood to the vertebrae, with bifurcating arteries supplying blood to the inferior margin of one end plate and the superior margin of the adjacent end plate. Consequently, when infection occurs, it generally follows this vascular pattern, involving bone in two adjacent vertebral bodies with invasion into their intervertebral disk (diskitis). Potential sources of hematogenous osteomyelitis include skin (injection drug users), urinary tract, or respiratory tract infection; endocarditis; or intravascular catheter-related infection. Patients with infectious diskitis are at risk for spinal epidural abscess. Because blood cultures are positive in up to 75% of patients with vertebral osteomyelitis, they should be obtained for all patients in whom this condition is suspected. In patients with suspected vertebral osteomyelitis, diskitis, or spinal epidural abscess, urgent evaluation with imaging is warranted. MRI is the preferred imaging modality, because scans show changes of acute osteomyelitis within days of infection and are superior to and more sensitive (90%) and specific (80%) than plain films and CT scans; can detect soft tissue abscesses and epidural, paravertebral, or psoas abscesses possibly requiring surgical drainage; and can delineate anatomy before surgery. Nonetheless, false-positive MRI results may occur in patients with noninfectious conditions such as fractures, tumors, and healed osteomyelitis.

Antibiotic therapy, with or without surgery, is typically required to treat spine and related soft tissue infection. However, antibiotic therapy should be guided, whenever possible, by blood culture results; empiric antibiotic therapy without an attempt to confirm the underlying cause of the patient's pain and source of infection is inappropriate.

MRI is the preferred imaging modality for suspected vertebral osteomyelitis, because scans show changes of acute osteomyelitis within days of infection and are superior to plain films and CT scans.

Bibliography

Wilson JF. In the clinic. Low back pain. Ann Intern Med. 2008;148: ITC5-1-ITC5-16. [PMID: 18458275]

Item 30   Answer: A

Educational Objective: *Manage acute nonspecific low back pain with acetaminophen.*

The best initial management option for this patient is acetaminophen. This patient has acute low back pain resulting from a recent injury. He has no signs of neurologic compromise or potentially serious underlying conditions. Guidelines published by the American College of Physicians and the American Pain Society recommend acetaminophen or NSAIDs for first-line treatment of acute nonspecific low back pain. An opioid analgesic or tramadol is an option when used judiciously in patients with severe, disabling acute low back pain that is not controlled (or is unlikely to be controlled) with acetaminophen or NSAIDs. Patients should be informed that the prognosis for acute low back pain is generally good and that most patients improve within 1 month.

The patient has no signs of neurologic compromise or features suggesting a potentially serious condition; therefore, MRI would not be necessary. Even if there were signs of disk herniation (a positive straight leg raising test), an MRI would not be necessary unless the patient had evidence of motor impairment, had not responded to therapy, or symptoms were increasing.

Lumbar plain radiographs are generally not recommended in the evaluation of low back pain because there is no evidence that routine plain radiography in patients with nonspecific low back pain is associated with a greater improvement in patient outcomes than selective imaging. Plain radiographs would be appropriate if a vertebral compression fracture is suspected.

Studies have not demonstrated that bed rest is helpful in acute low back pain, and it may impair recovery time.

KEY POINT

Acetaminophen or NSAIDs are first-line therapy for acute nonspecific low back pain.

Bibliography
Wilson JF. In the clinic. Low back pain. Ann Intern Med. 2008;148(9): ITC5 1 ITC5 16. [PMID: 18458275]

Item 31   Answer: C
Educational Objective: *Diagnose spinal cord compression due to bone metastases with MRI scan.*

The next diagnostic study should be an MRI scan of the thoracolumbar spine. This patient most likely has spinal cord compression due to bone metastases from recurrent prostate cancer. The three most common malignancies responsible for spinal cord compression are prostate, breast, and lung cancer. His signs and symptoms are consistent with spinal cord compression. The initial symptom in patients with epidural spinal cord compression due to tumor usually is spinal or radicular pain that may precede the onset of neurologic symptoms, which may include weakness, numbness, or sphincter disturbances. Spinal cord compression is an oncologic emergency, and MRI of the thoracolumbar spine is needed to confirm the diagnosis and assist in treatment planning. Clinicians should have a low threshold of suspicion for spinal cord compression in a patient with known cancer or a risk for recurrent cancer. The absence of neurologic findings should not alter that strategy. Patients whose cord compression is discovered after developing neurologic deficits are more likely to remain functionally impaired after intervention.

Radionuclide bone scanning is very sensitive for detecting bone metastases and has the advantage of visualizing the entire skeleton, but it has a high false-positive rate and provides no information about thecal sac compression. Because a bone scan cannot confirm a diagnosis of spinal cord compression, it is an inappropriate diagnostic test in this emergent setting.

The clinical feature of bilateral lower extremity weakness accompanied by hyperreflexia localizes the process to the spinal cord. An MRI of the brain would therefore be an inappropriate diagnostic test.

Plain radiographs are used to diagnose compression fractures of the thoracic spine but cannot directly visualize spinal cord compression. In a patient such as this, major vertebral body collapse or pedicle erosion is approximately 80% predictive of spinal cord compression, but a false-negative result occurs in nearly 20% of patients with spinal cord compression. Therefore, plain radiography is not the best diagnostic test for this patient.

KEY POINT

The triad of back pain, muscle weakness, and loss of bowel or bladder control is suggestive of spinal cord compression.

Bibliography
Cole JS, Patchell RA. Metastatic epidural spinal cord compression. Lancet Neurol. 2008;7(5):459-66. [PMID: 18420159]

Item 32   Answer: E
Educational Objective: *Diagnose cough-variant asthma with a trial of inhaled albuterol.*

A trial of inhaled albuterol could help control the patient's symptoms and confirm the diagnosis of cough-variant asthma. The most common causes of chronic cough are asthma, postnasal drip syndrome (chronic sinusitis-rhinitis), and gastroesophageal reflux disease (GERD). Bronchoscopy and chest CT play no role in diagnosing cough due to these three causes. The diagnosis of cough-variant asthma is suggested by the presence of airway hyperresponsiveness and confirmed when cough resolves with asthma therapy.

The patient does not have postnasal drip, purulent nasal secretions, sinus congestion, or other symptoms suggestive of chronic or recurrent sinusitis and has not responded to treatment. Therefore, CT of the sinuses is not necessary. If the patient does not respond to albuterol, eosinophilic bronchitis should be considered as the cause of chronic cough, and bronchoscopy with biopsy should be performed to confirm that diagnosis. Otherwise, bronchoscopy is not a first-line diagnostic test in this patient.

There is little about the character and timing of chronic cough due to GERD that distinguishes it from other conditions; in addition, it often can be "silent" from a gastrointestinal standpoint. However, the patient did not benefit from 3 months of empiric gastric acid suppression therapy for GERD. Therefore, it is reasonable to rule out cough-variant asthma before pursuing 24-hour esophageal pH monitoring.

KEY POINT

The diagnosis of cough-variant asthma is suggested by the presence of airway hyperresponsiveness and confirmed when cough resolves with a trial of inhaled albuterol.

Bibliography

Abouzgheib W, Pratter MR, Bartter T. Cough and asthma. Curr Opin Pulm Med. 2007;13(1):44-48. [PMID: 17133124]

Item 33   Answer: A

Educational Objective: *Initiate empiric management for chronic cough with antihistamine/decongestant combination.*

The most appropriate treatment for this patient is a trial of an antihistamine/decongestant combination. The initial approach in patients with chronic cough (>8 weeks in duration) is to conduct a history and physical examination looking for identifiable causes, determine whether the patient is taking an angiotensin-converting enzyme (ACE) inhibitor, and obtain a chest radiograph. In the population of patients who do not smoke, do not take an ACE inhibitor, and have a normal chest radiograph, upper airway cough syndrome (UACS) (previously termed *postnasal drip*), asthma, and gastroesophageal reflux disease (GERD) are responsible for approximately 99% of cases of chronic cough. When the cause of a chronic cough is unclear, the American College of Chest Physicians recommends initial treatment with a first-generation antihistamine/decongestant combination to treat UACS. This is true even in the absence of evidence of a postnasal drip. The diagnosis of chronic cough is often based upon the patient's response to empiric therapy, and it may take weeks or even months for the cough to resolve with appropriate therapy.

In a nonsmoking patient with a normal chest radiograph and no systemic symptoms, CT scan of the chest is not indicated.

Asthma is a common cause for a chronic cough and may present only with a cough (cough-variant asthma). However, pursuing pulmonary function testing or initiating empiric β-agonist therapy or an inhaled corticosteroid such as fluticasone for asthma is premature unless the patient fails to respond to empiric treatment of UACS.

In the absence of GERD symptoms, proton-pump inhibitors should be reserved for patients with chronic cough who have a normal chest radiograph, are not taking an ACE inhibitor, do not smoke, and who have failed to improve with treatment for UACS, asthma, and nonallergic eosinophilic bronchitis.

In patients with chronic cough who have normal chest radiograph findings, normal spirometry, and a negative methacholine challenge test, the diagnosis of nonasthmatic eosinophilic bronchitis (NAEB) should be considered. This diagnosis is often considered after patients fail to respond to treatments directed at UACS, GERD, and asthma. Although confirmation of NAEB requires a bronchial biopsy, the response to empirically administered inhaled corticosteroids is often used to establish the diagnosis.

KEY POINT

Empiric treatment of chronic cough in a nonsmoking patient not taking an angiotensin-converting enzyme inhibitor who has a normal chest radiograph begins with an antihistamine/decongestant combination.

Bibliography

Pavord ID, Chung KF. Management of chronic cough. Lancet. 2008;371(9621):1375-1384. [PMID:18424326]

Item 34   Answer: A

Educational Objective: *Diagnose angiotensin-converting enzyme inhibitor chronic cough.*

The most appropriate management option for this patient is to discontinue the angiotensin-converting enzyme (ACE) inhibitor, lisinopril. This patient presents with a cough of longer than 8 weeks' duration and thus meets the definition for chronic cough. According to American College of Chest Physicians guidelines, the initial evaluation includes a history and physical examination to determine likely etiologies, followed by a chest radiograph to identify obvious abnormalities. If the chest radiograph is normal, one should recommend discontinuing ACE inhibitors and smoking, if these factors are identified in the history, or pursue empiric management of chronic cough if the patient is a nonsmoker and is not taking an ACE inhibitor. In some estimates, up to 20% of patients taking an ACE inhibitor develop a chronic cough. There may be no obvious temporal relationship between the initiation of ACE inhibitor therapy and the onset of cough. The median time to resolution is 26 days from withdrawal of the ACE inhibitor.

In patients with chronic cough and a normal chest radiograph, a chest CT is only indicated for those at high risk for lung cancer.

Upper airway cough syndrome (UACS) is a common cause of chronic cough. A trial of a first-generation antihistamine/decongestant combination for several weeks is appropriate treatment for UACS. In a nonsmoking patient who is taking an ACE inhibitor, however, the ACE inhibitor should be discontinued for several weeks before treating for UACS.

Asthma and nonallergic eosinophilic bronchitis may present without any symptoms other than cough. Spirometry would be indicated in the evaluation of chronic cough that has not resolved after the initial management measures (history, physical examination, chest radiograph, cessation of ACE inhibitor, treatment for upper airway cough syndrome).

Although empiric therapy for gastroesophageal reflux disease (GERD) is appropriate if prominent symptoms of GERD accompany the cough or if initial management measures fail, discontinuing the ACE inhibitor always should precede empiric therapy for GERD.

KEY POINT

In patients taking an angiotensin-converting enzyme inhibitor who present with a chronic cough and a normal chest radiograph, discontinuing the angiotensin-converting enzyme inhibitor may be both diagnostic and therapeutic.

Bibliography

Irwin RS, Baumann MH, Bolser DC, et al; American College of Chest Physicians (ACCP). Diagnosis and management of cough executive summary: ACCP evidence-based clinical practice guidelines. Chest. 2006;129(1 suppl):1S-23S. [PMID:16428686]

Item 35   Answer: A

Educational Objective: *Use chest CT to evaluate a patient with hemoptysis for lung cancer.*

The most appropriate next step in the management of this patient is chest CT. The most commonly encountered causes of hemoptysis in ambulatory patients are infection (bronchitis or pneumonia) and malignancy. All patients with hemoptysis should have a chest radiograph. Risk factors that increase the risk of malignancy include male sex, age older than 40 years, a smoking history of more than 40 pack-years, and symptoms lasting for more than 1 week. These patients should be referred for chest CT and fiberoptic bronchoscopy even if the chest radiograph is normal.

Sputum cytology examination alone is not effective in early diagnosis of lung cancer because of low sensitivity. Although pulmonary function testing can determine if the patient has chronic obstructive pulmonary disease and whether the patient is a surgical candidate, it is not indicated to establish a diagnosis of lung cancer. Follow up in 6 months is not an advisable strategy for a patient at high risk for lung cancer such as this patient; delayed diagnosis may result in suboptimal outcome.

KEY POINT

All patients with hemoptysis should have a chest radiograph; patients at high risk for lung cancer should be referred for chest CT and fiberoptic bronchoscopy even if the chest radiograph is normal.

Bibliography

Dudha M, Lehrman S, Aronow WS, Rosa J. Hemoptysis: diagnosis and treatment. Compr Ther. 2009;35(3-4):139-49. [PMID: 20043609]

Item 36   Answer: E

Educational Objective: *Treat acute bronchitis with symptomatic measures.*

The best management for this patient is symptomatic treatment. Treatment of acute bronchitis is usually symptomatic. There is no evidence to support the use of most over-the-counter and prescription antitussive medications. However, some studies have shown that NSAIDs, with or without an antihistamine, decrease cough severity. A trial of ibuprofen may be reasonable for this patient, provided there are no contraindications.

Albuterol in a metered-dose inhaler may help to decrease cough severity and duration in adults with acute bronchitis when there is evidence of wheezing. However, β-agonist inhalers have not been shown to be helpful in the absence of wheezing and, therefore, probably would not benefit this patient.

Approximately 50% of patients with acute bronchitis have purulent sputum, but this is not a reliable predictor of bacterial infection. Most studies fail to show that administration of antibiotics, such as azithromycin, significantly improves outcomes, including symptom resolution and early return to work, in patients with acute bronchitis. In patients with an acute exacerbation of chronic obstructive pulmonary disease, antibiotic therapy is most likely to be helpful in those with at least two of the following: increased sputum purulence (change in sputum color), increased sputum volume, or increased dyspnea. Antibiotics are appropriate for patients with pertussis in order to decrease disease transmission, although these agents have a limited effect on symptoms. Pertussis should be suspected when a community outbreak has been reported. Symptoms may include coughing paroxysms and posttussive vomiting but are not reliable indicators of infection.

A chest radiograph is not indicated in a patient with acute bronchitis who does not have signs or symptoms of pneumonia, such as fever, dyspnea, and pleuritic chest pain. Cough that persists for more than 3 weeks is atypical for acute bronchitis, and a chest radiograph is generally indicated as the initial diagnostic test.

Influenza virus culture is not needed in a patient without fever, myalgia, or malaise because the probability of influenza virus infection is very low.

KEY POINT

Antibiotics are not beneficial for patients with acute bronchitis.

Bibliography

Wenzel RP, Fowler AA 3rd. Clinical Practice. Acute bronchitis. N Engl J Med. 2006;355(20):2125-2130. [PMID:17108344]

Item 37   Answer: A

Educational Objective: *Treat chronic obstructive pulmonary disease with smoking cessation.*

Smoking cessation is the single most effective intervention to reduce the risk of developing chronic obstructive pulmonary disease and to stop its progression. Short-term tobacco dependence treatment is effective, and every tobacco user should be offered counseling and nicotine replacement (patch, gum, inhaler, and nasal spray) at every visit. Counseling should focus on establishing a quit date, emphasizing abstinence, using other family members, and avoiding alcohol and other drugs. Several effective pharmacotherapies for tobacco dependency are available and at least one of these medications should be added to counseling unless contraindicated. Data from the National Institutes of Health Lung Health Study revealed that more participants in the smoking intervention group quit compared with usual and customary therapy (year 1: 34.4% vs. 9.0%; year 5: 37.4% vs. 21.9%). The annual rate of decline in FEV_1 over 4 years for quitters was half that for continuing smokers.

This patient is already on therapeutic doses of a long-acting bronchodilator, an inhaled corticosteroid, ipratropium, and a short-acting β-agonist, and she does not exhibit oxyhemoglobin desaturation with exertion. Therefore, she does not need any changes in her inhaled medications or require supplemental oxygen therapy.

KEY POINT

Smoking cessation is the single most effective intervention to reduce the risk of developing chronic obstructive pulmonary disease and to stop its progression.

Bibliography
Wilson JF. In the clinic. Smoking cessation. Ann Intern Med. 2007;146: ITC2-1-ICT2-16. [PMID: 17283345]

Item 38   Answer: A
Educational Objective: *Know the effects of smoking cessation on lung function.*

This patient likely has chronic obstructive pulmonary disease (COPD), based on her clinical findings and pulmonary function results (FEV_1 <80% and FEV_1/FCV <0.7). In the Lung Health Study, 6000 smokers with mild to moderate COPD were randomized to receive smoking intervention plus ipratropium bromide, smoking intervention plus placebo, or no intervention. Lung function was monitored for 5 years. The smoking intervention arms were both associated with a decreased rate of decline in lung function. The use of a bronchodilator had a small beneficial effect on lung function. The benefit did not persist after patients stopped using the bronchodilator. In a subsequent study, the Lung Health Study II, inhaled corticosteroids did not improve the rate of decline in lung function.

Among those who quit smoking, lung function improved during the first year by an average of 2%. Women who successfully quit smoking improved by 3.7%, compared with men, who improved by 1.6%. In the smoking intervention group, among those who quit smoking, the subsequent rate of decline in lung function was 31 mL per year, a normal value, compared with continuing smokers, whose lung function declined at a rate of 63 mL per year.

KEY POINT

Smoking cessation is associated with a decreased rate of decline in lung function.

Bibliography
Wilson JF. In the clinic. Smoking cessation. Ann Intern Med. 2007; 146(3):ITC2-1-ICT2-16. [PMID: 17283345]

Item 39   Answer: B
Educational Objective: *Counsel the patient on smoking cessation to reduce the risk of cardiovascular disease.*

Smoking cessation will have the greatest impact on reducing this patient's risk of future cardiovascular disease. This woman has several risk factors for cardiovascular disease, including obesity (BMI >30), her family history, her sedentary lifestyle, and her smoking status. When faced with the possibility of multiple interventions for cardiovascular disease risk factor management, it is often important to counsel the patient regarding the relative benefit of each intervention and to address the risk factors and interventions sequentially. However, there are also data to suggest that addressing multiple risk factors sequentially is not superior to a simultaneous approach. Women who are current smokers have a threefold higher risk of cardiovascular disease compared with women who have stopped smoking or have never smoked. Surprisingly, the duration of smoking does not correlate with risk of future cardiovascular disease. (It does, however, correlate with risk of smoking-related cancers and lung disease.) In addition, the risk of cardiovascular disease drops rapidly after smoking cessation, with the greatest relative reduction occurring in the first 5 years after stopping. Therefore, although this patient has a 32-pack-year history of smoking, smoking cessation now will immediately and significantly reduce her risk of cardiovascular disease. With regard to her risk of having a cardiovascular event, the Framingham risk estimate is calculated to be 3% over the next 10 years (low risk) compared with less than 1% if she were a nonsmoker.

Other important lifestyle considerations include regular exercise, a healthy diet, and maintaining a healthy weight. While these interventions have been shown to reduce the risk of hypertension and diabetes, they have not conclusively been shown to reduce the risk of cardiovascular events.

KEY POINT

The risk of a cardiovascular event is reduced rapidly (within 5 years) of smoking cessation in women.

Bibliography
Kenfield SA, Stampfer MJ, Rosner BA, Colditz GA. Smoking and smoking cessation in relation to mortality in women. JAMA. 2008; 299(17):2037-2047. [PMID:18460664]

Item 40   Answer: D
Educational Objective: *Treat smoking addiction with varenicline.*

The most appropriate pharmacologic therapy for this patient is varenicline. The U.S. Public Health Service has recommended brief smoking cessation counseling interventions for smokers interested in quitting. Potential quitters should be warned of withdrawal symptoms (which will improve in several weeks), plan a coping strategy for cravings (such as chewing gum), avoid high-risk smoking situations, and anticipate some weight gain.

For this patient who would like to try an alternative to nicotine replacement therapy, varenicline would be the best option. Systematic reviews have addressed a number of pharmacologic approaches to smoking cessation treatment. Varenicline for 12 weeks increased the odds of long-term smoking cessation approximately threefold compared with placebo. When compared directly with bupropion, varenicline was the more effective drug. The main side effect was nausea, which usually subsided over time. Two trials tested varenicline for an additional 12 weeks without adverse effects. One randomized, open label trial found a modest effect of varenicline compared to nicotine replacement therapy. Generally, nicotine replacement therapy should not be combined with varenicline, since the combination may increase the risk of nausea, vomiting, headache, dizziness, and other adverse effects. In 2009, the FDA required boxed warnings on varenicline and bupropion noting the risk for serious neuropsychiatric symptoms including changes in behavior, hostility, agitation, depressed mood, suicidal thoughts and behaviors, and attempted suicide.

When used as sole pharmacotherapy, bupropion and nortriptyline doubled the odds of cessation compared with placebo. However, although bupropion and nortriptyline appear to be equally effective and of similar efficacy to nicotine replacement therapy, they appear to be less effective than varenicline. There is a risk of 1 in 1000 of seizures associated with bupropion use, making bupropion a poor choice for this patient. Adverse effects of bupropion include insomnia, dry mouth, nausea and serious psychiatric symptoms (as noted above); those of nortriptyline include dry mouth, constipation, nausea, and sedation.

Trials of selective serotonin reuptake inhibitors, including sertraline, have shown no evidence of significant benefit for smoking cessation.

KEY POINT

For smoking cessation, bupropion and nortriptyline appear to be equally effective and of similar efficacy to nicotine replacement therapy but less effective than varenicline.

Bibliography
Wilson JF. In the clinic. Smoking cessation. Ann Intern Med. 2007; 146(3):ITC2-1-ICT2-16. [PMID: 17283345]

Item 41   Answer: B
Educational Objective: *Treat obesity with bariatric surgery.*

Surgical treatment should be considered for patients with BMI of 35 or greater and serious obesity-related medical comorbidities (such as hypertension, diabetes, dyslipidemia, coronary artery disease, or sleep apnea) or BMI of 40 or greater without comorbidities in whom attempts at weight loss, including drug therapy, were unsuccessful. Surgery produces long-term weight loss that can be more than 25% of body weight at 1 year, and lost weight is regained slowly, if at all. Surgery may also be recommended to persons with progressive obesity, such as continuing weight increases of more than 5 kg/year before age 30 years. After bariatric surgery, many patients have significant improvement or resolution of obesity-related diseases, including diabetes, hypertension, sleep apnea, and hyperlipidemia, and recent studies suggest decreased overall mortality.

Low carbohydrate diets produce slightly more weight loss than other diets, and may have a slightly more favorable effect on lipid panel and blood pressure. Unfortunately, this patient has had continued weight gain despite her diet attempts and a trial of a different diet is unlikely to produce different results.

Increasing physical activity increases energy expenditure. Recommending exercise for 30 to 60 minutes 5 or more days a week by increasing walking or other comparable activities is useful. Exercise is particularly helpful in maintaining a lower weight once achieved. Reducing calories, however, is essential for weight loss. Exercise alone is rarely a successful weight loss program.

KEY POINT

Surgical treatment should be considered for patients with BMI of 35 or greater and serious obesity-related medical comorbidities or BMI of 40 or greater without comorbidities in whom attempts at weight loss, including drug therapy, were unsuccessful.

Bibliography
Bray GA, Wilson JF. In the clinic. Obesity. Ann Intern Med. 2008; 149(7):ITC4-1-ITC4-15. [PMID: 18838723]

Item 42   Answer: C
Educational Objective: *Screen for obesity-related complications.*

The most appropriate evaluation for this patient includes fasting blood glucose, lipid panel, and serum creatinine evaluation. Abnormal waist circumference (>102 cm [40 in] for males or >88 cm [35 in] for females) is a measure for central obesity, a surrogate estimate for visceral fat. Visceral fat is a more metabolically active fat that releases free fatty acids into the portal system, which contributes to hyperlipidemia, hyperinsulinemia, and atherogenesis. BMI has a good correlation with risks associated with obesity and body fat, such as diabetes mellitus, heart disease, osteoarthritis, gallbladder disease, gastroesophageal reflux, and certain types of cancer (e.g., breast, endometrium, prostate, colon, kidney, and gallbladder). In adults with a BMI of 25 to 34.9, an abnormal waist circumference is associated with a greater risk than that determined by BMI alone. Patients identified as overweight (BMI, 25-29.9), obese (BMI, ≥30), or having an abnormal waist circumference are assessed for obesity-associated conditions such as hypertension, metabolic syndrome, endocrinopathies (i.e., hypothyroidism, diabetes, and Cushing syndrome), and reproductive disorders such as polycystic ovary disease. In all patients with a BMI greater than 25, obtain a blood glucose level, serum creatinine level, and fasting lipid profile (HDL cholesterol, triglycerides, and LDL cholesterol) to assess for comorbidities.

Screening asymptomatic patients with complete blood count and serum electrolytes (in the absence of conditions known to alter electrolytes) does not provide measureable health care benefits. Screening electrocardiograms are not recommended in asymptomatic patients because abnormalities of the resting electrocardiogram are rare, are not specific for coronary artery disease, and do not predict subsequent mortality from coronary disease. Similarly, screening chest x-rays are not helpful in asymptomatic persons. A sleep study may be indicated to confirm sleep apnea in patients with daytime fatigue, somnolence, hypertension, or history of snoring, but this patient is asymptomatic and does not require a sleep study or pulse oximetry to determine oxygen saturation.

KEY POINT

In all patients with a BMI greater than 25, obtain a blood glucose level, serum creatinine level, and fasting lipid profile (HDL cholesterol, triglycerides, and LDL cholesterol) to assess for comorbidities.

Bibliography

Bray GA, Wilson JF. In the clinic. Obesity. Ann Intern Med. 2008; 149(7):ITC4-1-ITC4-15. [PMID: 18838723]

Item 43   Answer: A
Educational Objective: *Treat obesity with orlistat.*

The best management option for this patient is to add a weight loss medication such as orlistat with meals, with continued encouragement of diet and exercise. A meta-analysis of orlistat trials demonstrated an average weight loss of 2.9 kg (6.4 lb) compared with placebo. Repeated attempts at dietary modification and exercise have failed to treat this patient's obesity, which is likely a contributing factor to her hyperlipidemia, hypertension, and type 2 diabetes mellitus. According to the American College of Physicians clinical guideline, drug therapy can be offered to obese patients who have failed to achieve their weight loss goals through diet and exercise alone. Before initiating drug therapy, it is important to have a frank discussion with the patient regarding the drugs' side effects, safety data, and the temporary nature of the weight loss achieved with medications.

Sibutramine is a sympathomimetic agent that suppresses appetite and food intake. Like orlistat, it is an effective drug for weight loss. However, sibutramine increases systolic blood pressure and pulse. It is also associated with in increase in nonfatal myocardial infarction and stroke in patients with preexisting cardiac disease. In October 2010, sibutramine was voluntarily withdrawn from the U.S. and Canadian markets for safety concerns.

Medications are a common contributing factor to obesity, and sulfonylureas such as glipizide have been associated with weight gain. However, insulin is also associated with weight gain, and switching the patient's medication from glipizide to insulin is unlikely to be of benefit.

Referring the patient for bariatric surgery is not indicated, as the patient does not meet commonly established referral guidelines (BMI ≥40 or BMI ≥35 with medical comorbidities such as sleep apnea, obesity-related cardiomyopathy, severe arthritis, hyperlipidemia, diabetes, or glucose intolerance).

KEY POINT

Pharmacologic treatment may be considered when obese patients fail to lose weight after an adequate trial of diet and exercise and treatment of any contributing comorbidities.

Bibliography

Bray GA, Wilson JF. In the clinic. Obesity. Ann Intern Med. 2008; 149(7):ITC4-1-15; quiz ITC4-16. [PMID: 18838723]

Item 44   Answer: D
Educational Objective: *Diagnose a stomal stenosis after gastric bypass surgery.*

The patient should undergo upper endoscopy to rule out a complication from her recent laparoscopic gastric bypass surgery, especially stomal stenosis (a stricture at the anastomosis of the gastric pouch and jejunum) or marginal ulcerations or erosions. If a stricture is diagnosed at the time of endoscopy, dilation of the stricture endoscopically often results in relief of symptoms without the need for repeat surgery.

Stomal stenosis typically presents with symptoms of nausea, vomiting, and inability to eat. Either barium swallow or upper endoscopy can establish the diagnosis. Endoscopy may be more appropriate than barium swallow in this patient because of the possibility of stomal erosion, which is more difficult to diagnose with barium radiography. Because the patient has not had other signs of upper gastrointestinal bleeding or anemia with her persistent symptoms, stricture is more likely. However, the patient takes naproxen, and therefore, ulceration at the anastomotic site should also be excluded.

Marginal erosions or ulcerations can be treated with proton pump inhibitors, such as omeprazole, and cessation of the NSAID in most patients. However, this therapy is not indicated until a diagnosis is established.

A right upper quadrant ultrasound would be useful for the diagnosis of biliary colic. Gallstones are very common after gastric bypass surgery with rapid weight loss. However, the close proximity to the surgery, normal hepatic enzyme levels, and the prominent recurrent vomiting (rather than pain) associated with this patient's symptoms argue against this diagnosis.

Surgical laparotomy should not be performed unless endoscopy fails to diagnose a treatable cause of her symptoms that can be managed less invasively.

KEY POINT

Stomal stenosis is a cause of persistent nausea and vomiting occurring within the first few months after gastric bypass surgery.

Bibliography

Schneider BE, Villegas L, Blackburn GL, Mun EC, Critchlow JF, Jones DB. Laparoscopic gastric bypass surgery: outcomes. J Laparoendosc Adv Surg Tech A. 2003;13(4):247-255. [PMID:14561253]

Item 45   Answer: E

Educational Objective: *Manage involuntary weight loss.*

The most appropriate management step is to re-evaluate the patient in 6 months. Among patients with involuntary weight loss, approximately 50% will have a physical cause for the weight loss, and a significant proportion of those with a physical cause have a malignancy. However, among patients who have an initial normal laboratory evaluation, normal chest x-ray, normal abdominal ultrasound, and no focal symptoms to guide further testing, the proportion who are ultimately diagnosed with an occult malignancy is extremely low, perhaps less than 1%. In these patients, continued extensive testing is unlikely to yield a diagnosis, leads to significant patient inconvenience, and is not cost effective. In particular, CT scanning has particularly low yield after an initial negative evaluation. A watchful waiting strategy is the preferred approach.

This patient does not have focal symptoms, abnormal laboratory studies, or radiographic screening to suggest upper endoscopy, chest CT, or measurement of antinuclear antibodies are indicated. No evidence indicates dietary supplements improve quality of life or mortality in this population.

KEY POINT

Among patients with involuntary weight loss, lack of focal symptoms and a negative baseline evaluation predict the absence of malignancy.

Bibliography

Metalidis C, Knockaert DC, Bobbaers H, Vanderschueren S. Involuntary weight loss. Does a negative baseline evaluation provide adequate reassurance? Eur J Intern Med. 2008;19(5):345-9. [PMID: 18549937]

Item 46   Answer: B

Educational Objective: *Diagnose depression as a cause of weight loss.*

The most likely cause of this patient's weight loss is depression. Among community-dwelling patients with involuntary weight loss, approximately 10% to 20% will have a psychiatric disorder as the cause. This proportion may be as high as 60% among nursing home residents. This patient's loss of interest in his previous activities represents anhedonia; this paired with his sleep difficulty, in the setting of a major life stressor (unemployment), may be a sign of major depression and warrant further evaluation. Unexplained weight loss of 5% or more in 1 month is one of the diagnostic criteria for major depression, although some patients present with weight gain due to a decline in physical activity and increase in appetite.

Although prostate cancer can rarely cause weight loss in the absence of other symptoms, it is a much less likely cause than is depression, particularly in a patient with anhedonia and sleep disturbance. This patient does not have polyuria or polydipsia to suggest a diagnosis of type 2 diabetes, and the fasting blood glucose level is normal. Age-appropriate cancer screening, which would include a colonoscopy in this age group, was normal 6 months ago, making colon cancer unlikely as well.

KEY POINT

Psychiatric disorders are common causes of involuntary weight loss among patients who do not have a physical cause for weight loss.

Bibliography

Vanderschueren S, Geens E, Knockaert D, Bobbaers H. The diagnostic spectrum of unintentional weight loss. Eur J Intern Med. 2005;16:160-164. [PMID: 15967329]

Item 47   Answer: B

Educational Objective: *Manage unintentional weight loss by stopping bupropion.*

The most appropriate next step in the management of this patient's unintended weight loss is to stop bupropion. Many medicines can cause involuntary weight loss by inducing anorexia, dysgeusia, gastrointestinal symptoms, dry mouth, confusion or inattention, or a movement disorder. The patient's medication list should be reviewed with special attention to the presence of anticholinergic agents, antiparkinsonian agents, digoxin, iron and potassium supplements, aspirin and NSAIDs, opiates, certain antidepressants (bupropion and fluoxetine), thyroid hormone supplementation, and certain hypoglycemic agents (metformin and exenatide). In this patient, there is a possible temporal relationship between the initiation of bupropion and the onset of anorexia and weight loss. Because she has no other findings to suggest another cause of weight loss, stopping the bupropion and carefully observing the patient is the most reasonable option. Most experts recommend maintenance with an antidepressant drug for 4 to 9 months after remission of symptoms. This patient has been treated for 7 months, so it is not unreasonable to discontinue therapy with careful follow up.

Body imaging of the thorax and abdomen with CT or MRI in the absence of historical information or physical examination findings pointing to the thorax or abdomen has not been shown to help determine the cause of involuntary weight loss. In studies in which a cause of involuntary weight loss was aggressively pursued, a thorough history and physical examination and basic laboratory testing, rather than advanced imaging, provided the diagnosis in nearly all patients. Similarly, in the absence of symptoms, upper endoscopy is unlikely to reveal a cause of unintentional weight loss and is not indicated.

Appetite stimulant therapy for involuntary weight loss with megestrol acetate or similar agents has been studied mainly in patients with AIDS or cancer cachexia. In these patients, certain agents have been shown to promote weight gain; however, a survival advantage has not been shown. Furthermore, the use of an appetite stimulate does not address the underlying cause of weight loss.

KEY POINT

Medications can be a cause of involuntary weight loss in elderly patients.

Bibliography

Alibhai SM, Greenwood C, Payette H. An approach to the management of unintentional weight loss in elderly people. CMAJ. 2005;172(6):773-780. [PMID: 15767612]

Item 48   Answer: C
Educational Objective: *Diagnose chronic obstructive pulmonary disease as a cause of weight loss.*

Severe chronic obstructive pulmonary disease (COPD) can cause systemic effects, including unexplained weight loss, skeletal muscle dysfunction, increased cardiovascular morbidity and mortality, increased risk for type 2 diabetes mellitus, osteoporosis, fractures, and depression. Unexplained weight loss occurs in approximately half of the patients with severe COPD, mostly because of the loss of skeletal muscle mass. Unexplained weight loss carries a poor prognosis in COPD independent of other indicators, such as FEV_1 or PCO_2. The mechanisms underlying these systemic effects are unclear but are probably interrelated and multifactorial, including inactivity, systemic inflammation, tissue hypoxia, and oxidative stress. Increases in concentrations of inflammatory mediators indicating peripheral blood cell activation also have been found throughout the body and may mediate some of these systemic effects.

Although the weight loss of malignancy is a possibility in this patient, the absence of gastrointestinal symptoms or other localizing symptoms, the normal cancer screening test results within the last year, and the patient's history of severe COPD make the cachexia of COPD, not cancer, the most likely cause

in this patient. The patient's spirometry indicates severe COPD, and aggressive management of COPD is necessary. Evaluation for depression is also indicated.

KEY POINT

Severe chronic obstructive pulmonary disease can cause systemic effects, including unintentional weight loss, skeletal muscle dysfunction, and increased risk of cardiovascular disease, osteoporosis, and depression.

Bibliography

Agusti A, Soriano JB. COPD as a systemic disease. COPD. 2008;5(2):133-138. [PMID: 18415812]

Item 49   Answer: D
Educational Objective: *Treat heavy menstrual bleeding with oral medroxyprogesterone.*

The most appropriate next management step is oral medroxyprogesterone acetate. In patients who present with menorrhagia (heavy menstrual bleeding) with a known etiology, several therapeutic agents can decrease bleeding. For moderate bleeding that can be managed on an outpatient basis, a progestational agent such as medroxyprogesterone acetate can be given for 10 to 21 days. The progesterone will typically act to stabilize the endometrium and stop uterine blood flow. Alternatively, a monophasic oral contraceptive may be dosed four times a day for 5 to 7 days, and subsequently reduced to daily dosing for 3 weeks, followed by withdrawal bleeding.

Nonsteroidal anti-inflammatory drugs act by inhibiting prostaglandin synthesis and may decrease mild bleeding by approximately 30%. Once daily oral contraceptives are effective in decreasing menstrual blood loss by 50%; however, in bleeding that is as heavy as this case, neither of these medications would be as effective as medroxyprogesterone.

If the patient were orthostatic or dizzy from blood loss, intravenous estrogen would be appropriate. Parenteral conjugated estrogens are approximately 70% effective in stopping the bleeding entirely. Pulmonary embolism and venous thrombosis are complications of intravenous estrogen therapy.

Surgical options are reserved for cases when medical treatment fails, but it is likely in this case that medical treatment can provide a bridge until her scheduled surgical procedure. Monitoring her for a week will not be helpful, because it is likely she will sustain a great deal of additional blood loss during this time.

KEY POINT

Medroxyprogesterone acetate for 10 to 21 days is effective treatment for moderate menstrual bleeding.

Bibliography

Fazio SB, Ship AN. Abnormal uterine bleeding. South Med J. 2007;100(4):376-82; quiz 383, 402. [PMID: 17458397]

Item 50   Answer: C

Educational Objective: *Diagnose polycystic ovary syndrome.*

This patient has classic polycystic ovary syndrome (PCOS). PCOS affects 6% of women of child-bearing age and typically presents with oligomenorrhea and signs of androgen excess (hirsutism, acne, and occasionally alopecia). Insulin resistance is a major feature of the disorder, as are overweight and obesity, although only 50% of affected women are obese. Typically, there is a mild elevation in testosterone and dehydroepiandrosterone sulfate levels and a luteinizing hormone to follicle-stimulating hormone ratio of greater than 2:1. Diagnosis requires two of the three following features: (1) ovulatory dysfunction, (2) laboratory or clinical evidence of hyperandrogenism, and (3) ultrasonographic evidence of polycystic ovaries. This patient has ovulatory dysfunction and clinical evidence of hyperandrogenism.

This patient's total testosterone level (84 ng/dL [2.9 nmol/L]), although somewhat high, is not high enough to raise concerns about a tumor. Typically, the serum testosterone level in patients with PCOS rarely exceeds 150 ng/dL (5.2 nmol/L); higher levels warrant a search for an adrenal or ovarian tumor. In addition the patient lacks any signs of virilism that is commonly associated with androgen secreting tumors such as sudden onset of menstrual irregularity, hirsutism, acne, deepening of the voice, frontal (or crown) balding, increased muscle mass, or clitoromegaly.

The absence of galactorrhea and normal prolactin level eliminates a pituitary prolactinoma as the cause of the patient's oligomenorrhea. Additionally, hyperprolactinemia does not cause hirsutism.

KEY POINT

Polycystic ovary syndrome typically presents with oligomenorrhea and signs of androgen excess including hirsutism, acne, and occasionally alopecia.

Bibliography
Wilson JF. The polycystic ovary syndrome. Ann Intern Med. 2011; 154(3):ITC21. [PMID: 21282692]

Item 51   Answer: B

Educational Objective: *Treat perimenopausal symptoms with estrogen replacement therapy.*

The most appropriate treatment for this patient is estrogen replacement therapy (ERT). ERT provides significant relief for hot flushes associated with menopause in 50% to 90% of patients. There is no clear benefit of one estrogen-containing product over another. Relief of hot flushes is the primary (arguably the only) indication for ERT, although it also reduces the rate of postmenopausal bone density loss. However, the benefits of ERT must be weighed against the risks, which include potential increased rates of breast cancer, thromboembolic events, and cardiac events.

Contraindications to estrogen use include undiagnosed vaginal bleeding, breast cancer, other estrogen-sensitive cancers, current or previous history of venous or arterial thrombosis, and liver dysfunction or disease. The U.S. Food and Drug Administration recommends use of the smallest effective dose of hormone replacement therapy for the shortest duration possible to treat menopausal symptoms.

Although some studies have reported positive results with black cohosh, reports have been inconsistent, and the methodologically strongest studies have found no evidence of benefit. Conclusive evidence is similarly lacking for other alternative medicines such as soy proteins and red clover.

Prescription treatments for which there is some evidence of benefit in patients with hot flushes include the selective serotonin and norepinephrine reuptake inhibitors venlafaxine and selective serotonin reuptake inhibitors such as citalopram, paroxetine, fluvoxamine, and fluoxetine. These can be considered as second-line agents, especially in women who also have some symptoms of mood or anxiety disorders. It is hypothesized that hot flushes are pathophysiologically associated with increased noradrenergic activity and decreased serotonergic activity, so it is likely that the blockage of serotonin reuptake is responsible for the benefits with these agents. Other agents that may relieve hot flushes include mirtazapine and gabapentin.

Raloxifene is a selective estrogen receptor modulator that is approved for the prevention of postmenopausal bone mass loss, but it does not help with hot flushes or other postmenopausal symptoms, and may even worsen them.

KEY POINT

Estrogen replacement therapy provides effective relief of hot flushes, but its use must be weighed against the potential adverse effects.

Bibliography
Col NF, Fairfield KM, Ewan-Whyte C, Miller H. In the clinic. Menopause. Ann Intern Med. 2009;150(7):ITC4-1-15; quiz ITC4-16. [PMID: 19349628]

Item 52   Answer: D

Educational Objective: *Evaluate secondary amenorrhea with a progestin withdrawal challenge.*

The next step in the evaluation of this patient with secondary amenorrhea after stopping her oral contraceptive pill is a progestin withdrawal challenge. This patient has an unremarkable personal and family medical history and no evidence of androgen excess. Results of her screening laboratory studies are negative for thyroid disorders, ovarian dysfunction, and hyperprolactinemia. Given these data, the differential diagnosis of this patient's secondary amenorrhea includes anatomic defects and chronic anovulation, with or without estrogen. The differential diagnosis can be narrowed most effectively with a progestin withdrawal challenge. Menses after challenge excludes anatomic defects and chronic anovulation without estrogen. Therefore, a progestin withdrawal challenge is the most appropriate next step.

Polycystic ovary syndrome (PCOS) affects 6% of women of childbearing age and typically presents with oligomenorrhea and signs of androgen excess (hirsutism, acne, and occasionally alopecia). Insulin resistance is a major feature of the disorder, as is overweight and obesity (although only 50% of women with PCOS are obese). Typically, testosterone and dehydroepiandrosterone sulfate levels are mildly elevated, and the luteinizing hormone to follicle-stimulating hormone ratio is greater than 2:1. Measurement of dehydroepiandrosterone sulfate is rarely clinically useful.

Positive withdrawal bleeding after the progestin withdrawal challenge suggests an estradiol level of greater than 40 pg/mL (146.8 pmol/L) and thus obviates the need for measurement of serum estradiol levels.

An MRI of the pituitary gland is unnecessary at this point because her follicle-stimulating hormone, prolactin, and thyroid levels are all normal.

KEY POINT

Menstrual flow on progestin withdrawal indicates relatively normal estrogen production and a patent outflow tract, which limits the differential diagnosis of secondary amenorrhea to chronic anovulation with estrogen present.

Bibliography
Practice Committee of the American Society for Reproductive Medicine. Current evaluation of amenorrhea. Fertil Steril. 2006;86(5 Suppl 1):S148-S155. [PMID:17055812]

Item 53   Answer: B
Educational Objective: *Evaluate secondary amenorrhea with measurement of serum follicle stimulating hormone and prolactin levels.*

This patient's serum follicle-stimulating hormone (FSH) and prolactin levels should be measured. Secondary amenorrhea is defined by the absence of menses for 3 or more consecutive months in a woman who has menstruated previously. Menstrual failure can be complete amenorrhea or varying degrees of oligomenorrhea, the latter being much more common. Pregnancy should be excluded in all patients prior to other evaluations. Polycystic ovary syndrome is the most common cause of secondary amenorrhea, and hypogonadotropic hypogonadism (low FSH and low estrogen) is most commonly caused by hyperprolactinemia (elevated serum prolactin). In young women, secondary amenorrhea may be associated with hypergonatrophic hypogonadism. This group includes primary ovarian failure (often due to Turner syndrome mosaicism and autoimmune disorders) and in cancer survivors can be traced to chemotherapy or radiation treatments.

Laboratory evaluation is first directed toward ovarian failure, hyperprolactinemia, and thyroid disease. Therefore, FSH, pro-

lactin, thyroid-stimulating hormone, and free thyroxine (T₄) levels are generally measured. An FSH greater than 20 mU/mL (20 U/L) suggests ovarian failure.

If serum FSH and prolactin levels are normal on laboratory studies, the next step in the evaluation is a progestin withdrawal challenge. If the progestin challenge does not result in withdrawal bleeding, then assessment of the pelvic anatomy with ultrasonography or MRI would be appropriate. A high serum prolactin level requires additional pituitary evaluation, including MRI. Obtaining an MRI before this patient's serum prolactin level has been determined, however, is premature.

This patient has no symptoms of hyperandrogenemia. Therefore, measurement of her total serum testosterone level is of little value.

KEY POINT

After pregnancy is excluded, the initial evaluation of secondary amenorrhea includes measurement of follicle-stimulating hormone, thyroid-stimulating hormone, and prolactin levels.

Bibliography
Practice Committee of the American Society for Reproductive Medicine. Current evaluation of amenorrhea. Fertil Steril. 2006;86(5 suppl 1): S148-S155. [PMID:17055812]

Item 54   Answer: D
Educational Objective: *Diagnose abnormal uterine bleeding with an endometrial biopsy.*

The most appropriate next step in the management of this patient with abnormal uterine bleeding is to obtain an endometrial biopsy. Abnormal uterine bleeding can take many forms, including infrequent menses, excessive flow, prolonged duration of menses, intermenstrual bleeding, and postmenopausal bleeding. In all patients with abnormal bleeding, physical examination should include a pelvic examination and Pap smear. In pre- or perimenopausal patients, a urine pregnancy test is also appropriate. Further laboratory testing depends on the findings of the history and physical examination and may include cultures for gonorrhea and *Chlamydia trachomatis*, complete blood count, thyroid function tests, plasma glucose measurement, prolactin levels, and coagulation studies. After performing appropriate laboratory studies, an assessment of the endometrial lining with an endometrial biopsy is appropriate to rule out endometrial cancer or hyperplasia in patients older than 35 years of age with abnormal uterine bleeding.

Luteinizing hormone and follicle-stimulating hormone levels may be able to confirm the menopausal state, but these tests cannot exclude the possibility of endometrial carcinoma.

In patients with anovulatory bleeding, initiation of oral contraceptives or cyclic progestins can help to maintain regular cycles. However, this intervention would be inappropriate without first eliminating the possibility of endometrial cancer as the cause of the abnormal uterine bleeding in this patient.

Estrogen is the most effective treatment for the relief of hot flushes, with a 50% to 90% response rate, and evidence shows that even low doses provide effective symptom relief. Relief of hot flushes is now considered the primary reason for initiating estrogen replacement therapy. Estrogen replacement therapy is not indicated in the management of abnormal uterine bleeding and would be harmful if the bleeding is caused by an endometrial cancer.

KEY POINT

An assessment of the endometrial lining with an endometrial biopsy is appropriate to rule out endometrial cancer or hyperplasia in patients older than 35 years with abnormal uterine bleeding.

Bibliography

Fazio SB, Ship AN. Abnormal uterine bleeding. South Med J. 2007;100(4):376-382. [PMID:17458397]

Item 55　　Answer:　C
Educational Objective: *Diagnose cellulitis.*

This patient has cellulitis. Cellulitis is a rapidly spreading, deep (dermis), subcutaneous-based infection most frequently caused by *Staphylococcus aureus* or group A streptococci. It is characterized by a well-demarcated area of warmth, swelling, tenderness, and erythema that may be accompanied by lymphatic streaking and/or fever and chills. Risk factors for lower-extremity cellulitis include inflammation (eczema), tinea pedis, onychomycosis, skin trauma, chronic leg ulcerations, type 2 diabetes mellitus, and edema. Cellulitis is a clinical diagnosis; cultures are usually not necessary and are seldom positive. Treatment is based on the risk of methicillin-resistant *S. aureus* (MRSA) infection and the severity of illness and generally consists of oral antibiotics and analgesics; intravenous antibiotics may be necessary for unsuccessful outpatient treatment, in some patients with diabetes, or if signs of systemic toxicity are present.

Allergic contact dermatitis (ACD) is a delayed-type hypersensitivity reaction in which the skin is itchy, red, edematous, weepy, and crusted, sometimes with vesicles or bullae. Contact dermatitis can usually be differentiated from cellulitis by the presence of pruritus and the absence of fever. Atopic dermatitis, when acute, results in poorly demarcated, eczematous, crusted, erythematous papulovesicular plaques and excoriations that characteristically are pruritic and involve the antecubital and popliteal fossae and flexural wrists. Venous stasis dermatitis affects the skin on the lower legs, particularly around the medial malleoli, and results from venous hypertension, edema, chronic inflammation, and microangiopathy. Bilateral involvement, absence of fever or leukocytosis, hyperpigmentation due to hemosiderin deposition, and minimal pain help distinguish venous stasis dermatitis from cellulitis.

KEY POINT

The hallmark of cellulitis is a well-demarcated, rapidly spreading area of warmth, swelling, tenderness, and erythema that may be accompanied by fever.

Bibliography

Daum RS. Clinical practice. Skin and soft-tissue infections caused by methicillin-resistant *Staphylococcus aureus*. N Engl J Med. 2007;357(4):380-90. [PMID: 17652653]

Item 56　　Answer:　C
Educational Objective: *Diagnose seborrheic dermatitis*

This patient has seborrheic dermatitis. Seborrheic dermatitis affects areas of the scalp (dandruff) and face that are rich in sebaceous glands and is distinguished from other dermatoses primarily by its distribution. Lesions are erythematous, with dry or greasy scales and crusts, and may be pruritic. Common areas of involvement include the nasolabial folds, cheeks, eyebrows, eyelids, and the external auditory canals. Frequent remissions and exacerbations are common. Treatment consists of low-potency corticosteroids (face), ketoconazole cream (face), and medicated shampoos that contain tar, ketoconazole, or selenium sulfide (scalp).

Patients with systemic lupus erythematosus (SLE) almost exclusively develop acute cutaneous lupus erythematosus (LE), which is typically precipitated by sunlight. Acute cutaneous LE can present as the classic "butterfly rash," characterized by confluent malar erythema, or as generalized, red, papular or urticarial lesions on the sun-exposed skin. Other symptoms of SLE may be present.

Rosacea is a chronic inflammatory skin disorder of unknown etiology affecting the face, typically the cheeks and nose, and usually occurring after the age of 30 years. Erythema with telangiectasias, pustules, and papules without comedones are found on physical examination. Rosacea can be differentiated from seborrheic dermatitis by the presence of pustules. In early stages, rosacea can present with only facial erythema and resemble the butterfly rash of SLE; however, acute cutaneous LE typically spares the nasal labial folds and areas under the nose and lower lip.

Dermatomyositis is a condition with characteristic cutaneous manifestations combined with proximal inflammatory muscle weakness; cutaneous disease may sometimes be the only manifestation. The distinctive cutaneous features are the heliotrope rash characterized by a violaceous to dusky erythematous periorbital rash and Gottron papules appearing as slightly elevated, scaly, violaceous papules and plaques over bony prominences, particularly the small joints of the hands.

KEY POINT

Seborrheic dermatitis affects the scalp and face and is recognized by erythematous, dry, or greasy scales and crusts.

Bibliography

Naldi L, Rebora A. Clinical practice. Seborrheic dermatitis. N Engl J Med. 2009;360(4):387-96. [PMID: 19164189]

Item 57   Answer: D
Educational Objective: *Diagnose tinea cruris.*

This patient has tinea cruris. Superficial fungal infections, or tinea, are classified by body part. Tinea cruris is a subacute and chronic dermatophyte infection of the skin, involving the groin, pubic region, and inner thighs; in contrast to candidiasis, the scrotum is rarely involved. The condition is recognized as light pink to red papules and thin plaques with scaling borders. Occasionally the lesions may have an arciform or polycyclic pattern. The lesion has an "active border," meaning that the border has more redness and scaling than the inner portion of the lesion, which may have central clearing. The presence of fungi can be confirmed with a potassium hydroxide (KOH) slide preparation.

Cutaneous candidiasis is a superficial infection that occurs most frequently in warm, moist skin areas. Many patients with this infection have altered local immunity, such as increased moisture at the site of infection, diabetes, or altered systemic immunity. The infection begins with pustules on a red base that become eroded and confluent. Eventually, the rash evolves into a sharply demarcated, bright red patch (or patches), with small, pustular lesions at the periphery (satellite lesions).

Psoriasis can present on the trunk with red to salmon-colored papules and plaques that are covered with a heavy silver-white scale.

The lesions of seborrheic dermatitis are ill defined (lack a distinct border), are yellowish-red, vary in size, and are usually associated with a greasy or dandruff-like scale. Seborrheic dermatitis most commonly occurs on the scalp, central face, upper mid-chest, and other oily areas of the body.

KEY POINT

Tinea is recognized as light pink to red papules and thin plaques with scaling, "active" borders and central clearing.

Bibliography

Schwartz RA. Superficial fungal infections. Lancet. 2004;364:1173-82. [PMID: 15451228]

Item 58   Answer: D
Educational Objective: *Diagnose Stevens-Johnson syndrome.*

This patient has Stevens-Johnson syndrome, which is characterized by fever followed by the onset of erythematous macules and plaques that progress to epidermal necrosis and sloughing. Involvement is limited to less than 10% of the body surface area. Mucous membranes are affected in most patients, and ocular, oral, and genital surfaces may be involved. Toxic epidermal necrolysis is the more severe variant of this condition, and is defined as epidermal necrosis and sloughing involving more than 30% of the body surface area. A sulfonamide is the most likely causative drug, but Stevens-Johnson syndrome can be caused by other antibiotics, anti-epileptic drugs, and allopurinol, as well as certain systemic diseases.

Allergic contact dermatitis is a delayed-type hypersensitivity reaction. The first reaction to an antigen may occur several weeks after exposure, but subsequent reactions usually develop within 24 to 48 hours of reexposure. Allergic contact dermatitis is usually intensely itchy. In acute reactions, the skin is red, edematous, weepy, and crusted, and there may be vesicles or bullae. This patient's eruption, which involves many parts of his body (including the soft palate) and includes the presence of urticarial targetoid lesions, is not consistent with the diagnosis of allergic contact dermatitis.

Cellulitis is a rapidly spreading, deep, subcutaneous-based infection characterized by a well-demarcated area of warmth, swelling, tenderness, and erythema that may be accompanied by lymphatic streaking and/or fever and chills. It is not characterized by urticarial targetoid lesions or involvement of the oral mucosa.

The "red man syndrome" is the most common adverse reaction to vancomycin. This reaction does not appear to be antibody related and is characterized by flushing, erythema, and pruritus involving primarily the upper body, neck, and face. This patient has none of the clinical findings characteristic of red man syndrome and was not exposed to vancomycin, making this an unlikely diagnosis.

KEY POINT

Stevens-Johnson syndrome is an acute severe cutaneous reaction characterized by fever followed by the onset of erythematous macules and plaques that progress to epidermal necrosis and sloughing; involvement is limited to less than 10% of the body surface area.

Bibliography

Greenberger PA. 8. Drug allergy. J Allergy Clin Immunol. 2006;117(2 Suppl Mini-Primer):S464-S470. [PMID: 16455348]

Item 59   Answer: A
Educational Objective: *Diagnose erythema multiforme.*

The most likely diagnosis is erythema multiforme. Erythema multiforme is a mucocutaneous reaction characterized by targetoid lesions and, in most cases, both skin and mucosal involvement. The majority (up to 90%) of recurrent cases of erythema multiforme have been associated with infections, the most common of which is herpes simplex virus (both HSV-1 and HSV-2). It may also be idiopathic or drug related. No virus is routinely recovered with culture, and treatment with antiviral agents does not affect the outcome of an acute outbreak. Suppressive antiviral therapy, however, may minimize the number of erythema multiforme recurrences. It is important to recognize that recurrences of erythema multiforme can occur in the absence of apparent clinical reactivation of HSV; patients may not be aware that they are infected with HSV.

Erythema migrans (also called erythema chronicum migrans) is the hallmark cutaneous lesion of early Lyme disease. A centrifugally spreading ring of erythema that resembles a bull's eye usually develops at the site of infection 3 to 30 days after a tick bite. Erythema migrans lesions are most typically found near the axilla, inguinal region, popliteal fossa, or at the belt line, and palmar involvement is rare, if it occurs at all. Lesions slowly expand over days or weeks, with central clearing producing a target or bull's-eye appearance, and increase in size to 20 cm or more. Erythema migrans is distinguished from erythema multiforme by the lesion size, its location, and lack of associated mucosal involvement.

Rocky Mountain spotted fever (RMSF) is a tick-borne disease caused by *Rickettsia rickettsii*. RMSF may present with subtle, fine, pink, blanching macules and papules on the wrists and ankles that then spread centripetally and to the palms and soles. As the rash spreads, the characteristic petechial and purpuric "spots" appear. Most patients have fever, severe headache, and myalgia.

Streptococcal infections have been associated with erythema nodosum, flares of psoriasis, and several skin infections, including perianal cellulitis and blistering distal dactylitis; however, they are not commonly associated with erythema multiforme.

KEY POINT

Erythema multiforme is a mucocutaneous reaction characterized by targetoid lesions and, in most cases, both skin and mucosal involvement.

Bibliography

Aurelian L, Ono F, Burnett J. Herpes simplex virus (HSV)-associated erythema multiforme (HAEM): a viral disease with an autoimmune component. Dermatol Online J. 2003;9(1):1. [PMID:12639459]

Item 60   Answer: C

Educational Objective: *Treat acute herpes zoster infection with oral famciclovir.*

The most appropriate treatment for this patient is oral famciclovir. This patient has acute herpes zoster. When given within 72 hours of the onset of the herpetic rash, antiviral therapy with oral acyclovir, valacyclovir, or famciclovir decreases acute pain severity and duration, promotes more rapid healing of the lesions, and possibly decreases postherpetic neuralgia incidence and severity. These benefits appear to be greatest in patients older than 50 years. This patient's pain began more than 72 hours ago, but the rash has been present for just 24 hours. Therefore, antiviral therapy will likely be beneficial. Because of their improved bioavailability, valacyclovir and famciclovir are preferred to acyclovir, which is poorly absorbed and requires more pills daily.

Adding corticosteroids may help accelerate healing of lesions, decrease the time to acute pain resolution, decrease insomnia incidence, help patients return to normal daily activities sooner, and decrease analgesic pain medication needs. However,

corticosteroids do not appear to decrease postherpetic neuralgia incidence. Therefore, if corticosteroids are given, they should be used only as an adjunct to antiviral agents, never as the sole therapy.

The bioavailability of oral valacyclovir and famciclovir is excellent, so treatment of cutaneous herpes zoster infection with intravenous acyclovir is not necessary. It is reasonable to consider beginning therapy with intravenous acyclovir for patients with severe herpes zoster ophthalmicus or for those who develop central nervous systemic complications of herpes zoster, but this patient does not meet any of these criteria.

There is no role for antiviral topical creams or ointments, including topical acyclovir or penciclovir, in the management of herpes zoster because they are not as effective as systemic antiviral treatment, and their addition to systemic antiviral treatment does not enhance healing compared with systemic treatment alone.

KEY POINT

In patients with herpes zoster, administration of oral acyclovir, valacyclovir, or famciclovir within 72 hours of the development of the rash decreases acute pain severity and duration, promotes more rapid healing of the lesions, and possibly decreases postherpetic neuralgia incidence and severity.

Bibliography

Wilson JF. Herpes zoster. Ann Intern Med. 2011;154(5):ITC31. [PMID:21357905]

Item 61   Answer: C

Educational Objective: *Diagnose rosacea.*

This patient has rosacea, which is an inflammatory dermatitis characterized by erythema, telangiectasias, papules, pustules, and sebaceous hyperplasia that develops on the central face, including the nasolabial folds. Rhinophyma, or the presence of a bulbous, red nose, is a variant of this condition. Recurrent flushing in response to stimuli such as spicy food or alcohol is a common manifestation.

Dermatomyositis may be associated with various skin manifestations. Periungual erythema and malar erythema, consisting of a light purple (heliotrope) edematous discoloration of the upper eyelids and periorbital tissues, are the most common presentations. Dermatomyositis also may cause an erythematous, papular eruption that develops in a V-shaped pattern along the neck and upper torso; in a shawl-shaped pattern along the upper arms; and on the elbows, knees, ankles, and other sun-exposed areas. Involvement of the hands may include scaly, slightly raised, purplish papules and plaques that develop in periarticular areas of the metacarpal and interphalangeal joints and other bony prominences (Gottron sign or Gottron papules) and scaly, rough, dry, darkened, cracked, horizontal lines on the palmar and lateral aspects of the fingers (mechanic's hands).

Psoriasis usually involves the scalp, elbows, or other extensor areas but does manifest as an isolated facial rash. Characteristic findings of psoriasis include an erythematous plaque with an adherent, variably thick, silvery scale.

Seborrheic dermatitis causes white, scaling macules and papules on yellowish-red skin and may be greasy or dry. Sticky crusts and fissures often develop behind the ears, and significant dandruff or scaling of the scalp frequently occurs. Seborrheic dermatitis may develop in a "butterfly"-shaped pattern but also may involve the nasolabial folds, eyebrows, and forehead. This condition usually improves during the summer and worsens in the fall and winter.

Distinguishing rosacea from systemic lupus erythematosus can be difficult and is frequently a reason that patients are referred to a dermatologist. Systemic lupus erythematosus is unlikely in this patient because the malar rash associated with this condition is usually photosensitive and often spares the nasolabial folds and the areas below the nares and lower lip (areas relatively protected from the sun). Finally, the patient has no other supporting symptoms or signs of systemic lupus erythematosus.

> **KEY POINT**
> Rosacea is an inflammatory dermatitis characterized by erythema, telangiectasias, papules, pustules, and sebaceous hyperplasia that affects the central face, including the nasolabial folds.

Bibliography
Powell FC. Clinical practice. Rosacea. N Engl J Med. 2005;352(8):793-803. [PMID:15728812]

Item 62   Answer: C
Educational Objective: *Diagnose seborrheic keratoses.*

This patient has seborrheic keratoses, a benign skin condition. These lesions are common in adults and increase in number with age. They are characterized by sharply demarcated, tan to dark brown, warty papules, plaques, and nodules that have a waxy texture and appear to be "stuck on" the skin. While they can arise on any area of the skin, they are frequently located in the scalp and on the back and chest.

Skin cancers tend to occur on the sun-exposed parts of the body. Basal cell carcinoma is a pearly or translucent papule or nodule with associated telangiectasias. Melanomas, like seborrheic keratoses, are pigmented, but do not classically have a waxy, warty surface. Melanomas often have irregular borders, whereas seborrheic keratoses are usually well demarcated. Distinguishing between the two can be difficult, however, and a biopsy may be necessary if the diagnosis is in question. Squamous cell carcinoma presents as a scaly, hyperkeratotic, red or pink papule, patch, or plaque. It is not brown, tan, or black and does not have a warty appearance like seborrheic keratoses.

> **KEY POINT**
> Seborrheic keratoses are common, benign neoplasms that present as brown to black, well-demarcated, "stuck-on"–appearing papules with waxy surfaces.

Bibliography
Luba MC, Bangs SA, Mohler AM, Stulberg DL. Common benign skin tumors. Am Fam Physician. 2003;67(4):729-738. [PMID:12613727]

Item 63   Answer: A
Educational Objective: *Treat inflammatory acne with oral antibiotics.*

This patient has cystic and pustular acne and should be treated with oral antibiotics. Acne is classified by severity and type as noninflammatory and inflammatory acne. Noninflammatory acne consists of open comedos ("blackheads") or closed comedones ("whiteheads"). Subsequent inflammatory papules, pustules, or nodules may develop. Acne lesions most commonly develop in areas that have a high concentration of sebaceous glands, including the face, neck, chest, upper arms, and back. Exacerbating factors are mechanical obstructions (such as clothing) and medications (anabolic steroids such as danazol and testosterone, corticosteroids, isoniazid, lithium, and phenytoin). Noninflammatory acne can be treated with topical comedolytic agents such as benzoyl peroxide, salicylic acid, azelaic acid, and retinoids. Mild inflammatory acne consisting of comedones and a few papules and pustules can be treated with topical comedolytic agents combined with a topical antibiotic. If topical therapy is ineffective, oral antibiotic therapy is indicated. Oral antibiotic therapy may be the first line of therapy in cases where the cystic and pustular acne lesions are extensive and topical application would be impractical or in cases where the disease is so severe that there would be a high likelihood of failure with topical treatment alone, as in this patient. Isotretinoin is the only medication that alters the natural history of acne, and it is indicated for cystic and pustular acne that is unresponsive to antibiotics. Isotretinoin is highly teratogenic and has potentially severe side effects, including hypertriglyceridemia, pseudotumor cerebri, decreased bone mineral density, and possibly depression and psychosis; strict attention to informed consent and careful monitoring are mandatory if this medication is used.

> **KEY POINT**
> Oral antibiotic therapy is first line in cases where the cystic and pustular acne lesions are extensive and topical application would be impractical or in cases where the disease is so severe that there would be a high likelihood of failure with topical treatment alone.

Bibliography
Bershad SV. In the clinic. Acne. Ann Intern Med. 2008;149:ITC1-1-ITC1-16. [PMID: 18591631]

Item 64   Answer: A

Educational Objective: *Diagnose acute urticaria.*

This patient has acute urticaria. Urticaria, also known as hives, is a common skin finding that arises from a recurrent, but transient, cutaneous swelling with sudden erythema caused by vascular extravasation. This condition can signify a completely benign, almost evanescent nuisance, or a severe, life-threatening form of urticaria called angioedema. The hallmark of urticaria is the rapid appearance of the wheal, a superficial, itchy, sometimes painful, discrete swelling of the skin. Wheals can be multiple or isolated and usually involve the trunk and extremities, sparing the palms and soles. The hallmark of angioedema is self-limited, localized swelling of the skin or mucosa, usually the lips, face, hands, feet, penis, or scrotum. The skin is either normal or red in color and itching is absent unless associated with urticarial lesions. Concomitant angioedema and urticaria occur in 40% of patients; 40% have urticaria alone; and 20% have angioedema but no urticaria.

The clinical classification of urticaria depends on symptom duration and precipitating factors. By definition, the individual lesions of acute urticaria last less than 24 hours. Lesions can be observed carefully by drawing circles around them and observing their duration. Acute urticaria is generally related to environmental allergens, including drugs, foods, and occasionally inhalants. Penicillin, aspirin, NSAIDs, contrast dyes, and sulfonamides are the most common drug-related causes of acute urticaria. Other common exposures that precipitate acute urticaria are latex, nuts, fish, eggs, and chocolate. When chronic urticaria occurs, patient diaries are often helpful in determining the cause. An individual wheal in chronic urticaria lasts more than 24 hours and may occur several times per week for up to six weeks.

Erythema multiforme is recognized by the appearance of red papules, vesicles, and bullae distributed in round, often target-shaped patterns. They often have a bullous component in the center of the target.

KEY POINT

The hallmark of urticaria is the rapid appearance of the wheal, a superficial, itchy, sometimes painful, discrete swelling of the skin.

Bibliography

Frigas E, Park MA. Acute urticaria and angioedema: diagnostic and treatment considerations. Am J Clin Dermatol. 2009;10(4):239-50. [PMID: 19489657]

Item 65   Answer: D

Educational Objective: *Diagnose benign lympha-denopathy.*

The most appropriate management for this patient is reassurance and watchful waiting. This patient has none of the features to suggest a serious cause of her generalized lymphadenopathy. She is younger than 40 years of age, and the lymphadenopathy is less than 2 cm, mobile and rubbery in consistency, and is located in regions typical for benign lymphadenopathy. Her recent viral-like illness suggests that it is reactive lymphadenopathy. Usually, an evaluation is initiated in patients with systemic symptoms, progressively enlarging lymph nodes, or persistently enlarged nodes for more than 2 weeks. Therefore, this is a situation in which watchful waiting is the correct course of action.

If she had any signs or symptoms to suggest a pathological cause of lymphadenopathy (systemic symptoms, progressive enlargement, persistence beyond 3 weeks), then a complete blood count with a differential and a chest radiograph would be reasonable tests in addition to targeting the evaluation of localized signs or symptoms. Her illness 2 weeks ago could have been Epstein-Barr virus (EBV) infection or another infectious mononucleosis-like illness, such as cytomegalovirus infection. The early antigen antibody test for EBV may not become positive until a month after the illness. The capsid (anti-VCA) IgM antibody becomes positive earlier, as does the heterophile agglutination test (monospot), and these are the usual early tests ordered for EBV infection. No features in the history or examination suggest a pathological cause of the lymphadenopathy warranting biopsy. Although the inguinal lymph node was the largest, it was less than 2 cm, and furthermore, inguinal lymph nodes are frequently reactive and thus the least preferred for biopsy when other enlarged lymph nodes are present.

KEY POINT

Lymphadenopathy is usually evaluated in patients with systemic symptoms, progressively enlarging lymph nodes, or persistently enlarged nodes for greater than 2 weeks.

Bibliography

Habermann TM, Steensma DP. Lymphadenopathy. Mayo Clin Proc. 2000;75(7):723-32. [PMID: 10907389]

Item 66   Answer: C

Educational Objective: *Diagnose metastatic breast cancer in a woman with isolated axillary lymphadenopathy.*

The most appropriate initial step in the evaluation of this patient is lymph node biopsy. Although she lacks obvious risk factors for breast cancer, the size, location, and growth of the lymph node are all worrisome for malignancy. Breast cancer would also be the most likely malignancy given the location, lack of other symptoms, and her age and gender; therefore, she should have a lymph node biopsy as part of her initial evaluation. Pathologic confirmation of malignancy should be performed early in the diagnostic evaluation. Optimal pathologic evaluation, including special stains that might reveal tissue of origin, help to distinguish carcinoma from other cancer types, determine histologic type, and identify specific treatment target characteristics.

Because the lymph node is increasing in size and it is already larger than 2 cm, it does not make sense to follow it conservatively with a repeat examination. She does have a history of latent tuberculosis, and she received the appropriate course of treatment. This, in addition to the absence of any systemic symptoms, makes tuberculous lymphadenitis very unlikely. If suspicion were greater for tuberculous lymphadenitis, then a lymph node aspirate and subsequent stains and culture for *Mycobacterium tuberculosis* would be a reasonable initial test. Chest x-ray can evaluate for the presence of intrathoracic lymphadenopathy caused by conditions like sarcoidosis, lung cancer, and lymphoma, but she does not have any symptoms to suggest these diagnoses such as fever, night sweats, weight loss, or cough.

KEY POINT

Enlarging, firm axillary lymphadenopathy in a woman older than 40 years suggests the possibility of metastatic breast cancer.

Bibliography
Habermann TM, Steensma DP. Lymphadenopathy. Mayo Clin Proc. 2000;75(7):723-32. [PMID: 10907389]

Item 67   Answer: A
Educational Objective: *Diagnose and treat cystitis as the cause of urinary incontinence.*

The best management of the urinary incontinence is the initiation of ciprofloxacin. Patients with new-onset urinary incontinence should first be evaluated for transient, reversible causes, for which the mnemonic DIAPERS may be useful: Drugs, Infection, Atrophic vaginitis, Psychological (depression, delirium, dementia), Endocrine (hyperglycemia, hypercalcemia), Restricted mobility, and Stool impaction. Urinary tract infection is a very common cause of transient incontinence in the elderly, particularly if other contributing factors such as cognitive impairment or impaired mobility are present. The presence of significant pyuria in this setting generally justifies administration of empiric antibiotic therapy pending urine culture results.

Although some medications may induce transient incontinence, causative agents are most often diuretics or drugs that affect autonomic nervous system or bladder function. Oral hypoglycemic agents do not typically cause incontinence, and discontinuing these agents in a patient with diabetes mellitus could precipitate hyperglycemia and increased incontinence.

Indwelling catheterization is a treatment of last resort for patients who have chronic incontinence that is unresponsive to other therapy and in whom intermittent catheterization is not feasible.

This patient's confusion is more consistent with delirium in an elderly patient as a generalized response to an acute illness rather than a focal neurologic event. CT scan of the head is typically not helpful in such patients and is unlikely to provide an explanation for this patient's incontinence.

KEY POINT

Patients with new-onset urinary incontinence should first be evaluated for transient, reversible causes, for which the mnemonic DIAPERS may be useful: Drugs, Infection, Atrophic vaginitis, Psychological (depression, delirium, dementia), Endocrine (hyperglycemia, hypercalcemia), Restricted mobility, and Stool impaction.

Bibliography
Goode PS, Burgio KL, Richter HE, Markland AD. Incontinence in older women. JAMA. 2010;303(21):2172-2181. [PMID: 20516418]

Item 68   Answer: C
Educational Objective: *Screen for hearing impairment with the whispered voice test.*

The best way to screen for hearing loss is the whispered voice test. Screening for hearing loss is important in elderly persons because hearing impairment is prevalent but frequently underdiagnosed in this population. In addition, significant hearing loss is still possible despite a patient's denial of having trouble hearing. A recent systematic review evaluated the accuracy and precision of office clinical maneuvers for diagnosing hearing impairment. The whispered-voice test is a quick and easy assessment tool that has the best test characteristics among the office maneuvers. This test assesses the ability to hear a whispered voice with the examiner standing behind the patient 2 feet from the patient's ear while occluding and simultaneously rubbing the opposite external auditory canal and whispering three numbers or letters. Using a battery-powered handheld audioscope is an acceptable alternative screening modality.

The systematic review also found that the Screening Hearing Handicap Inventory and the Weber and Rinne tests did not perform as well as the whispered-voice test in detecting hearing impairment.

Referring patients for formal audiometry, although the gold standard for evaluating hearing loss, is expensive and time consuming. It is also unnecessary to do routinely, since a normal result on the whispered-voice test effectively rules out significant hearing loss.

KEY POINT

Elderly persons should be screened for hearing impairment with the whispered-voice test or the handheld audioscopy, even if they deny having a hearing problem.

Bibliography
Bagai A, Thavendiranathan P, Detsky AS. Does this patient have hearing impairment? JAMA. 2006;295(4):416-428. [PMID:16434632]

Item 69   Answer: B
Educational Objective: *Evaluate a fall in an elderly patient with the "get up and go" test.*

The next diagnostic study for this patient is the "get up and go test." Risk factors for falling include lower extremity weakness, gait deficit, arthritis, impaired activities of daily living, female sex, and age over 80 years. Other risk factors for falls include balance deficits, impaired vision, depression, cognitive impairment, psychotropic drug use, and use of an assistive device. Because falls often have multiple causes and more than one predisposing risk factor, there is no standard diagnostic evaluation for patients who fall or are at risk for falling. However, evaluations should begin with balance and gait screening, such as the "get up and go" test. The "get up and go" test is appropriate for screening because it is a quantitative evaluation of general functional mobility. A strong association exists between performance on this test and a person's functional independence in activities of daily living. Persons are timed in their ability to rise from a chair, walk 10 feet, turn, and then return to the chair. Most adults can complete this task in 10 seconds, and most frail elderly persons, in 11 to 20 seconds. Those requiring more than 20 seconds should undergo a fall evaluation. Typically, this consists of a focused history and physical examination, much of which has already been performed in this patient. Further evaluation, including measurement of 25-hydroxyvitamin D levels, should be directed according to findings of the evaluation. Interventions to prevent falls should be tailored to the patient's needs.

A CT scan of the head, 24-hour electrocardiographic monitoring, and echocardiography are not routine studies for fall evaluation and should not be done before balance and gait screening. A CT scan of the head is unlikely to be helpful in the absence of focal neurologic findings. The diagnostic value of echocardiography in the evaluation of falls is low in the absence of heart failure or murmurs. Electrocardiographic monitoring is unlikely to be helpful in a patient who falls in the absence of syncope or other cardiac symptoms such as palpitations.

KEY POINT

For elderly persons the "get up and go" test is a good screening test for gait and balance problems that may warrant further evaluation.

Bibliography
Tinetti ME, Kumar C. The patient who falls: "It's always a trade-off". JAMA. 2010 ;303(3):258-266. [PMID: 20085954]

Item 70   Answer: C
Educational Objective: *Treat urge urinary incontinence with oxybutynin.*

The most appropriate medication for this patient is oxybutynin. This patient's symptoms are most consistent with urge urinary incontinence (overactive bladder), which is manifested by involuntary leakage of large amounts of urine. The incontinence is frequently preceded by a sense of urgency but an inability to get to the bathroom in time. This patient's memory loss and findings on the Mini–Mental State Examination could indicate early dementia, which is a risk factor for urge incontinence.

An anticholinergic agent such as oxybutynin is effective in reducing episodes of urge incontinence. Tolterodine is an alternative agent in the same drug class with similar efficacy. Although this patient has no signs or symptoms of benign prostatic hyperplasia, he should be monitored for difficulty urinating or urinary retention following initiation of any anticholinergic agent. Oxybutynin appears to be safe in patients with mild to severe dementia.

Doxazosin, like other α-adrenergic blockers, is effective for the urinary symptoms associated with benign prostatic hyperplasia, such as slow urinary stream, urinary hesitancy, and nocturia. However, doxazosin is not indicated for the treatment of urge incontinence.

Although tricyclic antidepressants such as imipramine have been used to treat urge incontinence, there is no strong evidence from clinical trials supporting their effectiveness in this setting.

Adrenergic drugs (phenylpropanolamine, norepinephrine, clenbuterol) have been principally studied for treatment of stress urinary incontinence in women, but have not proved superior to placebo or pelvic floor muscle training.

KEY POINT

Tolterodine and oxybutynin are anticholinergic agents that are effective for treating urge urinary incontinence.

Bibliography
Goode PS, Burgio KL, Richter HE, Markland AD. Incontinence in older women. JAMA. 2010;303(21):2172-2181. [PMID: 20516418]

Item 71   Answer: C
Educational Objective: *Screen an older patient for depression.*

This asymptomatic elderly man should be screened for depression. Depression is common in later life. Risk factors include older age, neurologic conditions including stroke and Parkinson disease, stressful life events, a personal or family history of depression, and other medical illnesses. The U.S. Preventive Services Task Force (USPSTF) has documented that screening adults in primary care settings leads to accurate identification of depression, a disorder for which treatment is often effective. The USPSTF recommends that screening be restricted to primary care settings in which an accurate diagnosis of depression can be made, effective treatment can be provided, and follow-up care is available. Screening should be considered in patients with the risk factors listed above (such as the stressful life events in the patient discussed here) and in those with unexplained or unrelated somatic symptoms; other psychological conditions, such as anxiety or substance abuse; chronic pain; or lack of response to usually effective treatment of other medical conditions.

A two-item screening instrument has a sensitivity of 96% and specificity of 57% for diagnosing depression. A "yes" response to either of the following questions constitutes a positive screen: *"Over the past 2 weeks have you felt down, depressed, or hopeless?"* and *"Over the past 2 weeks have you felt little interest or pleasure in doing things?"* A positive result on either of these screening measures should be followed by a full diagnostic interview to determine the presence of a depressive disorder.

Although the USPSTF recommends one-time ultrasonographic screening for abdominal aortic aneurysm in men 65 to 75 years of age who are current or former smokers, it does not extend this recommendation to never-smokers because of the lower risk of large aneurysms in this population.

The USPSTF does not recommend for or against screening for the diagnosis of peripheral arterial disease (such as determination of the ankle-brachial index) because there is little evidence that treatment, other than therapy based on standard cardiovascular risk factor assessment, is beneficial during the asymptomatic phase of this disease.

The USPSTF does not recommend for or against screening for dementia with instruments such as the Mini–Mental State Examination because of the potential harm of inaccurate diagnosis and the modest benefits of drug therapy for this disorder.

KEY POINT

Screening adults for depressive disorders in the primary care setting is recommended by the U.S. Preventive Services Task Force.

Bibliography

Williams JW Jr, No'l PH, Cordes JA, Ramirez G, Pignone M. Is this patient clinically depressed? JAMA. 2002;287(9):1160-1170. [PMID: 11879114]

Item 72   Answer: C

Educational Objective: *Manage multifactorial dizziness in a geriatric patient with physical therapy.*

Physical therapy is the best management option for this patient. Disequilibrium in the elderly is often described as a vague sense of unsteadiness, most often occurring while standing or walking. It is different from orthostatic hypotension in that symptoms are not always temporally related to moving from a seated to a standing position and are not associated with a drop in blood pressure. Disequilibrium in the elderly is often multifactorial, with contributors including peripheral neuropathy, visual loss, decline in bilateral vestibular function, deconditioning, autonomic neuropathy, and medication side effects. Treatment of disequilibrium involves reducing polypharmacy, installing safety features in patients' homes, providing assistive devices such as walkers and canes, correcting eyesight and hearing if possible, and instituting physical therapy to improve muscle strength.

Neuroimaging should usually be reserved for patients with signs suggesting cerebellar or focal neurologic symptoms or vertical nystagmus. There is no evidence that this patient has a new neurologic lesion.

Meclizine can be of use in patients with prolonged or sustained vertigo such as in acute viral labyrinthitis; however, for intermittent episodes of unsteadiness, it is not likely to be of benefit and will add to her polypharmacy.

The combination of aspirin and dipyridamole is an effective strategy for the secondary prevention of ischemic stroke. There is no evidence, however, that such treatment improves disequilibrium in the elderly.

KEY POINT

Dizziness in geriatric patients is often multifactorial and caused by deficits in multiple sensory systems and medication side effects.

Bibliography

Eaton DA, Roland PS. Dizziness in the older adult, Part 2. Treatments for causes of the four most common symptoms. Geriatrics. 2003;58(4):46,49-52. [PMID:12708155]

Item 73   Answer: D

Educational Objective: *Manage hypertension in a young patient with lifestyle modifications.*

Lifestyle modifications are recommended for all patients with hypertension, including prehypertension. The Dietary Approaches to Stop Hypertension (DASH) study showed that 8 weeks of a diet of fruits, vegetables, low-fat dairy products, whole grains, poultry, fish, and nuts, along with a reduction in intake of fats, red meat, and sweets, caused an 11.4-mm Hg decrease in systolic pressure and a 5.5-mm Hg decrease in diastolic pressure. In addition, patients using the DASH diet who consumed less than 100 mmol/d of sodium had a systolic pressure 3 mm Hg and a diastolic pressure 1.6 mm Hg less than those who consumed high amounts of sodium.

Weight reduction in a patient whose weight is 10% above ideal body weight lowers blood pressure by an average of 5 to 7 mm Hg. Alcohol consumption should be limited to two drinks daily for men and one for women because excess amounts of alcohol may contribute to hypertension and resistance to antihypertensive medications. Regular aerobic exercise also modestly decreases blood pressure. In addition, this patient should be counseled about smoking cessation.

In patients with stage 1 hypertension (systolic pressure between 140 and 159 mm Hg or diastolic pressure between 90 and 99 mm Hg), lifestyle modifications should be tried before antihypertensive medication is initiated. In patients with stage 1 hypertension who do not have evidence of cardiovascular disease or target organ damage, therapeutic lifestyle changes can be tried for 6 to 12 months before initiating drug therapy.

KEY POINT

In young patients with stage 1 hypertension, lifestyle modifications should be tried before antihypertensive medication is initiated.

Bibliography
American College of Physicians. In the clinic. Hypertension. Ann Intern Med. 2008;149(11):ITC6(1-15). [PMID: 19047024]

Item 74 Answer: A

Educational Objective: *Treat hypertension in an elderly patient with the addition of hydrochlorothiazide.*

The most appropriate next step in this patient's management is the addition of low-dose chlorthalidone and follow-up in 1 week. Antihypertensive therapy has been shown to benefit patients age 60 to 80 years. Furthermore, antihypertensive therapy in patients older than 80 years is associated with a decrease in stroke and cardiovascular mortality.

Diuretics enhance the antihypertensive efficacy of multidrug regimens and are inexpensive. According to the Seventh Report of the Joint National Committee on Prevention, Detection, Evaluation, and Treatment of High Blood Pressure (JNC 7), thiazide diuretics should be used as initial therapy for most patients with hypertension, either alone or in combination with one of the other classes of antihypertensive agents. JNC 7 also recommends that older patients with hypertension should follow the same principles outlined for the general care of hypertension in younger patients. Because older patients with hypertension are more likely to be salt sensitive and responsive to a diuretic, low-dose chlorthalidone is appropriate for this patient. Follow-up evaluation in 1 week also is indicated to assess for electrolyte abnormalities or azotemia.

Adding an angiotensin-converting enzyme inhibitor (such as lisinopril), an angiotensin receptor blocker (such as losartan), or an α-blocker (such as terazosin) would be less likely than a diuretic to benefit an elderly patient.

KEY POINT

Low-dose diuretic therapy is appropriate in older patients with hypertension because these patients are more likely to be salt sensitive.

Bibliography
American College of Physicians. In the clinic. Hypertension. Ann Intern Med. 2008;149(11):ITC6(1-15). [PMID: 19047024]

Item 75 Answer: C

Educational Objective: *Identify the maximum blood pressure in a patient with diabetes as less than 130/80 mm Hg.*

The maximum target blood pressure for this patient is less than 130/80 mm Hg. The Seventh Report of the Joint National Committee on Prevention, Detection, Evaluation, and Treatment of High Blood Pressure (JNC 7) defines normal blood pressure as less than 120/80 mm Hg. Cardiovascular risk correlates directly with blood pressure stage, beginning at 115/75 mm Hg and doubling with each 20/10 mm Hg increment.

The goal of antihypertensive treatment in patients with essential hypertension is to reduce blood pressure to less than 140/90 mm Hg. However, patients with diabetes mellitus have an increased risk for cardiovascular morbidity and mortality. Therefore, the target blood pressure goal for these patients is less than 130/80 mm Hg, which is associated with a lower rate of cardiovascular outcomes.

A similar blood pressure target is appropriate for patients with chronic nondiabetic kidney disease not associated with significant proteinuria. A target blood pressure of less than 125/75 mm Hg is recommended for patients with kidney disease accompanied by a urine protein-creatinine ratio above 1 mg/mg. However, this level of blood pressure control is not indicated in this patient, because he does not meet the proteinuria criteria on the basis of his urine albumin-creatinine ratio.

KEY POINT

The target blood pressure in patients with type 2 diabetes mellitus and nondiabetic chronic kidney disease in the absence of proteinuria is less than 130/80 mm Hg.

Bibliography
Kidney Disease Outcomes Quality Initiative (K/DOQI). K/DOQI clinical practice guidelines on hypertension and antihypertensive agents in chronic kidney disease. Am J Kidney Dis. 2004;43(5 Suppl 1):S1-S290. [PMID:15114537]

Item 76 Answer: A

Educational Objective: *Diagnose coarctation of the aorta.*

This patient has classic features of aortic coarctation. He has a pulse delay between the upper and lower extremities (radial artery to femoral artery delay). The blood pressure in the lower extremities, when measured, will be lower than the blood pressure noted in the upper extremities. The patient also has an ejection click and an early systolic murmur consistent with a bicuspid aortic valve, which is present in more than 50% of patients with aortic coarctation. The systolic and diastolic murmurs noted over the back are related to collateral vessels, which also cause the sign of rib notching, seen on this patient's chest radiograph on the inferior surface of the posterior upper thoracic ribs bilaterally. Also, indentation of the aortic wall at the site of coarctation combined with pre- and post-coarctation dilatation produces the "3" sign.

Essential hypertension is the most common cause of systemic hypertension, but the physical examination features of this patient are not explained by this diagnosis. In addition, a family history of hypertension is common in patients with essential hypertension.

Pheochromocytoma causes paroxysmal hypertension in about half of affected patients; other pheochromocytomas present similarly to essential hypertension. The signs and symptoms of pheochromocytoma are variable. The classic triad of sudden severe headaches, diaphoresis, and palpitations carries a high degree of specificity (94%) and sensitivity (91%) for pheochromocytoma in hypertensive patients. The absence of all three symptoms reliably excludes the condition. Finally, the physical examination features in this patient do not reflect this diagnosis.

Renovascular hypertension due to fibromuscular disease of the renal arteries usually presents in patients younger than 35 years of age. Atherosclerotic renovascular disease is more common in older patients and is frequently associated with vascular disease in other vessels (carotid or coronary arteries and peripheral vessels). Azotemia is often observed in patients with atherosclerotic renovascular hypertension. Renal artery stenosis cannot explain this patient's cardiac and peripheral vascular examination findings.

KEY POINT

Coarctation of the aorta should be suspected in a young patient presenting with systemic hypertension, radial to femoral artery delay, and rib notching on chest radiography.

Bibliography

Tanous D, Benson LN, Horlick EM. Coarctation of the aorta: evaluation and management. Curr Opin Cardiol. 2009. [Epub ahead of print] [PMID: 19667980]

Item 77   Answer: B

Educational Objective: *Treat stage 2 hypertension with two-drug therapy.*

The most appropriate next step in management for this patient is initiation of lisinopril and hydrochlorothiazide. This patient has stage 2 hypertension (systolic blood pressure ≥160 mm Hg or diastolic blood pressure ≥100 mm Hg), and both lifestyle modifications and antihypertensive therapy are indicated. The guidelines proposed by the Seventh Report of the Joint National Committee on Prevention, Detection, Evaluation, and Treatment of High Blood Pressure (JNC 7) recommend initiating treatment with two medications in patients with stage 2 hypertension or those whose blood pressure is greater than 20 mm Hg systolic or 10 mm Hg diastolic above target. Low-dose hydrochlorothiazide and an angiotensin-converting enzyme (ACE) inhibitor, such as lisinopril, would be reasonable in this patient to ensure adequate blood pressure control. Careful follow-up and monitoring for signs of impaired fasting glucose or glucose intolerance also are recommended.

Monotherapy with hydrochlorothiazide, metoprolol, or terazosin would not be appropriate in a patient with stage 2 hypertension. Furthermore, evidence suggests that β-blockers do not perform as well as comparator drugs, particularly in preventing stroke, and thus they are no longer universally recommended as first-line single agents in the absence of a compelling indication, which may include a history of myocardial infarction and heart failure. Finally, thiazide diuretics appear to be superior to α-blockers (such as terazosin), ACE

inhibitors, and calcium channel blockers as initial therapy for reducing cardiovascular and kidney risk in patients with hypertension.

KEY POINT

Current guidelines recommend initiating treatment with two medications in patients with stage 2 hypertension or those whose blood pressure is greater than 20 mm Hg systolic or 10 mm Hg diastolic above target.

Bibliography

American College of Physicians. In the clinic. Hypertension. Ann Intern Med. 2008;149(11):ITC6(1-15). [PMID: 19047024]

Item 78   Answer: C

Educational Objective: *Treat prehypertension with lifestyle modification.*

The most appropriate next step in management is lifestyle modification. This patient has prehypertension, defined by the Seventh Report of the Joint National Committee on Prevention, Detection, Evaluation, and Treatment of High Blood Pressure (JNC 7) guidelines as a blood pressure of 120 to 139/80 to 89 mm Hg. Lifestyle modification consists of adhering to a Dietary Approaches to Stop Hypertension (DASH) diet, reducing sodium intake, regular aerobic exercise, and moderating alcohol intake. Lifestyle modifications can lower blood pressure, modify additional cardiovascular risk factors, and decrease the incidence of overt hypertension in patients with prehypertension.

Ambulatory blood pressure monitoring is primarily indicated for patients with white coat hypertension. Although no overall agreement exists about the diagnostic criteria, some experts define white coat hypertension as at least three separate office blood pressure measurements above 140/90 mm Hg with at least two sets of measurements below 140/90 mm Hg obtained in non-office settings.

Current data do not support pharmacologic treatment in patients with prehypertension with no other major risk factors for hypertension, such as diabetes mellitus, kidney disease, or evidence of target organ damage. Therefore, administration of hydrochlorothiazide or lisinopril is inappropriate.

KEY POINT

Lifestyle modifications, such as maintaining a normal body weight, regular aerobic physical activity, adhering to a Dietary Approaches to Stop Hypertension (DASH) diet, reducing sodium intake, and moderating alcohol intake, are indicated for patients with prehypertension who do not have other major risk factors for hypertension.

Bibliography

American College of Physicians. In the clinic. Hypertension. Ann Intern Med. 2008;149(11):ITC6(1-15). [PMID: 19047024]

Section 5

Hematology

Questions

Item 1 [Advanced]

A 50-year-old woman is evaluated for methotrexate therapy for her new-onset rheumatoid arthritis. She had a mild anemia attributed to rheumatoid arthritis. Low-dose methotrexate and folic acid therapy are initiated.

Five months later, her arthritis symptoms are improved, but her anemia has worsened. She feels well without fatigue. She continues to have menses every 28 days, with flow lasting 5 days. She has no other source of blood loss.

	5 Months Ago	Today
Hemoglobin	10.8 g/dL (108 g/L)	9.7 g/dL (97 g/L)
Reticulocyte count	0.7%	0.8%
Mean corpuscular volume	92 fL	93 fL
Serum iron	36 µg/dL (6.4 µmol/L)	15 µg/dL (2.7 µmol/L)
Total iron-binding capacity (calculated)	394 µg/dL (70.5 µmol/L)	394 µg/dL (70.5 µmol/L)
Serum ferritin	—	36 ng/mL (36 µg/L)
Serum creatinine	—	Normal
Serum haptoglobin	—	Normal
Serum lactate dehydrogenase	—	Normal
Vitamin B_{12}	—	Normal

Which of the following is the most likely diagnosis for her anemia?

(A) Iron deficiency
(B) Anemia of inflammation
(C) Anemia of inflammation plus iron deficiency
(D) Megaloblastic anemia

Item 2 [Basic]

A 28-year-old woman has a 3-month history of easy bruising and bleeding gums. She feels otherwise well. Medical and family histories are unremarkable, and she takes no medications.

On physical examination, vital signs are normal. Petechiae are present on the buccal mucosa and pretibial areas, and ecchymoses are noted on the upper thighs. There is no lymphadenopathy or splenomegaly.

Hemoglobin	10.4 g/dL (104 g/L)
Leukocyte count	2800/µL (2.8×10^9/L)
Absolute neutrophil count	1200/µL (1.2×10^9/L) (normal >1500/µL [1.5×10^9/L])
Platelet count	18,000/µL (18×10^9/L)
Reticulocyte count	0.9% of erythrocytes
Direct antiglobulin (Coombs) test	Negative

A peripheral blood smear shows no circulating blasts. The platelets are decreased in number but otherwise normal. Bone marrow examination shows hypoplastic marrow (<20% cellularity) with normal maturation of all cellular elements and normal iron stores. There are no findings suggesting an infiltrative disease and no fibrosis.

Which of the following is the most likely diagnosis?

(A) Aplastic anemia
(B) Autoimmune hemolytic anemia
(C) Immune thrombocytopenic purpura
(D) Iron deficiency anemia

Item 3 [Basic]

A 64-year-old man is evaluated in the office for a gradual decrease in exercise tolerance over the past 2 months. He has ostearthritis of the right knee but no other medical problems. His only medication is over-the-counter ibuprofen. Results of routine screening colonoscopy 4 months ago were normal.

On physical examination, heart rate is 90/min, respiration rate is 20/min, and blood pressure is 140/80 mm Hg.

Laboratory study findings include a hemoglobin level of 9.6 g/dL (96 g/L) and mean corpuscular volume of 76 fL. Results of routine serum chemistry analysis are normal. Serum iron, serum ferritin, and transferrin saturation levels are all low, and the total iron-binding capacity is elevated. Stool is positive for occult blood.

Upper endoscopy reveals chronic gastritis, and the ibuprofen is stopped.

Which of the following is the most appropriate treatment for this patient's anemia?

(A) Blood transfusion
(B) Erythropoietin
(C) Intravenous iron
(D) Oral iron

Item 4 [Advanced]

A 27-year-old man is evaluated in the office for dark urine. Four days ago, the patient began taking trimethoprim-sulfamethoxazole for bacterial sinusitis. He has a brother who developed hemolytic anemia when exposed to a sulfa-containing drug.

On physical examination, temperature is 37.8°C (100.2°F), blood pressure is 127/66 mm Hg, pulse rate is 112/min, and respiration rate is 25/min. Scleral icterus is noted. Tachycardia is heard on cardiac auscultation, but cardiac examination is otherwise unremarkable. Abdominal examination discloses no hepatosplenomegaly.

Hemoglobin	10.2 g/dL (102 g/L)
Reticulocyte count	11% of erythrocytes
Bilirubin	
Total	5.1 mg/dL (87.2 μmol/L)
Indirect	4.6 mg/dL (78.7 μmol/L)
Lactate dehydrogenase	1145 U/L
Urinalysis	3+ bilirubin

A peripheral blood smear is shown (Plate 11).

Which of the following is the most likely diagnosis?

(A) Glucose 6-phosphate dehydrogenase deficiency
(B) Hereditary spherocytosis
(C) Microangiopathic hemolytic anemia
(D) Warm antibody–mediated hemolytic anemia

Item 5 [Advanced]

A 14-year-old boy undergoing a routine evaluation is found to have mild microcytic anemia. His history and physical examination findings are normal.

Hemoglobin level is 10 g/dL (100 g/L), erythrocyte count is $5.9 \times 10^6/\mu L$ ($5.9 \times 10^{12}/L$), and mean corpuscular volume is 76 fL. The serum iron and ferritin levels are normal.

The peripheral blood smear is shown (Plate 12).

Which of the following is the most likely diagnosis?

(A) Hereditary spherocytosis
(B) Iron deficiency anemia
(C) Sickle cell anemia
(D) Thalassemia minor

Item 6 [Advanced]

An 86-year-old woman is evaluated for a 6-month history of increasing fatigue and paresthesias of the toes. Medical history is otherwise noncontributory. Her only medication is a daily aspirin.

On physical examination, vital signs are normal. Neurologic examination shows decreased vibratory sense and proprioception in the toes and fingers. Findings from the remainder of the neurologic and general physical examination are normal.

Hemoglobin	11.8 g/dL (118 g/L)
Mean corpuscular volume	106 fL
Platelet count	102,000/μL ($102 \times 10^9/L$)
Reticulocyte count	0.8% of erythrocytes
Vitamin B_{12}	220 pg/mL (162.4 pmol/L)
Folate (serum)	22 ng/mL (49.8 nmol/L)
Lactate dehydrogenase	470 U/L

A peripheral blood smear shows macro-ovalocytes but no other abnormality.

Which of the following is the most appropriate next diagnostic test?

(A) Bone marrow biopsy
(B) Erythrocyte folate measurement
(C) Methylmalonic acid and homocysteine measurements
(D) Parietal cell antibody assay

Item 7 [Basic]

A 56-year-old woman is evaluated during a routine follow-up examination. Six months ago, she underwent aortic valve replacement with a mechanical prosthesis. Her initial postoperative course has been uneventful, and she has no symptoms. Her hematocrit at discharge was 40%. Her only medication is warfarin.

On physical examination, vital signs are normal. Her cardiac examination reveals a normal S_1 and mechanical S_2 without an S_3 or S_4. There is a nonradiating grade 2/6 midpeaking systolic murmur heard best at the lower left sternal border. Other physical examination findings are normal.

Haptoglobin	8 mg/dL (80 mg/L)
Hematocrit	31%
INR	2.6
Platelet count	144,000/μL ($144 \times 10^9/L$)
Reticulocyte count	6% of erythrocytes
Creatinine	1.0 mg/dL (88.4 μmol/L)
Lactate dehydrogenase	440 U/L

The blood smear shows normocytic erythrocytes with schistocytes.

Which of the following is the most likely cause of her anemia?

(A) Autoimmune hemolytic anemia
(B) Disseminated intravascular coagulation
(C) Hemolytic anemia due to mechanical heart valve
(D) Thrombotic thrombocytopenic purpura

Item 8 [Basic]

A previously healthy 65-year-old man is evaluated for easy fatigability. He has no significant medical history, has never had a screening colonoscopy or other colon cancer screening, and does not drink alcohol. The patient takes no medications. His hemoglobin level 1 year ago was 14.3 g/dL (143 g/L).

Results of physical examination are normal except for the finding of pallor. Laboratory examination reveals a hemoglobin level of 8.6 g/dL (86 g/L). Testing of stool for occult blood is negative. A peripheral blood smear is shown (Plate 13).

Which of the following is the most likely diagnosis?

(A) Hereditary spherocytosis
(B) Iron deficiency anemia
(C) Sickle cell anemia
(D) Thalassemia minor

Item 9 [Basic]

A 57-year-old woman with chronic lymphocytic leukemia (CLL) is evaluated in the emergency department because of a 2-week history of increasing malaise, decreased exercise tolerance, and darkened urine. Her CLL was last treated 2 months ago with chemotherapy.

On physical examination, the patient has scleral icterus. Temperature is 37.3°C (99.2°F), blood pressure is 142/82 mm Hg, pulse rate is 117/min, and respiration rate is 18/min. Cardiopulmonary examination discloses a regular tachycardia. Splenomegaly is present.

Hemoglobin	6.9 g/dL (69 g/L)
Leukocyte count	6500/µL (6.5 × 10⁹/L)
Platelet count	250,000/µL (250 × 10⁹/L)
Reticulocyte count	10% of erythrocytes
Bilirubin	
Total	6.3 mg/dL (107.7 µmol/L)
Direct	0.5 mg/dL (8.6 µmol/L)
Lactate dehydrogenase	357 U/L
Direct antiglobulin (Coombs) test	Positive for IgG

A peripheral blood smear is shown (Plate 14).

Which of the following is the most likely diagnosis?

(A) Autoimmune hemolytic anemia
(B) Hereditary spherocytosis
(C) Microangiopathic hemolytic anemia
(D) α-Thalassemia

Item 10 [Advanced]

A 60-year-old man is evaluated in the hospital for esophageal variceal bleeding and easy bruising. He was admitted 2 hours ago and was initially stabilized with intravenous fluids and endoscopic band ligation, but he continues to bleed. He has a long history of alcohol abuse, is taking no medications, and has not recently consumed aspirin or nonsteroidal anti-inflammatory (NSAIDs) medications. There is no family history of bleeding. One year ago, he successfully underwent a partial colectomy for recurrent diverticulitis without excessive bleeding.

The patient is alert but tremulous. On physical examination, blood pressure is 90/60 mm Hg, pulse rate is 110/min, and respiration rate is 14/min. Cardiopulmonary examination is normal. Abdominal palpation reveals minimal tenderness. The spleen is palpable. Large ecchymoses are present at previous phlebotomy sites. No petechiae are present.

Hemoglobin	8.6 g/dL (86 g/L)

Serum creatinine	1.5 mg/dL (132.6 mmol/L)
Platelet count	105,000/µL (105 × 10⁹/L)
Prothrombin time	16.1 s
Activated partial thromboplastin time	40 s
Mixing study	Corrects to near normal

Which of the following is the most likely cause of his bleeding disorder?

(A) Acquired factor deficiency
(B) Acquired factor inhibitor
(C) Acquired platelet dysfunction
(D) Thrombocytopenia

Item 11 [Basic]

A 79-year-old woman is evaluated in the hospital for sepsis secondary to pyelonephritis. The patient was well before this illness and has no other medical problems.

On physical examination, temperature is 38.9°C (102.0°F), blood pressure is 90/50 mm Hg, pulse rate is 110/min, and respiration rate is 18/min. She has bleeding at phlebotomy sites and around her intravenous access insertion and many ecchymoses on her arms and legs.

Hemoglobin	9 mg/dL (90 g/L)
Platelet count	60,000/µL (60 × 10⁹/L)
Prothrombin time	15 s
Activated partial thromboplastin time	30 s
D-dimer	Elevated
Fibrinogen	Reduced

Examination of the peripheral blood smear shows many fragmented erythrocytes and diminished platelets.

Which of the following is the most likely cause of her bleeding disorder?

(A) Disseminated intravascular coagulation
(B) Hemolytic uremic syndrome
(C) Immune thrombocytopenic purpura
(D) Thrombotic thrombocytopenic purpura

Item 12 [Basic]

An 18-year-old man is evaluated for excessive bleeding. After a routine tooth extraction, he had 5 hours of bleeding that the dentist was able to control. The patient is healthy and takes no medications, including aspirin or NSAIDs. Medical history includes easy bruisability and occasional nose bleeds that are easily controllable. The patient was circumcised at birth, and his mother recalls that he had more bleeding than expected from the circumcision site. His father also has easy bruisability.

Physical examination is normal, with no evidence of petechiae, ecchymoses, or abnormal vasculature.

Hemoglobin	14.2 g/dL (142 g/L)
Platelet count	195,000/µL (195 × 10⁹/L)
INR	1.1
Activated partial thrombo- plastin time (aPTT)	41 s
aPTT mixing study	Corrects to normal
Thrombin time	16 s (control, 15 s)
Fibrinogen	Normal
D-dimer assay	Negative
Bleeding time	10 min (prolonged)
Factor VIII activity	60% (normal, 65%-120%)

Which of the following is the most likely diagnosis?

(A) Hemophilia A (factor VIII deficiency)
(B) Presence of a lupus inhibitor
(C) Vitamin K deficiency
(D) von Willebrand disease

Item 13 [Basic]

A 55-year-old woman undergoes preoperative evaluation before elective laparoscopic cholecystectomy. Medical history includes three pregnancies and full-term deliveries with no complications or health problems. She has had no previous surgeries. Physical examination findings are normal.

Which of the following is the best screening approach to detect any bleeding disorders in this patient?

(A) Clinical history
(B) INR
(C) INR, prothrombin time (PT), and partial thromboplastin time (PTT)
(D) INR, PT, PTT, and bleeding test

Item 14 [Advanced]

A 19-year-old man with sickle cell disease develops severe weakness and dyspnea. He has not had rash, fever, new joint or abdominal symptoms, bleeding from his mucous membranes, hemoptysis, hematemesis, or hematuria.

On physical examination, vital signs are normal except for a pulse rate of 148/min. His conjunctivae are very pale. There is no thrush or lymphadenopathy. A stool specimen is negative for occult blood. Hematocrit is 16% with no reticulocytes compared with his usual hematocrit of approximately 25% with 15% reticulocytes. The leukocyte and platelet counts are normal.

Which of the following is the most likely diagnosis?

(A) Acute myeloblastic leukemia
(B) Bleeding peptic ulcer
(C) Epstein–Barr virus infection
(D) Parvovirus B19 infection

Item 15 [Advanced]

A 46-year-old man is evaluated in the emergency department for swelling of the feet and ankles and a 2-month history of worsening dyspnea. The patient has homozygous sickle cell disease and a history of acute chest syndrome. Current medications are hydroxyurea and folic acid.

On physical examination, temperature is normal, blood pressure is 145/85 mm Hg, pulse rate is 98/min, and respiration rate is 28/min. Jugular venous pressure is elevated and is associated with large *a* and *v* waves. On cardiac examination, there is a heave, fixed splitting of S₂ with a palpable P₂, and a systolic murmur at the lower left sternal border that increases with respiration. The lungs are clear. Examination of the lower extremities shows 2+ edema bilaterally.

A chest radiograph shows enlargement of the central pulmonary arteries with clear lung fields. Echocardiographic findings include a normal left ventricular ejection fraction, right ventricular enlargement and hypertrophy, right atrial enlargement, and tricuspid regurgitation.

Which of the following is the most likely cause of this patient's findings?

(A) Aortic stenosis
(B) Hypertrophic cardiomyopathy
(C) Ischemic heart disease
(D) Pulmonary hypertension

Item 16 [Advanced]

A 31-year-old man with sickle cell disease is hospitalized because of right-sided pleuritic chest pain, a nonproductive cough, fever, and pain in his upper legs and pelvis.

On physical examination, temperature is 38.6°C (101.5°F), blood pressure is 130/85 mm Hg, pulse rate is 95/min, and respiratory rate is 20/min. Crackles and rhonchi are heard over the right lower lung field. There is no tenderness over the joints or bones. Hemoglobin is 6.7 g/dL (67 g/L), reticulocyte count is 18%, and leukocyte count is 17,000/µL (17 × 10⁹/L) with 65% neutrophils. No neutrophils are seen on a sputum smear. A chest radiograph shows a large infiltrate in the right lower lobe. His arterial Po₂ is 60 mm Hg (8 kPa) on ambient air. The patient is started on antibiotics and supplemental oxygen.

Which of the following should be performed next?

(A) Erythropoietin initiation
(B) Hydroxyurea initiation
(C) Red blood cell exchange transfusion
(D) Red blood cell transfusion

Item 17 [Advanced]

A 34-year-old woman with sickle cell disease is evaluated for a 2-week history of increasingly severe left groin pain. The pain awakens her at night and causes substantial difficulty in walking. There is no history of trauma, but she typically has 1 to 2 hospitalizations per year for treatment of sickle cell painful crisis. Her only medication is a folic acid supplement.

On physical examination, she has an obvious left leg limp. Vital signs are normal. There is restricted flexion and internal rotation of the left hip due to pain located in the groin. No tenderness to palpation over the lateral hip, sacroiliac joints, or sciatic notch is noted. There is no evidence of other joint involvement.

Plain radiographs of the pelvic region and hips are normal.

Which of the following is the best test to evaluate the hip pain?

(A) Arthrocentesis
(B) Bone densitometry
(C) MRI
(D) Radionuclide bone scan

Item 18 [Basic]

A 13-year-old girl is hospitalized because of the sudden development of left hemiparesis and aphasia. A peripheral blood smear is shown (Plate 15).

Which of the following is the most likely diagnosis?

(A) Hereditary spherocytosis
(B) Iron deficiency anemia
(C) Sickle cell disease
(D) Thalassemia minor

Item 19 [Advanced]

A 67-year-old woman is admitted to the hospital because of a deep venous thrombosis involving the left leg that developed during a 12-hour car trip. Medical history is significant for a 2-day hospitalization 14 weeks ago for a non–ST elevation myocardial infarction; she underwent cardiac catheterization at that time and was treated with low-molecular-weight heparin. Her current medications include aspirin, clopidogrel, pravastatin, and lisinopril.

On physical examination, vital signs are normal. The left leg is swollen and slightly tender to palpation. A complete blood count, electrolyte levels, and liver chemistry test findings are normal on laboratory studies; the platelet count is 150,000/μL (150 × 10⁹/L).

Unfractionated heparin is administered. Twelve hours later, the patient's platelet count is 87,000/μL (87 × 10⁹/L).

Which of the following is the most appropriate next step in treatment?

(A) Continue heparin and administer a platelet transfusion
(B) Continue heparin and initiate high-dose corticosteroid therapy
(C) Stop heparin and initiate argatroban
(D) Stop heparin and initiate warfarin

Item 20 [Advanced]

A 27-year-old woman is evaluated in the emergency department for a 2-day history of diffuse headache, fatigue, and gingival bleeding on brushing her teeth. She is otherwise healthy and takes no mediations.

On physical examination, she is alert and oriented but in considerable distress from the headache. Funduscopic examination is normal. A few scleral hemorrhages and mild icterus are noted. Petechiae are visible on the lower extremities. Cardiopulmonary and abdominal examination findings are normal.

Hemoglobin	8 g/dL (80 g/L)
Platelet count	34,000/μL (34 × 10⁹/L)
Reticulocyte count	12% of erythrocytes
Prothrombin time	Normal
Activated partial thrombo-plastin time	Normal
Thrombin time	Normal
Lactate dehydrogenase	2000 U/L
Serum creatinine	Normal

A peripheral blood smear is shown (Plate 16).

Which of the following is the most likely diagnosis?

(A) Autoimmune hemolytic anemia and thrombocytopenia
(B) Heparin-induced thrombocytopenia
(C) Immune thrombocytopenia
(D) Thrombotic thrombocytopenia purpura

Item 21 [Advanced]

A 28-year-old woman in the third trimester of an uncomplicated pregnancy has a complete blood count performed during a routine visit. She feels well and has no evidence of bleeding.

On physical examination, all findings are consistent with a normal seven month gestation.

Hemoglobin	13.5 g/dL (135 g/L)
Leukocyte count	5800/μL (5.8 × 10⁹/L)
Platelet count	12,000/μL (12 × 10⁹/L)

A peripheral blood smear is shown (Plate 17).

Which of the following is the most likely diagnosis?

(A) Gestational thrombocytopenia
(B) Immune thrombocytopenic purpura
(C) Pseudothrombocytopenia
(D) Thrombotic thrombocytopenic purpura

Item 22 [Advanced]

A 29-year-old woman is evaluated for a petechial rash of the lower extremities of 3 weeks' duration. The patient reports no bleeding problems except for recent, occasional bleeding from her gums after brushing her teeth. Medical history is otherwise unremarkable, and she takes no medications.

Physical examination reveals petechiae limited mainly to both lower extremities, with a few similar spots noted on her forearms and abdomen. Other examination findings are normal.

Hemoglobin	12.5 g/dL (125 g/L)
Leukocyte count	8500/μL (8.5 × 10⁹/L)
Platelet count	14,000/μL (14 × 10⁹/L)
Reticulocyte count	2.0% of erythrocytes
Antinuclear antibody assay	Negative
HIV antibody	Negative

A peripheral blood smear is shown (Plate 18).

Which of the following is the most appropriate next step in management?

(A) Admit for urgent splenectomy
(B) Initiate corticosteroids
(C) Initiate platelet transfusion
(D) Perform a bone marrow biopsy

Item 23 [Advanced]

A 27-year-old woman undergoes follow-up evaluation 5 months after diagnosis of an idiopathic pulmonary embolism for which she was prescribed a 6-month course of warfarin. Family history includes a maternal grandmother, a mother, and an older brother with a history of deep venous thrombosis, which was diagnosed in all three relatives before they were aged 50 years. The patient takes no oral contraceptives or other medications and is otherwise healthy. The complete blood count is normal, and the INR is 3.0.

Which of the following is the most appropriate next step in the evaluation of this patient?

(A) Immediate thrombophilic screening
(B) *JAK2* mutation analysis
(C) Thrombophilic screening 2 weeks after stopping warfarin
(D) No further evaluation needed

Item 24 [Advanced]

A 42-year-old woman is evaluated for swelling and discomfort of the right leg without an obvious precipitating event. She has no other medical problems.

On physical examination, vital signs are normal. Examination of the right lower extremity shows mild erythema, swelling, warmth, and tenderness to deep palpation of the calf. Cardiopulmonary and abdominal examination findings are normal.

Laboratory studies indicate a moderately elevated IgG anticardiolipin antibody level and the presence of a lupus inhibitor on coagulation testing.

An ultrasound shows a right proximal lower extremity deep venous thrombosis.

The patient is treated with anticoagulation therapy. Repeat anticardiolipin antibody testing 12 weeks later confirms the previous result.

Which of the following is the most appropriate anticoagulation management for this patient?

(A) Anticoagulation therapy indefinitely
(B) Anticoagulation therapy for a total of 12 months
(C) Anticoagulation therapy for a total of 6 months
(D) Cessation of anticoagulation therapy at 3 months

Item 25 [Advanced]

A 33-year-old woman who has been trying to become pregnant for 8 years is evaluated after receiving positive pregnancy test results. Medical history is significant for three miscarriages occurring 6 years ago, 3 years ago, and 1 year ago, each of which occurred early in her pregnancy. She had an unprovoked venous thromboembolism 18 months ago. Her last menstrual period was approximately 5 weeks ago.

Results of physical examination, including vital signs and abdominal examination, are normal.

Results of laboratory studies show a prolonged activated partial thromboplastin time (aPTT). A mixing study does not correct the aPTT

Testing for which of the following is the most appropriate next step?

(A) Factor V Leiden mutation
(B) Homocysteine level
(C) Lupus inhibitor and antiphospholipid antibody
(D) Prothrombin G20210A mutation

Item 26 [Basic]

A 70-year-old woman is evaluated because of malaise and anorexia for 1 week. She has hypertension treated with hydrochlorothiazide.

On physical examination, the supine blood pressure is 150/95 mm Hg, pulse rate is 80/min, respiration rate is 20/min, and temperature is 37.4°C (99.3°F). The blood pressure is 125/80 mm Hg and the pulse rate 96/min while standing. The remainder of the examination is unremarkable.

Hematocrit	29%
Blood urea nitrogen	62 mg/dL (22.1 mmol/L)
Serum creatinine	4.6 mg/dL (406.6 µmol/L)
Serum sodium	134 meq/L (134 mmol/L)
Serum potassium	5.0 meq/L (5.0 mmol/L)
Serum chloride	114 meq/L (114 mmol/L)
Serum bicarbonate	15 meq/L (15 mmol/L)
Serum calcium	12.5 mg/dL (3.1 mmol/L)
Serum phosphate	8.5 mg/dL (2.7 mmol/L)
Urinalysis	Specific gravity 1.007; trace proteinuria; no glucosuria or ketonuria

Which of the following is the most likely diagnosis?

(A) Hypercalcemia secondary to hydrochlorothiazide therapy
(B) Milk-alkali syndrome
(C) Multiple myeloma
(D) Primary hyperparathyroidism

Item 27 [Basic]

A 59-year-old man is evaluated for a 4-day history of progressively worsening fatigue, forgetfulness, constipation, excessive thirst, and increased urination. He has no pain. His only significant medical history is a diagnosis of right lower lobe pneumonia due to *Streptococcus pneumoniae* 3 months ago.

On physical examination, he appears somnolent but is arousable. Temperature is 37.1°C (98.8°F), blood pressure is 110/70 mm Hg, pulse rate is 120/min, and respiration rate is 17/min. The oral mucosa is dry, and the conjunctivae are pale. The lungs are clear.

Hemoglobin	8.9 g/dL (89 g/L)
Leukocyte count	2500/µL (2.5 × 10⁹/L)
Platelet count	150,000/µL (150 × 10⁹/L)
Calcium	13.6 mg/dL (3.4 mmol/L)
Creatinine	2.9 mg/dL (256.4 µmol/L)
Protein	
Total	7.6 g/dL (76 g/L)
Albumin	3.3 g/dL (33 g/L)
Urinalysis	Negative for protein

A peripheral blood smear shows normochromic, normocytic erythrocytes with rouleaux formation and no evidence of teardrop erythrocytes or immature myeloid and erythroid cells.

A chest radiograph shows osteopenia of all ribs. No pulmonary parenchymal infiltrates are seen.

The patient is hospitalized and responds to intravenous hydration with normal saline. The results of a bone marrow aspiration are shown (Plate 19).

Which of the following is the most likely diagnosis?

(A) Acute myeloid leukemia
(B) Chronic lymphocytic leukemia
(C) Metastatic small cell lung cancer
(D) Multiple myeloma

Item 28 [Advanced]

A 74-year-old woman is evaluated after a high serum total protein level was found during routine laboratory testing. Medical history is noncontributory.

On physical examination, vital signs are normal and examination findings are unremarkable, with no organomegaly or lymphadenopathy.

Hemoglobin	13.5 g/dL (135 g/L)
Leukocyte count	5500/µL (5.5 × 10⁹/L)
Platelet count	230,000/µL (230 × 10⁹/L)
Calcium	9.0 mg/dL (2.3 mmol/L)
Creatinine	1.0 mg/dL (88.4 µmol/L)
Protein	
Total	10.1 g/dL (101 g/L)
Albumin	4.0 g/dL (40 g/L)

Serum protein electrophoresis shows a monoclonal spike of 1.8 g/dL (18 g/L), which is further identified as IgG-κ by serum immunofixation. A bone marrow aspirate reveals 6% plasma cells. A skeletal survey does not show any lytic lesions.

Which of the following is the most likely diagnosis?

(A) AL (light chain) amyloidosis
(B) Lymphoplasmacytic lymphoma (Waldenström macroglobulinemia)
(C) Monoclonal gammopathy of undetermined significance (MGUS)
(D) Multiple myeloma

Item 29 [Basic]

A 60-year-old man comes to the office for follow-up evaluation 1 month after being seen for symptoms of an upper respiratory tract infection. Physical examination findings at his initial visit were normal; laboratory study results showed a leukocyte count of 18,000/µL (18 × 10⁹/L), with 60% lymphocytes. The patient's upper respiratory tract infection symptoms have since resolved completely, and he notes no other medical problems or symptoms.

Physical examination findings during this visit are again normal, with no evidence of lymphadenopathy or splenomegaly. The repeated leukocyte count remains the same, and the comprehensive metabolic profile and lactate dehydrogenase concentration are normal. Peripheral blood smear reveals morphologically mature–appearing lymphocytes.

Which of the following is the most likely diagnosis?

(A) Acute lymphocytic leukemia
(B) Acute myeloid leukemia
(C) Chronic lymphocytic leukemia
(D) Chronic myeloid leukemia

Item 30 [Basic]

A 57-year-old woman is evaluated in the emergency department for fever and shaking chills of 8 hours' duration. The patient has a 1-year history of myelodysplastic syndrome treated with azacitidine.

On physical examination, temperature is 39.2°C (102.6°F), blood pressure is 100/70 mm Hg, pulse rate is 110/min, and respiration rate is 20/min. Physical examination findings are otherwise unremarkable, with no rash, lymphadenopathy, costovertebral angle tenderness, abdominal tenderness, or splenomegaly.

Hemoglobin	10.6 g/dL (106 g/L)
Leukocyte count	33,600/µL (33.6 × 10⁹/L)
Platelet count	88,000/µL (88 × 10⁹/L)
Urinalysis	Normal

A chest radiograph is normal.

A peripheral blood smear is shown (Plate 20).

Which of the following is the most likely diagnosis?

(A) Acute lymphoblastic leukemia
(B) Acute myeloid leukemia
(C) Acute promyelocytic leukemia
(D) Chronic myeloid leukemia

Item 31 [Advanced]

A 58-year-old man is evaluated for increasing fatigue of 2 months' duration. He has no other medical problems and is not taking any medications.

On physical examination, vital signs are normal. There is no lymphadenopathy or peripheral edema. The spleen is palpable 4 cm below the left costal margin.

Hemoglobin	12.1 g/dL (121 g/L)
Leukocyte count	55,200/µL (55.2 × 10⁹/L)
Platelet count	105,000/µL (105 × 10⁹/L)

A peripheral blood smear shows an increased number of granulocytic cells in all phases of development but with a marked left shift and no Auer rods in the blasts. Bone marrow examination shows hypercellular marrow (80% cellularity) with marked granulocytic hyperplasia, a left shift in the granulocytes, and 3% myeloblasts. Cytogenetic testing reveals a *BCR/ABL* translocation.

Which of the following is the most likely diagnosis?

(A) Acute lymphoblastic leukemia
(B) Acute myeloid leukemia
(C) Acute promyelocytic leukemia
(D) Chronic myeloid leukemia

Section 5

Hematology
Answers and Critiques

Item 1 **Answer: C**

Educational Objective: *Diagnose iron deficiency in the setting of inflammatory anemia.*

This patient has anemia of inflammation and iron deficiency. She has rheumatoid arthritis, a cause of inflammatory anemia. Inflammatory cytokines block iron utilization, decrease transferrin (and total iron-binding capacity [TIBC]) levels, and increase ferritin levels. In contrast, the physiologic response to iron deficiency is to increase transferrin (and TIBC) levels and decrease ferritin levels. When inflammation accompanies iron deficiency, inflammatory cytokines always confound the expected pattern of serum iron chemistries for iron deficiency alone.

This patient's initial serum iron chemistries demonstrate a serum iron-to-TIBC ratio of 12%. Repeat serum iron chemistries 5 months later show an even lower iron-to-TIBC ratio of 4.7%, and her ferritin level is low-normal. Virtually all patients with serum ferritin levels lower than 10 to 15 ng/mL (10-15 µg/L) are iron deficient; however, 25% of menstruating women with absent stainable bone marrow iron have ferritin levels higher than 15 ng/mL (15 µg/L). Assuming absence of inflammation, higher ferritin cutoff limits of 30 to 41 ng/mL (30-41 µg/L) improve the efficiency of diagnosing iron deficiency in women during their reproductive years. Because this patient also has rheumatoid arthritis, serum ferritin levels are expected to rise (by as much as threefold) owing to the effects of inflammatory cytokines. Therefore, this patient's serum ferritin level of 36 ng/mL (36 µg/L) supports a diagnosis of iron deficiency, particularly in the setting of her inflammatory illness. As a rule of thumb, serum ferritin levels lower than 100 to 120 ng/mL (100-120 µg/L) may reflect iron deficiency in patients with inflammatory states.

Although monthly physiologic blood loss with menstruation is the most likely cause of iron deficiency in this patient, she should have age-appropriate cancer screening with colonoscopy (at a minimum) to exclude gastrointestinal causes of occult blood loss.

Methotrexate is an antimetabolite that inhibits dihydrofolate reductase and causes megaloblastic maturation; however, low-dose methotrexate is unlikely to cause significant megaloblastic anemia, whereas higher doses may do so with a significant rise in mean corpuscular volume (MCV). This patient's MCV is unchanged with low-dose methotrexate. Hence, megaloblastic anemia due to methotrexate is not a likely contributor to this patient's anemia.

KEY POINT

Serum ferritin levels lower than 100 to 120 ng/mL (100-120 µg/L) may reflect iron deficiency in patients with inflammatory states.

Bibliography

Weiss G, Goodnough LT. Anemia of chronic disease. N Engl J Med. 2005;352(10):1011-23. [PMID: 15758012]

Item 2 **Answer: A**

Educational Objective: *Diagnose aplastic anemia.*

This patient has aplastic anemia. Patients with this disorder have pancytopenia, a low reticulocyte count, and a hypoplastic bone marrow (<20% cellularity) with normal maturation of all cell lines. Aplastic anemia is a fatal disorder in which myeloid progenitor cells and stem cells are severely diminished or absent in the bone marrow because of either an intrinsic defect of the stem cells or immune-mediated stem cell destruction, which leads to transfusion-dependent anemia, thrombocytopenia, and severe neutropenia. In approximately 50% of cases of aplastic anemia, there is no obvious cause; chemicals, drugs, viral infections, collagen vascular diseases, and thymoma can be implicated in the remaining cases. Interferon-activated T lymphocytes are involved in autoimmune destruction of stem cells in a significant proportion of patients with the idiopathic or the acquired form of the disease; this fact explains why immunosuppressive therapy is effective in some patients. Initial management involves withdrawal of any potentially causative agents and a CT scan of the chest to rule out an associated thymoma.

Patients with immune thrombocytopenic purpura (ITP) have petechiae and ecchymoses but do not have a decreased leukocyte count. Most patients with ITP do not have anemia, but some of them may have an associated autoimmune hemolytic anemia or iron deficiency anemia due to bleeding. However, this patient's direct antiglobulin (Coombs) test was negative, and she had a low reticulocyte count, which together rule out hemolytic anemia. Finally, this patient does not have a clinical history of bleeding, and her iron stores are normal, which suggests that blood loss and iron deficiency is not the cause of her anemia.

KEY POINT

Patients with aplastic anemia have pancytopenia, a low reticulocyte count, and hypoplastic bone marrow.

Bibliography
Young NS, Scheinberg P, Calado RT. Aplastic anemia. Curr Opin Hematol. 2008;15(3):162-168. [PMID: 18391779]

Item 3   Answer: D

Educational Objective: *Treat iron deficiency anemia with oral iron.*

The most appropriate treatment for this patient is oral iron. This patient has iron deficiency anemia, as confirmed by the low mean corpuscular volume, low serum iron level, elevated total iron-binding capacity (TIBC), and low transferrin saturation (iron/TIBC). Iron deficiency is best treated by using oral iron salts; ferrous sulfate, 325 mg three times daily, is the least expensive preparation. Although there are alternative preparations of oral iron, none has conclusively been shown to increase oral tolerability and they deliver less elemental iron. Iron therapy is typically continued several months after normalization of the hemoglobin level. Patients who are unable to absorb iron orally (for example, patients with Crohn disease, celiac disease, or small bowel resection) instead may receive parenteral iron.

Because the patient is hemodynamically stable, there is no indication for a blood transfusion. This patient's signs, symptoms, and laboratory findings are not suggestive of renal disease, which may cause a low erythropoietin level, or of a bone marrow disorder, which would require administration of supraphysiologic levels of erythropoietin. Moreover, erythropoietin therapy would be ineffective in this patient until iron has become available for erythrocyte production. This patient has no evidence of malabsorption that would require parenteral administration of iron.

KEY POINT

Patients with iron deficiency anemia require oral iron replacement therapy.

Bibliography
Killip S, Bennett JM, Chambers MD. Iron deficiency anemia. Am Fam Physician. 2007;75(5):671-678. [PMID: 17375513]

Item 4   Answer: A

Educational Objective: *Diagnose glucose 6-phosphate dehydrogenase deficiency.*

This patient has glucose 6-phosphate dehydrogenase (G6PD) deficiency. G6PD deficiency is the most common disorder of erythrocyte metabolism. G6PD is necessary for generating adequate nicotinamide adenine dinucleotide phosphate–oxidase (NADPH) to prevent oxidant stress. G6PD is found on the X-chromosome, and, therefore, deficiency rarely occurs in women. The acute onset of symptoms and findings in patients with this deficiency can be precipitated by drugs, infection, or diabetic ketoacidosis. In this patient, hemolysis was likely precipitated by trimethoprim-sulfamethoxazole.

At 2 to 4 days after introduction of the oxidative stress in patients with G6PD deficiency, onset of jaundice and dark urine occurs, with or without abdominal and back pain. The hemoglobin level decreases by 3 to 4 g/dL (30 to 40 g/L), and there is an appropriate increase in reticulocytes. The hemolysis spontaneously resolves in approximately 1 week as the older enzyme-depleted cells are replaced by new cells with sufficient G6PD to prevent further hemolysis. Additional laboratory findings in patients with G6PD deficiency include a negative direct and indirect antiglobulin (Coombs) test and the presence of "bite" or "blister" cells, produced when accumulated oxidized hemoglobin remains adherent to the erythrocyte membrane with an adjacent membrane-bound clear zone. Such cells are visible on this patient's peripheral blood smear. Because reticulocytes can have normal G6PD levels, measuring G6PD levels during an acute episode may produce a false-negative result.

Patients with hereditary spherocytosis have spherocytes on the peripheral blood smear, as do patients with warm antibody–mediated hemolysis. The direct antiglobulin test is positive in patients with warm antibody–mediated hemolysis and negative in patients with hereditary spherocytosis. Patients with a microangiopathy have schistocytes on the peripheral blood smear and, typically, a low platelet count. Neither of these findings is present in the peripheral blood smear shown.

KEY POINT

In glucose-6-phosphate dehydrogenase deficiency, "bite" or "blister" cells are produced when accumulated oxidized hemoglobin remains adherent to the erythrocyte membrane, which creates an adjacent membrane-bound clear zone.

Bibliography
Cappellini MD, Fiorelli G. Glucose-6-phosphate dehydrogenase deficiency. Lancet. 2008;371:64-74. [PMID: 18177777]

Item 5   Answer: D

Educational Objective: *Diagnose thalassemia minor on the basis of a peripheral blood smear.*

The most likely diagnosis is thalassemia minor. Patients with thalassemia have a low mean cellular volume and target cells on the peripheral smear. Target cells are characterized by a central dense deposit of hemoglobin surrounded by a halo of pallor. This gives the erythrocytes a "bull's-eye" appearance. In normal erythrocytes, there is only central pallor. In thalassemia, the erythrocyte count is usually normal, or even slightly elevated. Iron studies are typically normal unless there is a coexisting iron deficiency anemia. The degree of poikilocytosis and anisocytosis is only modest but the hypochromia is striking and helps differentiate thalassemia from iron deficiency anemia.

Hereditary spherocytosis is characterized by uniformly small spherocytes that lack the typical central pallor of normal erythrocytes, and sickle cell anemia is characterized by sickled cells (crescent- or spindle-shaped cells) on the peripheral blood smear. These findings are absent in this patient's peripheral blood smear. Iron deficiency anemia is unlikely given the normal results of the iron studies. Additionally, a more striking variation in red blood cell size and shape would be expected with this degree of hypochromia in iron deficiency anemia.

KEY POINT

Patients with thalassemia have a low mean cellular volume and target cells on the peripheral blood smear and have normal results on iron studies.

Bibliography

Rund D, Rachmilewitz E. Beta-thalassemia. N Engl J Med. 2005; 353(11):1135-1146. [PMID: 16162884]

Item 6   Answer: C

Educational Objective: *Diagnose cobalamin deficiency in a patient with a low-normal vitamin B_{12} level with methylmalonic acid and homocysteine measurements.*

The most appropriate next diagnostic test is measurement of serum methylmalonic acid and homocysteine. This patient's findings of macrocytic anemia, thrombocytopenia, elevated lactate dehydrogenase level, and neurologic findings are very suggestive of vitamin B_{12} deficiency despite the low-normal B_{12} level. Levels of methylmalonic acid and homocysteine become elevated in patients with vitamin B_{12} deficiency before serum vitamin B_{12} levels decrease below the normal range. In contrast, only homocysteine is elevated in folate deficiency. Subclinical vitamin B_{12} deficiency in patients with subtle signs and symptoms of vitamin B_{12} deficiency can be detected by identification of elevated methylmalonic acid levels. This is particularly true for patients whose vitamin B_{12} level is in the "low-normal" range, as this patient's is.

Although bone marrow biopsy can be suggestive of vitamin B_{12} deficiency, it is not a specific test for confirming this disorder because there are other potential causes of megaloblastic marrow, including myelodysplasia.

Erythrocyte folate levels have been touted as a better indication of folate stores than serum folate levels are, but they are subject to problems of defining normal values and may not be that helpful clinically. Erythrocyte folate levels can also be depressed in patients with vitamin B_{12} deficiency. Additionally, folate deficiency would not cause the neurologic symptoms present in this patient.

Parietal cell antibodies are elevated in patients with pernicious anemia but may not be elevated in patients whose vitamin B_{12} deficiency is due to malabsorption, which is a very common cause of deficiency in the elderly.

KEY POINT

Methylmalonic acid levels become elevated before vitamin B_{12} levels decrease below the normal range in patients with vitamin B_{12} deficiency.

Bibliography

Cravens DD, Nashelsky J, Oh RC. Clinical inquiries. How do we evaluate a marginally low B_{12} level? J Fam Pract. 2007;56(1):62-63. [PMID: 17217902]

Item 7   Answer: C

Educational Objective: *Diagnose prosthetic valve hemolytic anemia.*

The most likely cause of this patient's anemia is hemolytic anemia due to mechanical destruction by the prosthetic heart valve. All patients with hemolytic anemia have common findings, which include an increased serum lactate dehydrogenase level, a decreased serum haptoglobin level, and reticulocytosis. Examination of the peripheral blood smear is often helpful in identifying the cause of the hemolytic anemia.

This patient's blood smear shows schistocytes (fragmented blood cells), which are found in patients with microangiopathic hemolytic anemia (for example, thrombotic thrombocytopenic purpura, hemolytic uremic syndrome, and disseminated intravascular coagulation) and with mechanical destruction due to prosthetic heart valves. Microangiopathic hemolytic anemia is an unlikely diagnosis for a patient who appears well, has no evidence of organ dysfunction, and has a normal platelet count. Patients with autoimmune hemolytic anemia have microspherocytes on their peripheral smear in addition to an increased reticulocyte count; schistocytes are notably absent.

Mild hemolytic anemia is common in patients with prosthetic heart valves, but the anemia can be more severe in up to 20% of patients. Symptomatic hemolytic anemia can usually be treated with oral iron and folate replacement, although more severe cases may warrant blood transfusion or recombinant human erythropoietin. Rarely, patients will require valve reoperation if hemolysis is due to significant valve dysfunction or progressive paravalvular regurgitation.

KEY POINT

Schistocytes (fragmented blood cells) are associated with microangiopathic hemolytic anemia (thrombotic thrombocytopenic purpura, hemolytic uremic syndrome, and disseminated intravascular coagulation) and with mechanical destruction due to prosthetic heart valves.

Bibliography

Shapira Y, Vaturi M, Sagie A. Hemolysis associated with prosthetic heart valves: a review. Cardiol Rev. 2009;17(3):121-124. [PMID: 19384085]

Item 8   Answer: B

Educational Objective: *Diagnose iron deficiency anemia on the basis of a peripheral blood smear.*

The findings on the peripheral blood smear are suggestive of iron deficiency anemia. The erythrocytes show hypochromia, anisocytosis (changes in size), and poikilocytosis (changes in shape) and are also likely to be microcytic. If a confirmatory test (for example, serum ferritin determination) supports the diagnosis of iron deficiency anemia, a source of gastrointestinal blood loss should be sought, regardless of whether the stool is positive or negative for occult blood. A gastrointestinal lesion, such as colon cancer or gastritis, is far more likely than dietary inadequacies or malabsorption in an otherwise healthy adult.

Hereditary spherocytosis, another cause of microcytosis, is associated with spherocytes (small cells with loss of the normal central pallor) and an enlarged spleen, and would be unlikely to present in a 65-year-old man. Sickle cell anemia would be associated with sickled cells (spindle- or crescent-shaped cells) on the peripheral blood smear, which are not present. Although the thalassemias are associated with hypochromic, microcytic erythrocytes, the diagnosis is unlikely in a patient who had a normal hemoglobin level 1 year ago. In addition, erythrocytes in thalassemia show less hypochromia, anisocytosis, and poikilocytosis and more target cells. Target cells are characterized by a concentration of dense hemoglobin in the center of the cell surrounded by a rim of pallor creating a "bull's-eye" appearance. Normal erythrocytes have an area of central pallor.

KEY POINT

Peripheral blood smear findings suggestive of iron deficiency anemia include microcytosis, hypochromia, anisocytosis (changes in size), and poikilocytosis (changes in shape).

Bibliography
Clark SF. Iron deficiency anemia: diagnosis and management. Curr Opin Gastroenterol. 2009;25(2):122-128. [PMID: 19262200]

Item 9   Answer: A

Educational Objective: *Diagnose autoimmune hemolytic anemia.*

This patient has autoimmune hemolytic anemia (AIHA). The hemolytic anemias are characterized by increased destruction of erythrocytes associated with reticulocytosis. Elevated levels of unconjugated bilirubin, lactate dehydrogenase, and uric acid and depressed levels of haptoglobin are characteristic of hemolysis. AIHA may be idiopathic or result from drugs, lymphoproliferative disorders, collagen vascular diseases, or malignancies. Warm antibody–mediated hemolytic anemia, the most common type of AIHA, is diagnosed by the direct antiglobulin (Coombs) test, which detects IgG or complement on the cell surface, and the presence of spherocytes on the peripheral blood smear. In this condition, IgG antibodies bind to Rh-type antigens on the erythrocyte surface at 37.0°C (98.6°F).

Hereditary spherocytosis is a congenital hemolytic anemia caused by abnormalities in erythrocyte membrane proteins and is characterized by spherocytic erythrocytes with increased osmotic fragility due to their large volume/surface area ratio. It would be very unusual for a congential hemolytic anemia to be first diagnosed at this patient's age. Additionally, hereditary spherocytosis is not associated with positive results on a

Coombs test. Spherocytes are small round cells that lack the typical central pallor of normal erythrocytes.

Microangiopathic hemolytic anemia is a nonimmune hemolytic anemia. As with other hemolytic anemias, it is characterized by reticulocytosis, elevated levels of unconjugated bilirubin, lactate dehydrogenase, and depressed levels of haptoglobin. Microangiopathic hemolysis may be associated with thrombocytopenia. Another distinguishing characteristic of microangiopathic hemolytic anemia is the presence of schistocytes on the peripheral blood smear. This finding was lacking on this patient's peripheral blood smear.

α-Thalassemia is a congenital hemolytic anemia. Patients with a two-α-gene defect have target cells and an absence of spherocytes on the peripheral blood smear and do not have positive results on a direct antiglobulin test.

KEY POINT

Warm antibody–mediated hemolytic anemia, a common complication of lymphoid malignancies, is characterized by spherocytes on the peripheral blood smear.

Bibliography
Hauswirth AW, Skrabs C, Schützinger C, Gaiger A, Lechner K, Jäger U. Autoimmune hemolytic anemias, Evans' syndromes, and pure red cell aplasia in non-Hodgkin lymphomas. Leuk Lymphoma. 2007;48(6): 1139-1149. [PMID:17577777]

Item 10   Answer: A

Educational Objective: *Diagnose an acquired coagulation factor deficiency.*

The patient most likely has an acquired coagulation factor deficiency. All coagulation factors are synthesized in the liver, and severe hepatic impairment leads to various factor deficiencies, and vitamin K deficiency may further increase the risk for deficient coagulation factors. Patients with liver disease, especially cirrhosis, have an enlarged spleen and a moderate reduction in the platelet count (50,000 to 100,000/µL [50-100 × 10^9/L]) caused by splenic sequestration (hypersplenism), which may increase the risk for bleeding. In addition, cirrhosis is often associated with esophageal varices, which also cause gastrointestinal bleeding. Coagulation usually does not become impaired until the cirrhosis is advanced, and the prothrombin time, activated partial thromboplastin time, and thrombin time are all prolonged (as in this patient). If results of any of these assays are prolonged and the diagnosis remains in doubt, an inhibitor mixing study should be done. This involves repeating the abnormal assay with a 1:1 mixture of the patient's plasma and normal plasma to detect either a factor deficiency or the presence of an inhibitor (that is, an antibody directed against a factor). The results of the mixing study will normalize in a patient with a factor deficiency (as they did in this patient) but will remain abnormal if an inhibitor is present.

The patient's platelet count is not low enough to cause significant bleeding. Acquired qualitative platelet disorders are most commonly caused by drugs, especially aspirin and NSAIDs. Other antiplatelet agents used to treat cardiovascular disease may also cause platelet disorders (for example, abciximab, eptifibatide, clopidogrel). Uremia is another common cause of a qualitative platelet disorder. The platelet defect in uremia has been attributed to impaired platelet–vessel wall adhesion. The patient is taking no medications and the serum creatinine is 1.5 mg/dL (132.6 mmol/L), making an acquired platelet function disorder unlikely.

KEY POINT

All coagulation factors are synthesized in the liver, and severe hepatic impairment leads to various factor deficiencies.

Bibliography

Caldwell SH, Sanyal AJ. Coagulation disorders and bleeding in liver disease: future directions. Clin Liver Dis. 2009;13(1):155-7. [PMID: 19150319]

Item 11   Answer: A
Educational Objective: *Diagnose disseminated intravascular coagulation.*

The most likely diagnosis is disseminated intravascular coagulation (DIC). DIC is the result of widespread activation of coagulation that leads to formation of fibrin clots. Some patients have a thrombotic disorder, but in most patients, secondary fibrinolysis dissolves the fibrin clot and consumption of platelets and coagulation factors causes thrombocytopenia, clotting factor deficiencies, bleeding, and vascular injuries. Erythrocyte consumption is manifested by a microangiopathic hemolytic anemia with fragmented erythrocytes seen on a peripheral blood smear. DIC most commonly occurs in patients with infections, cancer, and obstetrical complications. Gram-negative sepsis is the most common infection associated with DIC. The diagnosis of DIC is based on a prolonged prothrombin time, activated partial thromboplastin time, and thrombin time; a high D-dimer titer; a reduced serum fibrinogen level and platelet count; and microangiopathic hemolytic anemia. The degree of these abnormalities depends on the extent of consumption of platelets and coagulation factors and the ability of the patient to compensate for these findings.

Two thrombotic microangiopathies in the differential diagnosis of DIC are thrombotic thrombocytopenic purpura (TTP) and hemolytic uremic syndrome (HUS). The two syndromes overlap, and it is often difficult to distinguish between them. The pentad of TTP includes thrombocytopenia, microangiopathic hemolytic anemia, neurologic deficits, renal impairment, and fever. All five findings do not need to be present for the diagnosis to be established. HUS is a condition primarily of children and mainly affects the kidneys as a result of intrarenal platelet-fibrin thrombi. Neither TTP nor HUS is associated with elevations of the prothrombin or partial thromboplastin time or the D-dimer or depression of the fibrinogen level.

Immune thrombocytopenic purpura (ITP) may be autoimmune mediated or drug induced. The diagnosis is based on excluding other causes of thrombocytopenia, other systemic illnesses, and medications. The only laboratory disorder associated with ITP is thrombocytopenia.

KEY POINT

The diagnosis of disseminated intravascular coagulation is based on a prolonged prothrombin time, activated partial thromboplastin time, and thrombin time; a high D-dimer titer; a reduced serum fibrinogen level and platelet count; and microangiopathic hemolytic anemia.

Bibliography

Levi M, Toh CH, Thachil J, Watson HG. Guidelines for the diagnosis and management of disseminated intravascular coagulation. British Committee for Standards in Haematology. Br J Haematol. 2009;145(1):24-33. [PMID: 19222477]

Item 12   Answer: D
Educational Objective: *Diagnose von Willebrand disease.*

The most likely diagnosis is von Willebrand disease. This patient has abnormal bleeding on tooth extraction, a history suggestive of a bleeding tendency, and a family history of a potential bleeding problem. His laboratory studies support both a qualitative platelet defect (prolonged bleeding time) and a mild coagulopathy (borderline elevated activated partial thromboplastin time [aPTT] and low factor VIII level). These findings are suggestive of the most common inherited hemostatic disorder, namely, von Willebrand disease. von Willebrand disease is one of the few hemostatic disorders characterized by both a platelet and coagulation defect due to a reduction or defect in von Willebrand factor (vWF), which supports platelet adhesion and also serves as a carrier protein for factor VIII. The diagnosis is confirmed by measuring the vWF antigen level and activity.

Hemophilia A (factor VIII deficiency) is not associated with a prolonged bleeding time, nor is it transmitted from father to son (X-linked inheritance). The presence of a lupus inhibitor is generally associated with a thrombotic, not a bleeding, disorder; is an acquired disorder; does not prolong the bleeding time; and is not associated with decreased levels of factor VIII. Vitamin K deficiency can occur in patients receiving total parenteral nutrition or long-term antibiotics and in those who are malnourished, particularly in the setting of warfarin administration. This condition is characterized by a progressively prolonged prothrombin time (PT) and aPTT (with the PT proportionately more prolonged than the aPTT) and a normal thrombin time, findings not consistent with those in this patient.

KEY POINT

von Willebrand disease is an autosomal dominant disorder characterized by a personal and family history of a bleeding tendency, a prolonged bleeding time, a borderline-elevated activated partial thromboplastin time, and a low factor VIII level.

Bibliography

Kessler CM. Diagnosis and treatment of von Willebrand disease: new perspectives and nuances [erratum in Haemophilia. 2008;14(3):669]. Haemophilia. 2007;13 Suppl 5:3-14. [PMID: 18078392]

Item 13   Answer: A

Educational Objective: *Screen for bleeding disorders with a clinical history.*

The best screening approach to detect bleeding disorders is by taking a thorough clinical history. The clinical history should focus on the presence of any systemic illnesses and previous bleeding. If bleeding is reported, its severity should be determined, as should whether the bleeding is spontaneous or is an excessive response to normal bleeding after injury, surgery, or dental procedures; whether the bleeding pattern is lifelong or recently acquired; and whether the bleeding suggests a platelet or a coagulation defect. Platelet-related bleeding tends to occur immediately after injury and often affects the mucous membranes or the skin in the form of petechiae. Coagulation-related bleeding may be delayed in onset, is manifested more by deep tissue bruises (ecchymoses), and may produce hemarthroses in patients with congenital deficiencies. Women should be asked about the pattern of menstrual bleeding or, if postmenopausal, about whether any abnormal bleeding has occurred. Obtaining a detailed medication history and a family history of any bleeding disorders is imperative.

In the absence of a personal or family history of abnormal bleeding, liver disease, significant alcohol use, malabsorption, or anticoagulation therapy, the likelihood of a bleeding disorder is low, and no further preoperative testing is required. Patients with any of these risk factors should be screened further by obtaining a prothrombin time (PT/INR), an activated partial thromboplastin time, and a platelet count. In addition, plasma fibrinogen measurement and von Willebrand factor testing should be considered in patients with a history of bleeding problems.

KEY POINT

In the absence of a personal or family history of abnormal bleeding, liver disease, significant alcohol use, malabsorption, or anticoagulation therapy, the likelihood of a bleeding disorder is low, and no further preoperative testing is required.

Bibliography

Smetana GW, Macpherson DS. The case against routine preoperative laboratory testing. Med Clin North Am. 2003;87(1):7-40. [PMID: 12575882]

Item 14   Answer: D

Educational Objective: *Diagnose parvovirus B19 infection as the cause of aplastic crisis in sickle cell disease.*

Transient aplastic crisis in a patient with chronic hemolytic anemia is usually due to acute infection with parvovirus B19, a single-stranded DNA virus. The propensity of this virus to infect bone marrow erythroid progenitor cells can cause pro-

found anemia in someone who is dependent on rapid erythrocyte production. Acute infection can be diagnosed by finding serum IgM antibodies against parvovirus B19. Recovery usually occurs spontaneously in days to weeks.

Parvovirus B19 infection also causes erythema infectiosum (fifth disease), a common childhood illness characterized by a "slapped-cheek" appearance of the face followed by a lacy red rash on the trunk and limbs. This virus can also cause polyarthritis in adults (often after exposure to a child with erythema infectiosum), hydrops fetalis if infection occurs early during pregnancy, and chronic infection in immunocompromised persons, including patients infected with HIV.

Although leukemia may cause severe anemia, other hematopoietic lineages are also often involved, which was not evident in this patient. A bleeding ulcer should stimulate erythrocyte production and not depress reticulocyte production and most likely would be associated with melena or stool samples positive for occult blood. Epstein-Barr virus infection is unlikely to cause red cell aplasia. This viral infection may be associated with hemolytic anemia and reticulocytosis, lymphadenopathy, splenomegaly, hepatitis, and a variety of lymphoproliferative disorders.

KEY POINT

Transient aplastic crisis in patients with chronic hemolytic anemia is usually due to acute infection with parvovirus B19.

Bibliography

Servey JT, Reamy BV, Hodge J. Clinical presentations of parvovirus B19 infection. Am Fam Physician. 2007;75(3):373-376. [PMID: 17304869]

Item 15   Answer: D

Educational Objective: *Diagnose pulmonary hypertension in a patient with sickle cell anemia.*

The most likely diagnosis is pulmonary hypertension. Pulmonary hypertension is a newly recognized cause of morbidity and mortality in patients with homozygous sickle cell disease. Various studies suggest a prevalence of 20% to 60%. The presentation of pulmonary hypertension is characterized by right-sided heart failure with peripheral edema, abnormal venous waveforms, fixed splitting of S_2, loud or palpable pulmonic valve closure, tricuspid regurgitation, a right ventricular heave, and clear lungs. This patient's echocardiographic results are consistent with pulmonary hypertension.

The cardinal symptoms of aortic stenosis are angina, syncope, and dyspnea. The murmur of aortic stenosis is a midsystolic crescendo-decrescendo murmur heard best at the second right intercostal space; the murmur radiates toward the carotid arteries. The murmur does not vary with respiration and is not associated with fixed splitting of S_2; in aortic stenosis, splitting is often absent or reversed (heard during exhalation, not inspiration).

Most patients with hypertrophic cardiomyopathy are relatively asymptomatic; however, some may develop symptoms of pulmonary congestion (exertional dyspnea, orthopnea, and paroxysmal nocturnal dyspnea), chest pain, fatigue, palpitations, dizziness, and syncope. In affected patients, physical examination in the presence of left ventricular outflow obstruction shows a variable and dynamic systolic murmur that is increased by the Valsalva maneuver. There is no change in the murmur with respiration. Echocardiography in patients with hypertrophic cardiomyopathy delineates a pattern of left ventricular or septal hypertrophy, which is absent in this patient.

Ischemic heart disease can cause left ventricular dysfunction and signs of heart failure without chest pain. However, this patient's findings are most compatible with right-sided heart failure (peripheral edema and clear lungs) due to pulmonary hypertension, not left ventricular dysfunction (elevated central venous pressure, an S_3, and pulmonary crackles). Finally, the echocardiogram shows normal left ventricular function.

KEY POINT

Pulmonary hypertension is a common cause of morbidity and mortality in patients with sickle cell disease.

Bibliography

Gladwin MT, Vichinsky E. Pulmonary complications of sickle cell disease. N Engl J Med. 2008;359(21):2254-2265. [PMID: 19020327]

Item 16   Answer: C

Educational Objective: *Diagnose and treat acute chest syndrome.*

Acute chest syndrome in patients with sickle cell anemia should be managed by exchange transfusion. Red blood cell exchange transfusions are performed to increase the hemoglobin A level to at least 50% and thereby decrease the percentage of abnormal sickle cells and prevent hemoglobin S polymerization and sickling. In adolescents and adults, pulmonary crises usually start with infarctions that may become secondarily infected. With time, multiple infarctions predominate, and pulmonary congestion and intrapulmonary shunting develop and lead to more hypoxia and sickling.

Erythropoietin administration has a limited role in patients with sickle cell disease. Erythropoietin has been used to accelerate recovery from aplastic crises in some patients. However, this patient has a brisk reticulocyte response, which indicates that erythropoiesis is likely already under intense erythropoietin stimulation; the addition of extra exogenous erythropoietin is unlikely to be helpful. Hydroxyurea may reduce the frequency of painful crises and acute chest syndrome but is not used in the acute treatment of the sickling process. The drug works by increasing hemoglobin F production, which helps prevent hemoglobin S polymerization and sickling. Because of the increased blood volume resulting from red blood cell transfusions, it is not possible to increase the hemoglobin A to more than 50% without inducing volume overload; therefore, exchange transfusions are required.

KEY POINT

In patients with sickle cell disease, acute chest syndrome should be managed by exchange transfusion.

Bibliography

Swerdlow PS. Red cell exchange in sickle cell disease. Hematology Am Soc Hematol Educ Program. 2006:48-53. [PMID: 17124039]

Item 17   Answer: C

Educational Objective: *Diagnose osteonecrosis of the hip with MRI.*

The best test to evaluate the patient's hip pain is MRI. This patient most likely has osteonecrosis of the hip. Osteonecrosis (previously called avascular necrosis) of the femoral head in adults is often associated with trauma, sickle cell disease, alcohol abuse, gout, corticosteroid use, and hypercoagulable states; it can also be idiopathic. Pain is the most common symptom and is usually located in the groin; thigh and buttock pain is also common. Plain film radiography is often the initial diagnostic test, and early findings may include increased density, reflecting marrow infarction and calcification. However, changes on plain film radiography may take weeks to months to appear, and radiography is insensitive in the diagnosis of early osteonecrosis. MRI has a reported sensitivity for osteonecrosis that exceeds 90% and is positive when other studies are negative. It is the preferred imaging modality, particularly if initial plain radiographs are normal.

Septic arthritis should always be considered in a patient with acute monoarticular arthritis. However, in the absence of previous hip disease or prosthesis, septic arthritis of the hip is relatively rare. An arthrocentesis is thus not indicated at this time.

Localized osteoporosis may occur in patients with injuries and is a prominent feature of complex regional pain syndrome (reflex sympathetic dystrophy), which is characterized by pain in the extremities associated with swelling, limited range of motion, vasomotor instability, and skin changes. Bone densitometry is not indicated in this patient because she has no history of injury and none of the symptoms characteristic of complex regional pain syndrome.

A radionuclide bone scan is more sensitive than plain radiographs but not as sensitive as MRI in the diagnosis of osteonecrosis. A radionuclide bone scan is typically reserved for patients who have a contraindication for MRI (for example, metal implants).

KEY POINT

MRI is more than 90% sensitive in the diagnosis of osteonecrosis and is the preferred imaging procedure when plain radiographs are normal.

Bibliography

Jones LC, Hungerford DS. Osteonecrosis: etiology, diagnosis, and treatment. Curr Opin Rheumatol. 2004;16(4):443-449. [PMID: 15201609]

Item 18   Answer: C

Educational Objective: *Diagnose sickle cell disease on the basis of a peripheral blood smear.*

It is highly likely that this adolescent has homozygous sickle cell disease and has had occlusion of a major vessel in the distribution of the left middle cerebral artery causing right hemiparesis and aphasia. The peripheral blood smear shows characteristic sickle cells (elongated crescent- and spindle-shaped cells). Patients with sickle cell disease commonly have target cells characterized by a central dense area of hemoglobin surrounded by a rim of pallor, giving it a "bull's-eye" appearance. Normal erythrocytes have an area of central pallor. Strokes due to occlusion of a large vessel are not uncommon in patients with sickle cell disease and are an indication for chronic blood transfusion therapy to maintain the peripheral blood hemoglobin S level below 50%.

Hereditary spherocytosis, iron deficiency anemia, and thalassemia all cause microcytosis but are not associated with elongated sickled cells. Hereditary spherocytosis is associated with uniformly small erythrocytes that lack the normal central pallor. Iron deficiency anemia usually is associated with erythrocytes that have increased central pallor and variation in size (anisocytosis) and shape (poikilocytosis). Thalassemia minor is associated with many target cells on the peripheral blood smear.

KEY POINT

Sickle cell disease is characterized by a peripheral blood smear showing elongated crescent- and spindle-shaped cells (sickle cells) and target cells.

Bibliography

Inati A, Koussa S, Taher A, Perrine S. Sickle cell disease: new insights into pathophysiology and treatment. Pediatr Ann. 2008;37(5):311-321. [PMID: 18543542]

Item 19   Answer: C

Educational Objective: *Treat a patient with heparin-induced thrombocytopenia.*

The most appropriate next step is to stop heparin and administer argatroban. Up to 2% of patients treated with heparin (either unfractionated or low molecular weight heparin) develop heparin-induced thrombocytopenia (HIT), and approximately 30% of patients with HIT also develop thrombosis (HIT/T). HIT/T should be considered in any patient with an otherwise unexplained decrease in the platelet count and/or a new thrombotic event 5 to 10 days after initiation of heparin therapy. However, in patients with recent exposure to heparin (such as this patient), the onset of HIT may be rapid (median time, 10.5 hours), and a syndrome of delayed-onset HIT that develops as late as 3 weeks after discontinuation of heparin has also been recognized. Almost all patients with HIT/T have circulating antibodies to complexes containing platelet factor 4 (PF4) and heparin. Laboratory testing for HIT/T is considered confirmatory to clinical evaluation findings. Tests for the diagnosis of HIT/T rely on platelet activation or measure binding of antibodies to PF4/heparin complexes. The ^{14}C-serotonin release assay (SRA) is considered the "gold standard" for diagnosis, with a positive predictive value approaching 100% and a negative predictive value of approximately 20%; therefore, a negative SRA does not exclude HIT/T. Heparin must be discontinued promptly after the diagnosis of HIT is suspected and alternative anticoagulation initiated. Lepirudin and argatroban are direct thrombin inhibitors that have emerged as the agents of choice for treatment of HIT or HIT/T in the United States. Fondaparinux and bivalirudin have also been used.

Platelet transfusions are contraindicated in patients in whom thrombocytopenia is caused by a consumptive process, unless there is life-threatening bleeding. Corticosteroids would only be appropriate if the thrombocytopenia were thought to be typical for immune thrombocytopenic purpura, which is not likely in this patient given the relationship between the reexposure to heparin and the rapid development of thrombocytopenia. Warfarin should not be initiated in the absence of a concurrently administered parenteral anticoagulant because warfarin alone can potentiate a hypercoagulable state early in treatment.

KEY POINT

Heparin-induced thrombocytopenia and thrombosis should be considered in any patient with an otherwise unexplained decrease in the platelet count and/or a new thrombotic event 5 to 10 days after initiation of heparin therapy.

Bibliography

Prechel M, Walenga JM. The laboratory diagnosis and clinical management of patients with heparin-induced thrombocytopenia: an update. Semin Thromb Hemost. 2008;34(1):86-96. [PMID: 18393145]

Item 20   Answer: D

Educational Objective: *Diagnose thrombotic thrombocytopenic purpura.*

The most likely diagnosis is thrombotic thrombocytopenic purpura (TTP). This patient has the principal triad of TTP: microangiopathic hemolytic anemia (schistocytes, or erythrocyte fragments, on the peripheral blood smear); thrombocytopenia with normal coagulation; and central nervous system symptoms. The presence of renal failure and fever compose the pentad of TTP findings. Classic TTP occurs mainly in adults, and its pathogenesis appears to be related to deficient von Willebrand factor (vWF) cleavage. Patients with TTP often have increased levels of ultralarge vWF multimers (ULvWF), which are particularly active in binding to platelets and inducing platelet agglutination. Under normal conditions, ULvWF are not present in the circulation because of cleavage of vWF monomers by ADAMTS13, the vWF cleaving protease. A severe deficiency of ADAMTS13 has been shown in most patients with TTP. Plasma exchange is the principal treatment modality for TTP and should be initiated as soon as possible to decrease patient morbidity.

Idiopathic thrombocytopenic purpura is an immune-mediated disorder of platelet destruction. At presentation, affected patients typically have isolated thrombocytopenia, generally without splenomegaly or adenopathy. The peripheral blood smear in idiopathic thrombocytopenic purpura shows only decreased numbers of platelets with normal erythrocyte and leukocyte morphology. The presence of severe microangiopathic hemolytic anemia seen in this patient's blood smear is inconsistent with immune thrombocytopenic purpura.

Evans syndrome refers to the combination of Coombs-positive warm autoimmune hemolytic anemia and immune thrombocytopenic purpura. However, patients with autoimmune hemolytic anemia have microspherocytes on their peripheral smear (in addition to an increased reticulocyte count) rather than schistocytes, such as this patient has.

Heparin-induced thrombocytopenia (HIT) should be considered in any patient with an otherwise unexplained decrease in the platelet count of at least 50% and/or a new thrombotic event 5 to 10 days after initiation of heparin therapy. However, this patient has no history of heparin exposure, and HIT is not associated with microangiopathic hemolytic anemia.

KEY POINT

Microangiopathic hemolytic anemia, thrombocytopenia with normal coagulation, and central nervous system symptoms are the principal triad of thrombotic thrombocytopenic purpura; renal failure and fever compose the pentad of symptoms.

Bibliography

George JN. Clinical practice. Thrombotic thrombocytopenic purpura. N Engl J Med. 2006;354(18):1927-1935. [PMID:16672704]

Item 21   Answer: C
Educational Objective: *Diagnose pseudothrombocytopenia.*

This patient most likely has pseudothrombocytopenia, a condition in which platelets agglutinate and the clumped platelets are not recognized as such by automated blood counters. The diagnosis is suspected by finding large platelet clumps on the stained blood film. These clumps occasionally adhere to neutrophils but may also be unassociated with any other cell types. If platelet clumping is observed, the platelet count is repeated using an alternative anticoagulant to EDTA, such as heparin or sodium citrate.

Gestational thrombocytopenia is the most common cause of pregnancy-associated thrombocytopenia. Most pregnant women who do have a mild thrombocytopenia have platelet counts ranging between 70,000/μL (70 × 10^9/L) and 150,000/μL (150 × 10^9/L). This occurs in approximately 5% of pregnancies and appears in late gestation. The cause of gestational thrombocytopenia is unknown, although it is not

believed to have an immune basis. Specific therapy is not required. The diagnosis of gestational thrombocytopenia cannot be confirmed or excluded until a reliable platelet count is obtained.

Immune thrombocytopenic purpura is a disorder caused by antibodies reactive with platelet glycoproteins (particularly glycoprotein IIb-IIIa), the platelet fibrinogen receptor, and glycoprotein Ib. At presentation, affected patients have isolated thrombocytopenia, generally without splenomegaly or adenopathy. The peripheral blood smear shows only decreased numbers of platelets with normal erythrocyte and leukocyte morphology; occasionally, large (immature) platelets are seen. In this patient the diagnosis of ITP cannot be confirmed or excluded until the platelet count is repeated with an alternative anticoagulant to eliminate platelet clumping.

Microangiopathic hemolytic anemia, thrombocytopenia with normal coagulation, and central nervous system symptoms are the principal triad of thrombotic thrombocytopenic purpura; renal failure and fever compose the pentad of symptoms. Microangiopathic hemolytic anemia is suggested by the presence of schistocytes (erythrocyte fragments) on the peripheral blood smear, reticulocytosis, and an elevated lactate dehydrogenase level. These findings are not present.

KEY POINT

Pseudothrombocytopenia, in which platelets agglutinate and the clumped platelets are not counted by automated blood counters, is an artifactual cause of thrombocytopenia.

Bibliography

Sekhon SS, Roy V. Thrombocytopenia in adults: a practical approach to evaluation and management. South Med J. 2006;99(5):491-498. [PMID: 16711312]

Item 22   Answer: B
Educational Objective: *Initiate corticosteroids to manage immune thrombocytopenic purpura.*

The most appropriate next step in management is the initiation of corticosteroids. This healthy young woman has petechiae caused by her very low platelet count. Although most of her remaining laboratory studies are normal, her peripheral blood smear showing few, but large, platelets supports the presence of a young population of platelets, consistent with increased turnover. These findings are suggestive of immune thrombocytopenic purpura (ITP), and a bone marrow examination is not essential. Instead, a presumptive diagnosis of ITP should be established, and the patient should receive high-dose corticosteroids. Corticosteroids are generally indicated in patients with ITP who have symptomatic bleeding and platelet counts below 50,000/μL (50 × 10^9/L) or in those with severe thrombocytopenia and platelet counts below 15,000/μL (15 × 10^9/L).

Splenectomy is not indicated as first-line therapy for ITP but may be considered when other less-invasive therapies have failed. Platelet transfusions would not be indicated in this patient unless serious, life-threatening bleeding was present. A bone marrow biopsy also is not necessary in this setting given the absence of any other signs of a bone marrow stem cell disorder, such as leukopenia or the presence of nucleated erythrocytes; early myeloid forms suggest a myelophthisic process, which occurs in neoplastic and metastatic disease, lymphoma, granulomatous disease, and infections of the bone marrow.

KEY POINT

Corticosteroids are the first-line treatment for patients with immune thrombocytopenic purpura.

Bibliography

Stasi R, Evangelista ML, Stipa E, Buccisano F, Venditti A, Amadori S. Idiopathic thrombocytopenic purpura: current concepts in pathophysiology and management. Thromb Haemost. 2008;99(1):4-13. [PMID: 18217129]

Item 23   Answer: C

Educational Objective: *Evaluate a patient for thrombophilia after completion of a course of warfarin.*

The most appropriate next step in the evaluation of this patient is thrombophilic screening at least 2 weeks after she completes the 6-month course of warfarin. This patient with an idiopathic pulmonary embolism and a strong family history of venous thromboembolism has a high likelihood of having an underlying thrombophilic condition. Therefore, she should undergo testing for activated protein C resistance, the prothrombin gene mutation, antiphospholipid antibodies, factor V Leiden, antithrombin deficiency, protein C deficiency, protein S deficiency, and the lupus inhibitor. Screening for thrombophilia should not be performed during anticoagulant therapy because both heparin and warfarin will influence the results of certain tests. Neither should it be done during the acute presenting episode before anticoagulants are initiated because the thrombosis itself may influence the results of certain tests. Thus, thrombophilia testing is best done at least a few weeks after a course of therapy is completed.

Polycythemia vera and essential thrombocythemia predispose patients to venous and arterial thrombotic events, particularly when the red blood cell mass or platelet count is not controlled. Although the *JAK2* mutation is found in almost all patients who have polycythemia vera and in approximately 50% of patients with essential thrombocythemia, routine screening for this mutation is not recommended, except in patients in whom a myeloproliferative disease is suspected. Because this patient has a normal complete blood count, screening for the *JAK2* mutation would be inappropriate.

Performing no further testing in this patient, given her recent idiopathic pulmonary embolism and family history of thrombotic issues, would be inappropriate because the risk of recurrent venous thromboembolism and need for continued anticoagulation cannot be estimated without screening for inherited thrombophilia.

KEY POINT

Thrombophilic screening should be performed not at the onset of a thrombotic event or during anticoagulant therapy but rather a few weeks after completion of therapy.

Bibliography

Dalen JE. Should patients with venous thromboembolism be screened for thrombophilia? Am J Med. 2008;121(6):458-463. [PMID: 18501222]

Item 24   Answer: A

Educational Objective: *Treat a patient with antiphospholipid antibodies after a first deep venous thrombosis with anticoagulation indefinitely.*

The most appropriate anticoagulation management for this patient is anticoagulation therapy indefinitely. The absolute risk of new venous thromboembolism (VTE) in patients with antiphospholipid antibodies is low (less than 1% per year). However, this risk may be increased to up to 10% per year in women with antiphospholipid antibodies or antiphospholipid antibody syndrome and recurrent fetal loss and to more than 10% per year in patients with antiphospholipid antibodies and previous VTE who have discontinued anticoagulants within 6 months. Current recommendations are to treat these patients with anticoagulation indefinitely. The benefit of VTE prevention with long-term anticoagulation in these high-risk patients may outweigh the risk for bleeding complications.

Positive results for anticardiolipin antibody or lupus inhibitor assay should be confirmed over time to ensure that they are not transient, which can occur after viral infections. Ideally, at least two positive laboratory tests (anticardiolipin antibody or lupus inhibitor assay) at least 12 weeks apart should be documented to confirm the presence of an antiphospholipid antibody syndrome before a patient is committed to lifelong anticoagulation.

KEY POINT

Patients with an antiphospholipid antibody syndrome and deep venous thrombosis have a high risk for recurrence once anticoagulation therapy is discontinued and thus require anticoagulation therapy indefinitely.

Bibliography

Giannakopoulos B, Krilis SA. How I treat the antiphospholipid syndrome. Blood. 2009;114(10):2020-2030. Epub 2009 Jul 8. [PMID: 19587374]

Item 25   Answer: C

Educational Objective: *Diagnose lupus inhibitor and antiphospholipid antibody syndrome.*

The most appropriate next diagnostic step is testing for the lupus inhibitor and antiphospholipid antibody. The antiphospholipid antibody sometimes interferes with the coagulation cascade as measured by the activated partial thromboplastin time or prothrombin time and causes a prolongation that is not corrected with a corresponding mix that includes normal plasma. These antibodies, although they prolong in vitro coagulation tests, are associated with an increased risk of venous (approximately two thirds) and arterial thromboembolism. There also is a strong correlation between these antibodies and pregnancy loss, presumably due to placental insufficiency in affected patients secondary to thrombosis. The diagnosis of antiphospholipid antibody syndrome requires a history of a thrombotic event (including recurrent fetal loss) in association with a persistent lupus anticoagulant or persistently elevated levels of IgG anticardiolipin or β_2-glycoprotein I antibodies. Lupus anticoagulants or elevated levels of antiphospholipid antibodies are frequently present in patients with systemic lupus erythematosus; they also occur in patients with cancer or infections (such as HIV) and in association with the use of certain drugs (for example, hydralazine, procainamide, or phenothiazines); the latter cases are often associated with IgM antibodies and do not result in a hypercoagulable state.

The factor V Leiden mutation results in resistance to activated protein C. In heterozygotes with the prothrombin G20210A mutation, prothrombin antigen and activity measurements are elevated by approximately 30% over those of normal persons. Among unselected white patients presenting with an initial symptomatic episode of deep venous thrombosis, 12% to 20% are heterozygous for the factor V Leiden mutation and 6% heterozygous for the prothrombin G20210A mutation, compared with 6% and 2%, respectively, in asymptomatic control populations. Neither the factor V Leiden mutation nor the prothrombin G20210A mutation is associated with increased fetal loss.

Hyperhomocysteinemia is associated with an increased risk of venous and arterial thrombosis. Plasma homocysteine levels are determined by genetic and environmental factors, the latter including primarily dietary intake of folic acid, vitamin B_{12}, and vitamin B_6. Administration of these B vitamins can lower plasma homocysteine levels, but this intervention has not yet been shown to reduce the risk of recurrent vascular events. Hyperhomocysteinemia is not associated with recurrent fetal loss.

KEY POINT

Antiphospholipid antibody syndrome consists of a history of a thrombotic event (including recurrent fetal loss) in association with a persistent lupus anticoagulant or persistently elevated levels of anticardiolipin or β_2-glycoprotein I antibodies.

Bibliography

George D, Erkan D. Antiphospholipid syndrome. Prog Cardiovasc Dis. 2009;52(2):115-125. [PMID: 19732604]

Item 26   Answer: C

Educational Objective: *Diagnose multiple myeloma as the cause of renal failure, anemia, low-anion gap, and hypercalcemia.*

The decreased anion gap in the presence of anemia, proteinuria, hypercalcemia, and renal failure suggests multiple myeloma. Acute kidney injury is the initial presentation in as many as one half of patients with multiple myeloma. Except

in multiple myeloma, hypercalcemia in the presence of acute kidney injury is relatively unusual because hyperphosphatemia and a decrease in renal 1-α hydroxylation of 25-hydroxycholecalciferol both act to predispose to hypocalcemia. Hypercalcemia may cause renal insufficiency through several mechanisms, including hemodynamic effects of vasoconstriction that mediate renal sodium and water retention, and direct effects on renal tubular sodium and water handling, resulting in prerenal azotemia secondary to volume depletion. Normally, the anion gap is approximately 12 ± 2 meq/L (12 ± 2 mmol/L). Most unmeasured anions consist of albumin. Therefore, the presence of either a low albumin level or an unmeasured cationic light chain, which occurs in multiple myeloma, results in a low anion gap.

Although hydrochlorothiazide toxicity can present with volume depletion and prerenal azotemia, the presence of hematologic and metabolic complications makes this less likely as a unifying diagnosis. The hypercalcemia that characterizes the milk-alkali syndrome is not associated with anemia or proteinuria and is usually associated with metabolic alkalosis. Primary hyperparathyroidism should be associated with hypophosphatemia and not anemia or proteinuria.

KEY POINT

A decreased anion gap in the presence of anemia, proteinuria, hypercalcemia, and renal failure suggests multiple myeloma.

Bibliography

Raab MS, Podar K, Breitkreutz I, Richardson PG, Anderson KC. Multiple myeloma. Lancet. 2009;374:324-339. [PMID: 19541364]

Item 27   Answer: D

Educational Objective: *Diagnose multiple myeloma in a patient with hypercalcemia.*

This patient has hypercalcemia, diffuse osteopenia, anemia, leukopenia, renal insufficiency, and a history of encapsulated organism–related pneumonia, which is a characteristic presentation of multiple myeloma. The diagnosis is supported by the bone marrow aspirate, which shows clusters of plasma cells. These cells can easily be distinguished from megaloblastoid erythrocytes by their dispersed chromatin pattern and perinuclear halo (Golgi apparatus).

Acute myeloid leukemia rarely causes hypercalcemia. In addition, more severe bone marrow failure and a decreased platelet count would be likely, and the bone marrow aspirate would show leukemic blasts. Chronic lymphocytic leukemia (CLL) only rarely causes hypercalcemia and renal insufficiency; an elevated leukocyte count is typical. Moreover, the increased number of plasma cells in the bone marrow aspirate in this patient rules out a diagnosis of CLL. Metastatic small cell lung cancer in the bone marrow may cause cytopenia and hypercalcemia. However, the peripheral blood smear would show leukoerythroblastic features with teardrop erythrocytes and immature myeloid and erythroid cells. Furthermore, the morphologic findings of the bone marrow aspirate in this patient, which shows a proliferation of plasma cells, is inconsistent with metastasis from any other cancer.

Multiple myeloma is suggested by the presence of hypercalcemia, osteopenia, anemia, leukopenia, and renal insufficiency.

Bibliography

Raab MS, Podar K, Breitkreutz I, Richardson PG, Anderson KC. Multiple myeloma. Lancet. 2009;374(9686):324-339. Epub 2009 Jun 21. [PMID: 19541364]

Item 28   Answer: C

Educational Objective: *Diagnose monoclonal gammopathy of undetermined significance.*

This patient has monoclonal gammopathy of undetermined significance (MGUS), which is characterized by the presence of a low serum monoclonal protein (M-protein) level (<3.0 g/dL [30 g/L]), less than 10% plasma cells in the bone marrow, and the absence of lytic bone lesions, anemia, hypercalcemia, or renal insufficiency associated with a plasma cell proliferative process or related B-cell lymphoproliferative disorder. The incidence of MGUS increases with age, and more than 5% of persons older than 80 years may be affected. No specific treatment is required, except for close follow-up to identify progression to myeloma or other disorders and periodic measurement of serum M-protein levels. The risk of progression correlates best with the M protein level: the higher the level, the greater the risk.

AL (light-chain) amyloidosis is a monoclonal plasma cell dyscrasia in which secreted immunoglobulin is deposited as fibrils in kidneys, heart, and peripheral nerves, thereby producing progressive organ dysfunction. Common symptoms include fatigue, weight loss, and easy bruising. Kidney involvement produces nephrotic syndrome with large amounts of non–light-chain proteinuria; azotemia develops late in the disease course. Cardiac involvement can be detected as thickening of the septum and leads to heart failure and arrhythmias. Sensorimotor neuropathy is the manifestation of peripheral nerve involvement. Detection of monoclonal immunoglobulin in serum, blood, or tissues differentiates AL amyloidosis from other forms of amyloidosis.

Lymphoplasmacytic lymphoma is usually associated with a monoclonal serum paraprotein of immunoglobulin M type (Waldenström's macroglobulinemia), not IgG as seen in this patient. Most patients have bone marrow, lymph node, and splenic involvement, and some may develop hyperviscosity syndrome.

Major diagnostic criteria for multiple myeloma include the following: the finding of a plasmacytoma on tissue biopsy; greater than 30% clonal plasma cells in the bone marrow; high M-protein levels (IgG >3.5 g/dL [35 g/L] and IgA >2.0 g/dL [20 g/L]); and Bence Jones proteinuria (urine protein excretion >1.0 g/24h). Minor criteria include 10% to 30% plasma cells in the bone marrow; M-protein level less than 3.5 g/dL

(35 g/L); lytic bone lesions; and diminished levels of non-monoclonal proteins. A diagnosis is established with one major and one minor criterion or three minor criteria.

Monoclonal gammopathy of undetermined significance is characterized by a serum monoclonal protein level less than 3.0 g/dL (30 g/L) without the overt clinical features of myeloma and less than 10% plasma cells in the bone marrow.

Bibliography

Bladé J, Rosiñol L, Cibeira MT, de Larrea CF. Pathogenesis and progression of monoclonal gammopathy of undetermined significance. Leukemia. 2008;22(9):1651-1657. Epub 2008 Jul 31. [PMID: 18668131]

Item 29   Answer: C

Educational Objective: *Diagnose chronic lymphocytic leukemia.*

The most likely diagnosis for this patient is chronic lymphocytic leukemia (CLL), which is characterized by abnormal accumulation of morphologically mature–appearing lymphocytes with a characteristic immunophenotype (CD5+, CD20+, and CD23+ B cells) in the blood, bone marrow, or lymphatic tissues. The diagnosis often is established by flow cytometry to avoid the need for bone marrow aspiration or biopsy. CLL occurs in patients after age 40 years, with increasing frequency in successive decades of life. The disease is often found incidentally on routine blood workup as a lymphocytosis without other evident disease. Long periods of stability or very slow progression of disease may occur over many years.

Acute lymphoblastic leukemia (ALL) is an extremely aggressive disease of precursor T or B cells that is usually of explosive onset. Rapidly rising levels blast cells in the blood and bone marrow, bulky lymphadenopathy (especially in the mediastinum), a younger age at onset, and cytopenia secondary to bone marrow involvement are the usual presenting clinical features of ALL.

Acute myeloid leukemia (AML) typically presents with severe pancytopenia and circulating myeloid blasts. Infection and bleeding are common presenting problems of patients with AML.

Chronic myeloid leukemia (CML) is recognized by an elevated leukocyte count and increased numbers of granulocytic cells in all phases of development on the peripheral blood smear. Very immature cells or blasts represent 1% to 5% of the granulocytes, with increasing numbers of promyelocytes, myelocytes, and metamyelocytes. CML is discovered incidentally in many patients.

Chronic lymphocytic leukemia is characterized by abnormal accumulation of morphologically mature–appearing lymphocytes with a characteristic immunophenotype in the blood, bone marrow, or lymphatic tissues.

Bibliography

Yee KW, O'Brien SM. Chronic lymphocytic leukemia: diagnosis and treatment. Mayo Clin Proc. 2006;81(8):1105-1129. [PMID: 16901035]

Item 30   Answer: B

Educational Objective: *Diagnose acute myeloid leukemia on the basis of a peripheral blood smear.*

The most likely diagnosis is acute myeloid leukemia (AML). Myelodysplastic syndromes are clonal disorders of the hematopoietic stem cells in patients older than 50 years and are characterized by ineffective hematopoiesis and peripheral cytopenia. Although the natural history of distinct subtypes of myelodysplasia ranges from indolent chronic anemia to rapid death from progression to acute leukemia, most patients eventually progress to leukemic syndromes or die from complications of bone marrow failure. Patients with myelodysplastic syndrome treated with azacitidine have significantly delayed transformation to leukemia and improved quality of life. Despite treatment with azacitidine, this patient has AML, as indicated by the peripheral blood smear showing a myeloblast with Auer rods. Auer rods are clumps of azurophilic, needle-shaped crystals made from primary cytoplasmic granules. They occur most often in patients with AML and rarely in patients with myelodysplasia. Fever in patients with AML is almost always related to infection; therefore, this patient must be quickly and thoroughly evaluated for a source of infection and treated empirically with broad-spectrum antibiotics.

Acute lymphoblastic leukemia (ALL) is an extremely aggressive disease of precursor T or B cells, usually of explosive onset. Rapidly rising blast cells in the blood and bone marrow, bulky lymphadenopathy (especially in the mediastinum), and cytopenia secondary to bone marrow involvement are the usual presenting clinical features. Auer rods do not occur in patients with ALL.

Acute promyelocytic leukemia (APL) is a subtype of AML that accounts for 10% of patients with AML. The disorder is exquisitely sensitive to anthracycline cytotoxic therapy. The addition of all-*trans*-retinoic-acid and arsenic trioxide to the therapy has resulted in high cure and salvage rates. Patients with APL may have circulating blasts, but the predominant cell is a large immature granulocyte with multiple granules overlying the cytoplasm and nucleus.

Typically, chronic myeloid leukemia (CML) is diagnosed as a result of a routine blood count that shows leukocytosis with circulating myeloid precursors in all stages of development. Patients with CML may have circulating blasts but also will have more mature granulocytes and will not have Auer rods.

KEY POINT

A peripheral blood smear showing myeloblasts that contain Auer rods is diagnostic of acute myeloid leukemia.

Bibliography

O'Donnell MR, Appelbaum FR, Coutre SE, et al. Acute myeloid leukemia. J Natl Compr Canc Netw. 2008;6(10):962-993. [PMID: 19176196]

Item 31   Answer: D

Educational Objective: *Diagnose chronic myeloid leukemia.*

This patient has chronic myeloid leukemia (CML). The prototype of the myeloproliferative syndromes, CML results from a balanced translocation between chromosomes 9 and 22 [t(9;22), the Philadelphia chromosome], which creates a unique gene designated *BCR-ABL*; this gene codes a 210-kDa protein (p210) that functions as tyrosine kinase. A t(9;22) is not only diagnostic of CML but is also the causative genetic event and a therapeutic target. The diagnosis of CML in this patient is based on the presence of the *BCR/ABL* oncogene, peripheral blood smear findings showing increased granulocytes with a marked left shift, and hypercellular bone marrow with marked myeloid proliferation.

Patients with acute lymphoblastic leukemia (ALL) typically have lymphocytosis, neutropenia, anemia, thrombocytopenia, lymphadenopathy, and hepatosplenomegaly at presentation. An increased number of lymphoblasts found on bone marrow examination are suspicious for the diagnosis. Immunophenotyping is necessary to confirm the diagnosis of AML and determine if the lymphocytes are B cells, T cells, or biphenotypic cells with markers of both lymphoid and myeloid cells.

Acute myeloid leukemia (AML) should be considered when circulating blasts are present in the peripheral blood smear. The diagnosis of AML is confirmed by a bone marrow aspirate showing hypercellular marrow containing greater than 20% to 30% myeloblasts. Once the diagnosis of acute leukemia is established, the classification is based on the morphology of the immature cells. The presence of Auer rods confirms the myeloid nature of the leukemia.

Acute promyelocytic leukemia (APL) is a subtype of AML that accounts for 10% of cases. Patients with APL may have circulating blasts, but the predominant cell is a large immature granulocyte with multiple granules overlying the cytoplasm and nucleus.

KEY POINT

The diagnosis of chronic myeloid leukemia is based on the presence of the *BCR/ABL* oncogene, peripheral blood smear findings showing increased granulocytes with a marked left shift, and hypercellular bone marrow with marked myeloid proliferation.

Bibliography

Vardiman JW. Chronic myelogenous leukemia, BCR-ABL1+. Am J Clin Pathol. 2009;132(2):250-260. [PMID: 19605820]

Infectious Disease Medicine
Questions

Item 1 [Advanced]

A 62-year-old man who lives in Atlanta is evaluated in July for a 24-hour history of fever, myalgia, and a frontal headache. He is otherwise healthy and takes no medications.

Recent travel includes a 2-week camping trip to the Blue Ridge Mountains of Virginia 11 days ago. The patient does not recall a specific insect or tick bite.

On physical examination, the patient appears mildly ill. Temperature is 38.7°C (101.6°F), blood pressure is 125/65 mm Hg, pulse rate is 90/min, and respiration rate is 18/min. He has blanching erythematous macules located around the wrists. There is no lymphadenopathy. Cardiopulmonary and abdominal examinations are normal.

Laboratory tests, blood cultures, and chest radiograph are pending.

Which of the following is the most likely diagnosis?

(A) Babesiosis
(B) Influenza
(C) Lyme disease
(D) Rocky Mountain spotted fever

Item 2 [Advanced]

A 33-year-old woman is evaluated for fever, fatigue, myalgia, headaches, dyspnea, and abdominal pain of 1 month's duration. She has no history of travel, camping, or animal exposure. She takes no medications.

On physical examination, she appears healthy. The vital signs and complete physical examination are normal.

She is re-evaluated for the same symptoms 10 days later and no changes from her initial examination are evident.

Laboratory evaluation is normal, including complete blood count, erythrocyte sedimentation rate, comprehensive metabolic profile, and urinalysis. Serologic testing for antinuclear antibody and rheumatoid factor are negative. Testing for Epstein-Barr, cytomegalovirus, and HIV infection is negative. Urine culture and three sets of blood cultures are negative.

CT of the chest, abdomen, and pelvis is normal.

Review of her fever diary shows nondaily, random spikes to 40.3°C (104.5°F) lasting less than 1 hour. No diurnal temperature variation is noted, and no associated chills or sweats are reported.

Which of the following is the most likely diagnosis?

(A) Factitious fever
(B) Familial Mediterranean fever
(C) Infective endocarditis
(D) Systemic lupus erythematosus

Item 3 [Advanced]

A 65-year-old man is admitted to the intensive care unit for gram-negative sepsis. The patient's medical history is significant only for hyperthyroidism, for which he takes methimazole. On day 2 in the intensive care unit, he undergoes intubation following medication with propofol and succinylcholine for acute respiratory distress syndrome. The patient also receives intermittent lorazepam and fentanyl boluses intravenously for sedation. Several hours later, the patient becomes febrile (temperature 40°C [104°F]), hypertensive, and tachycardic. On examination, he is diaphoretic and has muscular rigidity. Arterial blood gas analysis shows a metabolic and respiratory acidosis, and laboratory results are significant for an elevated serum creatine kinase level.

Which of the following is the most likely cause of the fever?

(A) Malignant hyperthermia
(B) Neuroleptic malignant syndrome
(C) Serotonin syndrome
(D) Thyroid storm

Item 4 [Advanced]

A 23-year-old woman is admitted to the intensive care unit with sepsis. She reports sustaining a cut on her left leg 4 days ago while hiking. She takes no medications and has been otherwise healthy.

On physical examination, temperature is 38.5°C (101.3°F), blood pressure is 95/55 mm Hg, pulse rate is 115/min, and respiration rate is 22/min. On the lower left leg is a 3-cm purulent wound surrounded by 10 cm of marked erythema, induration, and crepitus under the skin. Skin mottling is present up to midthigh.

Leukocyte count is 22,000/μL (22 × 10^9/L) and serum creatinine is 1.9 mg/dL (168 mmol/L). Radiograph of the leg shows subcutaneous air.

Blood and wound culture specimens are taken, and high-volume intravenous fluid administration and empiric broad spectrum antibiotics are initiated.

Which of the following is the most appropriate immediate next step in management?

(A) Begin drotrecogin alfa (activated protein C)
(B) Begin renal (low-dose) dopamine
(C) Begin norepinephrine
(D) Surgical wound debridement

Item 5 [Basic]

A 71-year-old woman is brought to the emergency department from a nursing home because of confusion, fever, and flank pain. Her temperature is 38.5°C (101.3°F), blood pressure is 82/48 mm Hg, pulse rate is 123/min, and respiration rate is 27/min. Mucous membranes are dry, and there is costovertebral angle tenderness, poor skin turgor, and no edema. Hemoglobin concentration is 10.5 g/dL (105 g/L) and leukocyte count is 15,600/μL (15.6 × 10^9/L); urinalysis reveals 50 to 100 leukocytes/hpf and many bacteria/hpf. The patient has an anion gap metabolic acidosis. A central venous catheter is placed, and antibiotic therapy is started.

Which of the following is most likely to improve survival for this patient?

(A) Aggressive fluid resuscitation
(B) Hemodynamic monitoring with a pulmonary artery catheter
(C) Maintaining hemoglobin concentration above 12 g/dL (120 g/L)
(D) Maintaining P_{CO_2} below 50 mm Hg (6.7 kPa)

Item 6 [Advanced]

A 67-year-old man is evaluated in the surgical intensive care unit. He underwent laparotomy and diverting colostomy for a ruptured diverticulum 72 hours ago, and now has a temperature of 40.0°C (104.0°F) and a heart rate of 135/min. In the past 3 hours his mean arterial blood pressure has dropped to 58 mm Hg despite three 1-L boluses of normal saline; urine output was only 15 mL in the past hour. The patient's oxygen saturation is 85% on 100% oxygen by non-rebreather mask. Platelet count is 42,000/μL (42 × 10^9/L) and random glucose is 148 mg/dL (8.2 mmol/L).

A portable chest radiograph shows bilateral alveolar infiltrates. A central venous catheter is placed; invasive mechanical ventilation and broad-spectrum antibiotic therapy are begun.

Which of the following is most likely to improve survival of this patient?

(A) Activated protein C
(B) Colloid fluid infusion
(C) Insulin drip
(D) Low-dose dopamine

Item 7 [Advanced]

A 60-year-old woman is admitted to the intensive care unit because of upper abdominal pain, fever, nausea, and vomiting of 6 hours' duration. She has no other pertinent medical history and takes no medications.

On physical examination, her temperature is 39.1°C (102.4°F), blood pressure is 70/30 mm Hg, and heart rate is 120/min. She has right upper quadrant tenderness without rebound.

Abdominal ultrasonography shows a gallstone obstructing the common bile duct that is extracted during emergency endoscopic retrograde cholangiopancreatography. Post-procedure, her systolic blood pressure remains below 90 mm Hg despite two intravenous boluses of 500 mL of normal saline. Ampicillin, gentamicin, and metronidazole are begun.

Which of the following is the most appropriate next step in management?

(A) Central venous catheter placement and aggressive fluid resuscitation
(B) Methylprednisolone, intravenously
(C) Pulmonary artery catheter placement
(D) Recombinant human activated protein C (drotrecogin α), intravenously

Item 8 [Advanced]

A 75-year-old woman is brought to the emergency department because of a 2-day history of generalized weakness and fever. The patient is a nursing home resident and requires a chronic indwelling urinary catheter.

On physical examination, temperature is 38.4°C (101.1°F), blood pressure is 132/72 mm Hg, pulse rate is 95/min, and respiration rate is 22/min. Examination findings are otherwise normal.

The leukocyte count is 13,000/μL (13 x 10^9/L) with 11% immature band forms. Urinalysis shows 20–25 leukocytes/hpf. A complete metabolic profile is normal. Arterial oxygen saturation is 95% by pulse oximetry with the patient breathing ambient air. Urine culture and two sets of blood cultures obtained in the emergency department are growing *Escherichia coli*.

Which of the following terms best describes this patient's illness?

(A) Sepsis
(B) Septic shock
(C) Severe sepsis
(D) Systemic inflammatory response syndrome

Item 9 [Advanced]

A 21-year-old man is evaluated for 5 days of sore throat, anterior neck pain and fever. Four days ago he was treated for streptoccocal pharyngitis with penicillin. Despite antibiotic therapy, his symptoms progressed and now he has difficulty swallowing and managing his secretions. Medical history is otherwise unremarkable and his only medication is oral penicillin.

On physical examination his temperature is 38.9°C (102°F), blood pressure is 140/86 mm Hg, pulse rate is 110/min and respiration rate is 20/min. He spits frequently and drools. His oral pharynx is notable for enlarged tonsils, right significantly greater than the left. The right tonsil enlargement crowds the uvula to the left. He has tender right cervical lymphadenopathy.

Which of the following is the most appropriate management?

(A) Add azithromycin
(B) Change to clindamycin
(C) Change to intramuscular penicillin
(D) Emergency ENT consultation

Item 10 [Basic]

A 32-year-old woman is evaluated for an upper respiratory infection. She was well until 5 days ago when she developed a fever, sore throat, nonproductive cough, and runny nose. She has no ear pain or nasal congestion. Her medical history is otherwise unremarkable. She has no allergies and takes no medications. She lives at home with her husband and 8-year-old twin boys.

On physical examination, her vital signs are normal. Her ears, nose, and oropharynx appear normal. She has no lymphadenopathy and her lungs are clear to auscultation.

Which of the following is the best prevention strategy for her family?

(A) Echinacea
(B) Frequent hand washing
(C) Penicillin G
(D) Surgical facemask
(E) Vitamin C

Item 11 [Basic]

A 45-year-old man is evaluated because of the acute onset of right ear pain. The patient was well until 10 days ago, when he developed symptoms of an upper respiratory tract infection, including nasal congestion and a nonproductive cough. Although these symptoms are resolving, pain and some loss of hearing in the right ear first occurred last night. He does not have fever, sore throat, or drainage from the ear. Medical history is unremarkable. The patient has no allergies and takes no medications.

On physical examination, vital signs, including temperature, are normal. The right tympanic membrane is erythematous, opacified, and immobile, but the external auditory canal is normal. The left ear and posterior pharynx are normal. Examination of the chest is unremarkable.

Which of the following is the best initial antibiotic choice in this patient?

(A) Amoxicillin
(B) Amoxicillin-clavulanate
(C) Azithromycin
(D) Ceftriaxone

Item 12 [Basic]

A 28-year-old woman has a 3-day history of a sore throat, malaise, and fatigue without cough or fever. Medical history is unremarkable. She has no known drug allergies and takes no medications.

On physical examination, vital signs, including temperature, are normal. Bilateral tonsillar exudates are present. There is no cervical lymphadenopathy.

Which of the following is the most appropriate next management step?

(A) Begin erythromycin
(B) Begin penicillin
(C) Obtain a rapid streptococcal antigen test
(D) Obtain a throat culture

Item 13 [Basic]

A 32-year-old man has a 5-day history of persistent nasal congestion and pain in the right forehead area associated with a clear nasal discharge and mild cough. The patient reports that he has had similar episodes in the past that were helped in 2 to 3 days by antibiotics. Medical history is otherwise unremarkable, and he currently takes no medications.

On physical examination, vital signs, including temperature, are normal. Mild right suborbital ridge tenderness is present. The nares are patent with a clear mucoid discharge. There is no pharyngeal erythema or exudate. The lungs are clear to auscultation.

Which of the following is the best initial management?

(A) Amoxicillin
(B) CT scan of the sinuses
(C) Plain films of sinuses
(D) Symptomatic treatment
(E) Trimethoprim-sulfamethoxazole

Item 14 [Basic]

A 25-year-old woman who is 28 weeks pregnant has asymptomatic bacteriuria detected during a routine prenatal visit. She has not had fever, urinary frequency, or dysuria and is not taking any medications other than prenatal vitamins. She has never had a urinary tract infection before and has no medical problems.

On physical examination, vital signs, including temperature, are normal. There is no costovertebral angle tenderness.

Which of the following is the most appropriate management?

(A) Ampicillin
(B) Ciprofloxacin
(C) Trimethoprim
(D) Observation

Item 15 [Advanced]

A 69-year-old man is evaluated in the emergency department for a 2-day history of fever, confusion, vomiting, dysuria, and lower abdominal and perineal pain. He has a history of chronic kidney disease, and his last serum creatinine level was 2.5 mg/dL (221 mmol/L).

On physical examination, temperature is 39.9°C (103.8°F), blood pressure is 88/50 mm Hg, heat rate is 130/min.

Examination shows poor skin turgor and dry mucous membranes. The abdomen is soft, but suprapubic tenderness is present. Rectal examination reveals an enlarged and tender prostate.

Leukocyte count is 22,000/μL (22×10^9/L) with 80% segmented neutrophils and 10% band forms. Blood urea nitrogen is 35 mg/dL (12.5 mmol/L) and creatinine is 3.8 mg/dL (336 mmol/L). Urinalysis shows 150 leukocytes per high-power field and many bacteria.

Intravenous fluids and parenteral ciprofloxacin are started. Urine culture grows *Proteus mirabilis* sensitive to fluoroquinolones. After 3 days, the patient continues to have fever, abdominal and perineal pain, and persistent leukocytosis.

Which of the following is the most appropriate management for this patient?

(A) Discontinue ciprofloxacin and start gentamicin
(B) Add gentamicin
(C) Insert a catheter for bladder drainage
(D) Obtain a transrectal ultrasound

Item 16 [Advanced]

A 77-year-old woman is evaluated during a routine physical examination. She is asymptomatic and has a history of hypertension, type 2 diabetes mellitus, and hyperlipidemia. Medications are aspirin, lisinopril, hydrochlorothiazide, a glyburide, and lovastatin. She has no allergies.

Her physical examination is unremarkable. Laboratory studies including serum creatinine, blood urea nitrogen, electrolytes, liver function tests, and a fasting lipid panel are normal. Her hemoglobin A_{1c} is 6.3%.

Urinalysis shows 15 leukocytes per high-power field and bacteria; no erythrocytes, protein, or glucose are noted. Urine culture grows *Escherichia coli* of at least 10^5 colony-forming units (cfu)/mL.

Repeat urinalysis and urine culture confirm these results.

Which of the following is the most appropriate next step in management of this patient?

(A) Ciprofloxacin for 3 days
(B) Ciprofloxacin for 7 days
(C) Trimethoprim-sulfamethoxazole for 3 days
(D) No treatment

Item 17 [Advanced]

A 32-year-old woman is evaluated for a 2-day history of fever, urinary frequency, left-sided flank pain, and nausea without vomiting. She also has diet-controlled type 2 diabetes mellitus.

On physical examination, temperature is 38.3°C (100.9°F), blood pressure is 122/82 mm Hg, pulse rate is 102/min, and respiration rate is 18/min. Left-sided costovertebral angle tenderness is present. Results of abdominal and pelvic examinations are normal.

Leukocyte count	14,000/μL (14×10^9/L)
Creatinine	1.1 mg/dL (97.2 μmol/L)
Urinalysis	Positive for leukocyte esterase and nitrites
Pregnancy test	Negative
Urine culture	Pending

Which of the following is the most appropriate treatment?

(A) Ampicillin
(B) Ciprofloxacin
(C) Nitrofurantoin
(D) Trimethoprim-sulfamethoxazole

Item 18 [Advanced]

An otherwise healthy 28-year-old woman has had two episodes of acute cystitis within the past 6 months. The patient is sexually active and has intercourse with her husband on average 2 times per week and says her cystitis does not seem to be intercourse related. Each time, symptoms remit after a single course of trimethoprim-sulfamethoxazole. The patient is currently asymptomatic but will be traveling abroad for the next 2 months and is concerned about recurrent infections. Her only medication is an oral contraceptive for birth control. She reports no allergies.

Which of the following is the most appropriate management?

(A) Ciprofloxacin after intercourse
(B) Ciprofloxacin for 10 days when symptoms develop
(C) Trimethoprim chronic suppressive therapy
(D) Trimethoprim-sulfamethoxazole for 3 days when symptoms develop

Item 19 [Basic]

A 24-year-old woman is evaluated during a new patient visit. She is not currently sexually active, but has been in the past; she has had two lifetime partners, and has always used condoms. She has no medical problems and takes no medications. She was last seen by a physician 3 years ago.

In addition to obtaining a Pap smear, screening for which of the following sexually transmitted diseases should be preformed?

(A) Chlamydia and gonorrhea
(B) Chlamydia, gonorrhea, and HIV
(C) Chlamydia, gonorrhea, and syphilis
(D) Chlamydia, gonorrhea, HIV, and syphilis
(E) HIV and syphilis

Item 20 [Basic]

A 34-year-old woman is evaluated for vaginal discharge and intermenstrual bleeding. She is gravida 4, para 2, with one spontaneous pregnancy loss and one termination. She had been living intermittently with the father of her children, though recently the two have been apart, and she is in the process of moving out of town. Her last menstrual period was 3 weeks ago. She takes no medications and has no allergies.

Vital signs are normal. On pelvic examination, a yellow-tinged cervical discharge is noted, and bleeding is easily induced when obtaining a culture from the os. Bimanual examination is unremarkable, with no adnexal or cervical motion tenderness.

Examination of the discharge under microscopy reveals no pseudohyphae or clue cells, and Gram stain is unremarkable. Pregnancy test is negative.

Which of the following conditions should receive empiric antibiotic treatment at this time?

(A) Bacterial vaginosis
(B) Chlamydia
(C) Gonorrhea and chlamydia
(D) Pelvic inflammatory disease (PID)

Item 21 [Basic]

An 18-year-old woman is evaluated in the emergency department for a 3-day history of fever and rash accompanied by joint pain and swelling that initially involved only the left elbow before progressing to the left wrist. Medical history is unremarkable. She takes a depot medroxyprogesterone acetate injection every 12 weeks for contraception.

On physical examination, temperature is 38.1°C (100.6°C); other vital signs are normal. The left wrist is erythematous and swollen, and pain is induced with active range of motion. The left elbow is also swollen and painful. Scattered lesions are present on the left hand and both feet. Skin examination findings of the left hand are shown (Plate 21).

Appropriate cultures are taken.

Which of the following is the most appropriate treatment?

(A) Acyclovir
(B) Ceftriaxone
(C) Ciprofloxacin
(D) Gentamicin

Item 22 [Basic]

An 18-year-old woman has a 3-day history of fever, headache, and painful sores in the genital area. The patient has no previous history of genital lesions. Medical history is unremarkable, and her only medication is an oral contraceptive agent. She does not use condoms.

On physical examination, temperature is 38.1°C (100.6°F); other vital signs are normal. There are no signs of meningismus. Tender ulcerative lesions with a yellow crusted roof cover the labia bilaterally and the vaginal introitus.

Which of the following is the most likely diagnosis?

(A) Chancroid
(B) Herpes simplex virus infection
(C) Primary syphilis
(D) Vulvovaginal candidiasis

Item 23 [Advanced]

An 18-year-old woman is evaluated in the emergency department because of a 3-day history of lower abdominal pain. She does not have urinary frequency, dysuria, flank pain, nausea, or vomiting. Her only medication is an oral contraceptive agent.

On physical examination, temperature is 38.3°C (101.0°F), blood pressure is 118/68 mm Hg, pulse rate is 104/min, and respiration rate is 16/min. Abdominal examination is normal. There is no flank tenderness. Pelvic examination shows cervical motion tenderness, fundal tenderness, and bilateral adnexal tenderness on bimanual examination.

The leukocyte count and urinalysis results are normal. Urine and serum pregnancy tests are negative.

Which of the following is the most appropriate treatment?

(A) Ampicillin and gentamicin, intravenously
(B) Azithromycin, orally
(C) Cefoxitin, intramuscularly
(D) Ceftriaxone, intramuscularly, and doxycycline, orally

Item 24 [Advanced]

A 38-year-old man is admitted to the hospital with a 1-week history of progressive dyspnea, cough, and low-grade fever. He has a history AIDS and has found it difficult to take all of his medications. His CD4 count measured 6 months ago was 80/μL. He has no allergies.

On examination, he appears dyspneic. Temperature is 39.2°C (102.5°F), blood pressure is 110/70 mm Hg, pulse rate is 110/min, and respiration rate is 32/min. Oxygen saturation by pulse oximetry is 82% on ambient air. Cardiopulmonary examination is normal.

Arterial blood gas results are: pH, 7.41; Po$_2$, 58 mm Hg (7.7 kPa); Pco$_2$, 32 mm Hg (4.3 kPa); HCO$_3$, 20 meq/L (22 mmol/L). Chest x-ray revealed bilateral interstitial infiltrates. A silver stain of induced sputum is positive for *Pneumocystis jirovecii*.

Which of the following is the best initial treatment regimen for this patient?

(A) Dapsone
(B) Dapsone plus corticosteroids
(C) Trimethoprim-sulfamethoxazole
(D) Trimethoprim-sulfamethoxazole plus corticosteroids

Item 25 [Advanced]

A 28-year-old woman is evaluated following the diagnosis of HIV infection discovered during a routine screening examination.

On examination, the patient appears well. Temperature is 37.1°C (98.8°F), blood pressure is 105/70 mm Hg; pulse rate is 88/min, and respiration rate is 10/min. The remainder of her examination is normal.

Her CD4 cell count is 77/μL and her HIV-1 RNA level is 200,000/mL. Her toxoplasma antibody is positive, and her tuberculin skin test is negative. All of her immunizations are up to date.

The patient agrees to begin antiretroviral drug therapy.

Which of the following treatments is also indicated at this time?

(A) Trimethoprim-sulfamethoxazole
(B) Trimethoprim-sulfamethoxazole plus azithromycin
(C) Trimethoprim-sulfamethoxazole plus fluconazole
(D) Trimethoprim-sulfamethoxazole plus isoniazid
(E) Trimethoprim-sulfamethoxazole plus valganciclovir

Item 26 [Advanced]

A 37-year-old man is evaluated for a 6-day history of a painful eruption on his left posterior thorax. He had an episode of shingles 1 year ago that was treated with famciclovir. He has a history of alcoholism and intermittent injection drug use. He has lost approximately 3.0 kg (6.6 lb) over the past 3 months. He has had increased fatigue but denies fever, chills, lymphadenopathy, jaundice, or change in his bowel habits. He takes no medications.

On physical examination, temperature is 37.0°C (98.6°F), and BMI is 28. The skin findings are shown (Plate 22).

Which of the following is the most likely underlying disease?

(A) Cirrhosis
(B) Diabetes mellitus
(C) Hepatitis B
(D) Hepatitis C
(E) HIV infection

Item 27 [Advanced]

A 28-year-old man is evaluated at a community health center for a 10-day history of sore throat, headache, fever, anorexia, and muscle aches. Two days ago, a rash developed on his trunk and abdomen. He had been previously healthy and has not had any contact with ill persons. He has had multiple male and female sexual partners and infrequently uses condoms. He has been tested for HIV infection several times, most recently 8 months ago; all results were negative.

On physical examination, temperature is 38.6°C (101.4°F). There are several small ulcers on the tongue and buccal mucosa and cervical and supraclavicular lymphadenopathy. A faint maculopapular rash is present on the trunk and abdomen.

A rapid plasma reagin test is ordered.

Which of the following diagnostic studies should also be done at this time?

(A) CD4 cell count measurement
(B) Epstein-Barr virus IgG measurement
(C) HIV RNA viral load and HIV antibody measurements
(D) Skin biopsy

Item 28 [Advanced]

A 38-year-old man is evaluated for a 3-week history of progressive right-sided weakness of the upper and lower extremities, difficulty with balance, and slurred speech. Medical history includes syphilis 12 years ago that was treated with benzathine penicillin G.

On physical examination, vital signs are normal. The Mini–Mental State Examination score is 22 (normal >24/30). Speech is dysarthric. There is right-sided hemiparesis with increased muscle tone on the right. Serologic testing for HIV antibodies is positive. CD4 cell count is 80/μL.

MRI of the brain reveals numerous ring-enhancing lesions in the basal ganglia and the corticomedullary junction, predominantly on the left side, with mass effect.

Which of the following is the most likely diagnosis?

(A) Cryptococcal meningitis
(B) *Mycobacterium avium* complex infection
(C) Progressive multifocal leukoencephalopathy
(D) Toxoplasmosis encephalitis

Item 29 [Basic]

A 69-year-old man is admitted to the cardiac intensive care unit with an exacerbation of heart failure.

Notable clinical findings include elevated central venous pressure, an S_3, pulmonary crackles, and pedal edema. Intravenous furosemide and lisinopril are initiated, and a urinary catheter is placed to measure urine output.

In addition to meticulous hand hygiene, which of the following measures is most effective in preventing a catheter-associated urinary tract infection?

(A) Antibiotic prophylaxis
(B) Changing the urinary catheter every 72 hours
(C) Minimizing manipulation and irrigation of the catheter
(D) Promptly discontinuing urinary catheter use
(E) Using silver impregnated urinary catheters

Item 30 [Advanced]

A 36-year-old woman is admitted to the intensive care unit from the emergency department after intentionally ingesting an overdose of a long-acting barbiturate. Endotracheal intubation was performed in the emergency department and the patient was placed on mechanical ventilation. Other than being minimally arousable and mechanically ventilated, the patient is stable.

Which of the following measures will reduce the risk of ventilator-associated pneumonia?

(A) Changing the endotracheal tube every 2 days
(B) Nasal placement of the endotracheal tube
(C) Prophylactic antibiotics
(D) Semi-erect (45°) positioning in bed

Item 31 [Advanced]

A 68-year-old man is diagnosed with *Clostridium difficile* infection 5 days after elective hip replacement surgery. This hospital has recently reported a high incidence of *C. difficile* infections. The patient was in a two-bed hospital room.

In addition to bleach for enhanced room cleaning, which of the following "bundled" measures would be most effective in preventing the spread of *C. difficile* in this hospital setting?

(A) Airborne precautions and alcohol hand sanitizer
(B) Airborne precautions and soap and water for hand hygiene
(C) Barrier precautions and alcohol hand sanitizer
(D) Barrier precautions and soap and water for hand hygiene
(E) Droplet precautions and soap and water for hand hygiene

Item 32 [Advanced]

A 19-year-old female college freshman is evaluated for possible meningitis. Cerebrospinal fluid analysis shows a leukocyte count of $13,259/\mu L$ ($13,259 \times 10^6/L$) with 85% neutrophils, a glucose concentration of 40 mg/dL (2.2 mmol/L) and a protein level of 230 mg/dL (2300 mg/L). Gram stain shows many neutrophils and gram-negative diplococci.

The patient is placed in a private room and intravenous antibiotics are initiated.

Which of the following is the most appropriate next step in infection-control management?

(A) Face mask
(B) High-filter mask
(C) Nonsterile gloves and gown
(D) Sterile gloves and gown

Item 33 [Basic]

A 65-year-old man recently immigrated to the United States from Africa. He is evaluated in the emergency department for a 3-week history of cough and dyspnea, now with hemoptysis. He has also had fevers, night sweats, and a 13.6-kg (30-lb) weight loss over the past 3 months.

On physical examination, he is thin and coughs frequently. Temperature is 38.3°C (101.0°F), blood pressure is 100/60 mm Hg, pulse rate is 101/min, and respiration rate is 30/min. Pulmonary examination reveals crackles over the right upper lung field.

Which of the following is the most important initial infection-control option in this setting?

(A) Chest radiograph
(B) Institution of airborne precautions
(C) Sputum for acid-fast bacilli stain and culture
(D) Tuberculin skin testing

Item 34 [Advanced]

A 45-year-old woman is evaluated because of a tuberculin skin test result of 11-mm induration discovered yesterday following a hospital pre-employment examination. She is otherwise healthy. Her HIV test result is negative. She relocated 3 months ago to the United States from El Salvador where she worked as a bank teller. She feels well and reports no fever, cough, or weight loss. She takes no medications.

On physical examination, the vital signs and cardiopulmonary examinations are normal.

Which of the following is the most appropriate next management step?

(A) Chest radiograph
(B) Four-drug antituberculous therapy
(C) Isoniazid therapy
(D) Clearance for employment

Item 35 [Advanced]

A 32-year-old healthy female physician is beginning a postgraduate fellowship at a university hospital and must undergo tuberculin skin testing. She grew up in Africa and completed medical school and residency training in London. She received the bacille Calmette-Guérin (BCG) vaccine at age 6 years.

Tuberculin skin testing indicates a 16-mm area of induration at the tuberculin skin testing site.

Physical examination is normal.

Which of the following is the most appropriate next step in the management of this patient?

(A) Chest radiograph
(B) Isoniazid, rifampin, pyrazinamide, and ethambutol
(C) Repeat tuberculin skin testing in 2 weeks
(D) No additional therapy or evaluation

Item 36 [Basic]

A 32-year-old man is evaluated in the office for a 2-month history of fever, night sweats, weight loss, and cough. He works as a pharmacy technician in an extended care facility for veterans.

On physical examination, he has a prominent cough and appears ill. Temperature is 38°C (100.4°F); other vital signs are normal. Fine crackles are auscultated over the right posterior thorax. The remainder of the physical examination is normal.

A chest radiograph shows a right upper lobe infiltrate with a small cavity. A stained sputum specimen is positive for acid-fast organisms; sputum culture results are pending. HIV testing is negative.

Which of the following is the most appropriate initial therapy for this patient?

(A) Isoniazid
(B) Isoniazid, pyrazinamide, and ethambutol
(C) Isoniazid, rifampin, pyrazinamide, and ethambutol
(D) No therapy until cultures confirm *Mycobacterium tuberculosis*

Item 37 [Advanced]

A 39-year-old woman is recently diagnosed with systemic lupus erythematosus after investigation of a fever, fatigue, arthralgia, a Coombs-positive hemolytic anemia, and leukopenia. She requires treatment with prednisone at an initial dosage of 1 mg/kg/day. She weighs 60 kg (132 lbs).

Hemoglobin is 7.5 g/dL (750 g/L) and leukocyte count is 1900/μL (1.9 x 10⁹/L). Chest radiograph is normal. Tuberculin skin testing reveals 8 mm of induration.

Which of the following is the most appropriate next step in this patient's management?

(A) Isoniazid for 9 months
(B) Isoniazid, pyrazinamide, rifampin, and ethambutol for 12 months
(C) Rifampin for 1 month
(D) No antituberculous therapy

Item 38 [Advanced]

A 35-year-old woman is evaluated in the office before the initiation of infliximab for rheumatoid arthritis. She was diagnosed with rheumatoid arthritis 5 years ago, and her disease is inadequately controlled on methotrexate and naproxen. She has no other complaints or medical problems and has no risk factors for tuberculosis. She has never been screened for tuberculosis.

Her physical examination is unremarkable except for changes compatible with active rheumatoid arthritis involving her hands and feet. A chest radiograph is normal. Forty-eight hours after administering the tuberculin skin test, there is 7 mm of induration at the injection site.

Initiation of which of the following is the most appropriate next step in this patient's treatment?

(A) Infliximab
(B) Isoniazid
(C) Isoniazid and infliximab
(D) Isoniazid, rifampin, pyrazinamide, and ethambutol

Item 39 [Advanced]

A 65-year-old man is evaluated during a routine examination. Medical history is significant for hypertension, asthma, and type 2 diabetes mellitus; three years ago, he was admitted to the hospital with respiratory failure and was treated for pneumonia. He received pneumococcal immunization upon his hospital discharge. He is a current smoker with a 50 pack-year history. His medications are lisinopril, metformin, aspirin, and an albuterol inhaler that he uses as needed. He has no allergies.

Vital signs are normal. The results of the physical examination are normal.

Which of the following pneumococcal immunization strategies is the most appropriate for this patient?

(A) Administer one dose of pneumococcal vaccine now
(B) Administer one dose of pneumococcal vaccine in 2 years
(C) Administer a dose of pneumococcal vaccine now and every 5 years thereafter
(D) No need for additional pneumococcal vaccination

Item 40 [Advanced]

A 35-year-old woman is evaluated in the emergency department in December because of fever, confusion, and shortness of breath. Three days ago, she became ill with fever, sore throat, myalgias, and cough. Her symptoms rapidly worsened. Her medical history is unremarkable. Influenza infection has been reported in the community.

On physical examination, temperature is 40.0°C (104.0°F), blood pressure is 82/48 mm Hg, heart rate is 130/min, respiration rate is 36/min, and pulse oximetry is 86% on ambient air. Pulmonary examination reveals bilateral diffuse crackles. The patient is intubated and receives mechanical ventilation and is admitted to the intensive care unit.

The leukocyte count is 2200/μL (2.2 × 10⁹/L) with 82% segmented neutrophils and 10% band forms. The chest radiograph shows multilobar pneumonia. Sputum and blood cultures are sent, and intravenous fluids are started.

Which of the following is the most appropriate empiric antibiotic therapy for this patient?

(A) Ceftriaxone and azithromycin
(B) Clindamycin
(C) Cefotaxime, levofloxacin, and vancomycin
(D) Piperacillin-tazobactam

Item 41 [Basic]

A 60-year-old woman is evaluated for the acute onset of fever, chills, nonproductive cough, diarrhea, and altered mental status. Medical history is significant for a 10-year history of type 2 diabetes mellitus controlled with diet and metformin therapy.

On physical examination, temperature is 39.4 °C (103.0 °F), blood pressure is 100/56 mm Hg, pulse rate is 100/min, and respiration rate is 32/min. Crackles are heard at the left lung base. On neurologic examination, the patient is oriented only to person.

Laboratory studies indicate a hematocrit of 34%, a leukocyte count of 18,000/μL (18 × 10⁹/L), a platelet count of 149,000/μL (149 × 10⁹/L), and a serum sodium concentration of 125 meq/L (125 mmol/L). Chest radiograph reveals an alveolar infiltrate in the left lower lobe and a small left pleural effusion.

Which of the following studies is most likely to be helpful in determining the cause of pneumonia in this patient?

(A) Acid-fast bacilli sputum smear
(B) Blood culture
(C) *Legionella* urinary antigen test
(D) Thoracentesis

Item 42 [Basic]

A 22-year-old woman is evaluated in September for the acute onset of fever, myalgia, arthralgia, and nonproductive cough. Medical history is noncontributory.

On physical examination, the patient is not ill-appearing. Temperature is 38.0°C (100.5°F), blood pressure is 114/62 mm Hg, pulse rate is 90/min, and respiration rate is 18/min. A few crackles are heard at the right lung base.

The leukocyte count is 12,000/μL (12 × 10⁹/L), and the remaining laboratory studies are normal. Chest radiograph reveals a right middle lobe infiltrate.

Which of the following oral antimicrobial agents should be initiated?

(A) Azithromycin
(B) Moxifloxacin
(C) Penicillin
(D) Zanamivir

Item 43 [Advanced]

A 45-year-old woman is evaluated for fever, diminished appetite, weight loss, and cough productive of foul-smelling sputum of 2 weeks' duration. She has a history of chronic alcoholism and frequent hospital admissions for alcohol-withdrawal seizures, with the most recent episode occurring 3 weeks ago.

On physical examination, temperature is 38.3 °C (101.0 °F), blood pressure is 130/84 mm Hg, pulse rate is 80/min, and respiration rate is 18/min. Her breath is foul smelling and dentition is poor. Pulmonary examination reveals crackles and rhonchi in the right anterior chest.

Laboratory studies indicate a leukocyte count of 12,500/μL (12.5 × 10⁹/L) with 8% band forms. The chest radiograph is shown.

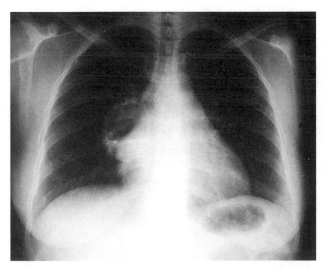

Sputum Gram stain results indicate gram-positive cocci in chains, gram-negative bacilli, and gram-positive bacilli.

Which of the following empiric antimicrobial regimens should be initiated?

(A) Ampicillin-sulbactam
(B) Aztreonam
(C) Ceftriaxone
(D) Levofloxacin
(E) Metronidazole

Item 44 [Advanced]

A 38-year-old man is scheduled to have a root canal. He has a history of a heart murmur. On physical examination, there is a normal S₁, an ejection sound, and a physiologically split S₂. There is a grade 2/6 midsystolic murmur heard best at the second right intercostal space that radiates to the right carotid artery. He has no other pertinent medical history.

A previous transthoracic echocardiogram demonstrated a bicuspid aortic valve with normal left ventricular function.

Which of the following is the most appropriate antibiotic prophylaxis for this patient before his dental procedure?

(A) Amoxicillin, orally
(B) Ampicillin, orally
(C) Clindamycin, orally
(D) Vancomycin, intravenously
(E) No antibiotic prophylaxis

Item 45 [Advanced]

A 56-year-old woman is scheduled to undergo a root canal procedure. Medical history is significant for mitral valve infective endocarditis treated 10 years ago. She has no other known medical problems. She is allergic to penicillin and developed hypotension and respiratory failure the last time she was given this antibiotic.

Which of the following is the most appropriate endocarditis prophylaxis for this patient?

(A) Amoxicillin, orally
(B) Ampicillin, intravenously
(C) Cefazolin, intravenously
(D) Clindamycin, orally
(E) No antibiotic prophylaxis

Item 46 [Basic]

A 26-year-old man is evaluated in the emergency department for the acute onset of a nonproductive cough and right-sided pleuritic chest pain of 2 days' duration. The patient is an injection drug user, with his last use approximately 4 days ago. Results of his most recent HIV test 2 months ago were negative. The remainder of the medical history is noncontributory, and he takes no medications.

On physical examination, temperature is 39.4°C (103.0 °F), blood pressure is 120/80 mm Hg, pulse rate is 100/min, and respiration rate is 20/min. Cardiopulmonary examination reveals clear lungs and a grade 3/6 holosystolic murmur heard best at the right sternal border that increases on inspiration.

Laboratory studies indicate a hematocrit of 39%, a leukocyte count of 17,000/μL (17 × 10⁹/L) with 15% band forms, and a platelet count of 160,000/μL (160 × 10⁹/L). Chest radiograph reveals small infiltrates in the left upper lobe, right upper lobe, and right lower lobe. Blood cultures are obtained.

Which of the following empiric antimicrobial regimens should be initiated?

(A) Azithromycin plus ceftriaxone
(B) Levofloxacin plus clindamycin
(C) Piperacillin/tazobactam plus aztreonam
(D) Trimethoprim-sulfamethoxazole plus prednisone
(E) Vancomycin plus cefepime

Item 47 [Basic]

A 54-year-old man is evaluated because of fatigue, backache, and intermittent fever of 3 months' duration. He has no history of cardiac disease or drug allergies.

On physical examination, there are no abnormalities of his skin. Ophthalmologic examination reveals a right conjunctival hemorrhage. Funduscopic examination is normal. The lungs are clear. Cardiac examination discloses a new murmur of aortic insufficiency. The remainder of the examination is normal.

A transthoracic echocardiogram shows a thickened bicuspid aortic valve, with evidence of mild aortic insufficiency. A transesophageal echocardiogram confirms these findings and also shows an oscillating mass on the aortic valve. Four sets of blood cultures grow a microorganism of the viridans streptococci group that is sensitive to penicillin.

Which of the following is the most appropriate initial antibiotic therapy for this patient?

(A) Penicillin G
(B) Vancomycin
(C) Vancomycin plus ceftriaxone
(D) Vancomycin plus gentamicin

Item 48 [Basic]

A 29-year-old woman is hospitalized because of a 4-day history of fever, chills, myalgia, and a nonproductive cough. The patient has a 10-year history of heroin use. Medical history is otherwise unremarkable, including no allergies.

Temperature is 39.0°C (102.0°F); other vital signs are normal. Cardiac examination discloses an early grade 2/6 systolic murmur at the base. The remainder of the examination is normal.

An electrocardiogram is normal, and a transthoracic echocardiogram shows changes compatible with a tricuspid valve vegetation.

After blood culture specimens are obtained, vancomycin, 1 g intravenously every 12 hours, is begun. Within 48 hours, all the initial blood cultures are growing *Staphylococcus aureus* that is susceptible to oxacillin, the cephalosporins, tetracycline, clindamycin, and the fluoroquinolones and is resistant to penicillin G, ampicillin, and erythromycin.

Which of the following is most appropriate at this time?

(A) Continue vancomycin
(B) Switch to clindamycin
(C) Switch to linezolid
(D) Switch to oxacillin

Item 49 [Advanced]

A 75-year-old man with type 2 diabetes mellitus is evaluated in the emergency department for a draining chronic ulcer on the left foot, erythema, and fever. Drainage initially began 3 weeks ago. Current medications include metformin and glyburide.

On physical examination, he does not appear ill. Temperature is 37.9°C (100.2°F); other vital signs are normal. The left foot is slightly warm and erythematous. A plantar ulcer that is draining purulent material is present over the fourth metatarsal joint. A metal probe makes contact with bone. The remainder of the examination is normal.

The leukocyte count is normal, and an erythrocyte sedimentation rate is 70 mm/h. A plain radiograph of the foot is normal.

Gram stain of the purulent drainage at the ulcer base shows numerous leukocytes, gram-positive cocci in clusters, and gram-negative rods.

Which of the following is the most appropriate management now?

(A) Begin imipenem
(B) Begin vancomycin and ceftazidime
(C) Begin vancomycin and metronidazole
(D) Perform bone biopsy

Item 50 [Advanced]

A 75-year-old man has a 2-month history of gradually increasing severe low back pain that is not related to trauma. The patient often feels warm and diaphoretic. He has no urine or stool incontinence. Ten weeks ago, he was discharged from the hospital after a prolonged intensive care unit stay for the treatment of community-acquired pneumonia–associated sepsis. During his stay, he required mechanical ventilation, enteral nutrition, and prolonged central venous access.

On physical examination, temperature is 38.1°C (100.5°F); other vital signs are normal. There is mild tenderness to palpation over the lower back with no definitive point of maximum tenderness. Neurologic examination is normal.

Complete blood count and urinalysis are normal. Erythrocyte sedimentation rate is 90 mm/h. Blood cultures are drawn.

Which of the following is the optimal diagnostic test?

(A) CT scan of the lumbar spine
(B) MRI of the lumbar spine
(C) Plain radiograph of the lumbar spine
(D) Three-phase bone scintigraphy

Item 51 [Advanced]

A 64-year-old woman is hospitalized because of a nonpainful draining ulcer on the plantar aspect of the left foot. She has a 10-year history of type 2 diabetes mellitus. The ulcer is chronic and nonhealing but over the past 3 days has begun draining foul-smelling material. Yesterday, the patient developed fever, and the area around the ulcer became erythematous. Medications include metformin and pioglitazone.

On physical examination, she does not appear ill. Temperature is 38.3°C (101.0°F); other vital signs are normal. A 3-cm by 2-cm deep plantar ulcer that is draining a purulent green exudate is present at the base of the fourth metatarsal. The entire foot is warm, erythematous, and edematous. Pulses in the foot are palpable. No bone is visible or detected with a metal probe. A plain radiograph of the foot shows only soft tissue swelling.

Which of the following imaging studies of the foot should be performed next?

(A) CT scan
(B) Indium-labeled leukocyte scan
(C) MRI
(D) Triple-phase technetium bone scan

Item 52 [Advanced]

A 65-year-old man is evaluated in the emergency department for a 3-day history of gradually worsening low back pain and fever.

On physical examination, temperature is 38.0°C (100.4°F); other vital signs are normal. General examination, including neurologic examination, is normal. MRI of the spine shows enhancement of the L3-L4 end plates and inflammation of the disk space. No epidural enhancement or paravertebral collections are seen. The patient is hospitalized.

Which of the following is the most appropriate next management step?

(A) Begin ceftriaxone
(B) Begin nafcillin
(C) Obtain blood cultures
(D) Obtain bone biopsy

Section 6

Infectious Disease Medicine
Answers and Critiques

Item 1　　**Answer: D**
Educational Objective: *Diagnose Rocky Mountain spotted fever.*

This patient most likely has Rocky Mountain spotted fever (RMSF). He presents with a flu-like illness during the summer. Because of the nonspecific nature of its symptoms, RMSF should be strongly considered in patients such as this one with a nonspecific febrile illness within 3 weeks of potential tick exposure, and immediate treatment with doxycycline should be given pending results of diagnostic studies. Many people with tick-borne infection do not recall a specific tick bite. Up to 90% of patients eventually develop the characteristic blanching erythematous macules located around the wrists and ankles that spread centripetally. The most commonly available diagnostic test for RMSF is a convalescent serology.

Babesiosis is caused by *Babesia microti*, an intracellular protozoan parasite. Babesiosis is transmitted to humans by ticks and occurs primarily in the northeastern United States with an epicenter in Cape Cod, Massachusetts, and the associated islands. Most infections are subclinical, but a nonspecific febrile illness can occur. Babesiosis should be considered in patients who have traveled to endemic areas and now have a nonfocal febrile illness with chills, sweats, myalgia, arthralgia, nausea, vomiting, or fatigue. On physical examination, fever, splenomegaly, hepatomegaly, and jaundice may be present.

Although this patient's presentation is compatible with influenza, this disease does not generally occur in temperate regions of the world during the summer.

Most early localized Lyme disease occurs in the summer and fall and is characterized by the erythema migrans rash, an expanding erythematous patch appearing 5 to 14 days after inoculation by an infected tick. Early Lyme disease is usually diagnosed clinically because serologic test results are often negative at presentation.

> **KEY POINT**
>
> **Rocky Mountain spotted fever should be strongly considered in patients with a nonspecific febrile illness within 3 weeks of potential tick exposure and blanching erythematous macules located around the wrists and ankles.**

Bibliography

Sexton DJ, Kaye KS. Rocky Mountain spotted fever. Med Clin North Am. 2002;86(2):351-60, vii-viii. [PMID: 11982306]

Item 2　　**Answer: A**
Educational Objective: *Diagnose factitious fever.*

This patient most likely has factitious fever. Factitious fever was the diagnosis in 9% of a National Institute of Health cohort of 343 referrals for evaluation of fever of unknown origin (a highly selected population). Factitious fever usually is diagnosed in young women, generally shows unusual fever patterns such as very high or brief spikes and rapid defervescence without chills, and diaphoresis. A fever diary will typically demonstrate a lack of normal diurnal temperature variation. Like this patient, physical and laboratory findings of infection or inflammation are lacking during the febrile illness.

Familial Mediterranean fever is an autosomal recessive disorder prevalent in people of Jewish, Turkish, Arabic, and Armenian heritage. Most patients have the onset of illness before age 10 years, 95% before the age of 20 years. The key feature is short periods of fever (1-3 days) associated with serositis; 90% of patients have abdominal pain, and pleuritis and synovitis are also common. Episodes of fever are accompanied by elevated markers of inflammation such as leukocytosis and erythrocyte sedimentation rate.

Endocarditis should be suspected if an abnormal murmur is heard on examination, particularly in patients with a compelling history or concurrent fever. Endocarditis is unlikely in this patient with normal physical findings and negative blood cultures.

Approximately 80% of patients with systemic lupus erythematosus (SLE) have cutaneous involvement at some point in their disease course. Most rashes associated with SLE occur in areas exposed to the sun. More than 90% of patients with SLE develop joint involvement that can manifest as arthralgia or true arthritis. Joint pain is often migratory and can be oligoarticular or polyarticular, or asymmetric or symmetric. More than 99% of untreated patients with SLE have high titers of antinuclear antibodies; a negative antinuclear antibody test effectively rules out the diagnosis of SLE.

> **KEY POINT**
>
> **Factitious fever usually is diagnosed in young women; generally shows unusual fever patterns such as very high or brief spikes, absent diurnal variation, and rapid defervescence without chills; and diaphoresis.**

Bibliography

Cunha BA. Fever of unknown origin: focused diagnostic approach based on clinical clues from the history, physical examination, and laboratory tests. Infect Dis Clin North Am. 2007;21(4):1137-87, xi. [PMID: 18061092]

Item 3   Answer: A
Educational Objective: *Diagnose malignant hyperthermia.*

This patient most likely has malignant hyperthermia, which is an inherited skeletal muscle disorder characterized by a hypermetabolic state precipitated by exposure to volatile inhalational anesthetics (halothane, isoflurane, enflurane, desflurane, sevoflurane) and the depolarizing muscle relaxants succinylcholine and decamethonium. It usually occurs on exposure to the drug but can occur several hours after the initial exposure and can develop in patients who were previously exposed to the drug without effect. Increased intracellular calcium leads to sustained muscle contractions, with skeletal muscle rigidity and masseter muscle spasm, tachycardia, hypercarbia, hypertension, hyperthermia, tachypnea, and cardiac arrhythmias. Rhabdomyolysis (elevated creatine kinase) and acute renal failure can develop. Malignant hyperthermia should be suspected in patients with a family history of problems during anesthesia.

The neuroleptic malignant syndrome is a life-threatening disorder caused by an idiosyncratic reaction to neuroleptic tranquilizers (dopamine D_2-receptor antagonists) and some antipsychotic drugs. The most common offending neuroleptic agents are haloperidol and fluphenazine. The syndrome occurs with all drugs that cause central dopamine receptor blockade, usually soon after starting a new drug or with dose escalation. It has been reported in patients with Parkinson disease who abruptly discontinue levodopa or anticholinergic therapy. Most patients with the syndrome develop muscle rigidity, hyperthermia, cognitive changes, autonomic instability, diaphoresis, sialorrhea, seizures, arrhythmias, and rhabdomyolysis within 2 weeks after initiating the drug. Because this patient did not receive a neuroleptic agent, neuroleptic malignant syndrome is unlikely.

Like the neuroleptic malignant syndrome, the serotonin syndrome presents with high fever, muscle rigidity, and cognitive changes. Findings unique to the serotonin syndrome are shivering, hyperreflexia, myoclonus, and ataxia. The serotonin syndrome is caused by the use of selective serotonin reuptake inhibitors, a category of drug that this patient has not been exposed to.

Thyroid storm is a potential cause of hyperthermia in hospitalized patients, but thyroid storm does not cause muscle rigidity or elevations of the creatine kinase level and is unlikely in a patient receiving adequate treatment for hyperthyroidism.

KEY POINT

Malignant hyperthermia is an inherited skeletal muscle disorder characterized by a hypermetabolic state precipitated by exposure to volatile inhalational anesthetics and depolarizing muscle relaxants.

Bibliography
Chamorro C, Romera MA, Balandin B. Fever in critically ill patients. Crit Care Med. 2008;36(11):3129-3130. [PMID: 18941337]

Item 4   Answer: D
Educational Objective: *Treat sepsis with infection source identification and control.*

In septic patients with identifiable or potential sources of infection, source control, including the removal of sources of infection such as indwelling catheters, drainage of abscesses, and surgical debridement of wounds should be done promptly upon diagnosis. In this patient with evidence of tissue destruction and infection with gas-forming organisms, early surgical debridement is an urgent necessity.

Therapy with drotrecogin alfa (activated protein C) is not indicated, because the patient does not meet the high-risk mortality threshold determined by a severity-of-illness scoring system such as APACHE (Acute Physiology and Chronic Health Evaluation) II with a score of greater than 25 or the presence of septic shock requiring vasopressors, sepsis-induced acute respiratory distress syndrome (ARDS) requiring mechanical ventilation, or two or more sepsis-induced organ dysfunctions. Drotrecogin alfa has not been shown to directly neutralize inflammatory mediators.

Low-dose dopamine is not indicated. A randomized controlled trial showed no benefit from "renal doses" of dopamine on renal or other clinical outcomes in early renal dysfunction. In sepsis, vasopressors can be added as part of early goal-directed therapy if a fluid challenge fails to achieve a mean arterial pressure (diastolic pressure plus one-third the pulse pressure) greater than 65 mm Hg despite adequate fluid resuscitation. In this patient, vasopressors may be considered after a fluid challenge of at least 4 to 6 liters but is premature at this time.

KEY POINT

In septic patients with identified sources of infection, efforts should be made to remove the source as early as possible

Bibliography
Jimenez MF, Marshall JC; International Sepsis Forum. Source control in the management of sepsis. Intensive Care Med. 2001;27(suppl 1):S49-62. [PMID: 11307370]

Item 5   Answer: A
Educational Objective: *Treat severe sepsis with aggressive fluid resuscitation.*

The additional intervention that is most likely to improve survival in this patient is aggressive fluid resuscitation. The patient has severe urosepsis. Aggressive fluid resuscitation with resolution of lactic acidosis within 6 hours will have a beneficial effect on this patient's survival. Fluid resuscitation should target central venous oxygen saturation (S_{CVO_2}) or mixed venous oxygen saturation (S_{VO_2}) of at least 70%. Other reasonable goals include a central venous pressure of 8 to 12 mm Hg, a mean arterial pressure of at least 65 mm Hg, and a urine output of at least 0.5 mL/kg/h. This often translates into administration of 5 to 6 L of fluid over 6 hours. Timing of resuscitation matters to survival. Early goal-directed therapy that includes interventions within the first 6 hours to maintain a Scvo$_2$ of greater than 70% and to resolve lactic acidosis results in higher survival rates than more delayed resuscitation attempts.

Blood transfusion may be part of resuscitation for anemic patients in shock, but maintaining hemoglobin levels above 12 g/dL (120 g/L) is not supported by evidence. In stable patients who are not in shock, a transfusion threshold of 7 g/dL (70 g/L) is an acceptable conservative approach. There are no data to support that maintaining a lower Pco$_2$ or using a pulmonary artery catheter would help to increase survival in this patient.

KEY POINT

In patients with severe sepsis, aggressive fluid resuscitation with resolution of lactic acidosis within 6 hours has a beneficial effect on survival.

Bibliography
Rivers E, Nguyen B, Havstad S, et al; Early Goal-Directed Therapy Collaborative Group. Early goal-directed therapy in the treatment of severe sepsis and septic shock. N Engl J Med. 2001;345(19):1368-1377. [PMID: 11794169]

Item 6   Answer: A
Educational Objective: *Treat a patient with severe sepsis with activated protein C.*

The administration of activated protein C is the most appropriate next step. Activated protein C (drotrecogin alfa activated) is a time-sensitive intervention that can improve survival in patients with severe sepsis at high risk of death. Improved survival has been demonstrated in patients with severe sepsis who have an APACHE score of 25 or greater. Patients with either a single failing organ system or an APACHE score less than 25 do not appear to benefit and are at risk of bleeding complications. Although activated protein C is an anticoagulant, when administered to patients with a platelet count between 30,000/μL (30 × 10^9/L) and 50,000/μL (50 × 10^9/L), there was a relative risk reduction in mortality of more than 30%. Platelet counts below 30,000/μL (30 × 10^9/L) are considered a relative contraindication. The patient is more than 12 hours out of surgery, with no ongoing active bleeding, a platelet count of 42,000/μL (42 × 10^9/L), and a high risk of death; therefore, activated protein C is an excellent consideration.

The goals of fluid resuscitation are a central venous pressure of 8 to 12 mm Hg, mean arterial pressure greater than 65 mm Hg, urine output greater than 0.5 mL/kg/h, and central venous oxygen saturation greater than 70%. Randomized controlled trials have shown no benefit to the use of colloid compared with crystalloid fluids.

Hyperglycemia is associated with poor clinical outcomes in critically ill patients. However, the benefit of tight glycemic control (≤110 mg/dL [6.1 mmol/L]) is controversial in critically ill postsurgical patients, and no benefit has been shown in critically ill medical patients.

Vasopressors are part of early goal-directed therapy if the mean arterial pressure is less than 65 mm Hg after initial adequate fluid resuscitation. The most commonly used vasopressor for septic shock is norepinephrine, a potent peripheral vasoconstrictor that reverses the endotoxin-induced vasodilation that is the hallmark of septic shock. Dopamine is also acceptable but is associated with more tachycardia and arrhythmia. Low-dose dopamine, however, is not indicated. A randomized controlled trial showed that there is no benefit from low-dose dopamine on renal or other clinical outcomes in early renal dysfunction.

KEY POINT

Activated protein C has been shown to improve survival in patients with severe sepsis with an APACHE score of 25 or greater.

Bibliography
Toussaint S, Gerlach H. Activated protein C for sepsis. N Engl J Med. 2009;361(27):2646-52. [PMID: 20042756]

Item 7   Answer: A
Educational Objective: *Treat sepsis with fluid resuscitation.*

The placement of a central venous line and aggressive fluid resuscitation will have the greatest impact on improving this patient's chances of survival. Sepsis is known to result in tissue hypoperfusion. Most patients need at least 4 to 6 L of intravascular volume replacement within the first 6 hours, and one of the biggest pitfalls of management is underestimating the intravascular volume deficit. Vasopressor therapy with norepinephrine, vasopressin, or dopamine may be necessary when appropriate fluid challenge fails to restore adequate tissue perfusion or during life-threatening hypotension, but no trials have established a single superior approach to handling initial vasopressor choice.

Replacement-dose hydrocortisone is no longer recommended routinely for patients with septic shock who achieve a systolic blood pressure of at least 90 mm Hg with fluids and vasopressors, although corticosteroids may be useful for patients with more profound, refractory shock.

Placement of a pulmonary artery catheter in a patient with clinical evidence of sepsis and hypoperfusion has not been shown to improve outcomes.

Drotrecogin alfa (activated protein C) is approved by the U.S. Food and Drug Administration and international regulatory authorities for patients with severe sepsis who are at high risk for death. Drotrecogin alfa therapy increases bleeding risk at rates similar to those of heparin. Serious bleeding increases by 1.5% to 2.5% above that expected with placebo, and intracerebral hemorrhage occurs in 0.6% of treated patients. Drotrecogin alfa is contraindicated in the presence of active bleeding, concurrent therapy with other anticoagulant drugs, and platelet counts less than 30,000/μL (30×10^9/L), and in patients with risks of uncontrollable or central nervous system bleeding. Drotrecogin alfa therapy should be considered in patients with all of the following criteria: septic shock requiring vasopressors despite fluid resuscitation, sepsis-induced acute respiratory distress syndrome (ARDS) requiring mechanical ventilation; and any two sepsis-induced dysfunctional organs. This patient does not meet the criteria for treatment with activated protein C.

KEY POINT

Most patients with sepsis need at least 4 to 6 L of intravascular volume replacement within the first 6 hours.

Bibliography

Rivers E, Nguyen B, Havstad S, Ressler J, Muzzin A, Knoblich B, et al. Early goal-directed therapy in the treatment of severe sepsis and septic shock. N Engl J Med. 2001;345:1368-77. [PMID: 11794169]

Item 8   Answer: A
Educational Objective: *Diagnose sepsis.*

The term that best describes this patient's illness is sepsis. The diagnostic criteria for sepsis include either a culture-proven infection or visual identification of an infection (for example, a wound with purulent drainage) and at least two criteria fulfilling the definition of a systemic response to infection (fever, tachycardia, tachypnea, and an elevated leukocyte count with immature band forms). She does not have organ dysfunction or perfusion abnormalities (hypotension and lactic acidosis), which occur in patients with severe sepsis or septic shock. Therefore, the term that best defines her illness is sepsis.

Definitions of systemic inflammatory response syndrome, sepsis, severe sepsis, septic shock, and multiple organ dysfunction syndrome are as follows:

Systemic inflammatory response syndrome (SIRS): The systemic inflammatory response to a wide variety of severe clinical insults, manifested by at least two of the following conditions: temperature greater than 38.0°C (100.4°F) or less than 36.0°C (96.8°F), heart rate greater than 90/min, respiration rate greater than 20/min or arterial blood P_{CO_2} less than 32 mm Hg (4.3 kPa), leukocyte count greater than 12,000/μL (12×10^9/L) or less than 4000/μL (4×10^9/L) or with greater than 10% immature band forms.

Sepsis: The systemic inflammatory response to a documented infection. In association with infection, manifestations of sepsis are the same as those described for SIRS.

Severe sepsis: Sepsis associated with organ dysfunction, hypoperfusion, or hypotension.

Septic shock: A subset of severe sepsis, defined as sepsis-induced hypotension despite adequate fluid resuscitation plus the presence of perfusion abnormalities. Patients receiving inotropic or vasopressor agents may no longer be hypotensive by the time they develop hypoperfusion abnormalities or

organ dysfunction; however, they would still be considered to have septic shock.

KEY POINT

The diagnostic criteria for sepsis include a culture-proven infection or visual identification of an infection and evidence of a systemic response to infection (fever, tachycardia, tachypnea, and an elevated leukocyte count with immature band forms).

Bibliography

Levy MM, Fink MP, Marshall JC, Abraham E, Angus D, Cook D, Cohen J, Opal SM, Vincent JL, Ramsay G; SCCM/ESICM/ACCP/ATS/SIS. 2001 SCCM/ESICM/ACCP/ATS/SIS International Sepsis Definitions Conference. Crit Care Med. 2003;31(4):1250-6. [PMID: 12682500]

Item 9   Answer: D
Educational Objective: *Diagnose and treat peritonsillar abscess.*

The most appropriate management for this patient is emergent ENT consultation. The patient is not responding to antibiotics. He most likely has a peritonsillar abscess. Complications of untreated group A β-hemolytic streptococcal (GABHS) infection include peritonsillar abscess ("quinsy"), poststreptococcal glomerulonephritis, and rheumatic fever. About half of patients with peritonsillar abscess present first with this complication rather than with pharyngitis. Among those who present first with sore throat and then develop peritonsillar abscess, only one quarter have GABHS pharyngitis. Patients who present first with sore throat, such as this patient, are distinguished by worsening sore throat despite antibiotic therapy, fever dysphagia, pooling of saliva, possible drooling, and muffled voice. On physical examination, the patient is ill-appearing and often has enlarged tonsils with deviation of the uvula to the unaffected side. The more serous complications include airway obstruction, dissection of the infection to the parapharyngeal space, spontaneous abscess drainage and aspiration of pus (usually while sleeping) and sepsis. Treatment consists of needle drainage or surgical incision and drainage of the abscess.

Antibiotic selection is informed by culture results. However, cultures are not frequently obtained in this setting and are difficult to interpret because of the presence of mouth flora. Penicillin alone, by any route, is unlikely to be successful due to the emergence of penicillin-resistant oral anaerobes associated with this infection. Recommended treatment is ampicillin-sulbactam or the combination of parenteral penicillin G and metronidazole. Surgical drainage may be necessary. Clindamycin is reserved for penicillin allergic patients. Azithromycin does not provide anaerobic coverage and is therefore not indicated in this infection.

KEY POINT

A serious complication of untreated group A β-hemolytic streptococcal (GABHS) infection is peritonsillar abscess.

Bibliography

Steyer TE. Peritonsillar abscess: diagnosis and treatment. Am Fam Physician. 2002;65(1):93-6. Erratum in: Am Fam Physician 2002;66(1):30. [PMID: 11804446]

Item 10   Answer: B
Educational Objective: *Prevent upper respiratory tract infection with hand washing.*

Handwashing with soap and water has proven efficacy in removing viruses from the hands and helps prevent the spread of infections. Contact with secretions is probably the principle mode of upper respiratory viral infection transmission. A meta-analysis of 30 studies assessing hand hygiene showed a reduction in respiratory illness of 21%.

Although commonly used to prevent upper respiratory tract infections, prevention studies using echinacea have failed to show consistent benefit and it cannot be recommended. Antibiotics, such as penicillin G, are ineffective in the treatment or prevention of viral diseases. In addition, the inappropriate use of antibiotics increases the risk of bacterial resistance and exposes the patient to unnecessary risks, such as allergic reactions, and complications, such as vaginal yeast infection and gastrointestinal upset, including the possibility of *Clostridium difficile* infection. Commonly used in Asia to prevent respiratory infections, the benefit of face masks is undocumented. In one trial in Japan, use of surgical face masks did not result in a lower incidence of upper respiratory tract infections but was associated with a greater incidence of headache. Prevention studies using vitamin C have failed to show consistent benefit in the general community; however, a subgroup of studies that included persons exposed to significant cold or physical stress showed a reduction in the incidence and duration of colds. Multivitamin and multimineral supplementation are commonly used in men and women aged 65 years or older; however, prevention studies using daily multivitamin and multimineral supplementation in this population have failed to show consistent benefit on the incidence of upper respiratory tract infections.

KEY POINT
Handwashing with soap and water has proven efficacy in removing viruses from the hands and helps prevent the spread of infections.

Bibliography
Pratter MR. Cough and the common cold: ACCP evidence-based clinical practice guidelines. Chest. 2006;129(1 suppl):72S-74S. [PMID: 16428695]

Item 11   Answer: A
Educational Objective: *Treat otitis media with amoxicillin.*

The best initial antibiotic for this patient is amoxicillin. Although otitis media is the most frequent bacterial infection in children, it is much less common in adults. In most cases of acute otitis media, a viral upper respiratory tract infection precedes the ear infection. Eustachian tube obstruction occurs secondary to inflammation. Bacteria subsequently enter the middle ear by means of a compliant eustachian tube, aided by other factors, including nose blowing, sniffing, and negative middle ear pressure. The microbiology of otitis media in adults is similar to that of children: *Streptococcus pneumoniae*, 21% to 63%; *Haemophilus influenzae*, 11% to 26%; *Staphylococcus aureus*, 3% to 12%; and *Moraxella catarrhalis*, 3%. Thirty percent of bacterial cultures of the middle ear show no growth.

Antibiotic therapy should be reserved for patients in whom evidence of purulent otitis exists. Guidelines for antibiotic use are the same in children and adults. Amoxicillin is the recommended initial antibiotic because of its proven efficacy, safety, relatively low cost, and narrow spectrum of activity. If symptoms do not improve after 48 to 72 hours of amoxicillin therapy, initiation of amoxicillin-clavulanate, cefuroxime, or ceftriaxone is recommended. Alternative agents for patients with penicillin allergy are oral macrolides (azithromycin, clarithromycin). Follow-up of these patients is not necessary unless symptoms persist or progress.

KEY POINT
Amoxicillin is the recommended antibiotic for treating acute otitis media in adults because of its proven efficacy, safety, relatively low cost, and narrow spectrum of activity.

Bibliography
Ramakrishnan K, Sparks RA, Berryhill WE. Diagnosis and treatment of otitis media [erratum in Am Fam Physician. 2008;78(1):30]. Am Fam Physician. 2007;76(11):1650-1658. [PMID: 18092706]

Item 12   Answer: C
Educational Objective: *Manage acute pharyngitis using the Centor criteria.*

The best management step is rapid streptococcal antigen testing. Managing patients with pharyngitis includes estimating the probability of the presence of group A β-hemolytic streptococcal (GABHS) infection. The four-point Centor criteria (fever, tonsillar exudates, tender anterior cervical lymphadenopathy, and absence of cough) are often used as a prediction rule in patients with suspected GABHS infection. Patients with two Centor criteria, such as the patient described here, have an intermediate probability for GABHS infection, and rapid streptococcal antigen testing (sensitivity of 88% and specificity of 94%) is a reasonable strategy for these patients. Patients with 0 or 1 criterion have a low (<3%) probability of GABHS, and neither testing nor antibiotic treatment is recommended. Empiric antibiotic therapy is recommended for patients who meet all four Centor criteria because the probability of GABHS is 40% or greater. Opinion differs regarding the management of patients with three criteria, and either empiric antibiotic treatment or testing and then treating only if test results are positive is acceptable. Patients with Centor scores of 3 or 4 who have negative rapid antigen testing should then undergo throat cultures to guide treatment decisions. An initial throat culture rather than a rapid antigen test would be unnecessarily expensive.

Antibiotics are not indicated for this patient before rapid streptococcal antigen testing is done to determine whether they are needed. If treatment is indicated, the antibiotic of choice is penicillin. Macrolide antibiotics and first- and second-generation cephalosporins are alternative choices for penicillin-allergic patients.

KEY POINT

Rapid streptococcal antigen testing is a reasonable strategy for patients with pharyngitis who have two of the four Centor criteria (fever, tonsillar exudates, tender anterior cervical lymphadenopathy, and absence of cough).

Bibliography
Wessels MR. Clinical practice. Streptococcal pharyngitis. N Engl J Med. 2011;364(7):648-55. [PMID: 21323542]

Item 13   Answer: D
Educational Objective: *Treat acute sinusitis with symptomatic measures.*

Symptomatic management is best for this patient. He most likely has acute sinusitis. Most cases of acute sinusitis are caused by a virus; only 0.5% to 2% are caused by bacteria. Signs and symptoms are not reliable for diagnostic purposes. A meta-analysis found that no symptoms or signs, including unilateral facial pain, pain in the teeth, pain on bending, or purulent nasal discharge, were precise enough to establish the diagnosis. In most patients, symptoms last up to 2 weeks and resolve without additional diagnostic studies or administration of antibiotics.

Antibiotics are not indicated for this patient. Even though most patients with suspected acute sinusitis do receive antibiotics, there is little evidence to support the effectiveness of this practice. A randomized trial found that the duration of symptoms did not differ between patients who did and did not receive antibiotics. A meta-analysis found that although patients with more severe symptoms had a longer period of illness, antibiotics did not decrease symptom severity or duration of infection. However, some guidelines still recommend administration of antibiotics. If these agents are used, they should be limited to patients with at least two of the following findings: symptoms lasting longer than 7 days, facial pain, and purulent nasal discharge. The data as a whole suggest that if antibiotics are to be used, amoxicillin or doxycycline are adequate first-line agents. Trimethoprim-sulfamethoxazole is acceptable for β-lactam–allergic adults. The patient described here does not meet the criteria for antibiotic administration by most guidelines.

Imaging studies, including CT scans or plain films of the sinuses and sinus aspiration, should be considered only in patients with predisposing factors for atypical microbial causes (for example, pseudomonal or fungal infection) and in patients with AIDS or who are otherwise immunocompromised.

KEY POINT

Antibiotics are unlikely to be effective for most patients with suspected acute sinusitis.

Bibliography
Wilson JF. Acute Sinusitis. Ann Intern Med. 2010;153(5):ITC31. [PMID: 20820036]

Item 14   Answer: A
Educational Objective: *Treat asymptomatic bacteriuria in a pregnant patient with ampicillin.*

The most appropriate management is to begin ampicillin. Pregnant women are screened for asymptomatic bacteriuria, which is associated with low birth weight, prematurity, and an increased risk for pyelonephritis. This pregnant woman has asymptomatic bacteriuria that now requires treatment. An appropriate antibiotic for this patient is ampicillin, amoxicillin, or nitrofurantoin. These antibiotics are Food and Drug Administration pregnancy risk category B drugs. Ciprofloxacin and trimethoprim are both pregnancy risk category C drugs and are therefore not indicated.

Urine cultures should be obtained after treatment in pregnant women with asymptomatic bacteriuria to confirm eradication of bacteria. Confirming the sterility of the urine can be done by repeating urine cultures at intervals until delivery.

KEY POINT

Asymptomatic bacteriuria during pregnancy should be treated with ampicillin, amoxicillin, or nitrofurantoin.

Bibliography
Drekonja DM, Johnson JR. Urinary tract infections. Prim Care. 2008;35(2):345-367. [PMID: 18486719]

Item 15   Answer: D
Educational Objective: *Diagnose prostatic abscess.*

The most appropriate management for this patient is a transrectal ultrasound. The patient presents with acute prostatitis and appropriately has intravenous ciprofloxacin initiated. The failure of clinical improvement after 36 to 72 hours is most likely due to a complication such as a prostatic abscess and further evaluation with a transrectal ultrasound (TRUS) or abdominal/pelvic CT is indicated. The TRUS might be the preferred diagnostic modality in this patient because of his chronic kidney disease. Contrast-enhanced CT should be avoided in patients with reduced kidney function.

Parenteral administration of empiric antibiotics is appropriate for a patient who presents with systemic signs of illness and requires hospital admission. Intravenous antibiotic therapy may be changed to oral when the patient shows clinical improvement and can tolerate oral intake. Adding or starting an aminoglycoside should be avoided in this patient with reduced kidney function. Also, substituting aminoglycoside for ciprofloxacin would not be indicated. The urine culture shows an organism that is sensitive to fluoroquinolones. Furthermore, fluoroquinolones have excellent prostate penetration, favorable pharmacokinetic properties, a good safety profile, and a broad spectrum of antibacterial activity against gram-negative pathogens, including *Proteus mirabilis.*

Transurethral catheterization should be avoided in acute prostatitis. If bladder drainage is necessary, it should be suprapubic to reduce the risk of prostatic abscess and septicemia. Furthermore, there is no indication for placement of a bladder catheter such as outflow obstruction.

KEY POINT

Patients with acute prostatitis who fail to respond to appropriate antibiotic therapy within 36 to 72 hours may have a complication such as a prostatic abscess.

Bibliography

Ramakrishnan K, Salinas RC. Prostatitis: acute and chronic. Prim Care. 2010;37(3):547-63, viii-ix. [PMID: 20705198]

Item 16   Answer: D

Educational Objective: *Recognize that asymptomatic bacteriuria does not require treatment.*

The most appropriate management for this patient's asymptomatic bacteriuria is no treatment. For asymptomatic women, bacteriuria is defined as 2 consecutive voided urine specimens with isolation of the same bacterial strain in quantitative counts of at least 10^5 cfu/mL. *Escherichia coli* remains the single most common organism isolated from women, but other organisms, such as *Proteus mirabilis,* are more common in men. Treatment of asymptomatic bacteriuria in women with diabetes is not indicated. A randomized, controlled trial of antibiotic therapy or no therapy for women with diabetes and asymptomatic bacteriuria showed antibiotic therapy did not delay or decrease the frequency of symptomatic urinary tract infection, nor did it decrease the number of hospitalizations for urinary infection or other causes. However, women who received antibiotic therapy had significantly more adverse antimicrobial effects.

Screening for asymptomatic bacteriuria is recommended only for pregnant women and before transurethral resection of the prostate, urinary tract instrumentation involving biopsy, or other tissue trauma resulting in mucosal bleeding. Women with diabetes, premenopausal nonpregnant women, older persons living in the community, elderly institutionalized persons, persons with spinal cord injury, and patients with catheters while the catheter remains in situ should not be screened or treated for asymptomatic bacteriuria. Screening is also not recommended for simple catheter placement or cystoscopy without biopsy. Unless indicated, screening and treatment for asymptomatic bacteriuria should be discouraged.

KEY POINT

Screening or treatment of asymptomatic bacteriuria is not recommended for most nonpregnant women.

Bibliography

Nicolle LE, Bradley S, Colgan R, Rice JC, Schaeffer A, Hooton TM; Infectious Diseases Society of America; American Society of Nephrology; American Geriatric Society. Infectious Diseases Society of America guidelines for the diagnosis and treatment of asymptomatic bacteriuria in adults [erratum in Clin Infect Dis. 2005;40(10):1556]. Clin Infect Dis. 2005;40(5):643-54. [PMID: 15714408]

Item 17   Answer: B

Educational Objective: *Treat pyelonephritis with a fluoroquinolone antibiotic.*

This patient has pyelonephritis and should be treated with a fluoroquinolone antibiotic, such as ciprofloxacin or levofloxacin. Pyelonephritis is associated with the abrupt onset of fever, chills, sweats, nausea, vomiting, diarrhea, and flank or abdominal pain; hypotension and septic shock may occur in severe cases. The presence of bacteriuria and pyuria is the gold standard for diagnosing pyelonephritis if these findings are associated with a suggestive history and physical examination findings. Leukocyte casts in the urine are suggestive of pyelonephritis but are uncommonly detected. Blood cultures should be obtained in patients who appear ill. Hypotensive patients with pyelonephritis should receive intravenous fluids.

Treatment of pyelonephritis consists of antibiotics for 7 to 14 days. Patients who are acutely ill, nauseated, or vomiting should receive parenteral therapy initially and can begin receiving oral therapy once oral intake is tolerated. The standard therapy in nonpregnant women is a fluoroquinolone. Alternatives to fluoroquinolone antibiotics include extended-spectrum cephalosporins or penicillins, but oral options may be more limited for patients with a contraindication to fluoroquinolones. Eradication of bacteriuria in patients treated for pyelonephritis can be confirmed through repeat urinalysis and urine culture. Imaging studies should be used only if an alternative diagnosis or a urologic complication is suspected.

Ampicillin and amoxicillin are not used as initial therapy of acute pyelonephritis because of the high rates of resistance to these agents. Nitrofurantoin does not achieve levels sufficiently high for pyelonephritis treatment.

Until recently, trimethoprim or the combination of trimethoprim-sulfamethoxazole was highly effective for treating acute pyelonephritis. The increased frequency of resistant strains of *Escherichia coli* and other gram-negative bacteria to these antimicrobial agents has led to a preference for initial therapy with fluoroquinolones except in pregnant women, because fluoroquinolone antibiotics are Food and Drug Administration pregnancy risk category C drugs.

KEY POINT

Standard outpatient management for pyelonephritis in women who are not pregnant is an oral fluoroquinolone.

Bibliography

Drekonja DM, Johnson JR. Urinary tract infections. Prim Care. 2008;35(2):345-367. [PMID: 18486719]

Item 18   Answer: D

Educational Objective: *Manage recurrent cystitis with patient-initiated trimethoprim-sulfamethoxazole.*

The most appropriate management is trimethoprim-sulfamethoxazole for 3 days when symptoms develop. This patient most likely has a recurrent urinary tract infection (UTI). Self-treatment with trimethoprim-sulfamethoxazole on development of symptoms is appropriate. Recurrent UTIs are common in women and are believed to represent new infection rather than a relapse of a previous episode. Although evaluation for subtle predisposing factors such as anatomic urinary tract abnormalities is seldom useful, inquiring about behavioral practices can be helpful. Sexual intercourse is a risk factor for acute and recurrent UTIs, as is the use of spermicides or spermicides plus a diaphragm.

Most women are able to diagnose a UTI accurately and begin antimicrobial treatment without being seen by a physician. Self-treatment is highly effective in compliant women. One study found that women correctly diagnosed more than 90% of recurrent infections, and that self-treatment was effective in more than 95% of patients—numbers that rival those of physician-initiated therapy. Self-management at first onset of symptoms is a feasible, safe, and convenient option for this young, otherwise healthy woman with recurrent cystitis. Trimethoprim-sulfamethoxazole, 160 mg/800 mg twice daily for 3 days, is effective for treating uncomplicated cystitis. In addition, the reported 12% resistance of *Escherichia coli* to this agent is low enough that other antibiotics do not need to be considered.

This patient's recurrent infections do not seem to be related to sexual intercourse; therefore, postcoital prophylactic ciprofloxacin therapy would not be indicated. A 10-day course of ciprofloxacin is indicated only if pyelonephritis is documented. Some sources may recommend chronic suppressive therapy for patients with more than two UTIs per year; however, this approach may increase the risk of infection with antibiotic-resistant bacteria.

KEY POINT

Short-course antibiotic self-treatment is appropriate for young, otherwise healthy women with recurrent cystitis.

Bibliography

Drekonja DM, Johnson JR. Urinary tract infections. Prim Care. 2008;35(2):345-367. [PMID: 18486719]

Item 19   Answer: B

Educational Objective: *Screen for HIV, chlamydia, and gonorrhea.*

According to Centers for Disease Control and Prevention (CDC) guidelines, all sexually active women aged 24 years and younger should be screened for chlamydial infection, either with nucleic acid amplification of a cervical swab if a pelvic examination is being performed or of a urine sample, which has a very similar sensitivity. The United States Preventative Services Task Force recommends screening for gonorrhea in high-risk persons, including women who have a history of sexually transmitted disease (STD) infection, have multiple sexual partners, are pregnant, or are under the age of 25 years, because this is the population with the highest prevalence. Gonorrhea testing can only be performed on a cervical swab. The American College of Physicians and the CDC recommend HIV screening for patients in all health care settings. They recommend "opt-out screening," in which the patient is notified that testing will be performed unless the patient declines. In addition, pregnant women at increased risk or in areas of high prevalence should have an additional HIV test during their third trimester.

Persons at risk and all pregnant women should be screened for syphilis. Pregnant women are screened during the first prenatal visit and during the third trimester and, for women at high risk, at the time of delivery. Other high-risk persons include commercial sex workers, prisoners, any person diagnosed with another STD, men who have sex with men, and those who engage in other high-risk behaviors. Screening is not recommended in the general population because a positive test result will most likely be a false-positive test result.

KEY POINT

Routinely screen sexually active women under the age of 25 years for chlamydia, gonorrhea, and HIV.

Bibliography

Centers for Disease Control and Prevention, Workowski KA, Berman SM. Sexually transmitted diseases treatment guidelines, 2006 [erratum in MMWR Recomm Rep. 2006;55(36):997]. MMWR Recomm Rep. 2006;55(RR-11):1-94. [PMID: 16888612]

Item 20   Answer: C

Educational Objective: *Diagnose and empirically treat cervicitis.*

This patient has cervicitis and should be treated empirically for gonorrhea and chlamydia. Cervicitis is the presence of a mucopurulent cervical discharge or endocervical bleeding easily induced by gentle passage of a cotton swab through the cervical os. Cervicitis is commonly caused by either gonorrhea or chlamydial infection, and although gonorrhea infection is often symptomatic, either may be asymptomatic or only mildly symptomatic. In patients with cervicitis, an abnormal vaginal discharge or intermenstrual bleeding is not uncommon. The absence of gram-negative intracellular diplococci on Gram stain does not rule out gonorrhea, because it is observed in only 50% of women with this infection.

In a woman with a high pretest probability for cervicitis who may easily be lost to follow-up, it is best to treat empirically for gonorrhea and chlamydia rather than wait for specific testing to return. Ceftriaxone with either doxycycline or azithromycin is an appropriate regimen. In the presence of a documented gonorrhea infection by nucleic acid or culture, chlamydia is always treated even in the absence of positive test results for chlamydia infection.

(PID) includes a spectrum of disorders of the female upper genital tract, including endometritis, salpingitis, tubo-ovarian abscess, and pelvic peritonitis. Diagnosis is established clinically with suggestive findings, including cervical motion tenderness, uterine tenderness, or adnexal tenderness on pelvic examination.

Bacterial vaginosis is not a sexually transmitted disease and does not cause cervicitis. On vaginal examination, inflammation is not evident, but a homogeneous, white, noninflammatory discharge coats the vaginal walls. The vaginal pH is higher than 4.5, the "whiff test" is positive (a fishy odor is present when potassium hydroxide is added to vaginal secretions), and "clue cells" (squamous epithelial cells covered with bacteria obscuring the edges of the epithelial cells) are found on wet mount.

KEY POINT

Cervicitis is defined by either the presence of a mucopurulent cervical discharge or endocervical bleeding and is caused by chlamydial and/or gonococcal infection.

Bibliography

Wilson JF. In the clinic. Vaginitis and cervicitis. Ann Intern Med. 2009;151(5):ITC3-1-ITC3-15; Quiz ITC3-16. [PMID: 19721016]

Item 21   Answer: B

Educational Objective: *Treat disseminated gonococcal infection.*

This patient most likely has disseminated gonococcal infection (DGI) and initial treatment should include parenteral therapy with ceftriaxone or a comparable third-generation cephalosporin.

DGI may cause septic or sterile immune-mediated arthritis and tenosynovitis and frequently involves the knees, hips, and wrists but not the spine. Dermatitis associated with sparse peripheral necrotic pustules also is common. A characteristic prodrome of migratory arthralgia and tenosynovitis may precede the settling of the synovitis in one or several joints.

Genitourinary symptoms associated with DGI usually are absent in women, and genital infection in women may have occurred long before systemic dissemination. Patients with rectal and pharyngeal colonization of *Neisseria gonorrhoeae* in the setting of DGI are commonly asymptomatic. In all patients in whom DGI is clinically suspected, routine culture of the rectum and pharynx, as well as the blood and the joints, is indicated.

On diagnosis of DGI, prompt evaluation for additional sexually transmitted diseases, including syphilis and HIV, is indicated. Empiric treatment for *Chlamydia trachomatis* infection with doxycycline also should be considered, because coinfection with *N. gonorrhoeae* and *C. trachomatis* is common. Patients with DGI are frequently asymptomatic, and this condition can cause infertility if untreated. Sexual partners of patients with DGI also should be treated.

Acyclovir is an effective treatment for herpes simplex infection. However, herpes simplex is most likely to cause painful vesicular and erosive disease of the genitalia, not papules and necrotic pustules on the cutaneous surfaces, and herpes simplex is not associated with a migratory arthritis.

Fluoroquinolones such as ciprofloxacin are no longer recommended by the Centers for Disease Control and Prevention for the treatment of gonorrhea because of the high resistance rate. Gentamicin is not indicated because *N. gonorrhoeae* is not consistently susceptible to this agent.

KEY POINT

Disseminated gonococcal infection may cause arthritis and tenosynovitis and is often associated with sparse peripheral necrotic pustules.

Bibliography

Centers for Disease Control and Prevention, Workowski KA, Berman SM. Sexually transmitted diseases treatment guidelines, 2006. MMWR Recomm Rep. 2006;55(RR-11). [PMID: 16888612]

Item 22   Answer: B

Educational Objective: *Diagnose genital herpes simplex virus infection.*

This patient has the classic findings of primary genital herpes simplex virus (HSV) infection. HSV-1 or HSV-2 may cause the infection, but HSV-2 is the more common pathogen. Genital herpes lesions typically begin as vesicles that ulcerate and are quite painful. The initial infection is often the most severe and can be accompanied by local lymphadenopathy and systemic symptoms. Recurrences vary in frequency and are typically less severe than the initial episode. Many recurrences are subclinical but are nonetheless contagious. The diagnosis of genital herpes is often suspected on clinical grounds but may be confirmed by viral culture or serologic testing if the diagnosis is in doubt. Viral culture for HSV-1 and HSV-2 is a rapid test, with results often available by the next day. The specificity of viral culture approaches 100%, but the sensitivity varies with the quality of specimen handling and the age of the lesion (older, crusted lesions have lower yield).

Chancroid is a relatively uncommon sexually transmitted disease caused by *Haemophilus ducreyi*. Infection is characterized by the presences of ragged, purulent, painful ulcers associated with tender lymph nodes that may suppurate. The superficial vesicles and erosions of herpes simplex virus infection are not easily mistaken for the deep, ragged ulcers of chancroid.

The primary ulcerative lesion (chancre) in patients with syphilis develops approximately 3 weeks after infection occurs, has a clean appearance with heaped-up borders, and is usually painless and often unrecognized, particularly in women. Multiple small painful vesicles and erosions argue strongly against this diagnosis.

Symptoms of vulvovaginal candidiasis include pruritus, external and internal erythema, and nonodorous, white, curd-like discharge. Lack of pruritus makes vulvovaginal candidiasis less likely, and candidal infection does not cause painful genital ulcers.

KEY POINT

Primary genital herpes simplex virus infection is characterized by fever, headache, and painful, ulcerated, vesicular lesions.

Bibliography

Cernik C, Gallina K, Brodell RT. The treatment of herpes simplex infections: an evidence-based review. Arch Intern Med. 2008;168(11):1137-1144. [PMID: 18541820]

Item 23   Answer: D

Educational Objective: *Treat a patient with pelvic inflammatory disease with ceftriaxone and doxycycline.*

This patient's clinical findings are compatible with pelvic inflammatory disease (PID), and she should receive intramuscularly delivered ceftriaxone and oral doxycycline. PID is a polymicrobial infection of the endometrium, fallopian tubes, and ovaries; diagnosis is based on the presence of abdominal discomfort, uterine or adnexal tenderness, or cervical motion tenderness. Other diagnostic criteria include temperature higher than 38.3°C (101.0°F), cervical or vaginal mucopurulent discharge, leukocytes in vaginal secretions, and documentation of gonorrheal or chlamydial infection. PID is most likely to occur within 7 days of the onset of menses. All women with suspected PID should be tested for gonorrhea, chlamydia, and HIV infection, and undergo pregnancy testing. In severe cases, imaging should be performed to exclude a tubo-ovarian abscess. Ambulatory patients are treated with ceftriaxone and doxycycline with or without metronidazole. Duration of treatment is 14 days. Patients with PID should be hospitalized if there is (1) no clinical improvement after 48 to 72 hours of antibiotics; (2) an inability to tolerate oral antibiotics; (3) severe illness with nausea, vomiting, or high fever; (4) suspected intra-abdominal abscess; (5) pregnancy; or (6) noncompliance with outpatient therapy.

Ampicillin and gentamicin do not reliably treat gonorrhea and chlamydial infection and therefore are not adequate antibiotic therapy for a patient with PID. Azithromycin alone is sufficient treatment for chlamydial infection but is no longer recommended as initial treatment for gonorrheal infection owing to the high prevalence of gonorrhea strains with decreased susceptibility. Cefoxitin alone is insufficient treatment for PID and combination with oral doxycycline is recommended.

KEY POINT

The treatment for ambulatory patients with pelvic inflammatory disease is intramuscular ceftriaxone and oral doxycycline.

Bibliography

Centers for Disease Control and Prevention (CDC). Update to CDC's sexually transmitted diseases treatment guidelines, 2006: fluoroquinolones no longer recommended for treatment of gonococcal infections. MMWR Morb Mortal Wkly Rep. 2007;56(14):332-336. [PMID: 17431378]

Item 24   Answer: D

Educational Objective: *Treat Pneumocystis jirovecii pneumonia with trimethoprim-sulfamethoxazole plus corticosteroids.*

The best initial treatment regimen for this patient is trimethoprim-sulfamethoxazole plus corticosteroids. *Pneumocystis jirovecii* pneumonia remains the most common AIDS-defining illness and cause of death in patients with AIDS. The diagnosis should be considered in any patient with a CD4 cell count of less than 200/μL who presents with fever, dry cough, and dyspnea developing over several days or weeks. The chest radiograph typically shows bilateral interstitial infiltrates, but findings can vary from a normal film to consolidation or a pneumothorax. The diagnosis is established by silver stain examination of induced sputum or a bronchoscopic sample showing characteristic cysts. A 3-week course of trimethoprim-sulfamethoxazole is the standard treatment. Corticosteroids are required for patients with evidence of hypoxia (arterial P_{O_2} <70 mm Hg [9.3 kPa] or an alveolar-arterial gradient >35 mm Hg [4.7 kPa]) and should be continued for the entire course of treatment.

Dapsone can be an adjunctive treatment to trimethoprim in acute *Pneumocystis jirovecii* and can be used alone as a prophylactic agent for patients with a CD4 count less than 200/μL in patients who are intolerant of trimethoprim sulfamethoxazole, but it is not recommended as single drug therapy for *Pneumocystis jirovecii* pneumonia.

KEY POINT

Trimethoprim-sulfamethoxazole plus corticosteroids is the preferred initial treatment for *Pneumocystis jirovecii* pneumonia and hypoxia (arterial P_{O_2} <70 mm Hg [9.3 kPa] or an alveolar-arterial gradient >35 mm Hg [4.7 kPa]).

Bibliography

Catherinot E, Lanternier F, Bougnoux ME, Lecuit M, Couderc LJ, Lortholary O. *Pneumocystis jirovecii* pneumonia. Infect Dis Clin North Am. 2010;24(1):107-38. [PMID: 20171548]

Item 25   Answer: A

Educational Objective: *Provide appropriate prophylactic therapy for a patient with HIV infection.*

This patient should receive trimethoprim-sulfamethoxazole. Several drugs have been shown to provide effective prophylaxis against opportunistic infections in patients with HIV infection and to prolong life in some patients. The CD4 cell count is an indicator of immune competence. Recommendations regarding when to initiate prophylaxis are based on CD4 cell count levels. The threshold for *Pneumocystis* and toxoplasmosis prophylaxis is 200/μL and 100/μL, respectively. The patient's CD4 cell count is 77/μL, and she should receive prophylaxis for *Pneumocystis* and for toxoplasmosis if her antibody titer is positive (demonstrating previous infection but not immunity). Trimethoprim-sulfamethoxazole is the first-line agent for both.

Azithromycin is used for prophylaxis against *Mycobacterium avium* complex in patients with a CD4 cell count less than 50/µL. This patient's CD4 cell count is not at this threshold and, therefore, prophylactic azithromycin therapy is not recommended. Fluconazole is not recommended for the primary prophylaxis of *Candida* infections despite its effectiveness in this role. The potential for drug resistance, numerous potential drug-drug interactions, the ease and effectiveness of treating infection when it does occur, and lack of survival benefit argue against prophylactic use. Isoniazid would be indicated if the patient were found to have a positive tuberculin skin test greater than 5 mm and a negative chest x-ray excluding active tuberculosis. There is no reason to provide prophylactic isoniazid therapy for patients who have not been exposed to *Mycobacterium tuberculosis*. Although valganciclovir is effective in preventing cytomegalovirus (CMV), infection, decisions regarding prophylaxis are complex. Valganciclovir is expensive, a theoretical concern about the development of drug resistance exists, it is toxic to the bone marrow, and treatment of early infection is very effective. Finally, no proven survival benefit is associated with CMV prophylaxis.

KEY POINT

In patients with HIV infection, prophylactic therapy for *Pneumocystis*, toxoplasmosis, and *Mycobacterium avium* complex are determined by the CD4 cell count.

Bibliography

Aberg JA, Kaplan JE, Libman H, Emmanuel P, Anderson JR, Stone VE, Oleske JM, Currier JS, Gallant JE; HIV Medicine Association of the Infectious Diseases Society of America. Primary care guidelines for the management of persons infected with human immunodeficiency virus: 2009 update by the HIV medicine Association of the Infectious Diseases Society of America. Clin Infect Dis. 2009;49(5):651-81. [PMID: 19640227]

Item 26   Answer: E

Educational Objective: *Understand the association between recurrent herpes zoster infection and HIV infection.*

This patient most likely has HIV infection. Herpes zoster infection is the reactivation of the varicella virus in a single cutaneous nerve. Recurrence of herpes zoster infection in the immunocompetent host is uncommon but does occur. When recurrent disease is present, the underlying cause is overwhelmingly HIV infection. In this patient, there is a band of crusts and blisters on an erythematous base along a dermatomal distribution on the left thorax. There is evidence of scarring in a dermatome several centimeters above the currently involved site, representing a previous herpes zoster infection. Almost half of all herpes zoster episodes diagnosed in patients with HIV are recurrences. The advent of highly active antiretroviral therapy has not lessened the incidence of recurrent herpes zoster infection in patients with HIV infection. Patients on chemotherapy and patients who have undergone organ transplant may also develop recurrent herpes zoster.

All patients with HIV infection and herpes zoster infection are treated with antiviral therapy regardless of the age of the zoster lesions. Most patients with HIV infection can be treated with an oral antiviral drug with good bioavailability, such as valacyclovir or famciclovir, but patients with severe disease, evidence of dissemination, or ophthalmologic involvement may have better outcomes if treated with intravenous acyclovir.

This patient's alcoholism is a risk factor for cirrhosis but not for recurrent herpes zoster infection. A patient with unexplained weight loss and fatigue may have an underlying metabolic disease such as diabetes mellitus, but diabetes is not associated with recurrent herpes zoster. Because of this patient's injection drug use, he is at risk for hepatitis B and hepatitis C, and screening for these infections is recommended. However, neither of these infections is associated with recurrent herpes zoster.

KEY POINT

Recurrent herpes zoster infection should trigger testing for possible associated HIV infection.

Bibliography

Gebo KA, Kalyani R, Moore RD, Polydefkis MJ. The incidence of, risk factors for, and sequelae of herpes zoster among HIV patients in the highly active antiretroviral therapy era. J Acquir Immune Defic Syndr. 2005;40(2):169-174. [PMID: 16186734]

Item 27   Answer: C

Educational Objective: *Diagnose acute HIV infection with HIV RNA viral load measurement.*

The most appropriate additional test is an HIV RNA viral load and HIV antibody measurement. This patient's prolonged febrile syndrome in the setting of HIV risk factors should raise concerns for recent infection with HIV. Detection of HIV RNA is the most sensitive test for detecting HIV infection during the acute symptomatic phase. Tests for HIV-specific antigens, such as p24, can also detect the presence of virus in the acute setting. Antibodies to HIV do not commonly occur until about 6 weeks after infection and may therefore be negative during the acute symptomatic phase. Patients diagnosed with acute HIV infection on the basis of an HIV viral load measurement should have confirmatory serologic antibody testing performed at a subsequent point in time.

In addition to the acute retroviral syndrome, this patient must be evaluated for secondary syphilis using the rapid plasma reagin test. Secondary syphilis and acute retroviral syndrome should always be considered in sexually active patients with rash, fever, and generalized lymphadenopathy. Other causes of a mononucleosis syndrome (for example, Ebstein-Barr virus and cytomegalovirus infections) should also be considered if these tests are inconclusive.

The CD4 cell count may be profoundly depressed in patients with acute HIV infection, but the CD4 cell count can be both insensitive in the diagnosis of acute infection and depressed by various other, non–HIV-1 infectious agents.

Although acute HIV infection can mimic the signs and symptoms of mononucleosis, testing for Epstein-Barr virus infection is a less immediate concern in this patient who has multiple risk factors for HIV infection. Furthermore, acute infection would be detected with an elevated IgM antibody titer, not IgG.

The histopathology of the rash in acute HIV infection is nonspecific and is not useful in diagnosis; therefore, a skin biopsy is not indicated.

KEY POINT

The measurement of HIV RNA viral load is the most sensitive test for infection during the acute stage.

Bibliography

Miles K. Primary HIV infection. Community Pract. 2005;78(9):331-3. [PMID: 16187668]

Item 28   Answer: D

Educational Objective: *Diagnose toxoplasmosis encephalitis.*

The most likely diagnosis is toxoplasmosis encephalitis. Toxoplasmosis almost always presents as reactivation disease in patients with HIV infection and typically occurs when the CD4 cell count is less than 100/μL. Additional findings are fever, neurologic deficits, and an MRI showing ring-enhancing lesions, often with associated edema. Sulfadiazine plus pyrimethamine and folinic acid are given initially. Follow-up MRI is critical to assess treatment response. If there is no therapeutic response after 14 days, stereotactic brain biopsy is recommended to rule out other causes, especially a primary central nervous system lymphoma.

Cryptococcal meningitis is the most common form of meningitis in patients with AIDS, who typically present with symptoms such as headache, irritability, and nausea that can mimic other disorders. Most patients have a CD4 cell count of less than 100/μL. The diagnosis is based on detection of cryptococcal antigen in the cerebrospinal fluid or culture of *Cryptococcus neoformans* in the cerebrospinal fluid. Cryptococcal meningitis is not usually associated with ring-enhancing lesions on brain MRI.

Disseminated *Mycobacterium avium* complex (MAC) infection is common in patients with advanced-stage HIV infection and a CD4 cell count of less than 50/μL. Symptoms include fever, weight loss, hepatosplenomegaly, lymphadenopathy, malaise, and abdominal pain. The diagnosis is generally confirmed by recovering the pathogen from sterile tissue (usually blood). MAC infection is not associated with ring-enhancing lesions on MRI. This patient's CD4 count also helps exclude this diagnosis.

Progressive multifocal leukoencephalopathy is a demyelinating disease of the central nervous system caused by the polyomavirus JC virus. It occurs almost exclusively in severely immunocompromised patients, including those with advanced HIV-1 infection. Clinical findings of progressive multifocal leukoencephalopathy include dementia, hemiparesis or paralysis of one extremity, ataxia, hemianopia, and diplopia. The characteristic MRI appearance of these lesions is hyperintense (white) areas on T2-weighted images and fluid-attenuated inversion recovery (FLAIR) sequences and hypointense (dark) areas on T1-weighted images. There is usually no mass effect.

KEY POINT

Toxoplasmosis encephalitis typically occurs in HIV-infected patients when the CD4 cell count is less than 100/μL and is associated with ring-enhancing lesions on brain MRI, often with mass effect.

Bibliography

Guidelines for prevention and treatment of opportunistic infections in HIV-infected adults and adolescents. Available at [http://aidsinfo.nih.gov/contentfiles/Adult_OI_041009.pdf]. Published April 10, 2009. Accessed on April 26, 2011.

Item 29   Answer: D

Educational Objective: *Prevent catheter-associated urinary tract infection.*

The most effective way to prevent catheter-associated urinary tract infections (UTIs) is to decrease catheter use. Devices should be used for specific indications, not for convenience and should be removed as soon as possible. Examples of appropriate use include diagnosing pathologic findings in the lower urinary tract or the cause of urinary retention, monitoring fluid status in acutely ill patients when this directly impacts medical treatment, and managing patients with stage 3 or 4 pressure ulcers on the buttocks. However, urinary catheters often are used for convenience, which significantly increases the risk for UTIs. If the catheter is needed, measures are required to decrease the risk of bacteriuria and subsequent infection. These include handwashing, using an aseptic technique and sterile equipment for catheter insertion and care, securing the catheter properly, maintaining unobstructed urine flow and closed sterile drainage, and considering use of antibacterial-coated catheters. Manipulation and irrigation should be minimized. Specimens should be collected using the drainage bag valve. Antibiotics should not be used as prophylaxis for the prevention of UTIs because such use promotes antibiotic resistance.

KEY POINT

The most effective way to prevent catheter-associated urinary tract infections is to decrease catheter use.

Bibliography

Lo E, Nicolle L, Classen D, et al. Strategies to prevent catheter-associated urinary tract infections in acute care hospitals. Infect Control Hosp Epidemiol. 2008;29(suppl 1):S41-50. [PMID: 18840088]

Item 30   Answer: D
Educational Objective: *Prevent ventilator-associated pneumonia with semi-erect positioning.*

Semi-erect position will most likely reduce the risk of ventilator-associated pneumonia (VAP). Even when a cuffed tube is in place, bacteria from the stomach can reach the lungs and cause pneumonia. Semi-erect positioning in bed at 45° is useful because it reduces the risk of excursion of bacteria from the stomach into the upper airways.

Changing endotracheal tubes seems logical, but reintubation is associated with certain risks (for example, intubating the esophagus or precipitating hypoxia during the procedure). Reintubation may also increase the risk of nosocomial pneumonia. Careful inspection and management of the tubing can help reduce infections slightly. Because the tubing has a tendency to collect water, careful drainage of accumulated condensate into patient-specific drainage containers is advocated.

Oral placement of endotracheal tubes is currently believed to be superior to nasal placement because nasogastric and nasotracheal tubes cause some degree of obstruction of the ostia in the nose, which can predispose to nosocomial sinusitis. Whether all nasal tubes should be replaced by oral tubes is unclear. However, no benefit will be gained by changing from an orotracheal tube to a nasotracheal tube to prevent a case of health-care associated pneumonia.

Reducing the density of gastric bacteria by use of prophylactic antibiotics is tempting. However, this approach is ineffective and serves to select for resistant strains.

KEY POINT

Semi-erect positioning reduces the risk of ventilator-associated pneumonia.

Bibliography

Barsanti MC, Woeltje KF. Infection prevention in the intensive care unit. Infect Dis Clin North Am. 2009;23(3):703-25. [PMID: 19665091]

Item 31   Answer: D
Educational Objective: *Use barrier precautions and soap and water for hand hygiene to prevent the spread of* Clostridium difficile *infection.*

The most effective bundled measures to prevent the spread of *Clostridium difficile* infection are barrier precautions and soap and water for hand cleaning. Environmental contamination with vegetative *C. difficile* and *C. difficile* spores frequently occurs. *C. difficile* is transmitted to other patients through the hands and clothes of health care workers and from common equipment that is used on patients without cleaning. A combination of interventions "bundled" together have been shown to be effective at reducing many hospital-acquired infections. The use of a *C. difficile* bundle consisting of barrier precautions, enhanced cleaning with bleach, and traditional soap-and-water hand hygiene is useful in preventing the spread of *C. difficile*. Soap and water are not sporicidal, but the mechanics of hand washing effectively removes spores. Alcohol-based hand hygiene products do not kill spores and are ineffective at removing them from hands.

Barrier precautions such as wearing nonsterile gloves and a gown and using dedicated equipment have been recommended for *C. difficile* control by the Centers for Disease Control and Prevention and have been shown to be effective.

Airborne precautions are recommended for patients with known or suspected illnesses transmitted by airborne droplet nuclei, such as tuberculosis, measles, varicella, or disseminated varicella zoster virus infection. Patients must be isolated in a private room with negative air pressure, the door must remain closed, and all entering persons must wear masks with a filtering capacity of 95%. Transported patients must wear masks.

Droplet precautions are recommended for patients with known or suspected illnesses transmitted by large-particle droplets, such as *Neisseria meningitidis* infections and influenza. Patients are isolated in private rooms, and hospital personnel wear face masks when within 3 feet of the patient.

KEY POINT

A *Clostridium difficile* "bundle" consisting of barrier precautions, enhanced cleaning with bleach, and traditional soap-and-water hand hygiene is useful in preventing the spread of *C. difficile*.

Bibliography

Hessen MT. In the clinic. Clostridium difficile Infection. Ann Intern Med. 2010;153(7):ITC41-15; quiz ITC416. [PMID: 20921540]

Item 32   Answer: A
Educational Objective: *Institute infection-control measures in a patient with* Neisseria meningitidis *meningitis.*

The most appropriate next step is the use of a face mask. This patient has *Neisseria meningitidis* meningitis. Droplet precautions should be initiated when this diagnosis is suspected and require that health care workers within 6 to 10 feet of the index patient wear a face mask. Appropriate infection control measures for all patients include hand hygiene and standard precautions.

The human nasopharynx is the only known reservoir for meningococcal meningitis. Meningococci are spread from person to person by respiratory droplets of infected nasopharyngeal secretions. Persons with significant exposure to the index patient (same household, day-care center, or anyone with direct contact with a patient's oral secretions) should receive chemoprophylaxis with appropriate antibiotics. Significant health care exposure includes personnel with potential for intimate contact (within 3 feet) of the patient's respiratory secretions.

For infection spread by direct contact with the patient (for example, vancomycin-resistant enterococci), additional infection control measures include patient placement into a private room or with those who have a similar infection and the use of nonsterile gloves and gowns for direct contact with the patient or any infective material. Airborne infection precautions are appropriate for illnesses transmitted by airborne droplet nuclei (for example, tuberculosis, measles, and varicella). Additional infection control measures include placement into a private room, typically in a pressure-negative room, and special masks with a filtering capacity of 95% of particulates (N-95 respirator or a powered air purifying respirator [PAPR]).

KEY POINT

Droplet precautions, which require that health care workers wear a face mask for close contact with infectious patients and don the mask on room entry, are indicated when meningococcal meningitis is suspected.

Bibliography
Siegel JD, Rinehart E, Jackson M, Chiarello L; The Healthcare Infection Control Practices Advisory Committee. Guideline for Isolation Precautions: Preventing Transmission of Infectious Agents in Healthcare Settings. www.cdc.gov/ncidod/dhqp/pdf/guidelines/Isolation2007.pdf. Published 2007. Accessed on April 28, 2011.

Item 33   Answer: B
Educational Objective: *Institute airborne precautions in the setting of suspected tuberculosis.*

The most important infection control measure is the institution of airborne precautions. This foreign-born patient most likely has reactivation of pulmonary tuberculosis. Tuberculosis is a communicable disease and is inhaled into the respiratory system via airborne droplets. A diagnosis of pulmonary tuberculosis should be considered in any patient with cough for longer than 3 weeks, loss of appetite, unexplained weight loss, night sweats, hoarseness, fever, fatigue, or chest pain. The index of suspicion should be substantially high for patients who have spent time in developing countries, geographic areas of the United States such as Miami or New York City, or in a correctional facility.

Initially, the most important management is protection from potential tuberculosis exposure with airborne precautions, including placement of the patient into a negative-pressure room and use of respiratory protection by health care workers. Acceptable protection includes a "respirator," which refers to an N95 or higher filtering facepiece respirator or a powered air-purifying respirator. Within health care settings, tuberculosis airborne precautions should be immediately initiated in patients with symptoms or signs consistent with tuberculosis or in those with documented infectious tuberculosis who have not completed antituberculosis treatment. Such patients should continue to be managed with airborne precautions until they are determined to be noninfectious (clinical response to a standard multidrug antituberculosis treatment regimen or until an alternative diagnosis is made).

Although chest radiograph and sputum acid-fast bacilli stain and culture would be performed in a setting such as this, they

would not be done before implementation of effective airborne precautions to reduce the risk for transmission of infection to health care workers and other patients. Performing tuberculin skin testing can help to establish a diagnosis of tuberculosis; however, such testing would not differentiate active from latent tuberculosis and should not be performed before airborne precautions are instituted.

KEY POINT

Airborne precautions should be immediately initiated for any patient with suspected tuberculosis to reduce risk of transmission to health care workers and other patients.

Bibliography
Jensen PA, Lambert LA, Iademarco MF, Ridzon R; CDC. Guidelines for preventing the transmission of Mycobacterium tuberculosis in health-care settings, 2005. MMWR Recomm Rep. 2005;54(RR-17):1-141. [PMID: 16382216]

Item 34   Answer: A
Educational Objective: *Manage latent tuberculosis with a chest radiograph.*

The most appropriate next management step is to obtain a chest radiograph. The most common tuberculosis testing procedure is the tuberculin skin test (TST). The procedure involves injecting purified protein derivative (PPD) intradermally and assessing the skin response to the antigen load. The induration—not the erythema—resulting within 48 to 72 hours is then measured. Various cutoff values are used, based on the patient's risk status, to increase the specificity of the test results. Because of her recent arrival from a high-prevalence area, an induration greater than10 mm is considered a positive test result and is indicative of latent or active tuberculosis infection. Consequently, this patient should receive a chest radiograph to exclude the presence of active tuberculous disease. If radiographic results are negative, treatment for latent tuberculosis infection consisting of isoniazid therapy with vitamin B_6 (pyridoxine) supplementation should be offered. A tuberculin skin test with an induration greater than10 mm is also considered positive in the following high-risk groups: injection drug users, residents or employees of high-risk congregate settings (such as prisons and jails, nursing and homeless shelters), mycobacteriology laboratory personnel, persons with clinical conditions that put them at high risk for active disease, children younger than 4 years or children exposed to adults in high-risk categories.

Standard therapy for active tuberculosis includes at least 6 months of three- to four-drug therapy (isoniazid, rifampin, pyrazinamide, and ethambutol). This therapy would be inappropriate if the patient has a normal chest radiograph and no symptoms of active infection.

Treatment of latent tuberculosis infection substantially reduces the risk that tuberculosis infection will progress to active disease; therefore, providing no additional evaluation or therapy and clearing the patient for employment would not be appropriate.

A positive tuberculin skin test is defined as an induration greater than 10 mm for patients who are recent arrivals from high-prevalence countries.

Bibliography

Escalante P. In the clinic. Tuberculosis [erratum in Ann Intern Med. 2009;151(4):292]. Ann Intern Med. 2009;150(11):ITC61-614. [PMID: 19487708]

Item 35   Answer: A

Educational Objective: *Diagnose latent tuberculosis in a patient who received bacille Calmette-Guérin (BCG) vaccination.*

This patient should receive a chest radiograph. She received bacille Calmette-Guérin (BCG) vaccination in Africa more than 20 years ago. Receipt of this vaccination should not influence interpretation of the tuberculin skin test. BCG vaccination is used in many countries with a high prevalence of tuberculosis to prevent childhood tuberculous meningitis and miliary disease. Tuberculin reactivity caused by BCG vaccination wanes with the passage of time and is unlikely to persist more than 10 years after vaccination in the absence of *Mycobacterium tuberculosis* infection; therefore, tuberculin skin testing reactions in persons vaccinated with BCG should be interpreted using the same criteria as used in those who have not received the vaccine. This patient's tuberculin skin testing result should be interpreted as positive (16 mm) and is indicative of latent or active tuberculosis infection. Consequently, she should receive a chest radiograph to exclude the presence of active tuberculous disease. If radiographic results are negative, treatment for latent tuberculosis infection consisting of isoniazid therapy should be initiated. Vitamin B$_6$ (pyridoxine) supplementation should also be considered as 2% of patients treated with isoniazid will develop peripheral neuropathy that is preventable with supplemental pyridoxine therapy. Supplemental pyridoxine is especially important in patients at high risk for neuropathy (those with diabetes, uremia, alcoholism, malnutrition, HIV infection, pregnancy, or seizure disorders).

Four-drug therapy (isoniazid, rifampin, pyrazinamide, and ethambutol), which is appropriate in patients with active tuberculosis, is not indicated in this patient.

Treatment of latent tuberculosis infection substantially reduces the risk that tuberculosis infection will progress to active disease; therefore, providing no additional evaluation or therapy would not be appropriate. Patients exposed to tuberculosis in the distant past may have an initial negative skin test; performing a second test 7 to 21 days after the first may be helpful in reducing the false-negative response rate. Such two-step testing often "boosts" a negative test result to positive as the immune system recalls its previous exposure, thus divulging a true-positive result. Two-step testing may be particularly helpful in older persons and in distinguishing new from old expo-

sures in annual employee-testing programs. Because this patient has a positive tuberculin skin test, repeating the tuberculin skin test is unnecessary and will not alter management.

Tuberculin skin testing reactions in persons who received the bacille Calmette-Guérin (BCG) vaccine should be interpreted using the same criteria as for those who have not received the vaccine.

Bibliography

Escalante P. In the clinic. Tuberculosis. Ann Intern Med. 2009;150(11):ITC61-614; quiz ITV616. Erratum in: Ann Intern Med. 2009;151(4):292. [PMID: 19487708]

Item 36   Answer: C

Educational Objective: *Treat* Mycobacterium tuberculosis *infection with four-drug therapy.*

The initial treatment of this patient with active tuberculosis must include four antituberculous drugs. Because of increasing concerns of drug resistance, all patients with suspected or confirmed tuberculosis are treated with four-drug therapy with the first-line agents isoniazid, rifampin, pyrazinamide, and ethambutol for 2 months, followed by de-escalation of antimicrobial therapy once drug susceptibility of isoniazid and rifampin is established. These agents are then continued for 7 months, totaling a 9-month treatment course.

Latent tuberculosis (positive tuberculin skin test result but no evidence of active disease) can be treated with a 9-month course of isoniazid. However, this patient has symptoms, an abnormal chest radiograph, and a positive sputum stain for acid-fast organisms, excluding latent tuberculosis. Three-drug therapy with isoniazid, pyrazinamide, and ethambutol is insufficient therapy for potentially drug-resistant tuberculosis. Therapy cannot be delayed until a definitive diagnosis of tuberculosis is made because this may take weeks, and the infection could worsen or spread to other persons in the interim.

When initiating antituberculous therapy, a four-drug regimen is used initially.

Bibliography

Escalante P. In the clinic. Tuberculosis. Ann Intern Med. 2009;150:ITC61-614; quiz ITV616. Erratum in: Ann Intern Med. 2009;151:292. [PMID: 19487708]

Item 37   Answer: A

Educational Objective: *Treat latent tuberculosis in an immunosuppressed patient.*

Isoniazid therapy for 9 months is recommended for this patient and pyridoxine (vitamin B$_6$) is typically added to prevent isoniazid-induced peripheral neuropathy. This patient was screened for tuberculosis because of concerns regarding immunosuppression due to her disease and her impending therapy with prednisone. Malnutrition, immunosuppressed states, and stress are risk factors for primary progression or reactivation of quiescent tuberculosis. Various cutoff values are used, based on the patient's risk status, to increase the specificity of tuberculin skin test results. Three cut-points have been defined for a positive tuberculin reaction: 5 mm, 10 mm, and 15 mm of induration. An induration of 5 mm or more is considered positive in persons at highest risk of developing active tuberculosis (HIV-infected patients, immunosuppressed patients, persons with close contact with anyone with active tuberculosis, or those with a chest radiograph consistent with prior tuberculosis). This patient is immunosuppressed, and the 5-mm threshold for initiating therapy for latent tuberculosis applies to her. In addition, the American Thoracic Society recommends that patients who use prednisone (≥15 mg/d) or any other immunosuppressive agent and who have a 5 mm or larger area of induration on tuberculin skin testing begin prophylactic therapy with isoniazid.

An induration of 10 mm or more is considered positive in persons who have immigrated to the United States from high-risk countries within the past 5 years; injection drug users; prisoners; health care workers; and patients with silicosis, diabetes mellitus, chronic renal failure, leukemia or lymphoma, carcinoma of the head or neck or lung, recent significant weight loss, or a history of gastrectomy or jejunoileal bypass. Healthy adolescents who are exposed to adults in high-risk categories should also be screened using this 10-mm cut-off. A cut-off point of 15 mm is used for all low-risk persons.

Because this patient has no evidence of active tuberculosis, four-drug treatment for 1 year is not needed. The use of rifampin for the treatment of latent tuberculosis has not been extensively studied. Rifampin for 3 months seems to be as effective as longer treatment with isoniazid; one month of rifampin therapy is insufficient. No antituberculous therapy places the patient at risk for reactivation tuberculosis because of her immunosuppressed state and would not be appropriate.

KEY POINT

Prophylactic isoniazid therapy is beneficial in patients who use prednisone (≥15 mg/d) or any other immunosuppressive agent and who have 5 mm or more of induration on tuberculin skin testing.

Bibliography

Escalante P. In the clinic. Tuberculosis. Ann Intern Med. 2009;150:ITC61-614; quiz ITV616. Erratum in: Ann Intern Med. 2009;151:292. [PMID: 19487708]

Item 38   Answer: B

Educational Objective: *Treat latent tuberculosis with isoniazid prior to the administration of a tumor necrosis factor α (TNF-α) inhibitor.*

The most appropriate next step in this patient's management is to initiate isoniazid. Screening for latent tuberculosis is indicated in patients prior to solid organ transplant, initiation of chemotherapy or tumor necrosis factor α (TNF-α) inhibitors, or in the presence of other major immunocompromising conditions. Adverse effects of TNF-α inhibitors include the risk for serious infection. Infliximab, adalimumab, and etanercept are associated with an increased incidence of reactivation tuberculosis, particularly extrapulmonary tuberculosis. Therefore, all patients being considered for such therapy should undergo screening for latent tuberculosis infection, which includes a full medical history, physical examination, and tuberculin skin testing with purified protein derivative (PPD) or an interferon-γ release assay. If screening is positive, appropriate treatment for latent tuberculosis is indicated before beginning therapy with a TNF-α inhibitor. The Centers for Disease Control and Prevention recommend treatment of latent tuberculosis infection for all patients planning to take a TNF-α inhibitor who have a PPD result of 5 mm or more of induration or a positive interferon-γ release assay. Therefore, the most appropriate treatment for this patient is isoniazid for 9 months. Although the most appropriate duration of treatment with isoniazid before beginning infliximab is unknown, most experts recommend at least 2 months of isoniazid therapy before initiating a TNF-α inhibitor.

Four-drug antituberculous therapy is indicated for active tuberculosis when a patient's drug resistance status is unknown but is not appropriate for this patient, who has no evidence of active tuberculosis.

KEY POINT

The Centers for Disease Control and Prevention recommend treatment of latent tuberculosis infection for all patients planning to take a tumor necrosis factor α inhibitor who have a tuberculin skin test result of 5 mm or more of induration or a positive interferon γ release assay.

Bibliography

Bellofiore B, Matarese A, Balato N, Gaudiello F, Scarpa R, Atteno M, Bocchino M, Sanduzzi A. Prevention of tuberculosis in patients taking tumor necrosis factor-alpha blockers. J Rheumatol Suppl. 2009;83:76-7. [PMID: 19661550]

Item 39   Answer: B

Educational Objective: *Immunize a patient to prevent invasive pneumococcal disease.*

This patient should receive a repeat pneumococcal vaccination in 2 years. A one-time revaccination 5 years after the first dose is recommended for adults age 65 years and older who received their first dose for any indication when they were younger than age 65 years. This patient received his first pneumococcal vaccination when he was 62 years old after being hospitalized with respiratory failure due to severe pneumonia. The Centers for Disease Control and Prevention (CDC) also recommends one-time revaccination 5 years after the first dose for adults younger than age 65 years at highest risk for serious pneumococcal infection or who are likely to have a rapid decline in antibody levels. Persons at highest risk include adults with anatomic or functional asplenia (including sickle cell disease), HIV infection, leukemia, lymphoma, Hodgkin disease, multiple myeloma, generalized malignancy, chronic kidney disease, nephrotic syndrome, or other conditions associated with immunosuppression (such as organ or bone marrow transplantation), and those receiving immunosuppressive chemotherapy, including long-term corticosteroids.

Adults who receive pneumococcal vaccine at or after age 65 years should receive only a single dose. The pneumococcal vaccine is a polysaccharide vaccine that does not boost well, and data do not indicate that more than two doses are beneficial. Neither the CDC nor the Advisory Committee on Immunization Practices recommends an every-5-year schedule.

KEY POINT

Persons who received pneumococcal vaccine before age 65 years for any indication should receive another dose of the vaccine at age 65 years or later if at least 5 years have passed since their previous dose.

Bibliography

Centers for Disease Control and Prevention (CDC); Advisory Committee on Immunization Practices. Updated recommendations for prevention of invasive pneumococcal disease among adults using the 23-valent pneumococcal polysaccharide vaccine (PPSV23). MMWR Morb Mortal Wkly Rep. 2010;59(34):1102-6. [PMID: 20814406]

Item 40 Answer: C
Educational Objective: *Treat severe community-acquired pneumonia.*

The most appropriate empiric antibiotic therapy for this patient is cefotaxime, levofloxacin, and vancomycin. Methicillin-resistant *Staphylococcus aureus* (MRSA) should be suspected in persons with severe, rapidly progressive pneumonia, especially during influenza season; in those with cavitary infiltrates on the chest radiograph; or in those with a history of MRSA infection. Administering cefotaxime and levofloxacin for a patient who is admitted to the intensive care unit (ICU) with pneumonia and no risk factors for *Pseudomonas aeruginosa* infection (for example, bronchiectasis, corticosteroid or broad-spectrum antibiotic use in the previous month, malnutrition) is appropriate. However, if MRSA pneumonia is suspected, vancomycin or linezolid should be added to this empiric antibiotic regimen. Community-acquired MRSA pneumonia often affects young, otherwise healthy persons and can be rapidly fatal.

Empiric treatment with ceftriaxone and azithromycin or piperacillin-tazobactam for a patient with suspected MRSA pneumonia is not appropriate. The majority of community-acquired MRSA infections typically are resistant to beta-lactams and macrolides. Little information is available about the use of clindamycin for community-acquired MRSA pneumonia and vancomycin is preferred.

KEY POINT

Methicillin-resistant *Staphylococcus aureus* community-acquired pneumonia should be suspected in persons with severe, progressive pneumonia, especially during influenza season.

Bibliography

Centers for Disease Control and Prevention (CDC). Severe methicillin-resistant *Staphylococcus aureus* community-acquired pneumonia associated with influenza—Louisiana and Georgia, December 2006–January 2007. MMWR Morb Mortal Wkly Rep. 2007;56(14):325-9. [PMID: 17431376]

Item 41 Answer: C
Educational Objective: *Diagnose* Legionella *pneumophila pneumonia with* Legionella *urinary antigen.*

The test most likely to establish a diagnosis is the *Legionella* urinary antigen test. Risk factors for legionnaires disease include smoking, diabetes mellitus, hematologic malignancy, other types of cancer, chronic kidney disease, and HIV infection. Symptoms of *Legionella* pneumonia may include cough with nonproductive, mildly productive, or blood-streaked sputum and chest pain. Gastrointestinal symptoms are prominent and often include diarrhea, abdominal pain, nausea, and vomiting. Most patients are lethargic and have headache, and some may be obtunded. High fever is common, and an oral temperature greater than 40.0°C (104.0°F) is suggestive of legionnaires disease. Hyponatremia is found more often in patients with legionnaires disease than it is in patients with pneumonia from other causes.

The urinary antigen test has a sensitivity of 70% to 90% and a specificity of nearly 99% for detection of *L. pneumophila* serogroup 1; the urine is positive on day 1 of illness and continues to be positive for weeks. However, urinary antigen tests do not detect other *Legionella* species. Therefore, a negative test result cannot be used to exclude the diagnosis of *Legionella* pneumonia.

Legionella species would not be isolated from blood cultures or thoracentesis fluid. While blood cultures are generally warranted in patients hospitalized with pneumonia, a blood culture is unlikely to be diagnostic in this patient.

Most patients with pulmonary tuberculosis present with a subacute or chronic presentation of cough, weight loss, low-grade fever, mild systemic symptoms, and, possibly, blood-tinged sputum. The radiographic changes of reactivation tuberculosis include upper pulmonary lobe infiltrates, cavitation, and volume loss, and pleural effusions may be indicative of pleural tuberculosis. This patient's clinical presentation and radiographic findings are not consistent with tuberculosis; therefore acid-fast bacilli testing for tuberculosis would not be appropriate.

KEY POINT

Urinary antigen tests for detection of *Legionella pneumophila* serogroup 1 have a sensitivity of 70% to 90% and specificity of nearly 99%, but these tests do not detect other *Legionella* species; therefore, a negative test cannot be used to exclude the diagnosis of *Legionella* pneumonia.

Bibliography

Murdoch DR. Diagnosis of *Legionella* infection. Clin Infect Dis. 2003;36(1):64-69. [PMID: 12491204]

Item 42   Answer: A

Educational Objective: *Treat community-acquired pneumonia in a patient with no comorbidities with azithromycin.*

Oral azithromycin should be initiated. The most common pathogens identified from recent studies of patients with mild community-acquired pneumonia (CAP) were *Streptococcus pneumoniae*, *Mycoplasma pneumoniae*, and *Chlamydophila pneumoniae*. Macrolides have long been commonly prescribed for treatment of outpatients with CAP, and numerous randomized clinical trials have demonstrated the efficacy of clarithromycin or azithromycin as monotherapy. Erythromycin is a less expensive macrolide but not generally recommended owing to the need for more frequent dosing, more gastrointestinal upset, and lack of coverage for *Haemophilus influenzae*.

The use of fluoroquinolones to treat ambulatory patients with CAP without comorbidities is discouraged because of the concern that widespread use would lead to the development of resistance.

Penicillin would not be effective in treating *M. pneumoniae* or *C. pneumoniae* and is therefore not appropriate in this patient.

Influenza virus symptoms typically consist of fever (usually high), headache, extreme fatigue, nonproductive cough, sore throat, nasal congestion, rhinorrhea, myalgia, and, occasionally, gastrointestinal symptoms, with most cases of influenza occurring from November through April in the Northern Hemisphere. Because the patient's symptoms and findings are more consistent with CAP than influenza virus infection, antiviral therapy with zanamivir is not indicated.

KEY POINT

Clarithromycin or azithromycin are recommended for treatment of mild community-acquired pneumonia.

Bibliography
Niederman M. In the clinic. Community-acquired pneumonia. Ann Intern Med. 2009;151(7):ITC4-2-ITC4-14; quiz ITC4-16. [PMID: 19805767]

Item 43   Answer: A

Educational Objective: *Treat a patient with lung abscess following aspiration with ampicillin-sulbactam.*

This patient should receive ampicillin-sulbactam. She has a history of alcohol abuse and alcohol-withdrawal seizures, which puts her at risk for aspiration pneumonia. She now presents with a lung abscess, characterized radiologically by a cavity with an air-fluid level, which probably occurred as a complication of aspiration pneumonia. Lung abscesses are polymicrobial infections caused by anaerobic bacteria that are normally present in the mouth; micro-aerophilic streptococci, viridans streptococci, and gram-negative enteric pathogens

have also been implicated. In studies using sample techniques that avoid oral contamination, anaerobes are found in about 90% of patients with lung abscess and are the only organisms isolated in about half. Possible anaerobes in patients with lung abscess as a complication of aspiration pneumonia include *Peptostreptococcus* species, *Fusobacterium nucleatum*, *Prevotella melaninogenica*, and *Bacteroides* species (including *B. fragilis*). Of the choices listed, only ampicillin-sulbactam would have a broad enough spectrum to cover the likely pathogens.

Of the other antimicrobial choices, levofloxacin and aztreonam would not be effective in treating oral anaerobes, and ceftriaxone would be effective in treating some oral anaerobic species but not β-lactamase–producing strains.

Although metronidazole is highly active in vitro against most anaerobes, it is not active against micro-aerophilic streptococci and some anaerobic cocci.

KEY POINT

Patients with lung abscess as a complication of aspiration pneumonia require treatment with an antimicrobial agent effective against β-lactamase–producing strains of oral anaerobes, such as ampicillin-sulbactam.

Bibliography
Niederman M. In the clinic. Community-acquired pneumonia. Ann Intern Med. 2009;151(7):ITC4-2-ITC4-14; quiz ITC4-16. [PMID: 19805767]

Item 44   Answer: E

Educational Objective: *Appropriately withhold infective endocarditis prophylaxis in a patient with a heart murmur associated with a native valve abnormality.*

This patient does not require antibiotic prophylaxis prior to his dental procedure. Evidence is clear that bacteremia resulting from normal, daily activities is much more likely to cause infective endocarditis than bacteremia associated with dental procedures, and that only an extremely small number of cases of infective endocarditis are prevented by prophylaxis. Therefore, antibiotic prophylaxis is now recommended only for patients with underlying conditions associated with the highest risk of adverse outcome from infective endocarditis, including patients with:

- Prosthetic cardiac valves
- History of prior infective endocarditis
- Unrepaired cyanotic congenital heart disease
- Completely repaired congenital heart disease for 6 months following repair
- Repaired congenital heart disease with residual defects or abnormalities
- Cardiac transplantation recipients with cardiac valvulopathy

This patient meets none of the criteria for antibiotic prophylaxis.

Antibiotic prophylaxis to prevent infective endocarditis is now recommended only for patients with underlying conditions associated with the highest risk of adverse outcome from infective endocarditis; this does not include heart murmurs associated with native valve abnormalities.

Bibliography

Duval X, Leport C. Prophylaxis of infective endocarditis: current tendencies, continuing controversies. Lancet Infect Dis. 2008;8(4):225-32. [PMID: 18353264]

Item 45   Answer: D

Educational Objective: *Provide infective endocarditis prophylaxis in a patient who is allergic to penicillin.*

The most appropriate endocarditis prophylaxis for this patient is oral clindamycin. Antibiotic prophylaxis is recommended before certain dental procedures (i.e., those involving perforation of the oral mucosa or manipulation of the periapical region of the teeth or gingival tissue) for patients with underlying conditions associated with the highest risk of adverse outcome from infective endocarditis. These patients include those with:

- Prosthetic cardiac valves
- History of prior infective endocarditis
- Unrepaired cyanotic congenital heart disease
- Completely repaired congenital heart disease for 6 months following repair
- Repaired congenital heart disease with residual defects or abnormalities
- Cardiac transplantation recipients with cardiac valvulopathy

The organisms associated with the development of infective endocarditis in this setting are viridans streptococci. For the non–penicillin-allergic patient, oral amoxicillin is the recommended prophylactic regimen administered 30 to 60 minutes before the procedure. In patients unable to take oral medications, ampicillin, cefazolin, or ceftriaxone intramuscularly or intravenously is recommended. This patient, however, has a history of anaphylaxis to penicillin; therefore, oral clindamycin, azithromycin, or clarithromycin is recommended.

Oral clindamycin, azithromycin, or clarithromycin is recommended for infective endocarditis prophylaxis in penicillin-allergic patients.

Bibliography

Nishimura RA, Carabello BA, Faxon DP, et al; American College of Cardiology/American Heart Association Task Force. ACC/AHA 2008 guideline update on valvular heart disease: focused update on infective endocarditis: a report of the American College of Cardiology/American Heart Association Task Force on Practice Guidelines: endorsed by the Society of Cardiovascular Anesthesiologists, Society for Cardiovascular Angiography and Interventions, and Society of Thoracic Surgeons. Circulation. 2008;118(8):887-96. [PMID: 18663090]

Item 46   Answer: E

Educational Objective: *Treat an injection drug user with tricuspid valve endocarditis and multilobar pneumonia with vancomycin plus cefepime.*

The best initial treatment for this patient is vancomycin plus cefepime. He most likely has tricuspid valve endocarditis as suggested by the right sternal border systolic murmur that increases with inspiration. He has developed septic pulmonary emboli to both lung fields leading to multilobar pneumonia. Septic pulmonary emboli are common in tricuspid endocarditis, occurring in up to 75% of patients. In this instance, the most likely infecting organism is *Staphylococcus aureus*, and treatment of a possible methicillin-resistant strain must be initiated pending culture and in vitro susceptibility results. Vancomycin plus cefepime provides appropriate coverage for endocarditis caused by *S. aureus*, gram-negative bacilli (for example, *Pseudomonas aeruginosa*), and other likely infectious causes of pneumonia, especially *Streptococcus pneumoniae*.

Azithromycin plus ceftriaxone, levofloxacin plus clindamycin, and piperacillin/tazobactam plus aztreonam do not provide appropriate coverage for methicillin-resistant *S. aureus* and are therefore not appropriate for this patient. Although trimethoprim-sulfamethoxazole plus prednisone would treat *Pneumocystis jirovecii* pneumonia, such a diagnosis is unlikely in this patient given his clinical presentation. In HIV-infected patients, *Pneumocystis* pneumonia typically has a subacute onset of cough, fever, and dyspnea. The most common radiographic abnormalities are diffuse, bilateral, interstitial infiltrates. This patient's acute onset of symptoms, multilobar pneumonia, and presence of a heart murmur are not compatible with *Pneumocystis* pneumonia.

Treatment for septic pulmonary emboli from an infected tricuspid valve in an injection drug user should include empiric therapy for methicillin-resistant *Staphylococcus aureus,* such as vancomycin plus cefepime.

Bibliography

Chambers HF, Korzeniowski OM, Sande MA. Staphylococcus aureus endocarditis: clinical manifestations in addicts and nonaddicts. Medicine (Baltimore). 1983;62(3):170-177. [PMID: 6843356]

Item 47   Answer: A

Educational Objective: *Diagnose and treat native valve endocarditis.*

The patient meets all three major clinical criteria for definite endocarditis. He has a typical microorganism grown on two blood cultures, echocardiographic evidence of endocardial involvement (an oscillating intracardiac mass), and a new valvular regurgitation murmur. His history also suggests endocarditis (several months of fever, fatigue and muscle aches). Also supporting the diagnosis are the presence of a bicuspid aortic valve, fever, and conjunctival hemorrhage, which fulfill three of the minor clinical criteria for endocarditis.

Endocarditis due to sensitive viridans streptococci on native valves can be treated for 4 weeks with penicillin or ceftriaxone or for 2 weeks when either agent is combined with synergistic low-dose gentamicin. In a patient with uncomplicated endocarditis, the addition of gentamicin decreases the total treatment course from 4 weeks to 2 weeks.

In the absence of penicillin allergy or penicillin resistance, vancomycin is inappropriate.

Endocarditis due to penicillin-sensitive viridans streptococci on native valves can be treated for 4 weeks with penicillin or ceftriaxone or for 2 weeks when either agent is combined with synergistic low-dose gentamicin.

Bibliography

Beynon RP, Bahl VK, Prendergast BD. Infective endocarditis. BMJ. 2006;333:334-9. [PMID: 16902214]

Item 48   Answer: D

Educational Objective: *Treat methicillin-susceptible* Staphylococcus aureus *right-sided endocarditis with oxacillin.*

The most appropriate treatment as this time is oxacillin. She has bacteremia most likely resulting from right-sided endocarditis. Treatment requires using the most effective drug with the fewest side effects, and vancomycin should therefore be changed to oxacillin. Penicillins have never been shown to be less effective than other antibiotics for treating susceptible strains of *Staphylococcus aureus*, their safety profile is well documented, and they are reasonably inexpensive. In the rare setting in which an isolate of *S. aureus* is susceptible to penicillin G, this would be the drug of choice.

Both vancomycin and daptomycin have been used to treat *S. aureus* bacteremia and endocarditis. Although both are effective for treating methicillin-resistant *S. aureus* (MRSA) strains, they show no clinical superiority for treating methicillin-susceptible *S. aureus* (MSSA). Patients with MSSA infections appear to have a slower response to vancomycin than to the semisynthetic penicillins such as oxacillin or to the cephalosporins, and this accounts for the preference of β-lactam versus vancomycin therapy in patients with MSSA.

Clindamycin may be effective in vitro; however, the failure rate is higher for clindamycin than for other drugs used to treat endocarditis, presumably owing to its bacteriostatic, rather than bactericidal, activity for many strains of susceptible *S. aureus*.

Linezolid has been used with some success and some failure in patients with staphylococcal bacteremia. Because of concerns about its efficacy, it is usually reserved for patients who do not respond to first-line therapy.

Synthetic penicillins, such as oxacillin and nafcillin, are appropriate for treating patients with methicillin-susceptible *Staphylococcus aureus* bacteremia and endocarditis.

Bibliography

Fowler VG Jr., Boucher HW, Corey GR, et al; The S. aureus Endocarditis and Bacteremia Study Group. Daptomycin versus standard therapy for bacteremia and endocarditis caused by Staphylococcus aureus. N Engl J Med. 2006;355(7):653-665. [PMID: 16914701]

Item 49   Answer: D

Educational Objective: *Diagnose osteomyelitis of the foot in a patient with diabetes with a bone biopsy.*

The most appropriate management is to perform a bone biopsy. Contact with bone (when using a sterile, blunt, stainless steel probe) in the depth of an infected pedal ulcer in patients with diabetes mellitus is strongly correlated with the presence of underlying osteomyelitis, with a positive predictive value of 90%. Patients with diabetes require bone biopsy to obtain deep pathogens, identification of which is the only way to establish a definitive diagnosis and guide therapy. Although it may seem intuitive that drainage from a superficial site such as an ulcer or a sinus tract would contain the causative pathogens, superficial cultures usually do not include the deep organisms responsible for the infection. Failure to identify the causative deep-bone pathogens may lead to spread of infection to adjacent bones or soft tissues and the need for extensive débridement or amputation. The one exception is *Staphylococcus aureus*, which, if found in superficial cultures, correlates well with findings on deep cultures.

This patient appears well enough to wait for the bone biopsy to be completed before starting empiric antibiotic therapy and adjusting the antibiotics based on culture results. Empiric therapy should include activity against streptococci, methicillin-resistant *S. aureus* (MRSA), aerobic gram-negative bacilli, and anaerobes. Therapy with imipenem alone will not adequately cover MRSA, vancomycin and ceftazidime will not adequately cover anaerobic bacteria, and vancomycin and metronidazole will not adequately cover gram-negative organisms.

Cultures obtained from a sinus tract or ulcer base often do not reflect the bacterial etiology of an underlying osteomyelitis; bone biopsy is indicated to identify the causative pathogens and guide antibiotic therapy.

Bibliography

Butalia S, Palda VA, Sargeant RJ, Detsky AS, Mourad O. Does this patient with diabetes have osteomyelitis of the lower extremity? JAMA. 2008;299(7):806-13. [PMID: 18285592]

Item 50   Answer: B
Educational Objective: *Evaluate a patient with vertebral osteomyelitis with a spine MRI.*

The next management step is MRI of the lumbar spine. Vertebral osteomyelitis is an infection of the spine that must be considered in any patient with new-onset back pain and fever. Patients with acute hematogenous osteomyelitis are more likely to present with acute pain and fever than are patients with chronic contiguous osteomyelitis (for example, foot ulcer–associated osteomyelitis). In adults, hematogenous osteomyelitis most often involves the intervertebral disk space and two adjacent vertebrae. Potential sources of hematogenous infection include the genitourinary tract (particularly following instrumentation), skin (injection drug use), infected intravascular devices (for example, a central venous catheter), and endocarditis, but often, the source of the infection cannot be identified. In patients with hematogenous osteomyelitis, the leukocyte count is typically normal, but the erythrocyte sedimentation rate is elevated in 80% to 90% of patients and is often greater than 100 mm/h.

MRI is the most appropriate imaging study for patients with suspected vertebral osteomyelitis and is a more sensitive study than CT scans or plain radiographs. In addition, MRI can detect an epidural abscess or a paravertebral or psoas abscess that may require surgical drainage. If MRI cannot be performed (for example, in patients with pacemakers or metal prosthetic devices) or if results are inconclusive, a gallium nuclear study is very sensitive and specific in this setting.

Three-phase bone scintigraphy using labeled technetium can occasionally be helpful in diagnosing osteomyelitis, but it is associated with false-positive results in patients with other causes of back pain, including fracture, as well as false-negative results if the infection is early. Three-phase bone scintigraphy is an inferior diagnostic test compared to MRI scanning but may be appropriate when the initial MRI imaging result is indeterminate.

KEY POINT
The diagnosis of vertebral osteomyelitis must be considered in any patient who presents with new-onset back pain and fever.

Bibliography
Zimmerli W. Clinical practice. Vertebral osteomyelitis. N Engl J Med. 2010;362(11):1022-9. [PMID: 20237348]

Item 51   Answer: C
Educational Objective: *Evaluate possible osteomyelitis with MRI.*

MRI is the preferred imaging study for patients such as this one with foot infection. Foot infections are a significant cause of morbidity in patients with diabetes mellitus and, if untreated, can progress to osteomyelitis that may require amputation for cure. Appropriate assessment of diabetic foot infections is therefore essential. Unless bone is visible, physical examination findings are often inconclusive for diagnosing osteomyelitis. Plain radiographs are insensitive and may show soft tissue swelling but no bony abnormalities for 2 or more weeks after infection has developed. In addition, this patient had a negative metal-probe test (a positive test has a predictive value of 90% for diagnosing osteomyelitis). Although her ulcer is limited to the plantar surface, the cellulitis is more diffuse, which implies a more extensive process requiring rapid assessment and treatment.

A CT scan is neither as sensitive nor specific as MRI and is indicated only when MRI cannot be performed (for example, in patients with pacemakers or metal prosthetic devices). Indium-labeled leukocyte scan and triple-phase technetium bone scan are very sensitive but not specific for diagnosing osteomyelitis and are associated with high false-positive rates, especially when an overlying cellulitis or soft tissue infection is present.

KEY POINT
MRI is the most sensitive and specific study for diagnosing foot infection–associated osteomyelitis.

Bibliography
Butalia S, Palda VA, Sargeant RJ, Detsky AS, Mourad O. Does this patient with diabetes have osteomyelitis of the lower extremity? JAMA. 2008;299(7):806-13. [PMID: 18285592]

Item 52   Answer: C
Educational Objective: *Diagnose the cause of vertebral osteomyelitis with blood cultures.*

Blood cultures are the most appropriate next step. In a patient with suspected vertebral osteomyelitis, a microbiologic diagnosis must be established to guide antibiotic therapy. Because the infection is often hematogenous, blood cultures should be obtained initially in all patients. Cultures are positive in up to 75% of patients, and identification of *Staphylococcus aureus*, which is the most frequent cause of vertebral osteomyelitis, may obviate the need for a bone biopsy. However, if the imaging studies suggest vertebral osteomyelitis but the blood cultures are negative, CT-guided percutaneous needle biopsy should be performed. Because this procedure is only about 50% sensitive, antibiotics should be withheld until a microbiologic diagnosis is made.

Empiric ceftriaxone will provide adequate coverage for most gram-negative and streptococcal organisms responsible for vertebral osteomyelitis but will provide no coverage for methicillin-resistant *S. aureus* (MRSA). Starting empiric nafcillin would be a good choice if the infective organism were a susceptible staphylococcus; however, nafcillin will not adequately cover infections caused by MRSA or gram-negative organisms.

KEY POINT
Blood cultures are positive in 75% of patients with vertebral osteomyelitis.

Bibliography
Zimmerli W. Clinical practice. Vertebral osteomyelitis. N Engl J Med. 2010;362(11):1022-9. [PMID: 20237348]

Section 7

Nephrology
Questions

Item 1 [Advanced]

A 19-year-old man is evaluated for proteinuria discovered during a routine sports preparticipation evaluation. He has been asymptomatic, has no other medical problems, and takes no medications.

On physical examination, temperature is 36.6°C (97.8°F) blood pressure is 110/72 mm Hg, pulse rate is 60/min, and respiration rate is 12/min. BMI is 18. The funduscopic, cardiopulmonary, and skin findings are normal. No peripheral edema is present.

Hemoglobin	15 mg/dL (150 g/L)
Albumin	4.1 g/dL (41 g/L)
Total cholesterol	130 mg/dL (3.4 mmol/L)
Creatinine	0.7 mg/dL (61.9 µmol/L)
Glucose	92 mg/dL (5.1 mmol/L)
Total protein	6.5 g/dL (65 g/L)
Spot urine protein–creatinine ratio	0.8 mg/mg
Urinalysis	Urine dipstick: protein, 2+; blood, negative; glucose, negative. Microscopic: rare hyaline cast, no cells or crystals.

Which of the following is the most appropriate next diagnostic test?

(A) 24-Hour urine protein excretion
(B) Evaluate for orthostatic proteinuria
(C) Kidney biopsy
(D) Protein electrophoresis of the serum and urine

Item 2 [Advanced]

A 62-year-old woman is evaluated for acute oliguric renal failure. She was admitted to the hospital 7 days ago for sepsis due to methicillin-sensitive *Staphylococcus aureus*; intravenous cefazolin was begun and she quickly improved. Today, her urine output is 10 mL/h.

On physical examination, temperature is 37.5°C (99.5°F), blood pressure is 138/88 mm Hg, pulse rate is 78/min, and respiration rate is 12/min. A macular erythematous rash is present over her anterior chest and abdomen. The remainder of the physical examination is normal.

	Day 1	Day 7
Blood urea nitrogen	8 mg/dL (2.9 mmol/L)	20 mg/dL (7.1 mmol/L)
Creatinine	0.6 mg/dL (53.0 µmol/L)	1.8 mg/dL (159.1 µmol/L)
Urinalysis	Normal	Dipstick: pH, 5; protein, 1+; blood, negative. Microscopic: 15-20 white blood cells per high power field; many leukocyte casts
Urine culture		No growth

Renal ultrasonography shows normal kidney size without hydronephrosis.

Which of the following is the most likely diagnosis?

(A) Acute interstitial nephritis
(B) Acute tubular necrosis
(C) Cholesterol crystal embolization
(D) Prerenal azotemia

Item 3 [Advanced]

A 65-year-old man comes for a follow-up office visit. Three weeks ago, he was admitted to the hospital for deep venous thrombosis of the left leg. He was treated with low-molecular-weight heparin followed by warfarin. He takes no other medications. He has a 30-pack-year history of cigarette smoking and currently smokes two packs of cigarettes daily.

Vital signs and physical examination are normal.

Urinalysis 3 weeks ago revealed trace protein and 1+ blood.

Laboratory studies obtained today:

INR	3.0
Serum creatinine	1.4 mg/dL (123.8 µmol/L)
Urinalysis	Specific gravity 1.015; no protein; 1+ blood; 5-10 non-dysmorphic erythrocytes/hpf; no casts

On kidney ultrasound, the right kidney is 10.4 cm and the left kidney is 9.0 cm. No masses, cysts, or stones are identified.

Which of the following is the most appropriate next management step?

(A) Cystoscopy
(B) Discontinuation of warfarin
(C) Kidney biopsy
(D) Repeat urinalysis in 3 months

Item 4 [Basic]

An 18-year-old man is evaluated in the emergency department after his mother found him unconscious in his bed at home. She reported that her son had gone to a party 24 hours ago, but she was not sure when he returned home. When she checked on him, he was unarousable. He has no significant medical history and takes no medications.

In the emergency department, he is afebrile, blood pressure is 110/70 mm Hg, pulse rate is 50/min, and respiration rate is 6/min; he is intubated.

Creatinine	3.2 mg/dL (282.9 µmol/L)
Aspartate aminotransferase	80 U/L
Alanine aminotransferase	46 U/L
Creatine kinase	18,400 U/L
INR	1.2

Complete blood count, alkaline phosphatase, bilirubin, and albumin are normal. Urine dipstick is 4+ positive for occult blood, negative for erythrocytes. Blood alcohol level is 0.8 g/dL (174 mmol/L). Toxicology testing is positive for opiates and cocaine. Bladder catheterization reveals only 30 mL of brown urine.

Which of the following is the most likely cause of the acute kidney injury?

(A) Hemolytic anemia
(B) Hemolytic-uremic syndrome
(C) Hepatorenal syndrome
(D) Rhabdomyolysis

Item 5 [Advanced]

A 72-year-old man is evaluated in the emergency department for a 2-day history of suprapubic abdominal pain. He has had difficulty urinating for the last 6 months, including urinary frequency and difficulty starting his urinary stream. He has nocturia four to five times per night. Medical history is otherwise nonsignificant, and he takes no medications.

On physical examination, the patient is uncomfortable. Temperature is 37.0°C (98.6°F), blood pressure is 162/90 mm Hg, pulse rate is 92/min, and respiration rate is 12/min. Suprapubic fullness to palpation is noted.

Blood urea nitrogen	30 mg/dL (10.7 mmol/L)
Creatinine	2.2 mg/dL (194.5 µmol/L)
Electrolytes	
Sodium	136 meq/L (136 mmol/L)
Potassium	5.2 meq/L (5.2 mmol/L)
Chloride	100 meq/L (100 mmol/L)
Carbon dioxide	20 meq/L (20 mmol/L)

Which of the following is the best diagnostic test for this patient?

(A) Kidney arteriography
(B) Kidney biopsy
(C) Kidney ultrasound
(D) Urine dipstick for protein

Item 6 [Advanced]

A 21-year-old woman is evaluated in the emergency department for a 2-day history of abdominal pain and bloody diarrhea. Before this episode she was healthy, and she takes no medications.

On physical examination, she appears ill and pale; temperature is 38.5°C (101.3°F), blood pressure is 97/70 mm Hg, pulse rate is 120/min, and respiration rate is 16/min. Bowel sounds are hyperactive, and the abdomen is tender without guarding. The remainder of the examination is normal.

Hematocrit	27%
Platelet count	42,000/µL (42 × 10⁹/L)
Blood urea nitrogen	42 mg/dL (15.0 mmol/L)
Creatinine	3.2 mg/dL (283 µmol/L)
Lactate dehydrogenase	1124 U/L
Urinalysis (microscopic and dipstick)	Normal

The peripheral blood smear reveals schistocytes.

Which of the following is the most likely diagnosis?

(A) Acute interstitial nephritis
(B) Acute tubular necrosis
(C) Hemolytic uremic syndrome
(D) Rhabdomyolysis

Item 7 [Basic]

A 29-year-old woman comes for a follow-up office visit. Six months ago, she underwent double-lung transplantation for cystic fibrosis. She was diagnosed with *Pseudomonas* bronchitis 14 days ago and began oral ciprofloxacin and intravenous tobramycin at that time. Today, she states that her cough has resolved, she has not had fever, and she feels well. Additional medications are acyclovir, mycophenolate mofetil, prednisone, tacrolimus, and trimethoprim-sulfamethoxazole.

On physical examination, temperature is 36.6°C (97.8°F), blood pressure is 132/80 mm Hg, pulse rate is 90/min, and respiration rate is 18/min. Cardiopulmonary examination is normal. Cutaneous examination is normal. There is no asterixis. There is no edema.

Hemoglobin	12.0 g/dL (120 g/L)
Leukocyte count	8400/µL (8.4 × 10⁹/L)
Platelet count	335,000/µL (335 × 10⁹/L)
Serum creatinine	2.3 mg/dL (203.3 µmol/L) (1.2 mg/dL [106.1 µmol/L] 6 weeks ago)
Urinalysis	Specific gravity 1.011; pH 5.5; 1+ protein; no blood; 2-5 erythrocytes/hpf; no leukocyte esterase

Urine sediment findings are shown.

Kidney ultrasound shows normal-sized kidneys and no hydronephrosis.

Which of the following is the most likely cause of this patient's findings?

(A) Acute interstitial nephritis
(B) Acute tubular necrosis
(C) Thrombotic thrombocytopenic purpura
(D) Urinary tract obstruction

Item 8 [Basic]

A 56-year-old woman is evaluated for a 1-week history of right upper-quadrant abdominal pain, anorexia, nausea, and vomiting and a 3-day history of increasing lethargy and weakness. She also has dark-colored urine and a decreased urine output. One year ago, she was diagnosed with stage IV breast cancer treated with mastectomy and hormonal and chemotherapy. Current medications are tamoxifen and trastuzumab.

On physical examination, temperature is normal, blood pressure is 90/50 mm Hg, pulse rate is 100/min, and respiration rate is 18/min. Cardiopulmonary examination is normal. The mucous membranes are dry. Abdominal examination reveals hepatomegaly. There is no edema.

Sodium	124 meq/L (124 mmol/L)
Potassium	5.7 meq/L (5.7 mmol/L)
Chloride	94 meq/L (94 mmol/L)
Bicarbonate	12 meq/L (12 mmol/L)
Uric acid	9.2 mg/dL (0.54 mmol/L)
Phosphorus	5.8 mg/dL (1.9 mmol/L)
Calcium	10.1 mg/dL (2.5 mmol/L)
Blood urea nitrogen	105 mg/dL (37.5 mmol/L)
Serum creatinine	5 mg/dL (442 µmol/L) (1 mg/dL [88.4 µmol/L] 1 month ago)
Urinalysis	Specific gravity 1.022; pH 5; trace protein; rare amorphous crystals
Urine sodium excretion	4 meq/L (4 mmol/L)

On abdominal ultrasound, the right kidney is 9.6 cm and the left kidney is 9.1 cm. There is no hydronephrosis, and no renal calculi or focal solid masses are seen. There is hepatomegaly with multiple liver metastases.

Which of the following is the most appropriate next management step?

(A) Dialysis
(B) Isotonic saline
(C) Midodrine and octreotide
(D) Rasburicase

Item 9 [Basic]

A 65-year-old man with a history of stage 4 chronic kidney disease and hypertension comes for a follow-up examination. Two days ago, he was discharged from the hospital after a 4-day stay for pneumonia. During his hospitalization, his blood pressure averaged 130/70 mm Hg and he was not exposed to radiocontrast agents. He was treated with ceftriaxone and azithromycin; on discharge, these agents were discontinued and he began oral levofloxacin. Since his discharge, he has had nausea, vomiting, and anorexia. He believes that his urine output over the past day has been less than 500 mL. Additional medications are lisinopril, calcium carbonate, and low-dose aspirin.

On physical examination, temperature is 35.8°C (96.4°F), blood pressure is 110/50 mm Hg standing and 100/80 mm Hg supine, pulse rate is 108/min standing and 96/min

supine, and respiration rate is 16/min. The remainder of the examination is normal except for crackles heard at the base of the lungs bilaterally.

Serum creatinine	6.0 mg/dL (530.4 µmol/L) (2.5 mg/dL [221.0 µmol/L] in the hospital)
Urinalysis	Specific gravity 1.016; no protein or blood; occasional hyaline casts

Which of the following is the most likely cause of this patient's acute kidney injury?

(A) Acute interstitial nephritis
(B) Acute tubular necrosis
(C) Prerenal azotemia
(D) Renal vein thrombosis

Item 10 [Basic]

A 55-year-old man with a 15-year history of type 2 diabetes mellitus and hypertension is evaluated during a new-patient visit. He reports no symptoms other than ankle edema. A review of his medical records documents the presence of microalbuminuria 5 years ago. His medications are amlodipine, chlorthalidone, simvastatin, metformin, and glargine insulin.

On physical examination, temperature is 37.1°C (97.8°F), blood pressure is 150/95 mm Hg, pulse is 80/min, and respiration rate is 12/min. Cardiopulmonary examination is normal. He has trace pretibial edema.

Potassium	4.2 meq/L (4.2 mmol/L)
Creatinine	1.8 mg/dL (186 µmol/L)
Urine protein-creatinine ratio	1 mg/mg

The patient is prescribed losartan 25 mg/d. He returns in 3 weeks for a repeat blood pressure check. The average of two blood pressure recordings is 145/88 mm Hg. The serum potassium level is 4.4 meq/L (4.4 mmol/L) and the serum creatinine level is 2.0 mg/dL (177 µmol/L).

Which of the following is the most appropriate next step in this patient's management?

(A) Add lisinopril
(B) Discontinue losartan
(C) Increase the dose of losartan
(D) Schedule a renal biopsy

Item 11 [Advanced]

A 60-year-old man is evaluated during follow-up for chronic kidney disease secondary to autosomal dominant polycystic kidney disease. He reports no chest pain, dyspnea, changes in his mental status, or excessive sleepiness. He has no anorexia, nausea, vomiting, weight loss, or itching. His medications are lisinopril, furosemide, low-dose aspirin, calcitriol, sevelamer, and ferrous sulfate. He has several family members who are being evaluated as potential kidney donors. Estimated glomerular filtration rate (GFR) 2 months ago was 18 mL/min/1.73 m²

On physical examination, he is mentally alert. Temperature is 37.0°C (98.7°F), blood pressure is 125/75 mm Hg, pulse rate is 75/min, and respiration rate is 14/min. Cardiac rhythm is normal without murmurs, extra sounds, or rubs. The estimated central venous pressure is 8 cm H_2O. The lungs are clear to auscultation. His abdominal examination is significant for large, nontender bilateral flank masses. No bleeding, ecchymosis, or petechiae is evident. He scores 29/30 on the Mini–Mental State Examination and no asterixis is evident. He has 1+ pretibial edema.

Hemoglobin	13.0 g/dL (130 g/L)
Albumin	3.9 g/dL (39 g/L)
Blood urea nitrogen	60 mg/dL (21.4 mmol/L)
Calcium	8.4 mg/dL (2.1 mmol/L)
Creatinine	4.9 mg/dL (433.1 micromol/L)
Electrolytes	
Sodium	140 meq/L (140 mmol/L)
Potassium	5.3 meq/L (5.3 mmol/L)
Chloride	100 meq/L (100 mmol/L)
Carbon dioxide	21 meq/L (21 mmol/L)
Phosphorus	5.2 mg/dL (1.7 mmol/L)
Estimated GFR	13 mL/min/1.73 m^2

Which of the following is the most appropriate next step in the management of this patient's disease?

(A) Initiation of dialysis
(B) Increase the dose of lisinopril
(C) Ultrasonography of the abdomen
(D) No change in management

Item 12 [Advanced]

A 35-year-old woman is evaluated for a 1-month history of progressive bilateral lower-extremity edema. She was diagnosed with type 1 diabetes mellitus 10 years ago. At her last office visit 4 months ago, the urine albumin-creatinine ratio was 40 mg/g. Medications are enalapril, insulin glargine, insulin aspart, and low-dose aspirin.

On physical examination, vital signs are normal except for a blood pressure of 162/90 mm Hg (baseline 130/70 mm Hg). Cardiopulmonary and funduscopic examinations are normal. There is 3+ pitting edema of the lower extremities to the level of the thighs bilaterally.

Hemoglobin A$_{1c}$	6.8%
Albumin	3 g/dL (30 g/L)
Serum creatinine	1.1 mg/dL (97.2 μmol/L)
Urinalysis	3+ protein; 2+ blood; 8-10 dysmorphic erythrocytes/hpf; 2-5 leukocytes/hpf; few erythrocyte casts
Urine protein-creatinine ratio	5.2 mg/mg

On kidney ultrasound, the right kidney is 12.2 cm and the left kidney is 12.7 cm. There is no hydronephrosis, and no kidney masses are seen.

Which of the following is the most appropriate next step in this patient's management?

(A) Cystoscopy
(B) Kidney biopsy
(C) Spiral CT of the abdomen and pelvis
(D) Observation

Item 13 [Advanced]

A 33-year-old woman comes for follow-up examination for a left fibula fracture due to a fall 1 week ago. She has hypertension and stage 5 chronic kidney disease treated with home hemodialysis. Medications are lisinopril, sevelamer, epoetin alfa, paricalcitol, and multivitamins.

On physical examination, temperature is normal, blood pressure is 130/70 mm Hg, pulse rate is 88/min, and respiration rate is 12/min. BMI is 29. Cardiopulmonary examination is normal. An arteriovenous fistula is present in the left forearm. Except for a cast on her left leg, musculoskeletal examination is normal and reveals no bone pain.

Hemoglobin	10.3 g/dL (103 g/L)
Albumin	3.5 g/dL (35 g/L)
Phosphorus	5.8 mg/dL (1.9 mmol/L)
Calcium	8.4 mg/dL (2.1 mmol/L)
Parathyroid hormone	700 pg/mL (700 ng/L)
Alkaline phosphatase	330 U/L

Which of the following is the most likely cause of this patient's bone disease?

(A) Adynamic bone disease
(B) Osteonecrosis
(C) Osteoporosis
(D) Secondary hyperparathyroidism

Item 14 [Advanced]

A 55-year-old woman is found in an alleyway by paramedics. She is obtunded, hypotensive and tachycardic. Her breath smells of alcohol.

Electrolytes	
Sodium	135 meq/L (135 mmol/L)
Chloride	92 meq/L (92 mmol/L)
Potassium	3.8 meq/L (3.8 mmol/L)
Carbon dioxide	12 meq/L (12 mmol/L)
Blood gases	
pH	7.08
Pco$_2$	42 mm Hg (5.6 kPa)

Which of the following acid-base disorders is most likely present?

(A) Metabolic acidosis, metabolic alkalosis, and respiratory acidosis
(B) Metabolic acidosis and respiratory alkalosis
(C) Metabolic alkalosis and respiratory acidosis
(D) Respiratory acidosis and metabolic acidosis
(E) Simple metabolic acidosis

Item 15 [Advanced]

A 40-year-old woman is evaluated in the hospital for metabolic acidosis.

Arterial blood gases
pH	7.30
P_{CO_2}	36 mm Hg (4.8 kPa)

Electrolytes
Sodium	140 meq/L (140 mmol/L)
Potassium	3.0 meq/L (3 mmol/L)
Chloride	113 meq/L (113 mmol/L)
Carbon dioxide	17 meq/L (17 mmol/L)

Urine electrolytes
Sodium	40 meq/L (40 mmol/L)
Potassium	10 meq/L (10 mmol/L)
Chloride	30 meq/L (30 mmol/L)

Which of the following is the most likely cause of this patient's acid-base disorder?

(A) Diabetic ketoacidosis
(B) Renal tubular acidosis
(C) Laxative abuse
(D) Viral gastroenteritis

Item 16 [Basic]

A 61-year-old man is evaluated in the emergency department because of a 3-day history of cough productive of yellow sputum. He has chronic obstructive pulmonary disease and he routinely uses supplemental oxygen, 2 L/min. He states that he is now short of breath at rest.

Physical examination shows that he is using accessory muscles of respiration and pursed-lipped breathing. He has prolonged expiratory-to-inspiratory phase on exhalation and scattered wheezes. He has tachycardia and bilateral pitting edema of the extremities.

His oxygen saturation is 91% on supplemental oxygen. Chest radiograph shows changes consistent with emphysema, but is otherwise unchanged from baseline. His arterial blood gas values are P_{O_2}, 59 mm Hg (7.8 kPa); P_{CO_2}, 64 mm Hg (8.5 kPa); and pH, 7.32. Other pertinent laboratory values include sodium, 140 meq/L (140 mmol/L); chloride, 100 meq/L (100 mmol/L); potassium, 3.5 meq/L (3.5 mmol/L); and bicarbonate, 32 meq/L (32 mmol/L).

Which of the following acid-base disorders is most likely present?

(A) Metabolic acidosis
(B) Respiratory acidosis
(C) Respiratory acidosis and metabolic acidosis
(D) Respiratory alkalosis

Item 17 [Basic]

A 28-year-old man is brought to the emergency department with the sudden onset of dyspnea following a stressful interview at work.

On physical examination, temperature is 36.7°C (98°F), heart rate is 99/min, respiration rate is 32/min, and blood pressure is 156/80 mm Hg. He is weak and in moderate respiratory distress. Cardiovascular and pulmonary examinations are normal.

Sodium	140 meq/L (140 mmol/L)
Potassium	4.9 meq/L (4.9 mmol/L)
Chloride	110 meq/L (110 mmol/L)
Bicarbonate	22 meq/L (22 mmol/L)

Arterial blood gas studies (on ambient air):
pH	7.49
P_{CO_2}	30 mm Hg (4.0 kPa)
P_{O_2}	99 mm Hg (13.2 kPa)

Which of the following best characterizes the patient's acid–base disorder?

(A) Mixed anion gap metabolic acidosis and respiratory alkalosis
(B) Mixed metabolic alkalosis and respiratory alkalosis
(C) Respiratory acidosis
(D) Respiratory alkalosis

Item 18 [Basic]

A 56-year old man with a history of alcoholism is found lying on the street. On arrival at the emergency department, he is confused.

On physical examination, temperature is 36.1°C (97.0°F), blood pressure is 126/80 mm Hg, and pulse rate is 70/min. Funduscopic examination shows no papilledema. Cardiac, pulmonary, and abdominal examinations are normal.

Glucose (fasting)	86 mg/dL (4.8 mmol/L)
Blood urea nitrogen	45 mg/dL (16.1 mmol/L)
Serum creatinine	2.8 mg/dL (247.5 µmol/L)
Sodium	138 meq/L (138 mmol/L)
Potassium	5.4 meq/L (5.4 mmol/L)
Chloride	98 meq/L (98 mmol/L)
Bicarbonate	14 meq/L (14 mmol/L)
Plasma osmolality	336 mosm/kg (336 µmol/kg)
Urinalysis	Calcium oxalate crystals

Arterial blood gas studies (with the patient breathing ambient air)
pH	7.32
P_{CO_2}	29 mm Hg (3.9 kPa)
P_{O_2}	80 mm Hg (10.6 kPa)

Which of the following is the most likely diagnosis?

(A) Alcoholic ketoacidosis
(B) Diabetic ketoacidosis
(C) Ethylene glycol poisoning
(D) Lactic acidosis

Item 19 [Advanced]

A 39-year-old man is evaluated in the emergency department because of severe left flank pain and hematuria after playing softball. The pain is sharp and radiates to the groin. He vomited eight times before presentation. He has a nonobstructing, calcium-containing kidney stone at the ureteropelvic junction on the left side.

On initial evaluation, his blood pressure was 130/90 mm Hg, respiratory rate was 30/min, and pulse rate was 110/min.

Serum sodium	141 meq/L (141 mmol/L)
Serum potassium	4.0 meq/L (4.0 mmol/L)
Serum chloride	100 meq/L (100 mmol/L)
Serum bicarbonate	34 meq/L (34 mmol/L)
Arterial blood gases	pH, 7.60; Pco_2, 36 mm Hg (4.8 kPa)

Which of the following best describes this patient's acid-base disorder?

(A) Metabolic acidosis and respiratory alkalosis
(B) Metabolic alkalosis
(C) Metabolic alkalosis and respiratory acidosis
(D) Metabolic and respiratory alkalosis
(E) Respiratory alkalosis

Item 20 [Basic]

A 66-year old man is evaluated in the emergency department for a 6-week history of dyspnea on exertion and a 3-day history of orthopnea. He reports no chest pain or palpitations. He has a 45-pack-year history of cigarette smoking. He takes no medications.

On physical examination, temperatures is 37.2°C (99.0°F), blood pressure is 150/90 mm Hg, pulse rate is 108/min, and respiration rate is 26/min. Oxygen saturation by pulse oximetry is 88% on ambient air. The patient has jugular venous distention to the angle of the jaw when sitting upright. A prominent S_3 and bibasilar crackles are heard on auscultation of the lungs, and pitting edema to the knees is present.

Blood urea nitrogen	56 mg/dL (20 mmol/L)
Creatinine	1.7 mg/dL (150.3 µmol/L)
Electrolytes	
Sodium	120 meq/L (120 mmol/L)
Potassium	5.3 meq/L (5.3 mmol/L)
Chloride	100 meq/L (100 mmol/L)
Carbon dioxide	22 meq/L (22 mmol/L)
Glucose	180 mg/dL (6.5 mmol/L)

Which of the following best describes this patient's plasma tonicity and serum sodium status?

(A) Hyperosmolar hyponatremia
(B) Hyposmolar hyponatremia
(C) Normal osmolar hypernatremia
(D) Normal osmolar hyponatremia
(E) Normal osmolar pseudohyponatremia

Item 21 [Advanced]

A 73-year-old woman is brought to the emergency department after falling at home. Her family states that she has been very confused and disoriented over the past 2 days and that she began therapy with a new medication 4 days ago. She has type 2 diabetes mellitus, hypertension, and glaucoma. A bag containing the patient's medications includes glyburide, metformin, hydrochlorothiazide, acetazolamide, and enalapril.

On physical examination, temperature is 37°C (98.6°F), heart rate is 68/min, respiration rate is 12/min, and blood pressure is 115/65 mm Hg. She is confused and unable to answer questions appropriately. Cardiac examination is normal. The lungs are clear. There is no edema.

Blood urea nitrogen	17 mg/dL (6.1 mmol/L)
Creatinine	1.1 mg/dL (97.2 µmol/L)
Sodium	107 meq/L (107 mmol/L)
Potassium	3.9 meq/L (3.9 mmol/L)
Chloride	76 meq/L (76 mmol/L)
Bicarbonate	24 meq/L (24 mmol/L)

Which of the following drugs is most likely responsible for the patient's findings?

(A) Acetazolamide
(B) Glyburide
(C) Hydrochlorothiazide
(D) Metformin

Item 22 [Advanced]

A 55-year-old man is seen during a routine evaluation. He was diagnosed with type 2 diabetes mellitus 15 years ago. He also has hypertension and a 1-year history of right knee osteoarthritis that is well controlled with maximal-dose ibuprofen. His other medications are losartan, metformin, and pravastatin.

On physical examination, temperature is 37.2°C (98.9°F), blood pressure is 146/92 mm Hg, pulse rate is 70/min, and respiration rate is 14/min. Cardiopulmonary examination is normal. There is bilateral lower-extremity edema to the mid shin.

Glucose (nonfasting)	230 mg/dL (12.8 mmol/L)
Sodium	142 meq/L (142 mmol/L)
Potassium	5.9 meq/L (5.9 mmol/L)
Chloride	108 meq/L (108 mmol/L)
Bicarbonate	18 meq/L (18 mmol/L)
Serum creatinine	2.5 mg/dL (221 µmol/L)
Urine protein-creatinine ratio	0.46 mg/mg
Urinalysis	Specific gravity 1.015; 3+ protein; 2+ glucose; no casts

Which of the following is the most appropriate initial management step?

(A) Begin hydrochlorothiazide
(B) Begin spironolactone
(C) Discontinue ibuprofen and begin furosemide
(D) Substitute lisinopril for losartan

Item 23 [Basic]

A 30-year-old man with type 1 diabetes mellitus and chronic kidney disease (serum creatinine, 5.3 mg/dL [468.5 μmol/L]) is evaluated in the emergency department for a 2-day history of muscle weakness and recent onset of light headedness. An electrocardiogram taken in the emergency department is shown.

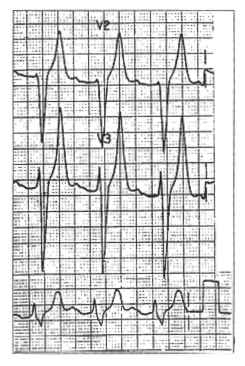

Which of the following is the best immediate treatment option?

(A) Calcium gluconate, intravenously
(B) 50% glucose, intravenously
(C) Hemodialysis
(D) Sodium polystyrene sulfonate in sorbitol, rectally

Item 24 [Advanced]

A 17-year-old girl is evaluated for weakness. On physical examination, the blood pressure is 124/74 mm Hg with no orthostatic changes, pulse rate 72/min, and respiration rate 15/min. BMI is 18. The rest of the physical examination is unremarkable.

Sodium	140 meq/L (140 mmol/L)
Potassium	2.8 meq/L (2.8 mmol/L)
Chloride	110 meq/L (110 mmol/L)
Bicarbonate	21 meq/L (21 mmol/L)

Blood urea nitrogen and serum creatinine are normal. A spot urine potassium concentration is 8 meq/L (8 mmol/L).

Which of the following is the most likely diagnosis?

(A) Laxative abuse
(B) Primary hyperaldosteronism
(C) Primary hypoaldosteronism
(D) Surreptitious diuretic use

Item 25 [Basic]

A 44-year-old man comes to the emergency department with polyuria and polydipsia. Over the past 3 days, he has noted increased urination with nearly constant thirst.

Physical examination is normal. Admission laboratory results included serum sodium of 155 meq/L (155 mmol/L), plasma glucose of 150 mg/dL (8.3 mmol/L), and urine osmolality of 117 mosm/kg (117 μmol/kg). He has significant increase in urine osmolality (greater than 50%) within 1 to 2 hours after injection of arginine vasopressin.

What is the most likely cause of the hypernatremia?

(A) Central diabetes insipidus
(B) Diabetes mellitus
(C) Nephrogenic diabetes insipidus
(D) Primary polydipsia

Item 26 [Advanced]

A 55-year-old woman is evaluated in the emergency department for a 2-day history of severe midepigastric pain radiating through to her back and of nausea with vomiting. Before this, she was well and had no medical problems; she does not take any medications or drink alcohol.

On examination, she is in distress from pain. Temperature is 37.8°C (98.9°F), blood pressure is 155/97 mm Hg, and pulse rate is 104/min. BMI is 29. Midepigastric tenderness to palpation is marked.

An abdominal ultrasound reveals a dilated common bile duct and multiple gallstones. Laboratory evaluation reveals elevated alkaline phosphatase, amylase, and lipase levels; total calcium level is 6.8 mg/dL (1.7 mmol/L).

What of the following is the most likely cause of the hypocalcemia?

(A) 1,25-dihydroxy vitamin D deficiency
(B) Autoimmune hypoparathyroidism
(C) Calcium chelation with free fatty acids
(D) Parathyroid gland injury

Item 27 [Advanced]

A 45-year-old man with stage 1 pulmonary sarcoidosis (hilar lymphadenopathy) is evaluated for abdominal pain and distention. He has chronic constipation, and his last bowel movement was 6 days ago.

On physical examination, temperature is 36.8°C (98.2°F), blood pressure is 152/80 mm Hg, pulse rate is 78/min, and respiration rate is 12/min. Bowel sounds are present but diminished. Tenderness to palpation is present and most prominent in the left lower quadrant without guarding. Rectal examination reveals firm stool but no masses.

Serum calcium level is 11.6 mg/dL (2.9 mmol/L); the reminder of the laboratory evaluation is normal, including thyroid-stimulating hormone level and free thyroxine. A plain film of the abdomen shows marked colonic distention with stool but no free air under the diaphragm or evidence of mechanical bowel obstruction. Enemas and laxatives are prescribed.

Which of the following is the most appropriate additional treatment for this patient?

(A) Cinacalcet
(B) Hydrochlorothiazide
(C) Intravenous normal saline
(D) Prednisone

Item 28 [Basic]

A 45-year-old man is evaluated for a 3-month history of fatigue, constipation, and polyuria. He also has a 5-year history of hypertension. Current medications are losartan and diltiazem.

Physical examination findings, including vital signs, are normal.

Calcium	11.4 mg/dL (2.9 mmol/L)
Creatinine	1.1 mg/dL (97.2 µmol/L)
Glucose, fasting	88 mg/dL (4.9 mmol/L)
Phosphorus	2.2 mg/dL (0.71 mmol/L)
Thyroid-stimulating hormone	1.2 µU/mL (1.2 mU/L)

Measurement of which of the following levels should be done next?

(A) Calcitonin
(B) 25-Hydroxy vitamin D
(C) Parathyroid hormone
(D) Parathyroid hormone–related protein

Item 29 [Advanced]

A 47-year-old man with a long-standing history of alcoholism is hospitalized for acute pancreatitis. His last drink was 6 days ago. He has lost approximately 10% of his body weight over the past 4 months due to drinking alcohol and not eating.

On physical examination, he is cachectic. Vital signs are normal. BMI is 17. He is not confused or tremulous. There is midepigastric tenderness without rebound. Neurologic examination is normal.

Sodium	130 meq/L (130 mmol/L)
Potassium	3.4 meq/L (3.4 mmol/L)
Chloride	90 meq/L (90 mmol/L)
Bicarbonate	20 meq/L (20 mmol/L)
Phosphorus	3.5 mg/dL (1.1 mmol/L)
Calcium	9.0 mg/dL (2.2 mmol/L)

The patient receives thiamine replacement, folic acid supplementation, and a multivitamin followed by vigorous intravenous fluid replacement with 5% dextrose and normal saline and potassium chloride. Morphine is used to control pain.

Eighteen hours later, the patient's abdominal pain has improved but he becomes restless, agitated, and extremely weak and is barely able to raise his extremities against gravity.

Which of the following is the most likely diagnosis?

(A) Hypercalcemia
(B) Hypokalemia
(C) Hyponatremia
(D) Hypophosphatemia

Section 7

Nephrology
Answers and Critiques

Item 1 **Answer: B**

Educational Objective: *Diagnose orthostatic protein-uria.*

The most appropriate next diagnostic test is to evaluate the patient for orthostatic proteinuria. This is done by obtaining separate upright (daytime) and supine (overnight) urine collections for protein quantitation. Orthostatic proteinuria is defined by an increase in urinary protein excretion only in the upright position; when supine, the urinary protein excretion rate is normal (<50 mg/8 h). The condition is seen most commonly in children or young adults. The total urine protein excretion rate is usually less than 1 g/24 h, and the urinalysis is otherwise normal. The etiology of the condition is uncertain; in some cases, mild alterations in glomerular histology have been reported. An association of orthostatic proteinuria with entrapment of the left renal vein between the aorta and the superior mesenteric artery ("nutcracker syndrome") also has been reported. The condition is benign; it often resolves spontaneously, and long-term follow-up studies in affected patients have shown renal function remains normal.

A kidney biopsy is not the most appropriate next step in this patient's management. His medical history provides no evidence of significant past or present illness, and his physical examination and initial laboratory studies do not suggest serious kidney disease. Specifically, he is normotensive and not edematous; the serum creatinine, albumin, and cholesterol are normal; and, the urinalysis is normal.

A single 24-hour urine collection would most likely only confirm the subnephrotic rate of urinary protein excretion, which is already evident from the spot urine protein–creatinine ratio of 0.8 mg/mg. More importantly, a single 24-hour urine collection would fail to differentiate the rates of upright versus supine proteinuria, which is essential in distinguishing orthostatic from persistent proteinuria.

Given the patient's age, normal hemoglobin, and serum protein, a dysproteinemia is very unlikely, and serum and urine protein electrophoresis studies are not needed. Should the patient prove to have persistent proteinuria, urine protein electrophoresis and immunofixation studies may be useful in determining whether the proteinuria reflects glomerular or tubular disease.

> **KEY POINT**
>
> Orthostatic proteinuria is defined by an increase in urinary protein excretion only in the upright position.

Bibliography

Sebestyen JF, Alon US. The teenager with asymptomatic proteinuria: think orthostatic first. Clin Pediatr. 2011;50(3):179-182. [PMID: 20837623]

Item 2 **Answer: A**

Educational Objective: *Diagnose acute interstitial nephritis.*

The most likely diagnosis is acute interstitial nephritis. This patient has acute kidney injury (AKI), as evidenced by the sudden onset of oliguria and an increase in her blood urea nitrogen (BUN) and serum creatinine values. Her urine (normal upon admission) is positive for leukocytes and leukocyte casts, but the culture is negative (sterile pyuria). This clinical picture is most consistent with tubulointerstitial inflammation caused by acute interstitial nephritis. Drugs, particularly β-lactam antibiotics, are the most common etiology of acute interstitial nephritis. Patients may also have fever, rash, and eosinophilia, although only a minority of patients will have all three features.

Acute tubular necrosis (ATN) is the most common form of intrarenal disease that causes acute kidney injury in hospitalized patients. Onset of this condition usually occurs after a sustained period of ischemia or exposure to nephrotoxic agents. Urinalysis in approximately 75% of patients with acute tubular necrosis reveals muddy brown casts; leukocytes and leukocyte casts are not associated with ATN.

Cholesterol crystal embolization may cause AKI in patients with aortic atherosclerotic plaques. This condition may occur spontaneously but most often develops after coronary or kidney angiography or aortic surgery. Kidney injury in patients with cholesterol crystal embolization usually has a subacute onset with a stuttering course over several weeks. Cutaneous manifestations develop in approximately 10% to 15% of patients and may include livedo reticularis, skin ulceration, and nodules. Patients with cholesterol crystal embolization typically have a bland urine sediment but may have dysmorphic hematuria and erythrocyte casts.

The absence of orthostatic hypotension, tachycardia, and the normal BUN-creatinine ratio of approximately 10:1, argue against prerenal azotemia as the cause of AKI.

> **KEY POINT**
>
> Acute interstitial nephritis is characterized by acute kidney injury, sterile pyuria, and leukocyte casts.

Bibliography

Perazella MA, Markowitz GS. Drug-induced acute interstitial nephritis. Nat Rev Nephrol. 2010;6(8):461-70. [PMID: 20517290]

Item 3   Answer: A

Educational Objective: *Evaluate persistent hematuria with cystoscopy.*

The most appropriate next step is cystoscopy. This patient has persistent hematuria, defined as the presence of three or more erythrocytes/hpf in the urine detected on two or more samples. Bleeding in patients with persistent hematuria may originate anywhere along the genitourinary tract, and differentiating between glomerular and nonglomerular hematuria helps to guide management. This patient's normal-appearing erythrocytes revealed on urine microscopy and absence of erythrocyte casts and protein in the urine are consistent with nonglomerular hematuria.

One possible cause of persistent nonglomerular hematuria is genitourinary tract malignancy. Risk factors for these malignancies include male sex, age greater than 50 years, tobacco use, and exposure to drugs such as cyclophosphamide and benzene and radiation. Because this patient has several risk factors, cystoscopy is indicated to exclude a malignancy.

Hematuria may develop in patients taking NSAIDs or anticoagulants but should not automatically be attributed to these agents; appropriate evaluation for glomerular or nonglomerular disorders should still be performed in this setting. In addition, discontinuation of warfarin may place him at risk for further thromboembolic disorders.

This patient's slightly increased serum creatinine level is suggestive of glomerular disease, which often manifests as a decrease in kidney function. However, glomerular hematuria is commonly associated with dysmorphic erythrocytes and erythrocyte casts. Glomerular disease also is unlikely in the absence of protein on urinalysis. Therefore, kidney biopsy, which is often used to evaluate patients with glomerular disease, would not be appropriate for this patient.

In a patient with persistent hematuria and at high risk for genitourinary tract malignancy, repeating the urinalysis in 3 months puts the patient at risk for progressive spread of cancer and is not an appropriate management option.

KEY POINT

In patients with nonglomerular hematuria, kidney ultrasonography and cystoscopy are indicated to exclude a genitourinary tract malignancy in individuals with risk factors for this condition.

Bibliography

Cohen R, Brown S. Microscopic hematuria. N Engl J Med. 2003;348 (23):2330-2338. [PMID:12788998]

Item 4   Answer: D

Educational Objective: *Diagnose rhabdomyolysis secondary to narcotic overdose.*

This patient most likely has rhabdomyolysis, which is caused by skeletal muscle damage that leads to release of intracellular components into the circulation. The syndrome was first identified in patients with traumatic crush injuries, but there are nontraumatic causes, such as alcohol (due to hypophosphatemia), drug use, metabolic disorders, and infections. The classic triad of findings includes muscle pain, weakness, and dark urine. The diagnosis is based on clinical findings and a history of predisposing factors (such as prolonged immobilization or drug toxicity) and confirmed by the presence of myoglobinuria, an increased serum creatine kinase level, and, in some cases, hyperkalemia. A positive urine dipstick for blood in the absence of erythrocytes also suggests rhabdomyolysis. The disorder usually resolves within days to weeks. Treatment consists of aggressive fluid resuscitation; fluids should be adjusted to maintain the hourly urine output at least 300 mL until the urine is negative for myoglobin. Acute kidney injury resulting from acute tubular necrosis occurs in approximately one third of patients. Dialysis is sometimes necessary.

Although fulminant hepatic failure may result in coma, dark urine, and renal failure, other tests of synthetic liver function in this patient are normal. Hemolytic anemia would not explain the patient's elevated creatine kinase level and usually does not cause renal failure. Hemolytic uremic syndrome is not consistent with the normal complete blood count, clinical findings of polysubstance overdose or the laboratory finding of the elevated serum creatine kinase level.

KEY POINT

Rhabdomyolysis is associated with muscle pain, weakness, and dark urine; laboratory findings include an elevated serum creatine kinase level and positive urine dipstick for blood in the absence of erythrocytes.

Bibliography

Talaie H, Pajouhmand A, Abdollahi M, et al. Rhabdomyolysis among acute human poisoning cases. Hum Exp Toxicol. 2007:26(7):557-561. [PMID: 17884958]

Item 5   Answer: C

Educational Objective: *Diagnose obstructive nephropathy as a cause of acute kidney injury.*

The best diagnostic test for this patient is kidney ultrasound to evaluate for urinary obstruction. The patient has lower urinary tract symptoms with difficulty voiding and suprapubic fullness. This is consistent with bladder outlet obstruction from prostatic hypertrophy. Obstruction can cause intrarenal vasoconstriction, ischemic tubular injury, and interstitial fibrosis that may lead to end-stage kidney disease if uncorrected. Although patients with complete obstruction have significantly decreased urine output, those with partial obstruction may have polyuria caused by loss of tubular function or excretion of excess retained solute. Kidney ultrasound in most patients with obstruction reveals hydronephrosis. Patients with acute kidney injury (AKI) caused by urinary tract obstruction have a favorable prognosis when obstruction is relieved within 1 week of onset. A kidney ultrasound would reveal a distended bladder and possible hydronephrosis. Insertion of a Foley catheter is initial treatment.

Kidney biopsy should be considered when the diagnosis of AKI remains unclear after excluding prerenal and postrenal disease. Biopsy is warranted to help guide therapy or provide prognostic information. Ultrasound duplex arteriography, CT arteriography, MRI, and angiotensin-converting enzyme inhibitor renography are used to evaluate renal vasculature in the presence of disrupted arterial or venous blood flow. In this patient with voiding symptoms and suprapubic fullness, non-invasive kidney ultrasoundy is the diagnostic test of choice.

Albumin is the only protein detected on dipstick urinalysis, and nothing in the patient's presentation suggests he has a primary glomerular disease causing AKI; dipstick evaluation would add little to this case. Quantitative measurements, rather than dipstick methodology, are recommended to detect albumin excretion less than 300 mg/24 h.

KEY POINT

Kidney ultrasound is indicated for all patients with acute kidney injury to define kidney anatomy and to exclude hydronephrosis.

Bibliography

Sharfuddin AA, Sandoval RM, Molitoris BA. Imaging techniques in acute kidney injury. Nephron Clin Pract. 2008;109(4):c198-c204. [PMID: 18802368]

Item 6   Answer: C

Educational Objective: *Diagnose hemolytic uremic syndrome.*

The most likely diagnosis is hemolytic uremic syndrome (HUS). HUS commonly manifests as acute kidney injury (AKI) accompanied by thrombocytopenia and microangiopathic hemolytic anemia (schistocytes on peripheral blood smear). The two most common causes are infection by Shiga toxin–producing *Escherichia coli* (*E. coli* O157:H7 and other serotypes) and familial deficiency of factor H. The toxin causes bloody diarrhea and enters the circulation and binds to platelets, glomerular capillary endothelial cells, mesangial cells, and glomerular and tubular epithelial cells. Shiga toxin binds to platelets by means of globotriaosylceramide receptors, which leads to platelet aggregation. Shiga toxin may also stimulate endothelial cells to release large von Willebrand factor multimers, which can further enhance platelet aggregation. Factor H, a protein in the complement pathway, normally protects cells from damage by the alternative complement pathway. A deficiency of factor H allows C3 to potentiate autoantibody-mediated or immune complex–mediated injury to

glomerular cells, leading to exposure of subendothelium and activation of both platelets and coagulation.

Acute interstitial nephritis (AIN) is most commonly caused by a hypersensitivity reaction to a medication or by certain infections or autoimmune conditions. Urinalysis findings in patients may include leukocyte casts and eosinophils. AIN does not cause hemolytic anemia or thrombocytopenia.

Acute tubular necrosis (ATN) usually occurs after a sustained period of ischemia or exposure to nephrotoxic agents. ATN may resolve in 1 to 3 weeks or result in permanent end-stage kidney disease, depending on the duration and severity of the ischemic or nephrotoxic insult. Urinalysis usually reveals muddy brown casts and is not associated with microangiopathic hemolytic anemia or thrombocytopenia.

Rhabdomyolysis develops when muscle injury leads to the release of myoglobin and other intracellular muscle contents into the circulation. Myoglobin is known to cause nephrotoxicity by induction of kidney ischemia and tubular obstruction. Rhabdomyolysis most commonly develops after exposure to myotoxic drugs, infection, excessive exertion, or prolonged immobilization. A diagnosis of rhabdomyolysis should be considered in patients with a serum creatine kinase level greater than 5000 U/L who demonstrate heme positivity on urine dipstick testing in the absence of hematuria.

KEY POINT

Hemolytic uremic syndrome commonly manifests as acute kidney injury accompanied by thrombocytopenia and microangiopathic hemolytic anemia.

Bibliography

Amirlak I, Amirlak B. Haemolytic uraemic syndrome: an overview. Nephrology (Carlton). 2006;11(3):213-8. [PMID: 16756634]

Item 7   Answer: B

Educational Objective: *Diagnose acute tubular necrosis–associated acute kidney injury.*

This patient's elevated serum creatinine level, minimal proteinuria, and muddy brown casts on urinalysis are most consistent with acute tubular necrosis. This condition usually develops after a sustained period of ischemia or exposure to nephrotoxic agents such as cisplatin, intravenous aminoglycosides, or radiocontrast.

Acute interstitial nephritis most commonly develops after exposure to certain medications, including trimethoprim. Manifestations of this condition may include rash, pruritus, eosinophilia, and fever. Urine sediment findings include pyuria, leukocyte casts, microscopic hematuria, and tubular-range proteinuria. These features are absent in this patient.

Manifestations of the thrombotic microangiopathies, including thrombotic thrombocytopenic purpura, may include acute kidney injury that is usually accompanied by microangiopathic hemolytic anemia and thrombocytopenia. Approximately 50%

of patients have low C3 levels. The urine sediment usually shows minimal or no abnormalities and is nondiagnostic; rarely, erythrocyte or muddy brown casts may be seen. This patient's normal hemoglobin concentration and platelet count exclude a thrombotic microangiopathy as the cause of the acute kidney injury.

Kidney ultrasonography in most patients with obstruction reveals hydronephrosis, which is absent in this patient. Furthermore, the urinalysis in patients with obstruction is benign and is not associated with the muddy brown casts found in this patient's urine.

KEY POINT

Acute tubular necrosis usually develops after a sustained period of ischemia or exposure to nephrotoxic agents and is associated with muddy brown casts on urinalysis.

Bibliography

Choudhury D, Ahmed Z. Drug-associated renal dysfunction and injury. Nat Clin Pract Nephrol. 2006;2(2):80-91. [PMID:16932399]

Item 8   Answer: B
Educational Objective: *Diagnose and treat prerenal azotemia with volume replacement.*

This patient most likely has prerenal azotemia, and the most appropriate next step in management is isotonic saline. Acute kidney injury in patients with malignancy is often due to prerenal disease, obstruction, or use of nephrotoxic agents. The presence of hypotension, hyponatremia, and a decreased urine sodium excretion accompanied by a bland urine sediment raises suspicion for prerenal azotemia.

Dialysis would be indicated if the azotemia persisted or worsened after correction of the hypovolemia, particularly if other uremic complications such as encephalopathy or refractory hyperkalemia were present. Dialysis is not indicated before this patient has undergone a trial of adequate volume replacement.

Therapy with midodrine and octreotide may be effective and safe for the treatment of hepatorenal syndrome in some patients. However, the absence of ascites or other signs of portal hypertension are not consistent with hepatorenal syndrome.

Tumor lysis syndrome may manifest as hyperkalemia, hyperphosphatemia, and hyperuricemia. Tumor lysis syndrome most likely occurs in patients with extremely rapidly progressive lymphoid neoplasms and in those who have bulky lymphoid neoplasms that respond rapidly to treatment. Rasburicase can be used to treat malignancy-related hyperuricemia in order to prevent tumor lysis syndrome in high-risk patients or as a component of therapy for established tumor lysis syndrome and associated hyperuricemia. However, this patient's serum electrolyte, phosphorus, and uric acid level abnormalities are most likely a result of hypovolemia and associated kid-

ney dysfunction and should improve with volume repletion; therefore, rasburicase therapy would not be warranted.

KEY POINT

The presence of hypotension, hyponatremia, and a decreased urine sodium excretion accompanied by a bland urine sediment should raise suspicion for prerenal azotemia.

Bibliography

Darmon M, Ciroldi M, Thiery G, Schlemmer B, Azoulay E. Clinical review: specific aspects of acute renal failure in cancer patients. Crit Care 2006;10:211. [PMID:16677413]

Item 9   Answer: C
Educational Objective: *Diagnose prerenal azotemia in a patient with chronic kidney disease.*

The most likely cause of this patient's acute kidney injury is prerenal azotemia. Prerenal azotemia develops when autoregulation of kidney blood flow can no longer maintain glomerular filtration rate (GFR). This condition generally occurs in patients with a mean arterial pressure below 60 mm Hg but may occur at higher pressures in individuals with chronic kidney disease (CKD) or in those who take medications that can alter local glomerular hemodynamics, such as NSAIDs. Patients with prerenal azotemia may have a history of fluid losses and decreased fluid intake accompanied by physical examination findings consistent with extracellular fluid volume depletion, such as postural hypotension. However, these findings are absent in up to 50% of patients with this condition. Nausea, vomiting, and anorexia accompanied by relatively low blood pressure in the absence of edema or urine sediment abnormalities strongly suggest prerenal azotemia.

Acute interstitial nephritis may be caused by use of certain drugs, including antibiotics and NSAIDs, and classically manifests as pyuria, leukocyte casts, or eosinophils on urinalysis. Fever, rash, and blood eosinophilia also may be present. The urine sediment in acute tubular necrosis usually shows muddy brown casts or tubular epithelial cell casts. Renal vein thrombosis is an uncommon cause of acute kidney injury associated with hematuria and nephrotic-range proteinuria. This condition is most often associated with membranous nephropathy, malignancy, trauma, or hypercoagulable states. The normal urinalysis helps exclude acute interstitial nephritis, acute tubular necrosis, and renal vein thrombosis as the cause of this patient's renal decompensation.

KEY POINT

Prerenal disease is usually associated with relative low blood pressure, oliguria, and normal urinalysis.

Bibliography

Kellum JA. Acute kidney injury. Crit Care Med. 2008;36(suppl 4):S141-S145. [PMID: 18382185]

Item 10   Answer: C
Educational Objective: *Treat diabetic nephropathy with an angiotensin receptor blocker.*

The most appropriate next management step is to increase the dose of the losartan. Uncontrolled hypertension and proteinuria are important modifiable risk factors for progressive kidney disease. Lowering blood pressure is critical regardless of the underlying disease. For patients with chronic kidney disease, guidelines recommend blood pressure targets of less than 130/80 mm Hg or less than 125/75 mm Hg when significant proteinuria is present. Angiotensin-converting enzyme inhibitors, such as lisinopril, and angiotensin receptor blockers (ARBs), such as losartan, are the preferred agents in chronic kidney disease and slow progression of kidney disease in patients with diabetes. These agents reduce efferent arteriolar resistance and lower intraglomerular pressure and, therefore, may be associated with increases in serum creatinine in patients with a reduced glomerular filtration rate. An increase in creatinine of up to 30% is acceptable. In this patient, blood pressure remains elevated and he has significant proteinuria. The most logical next step would be to increase losartan. It is not necessary to discontinue losartan, because the increase in creatinine is not unexpected and his potassium remains at an acceptable level.

Results from a recent study, which involved elderly patients at high risk for cardiovascular events, indicate the use of combination ACE inhibitor and ARB therapy does not reduce morbidity and mortality and furthermore increases adverse side effects compared with the use of ACE inhibitors alone. Further studies are warranted before combination therapy can be recommended.

The clinical course and long-standing diabetes progressing to microalbuminuria and then to overt proteinuria and loss of kidney function over a period of years strongly suggests diabetic nephropathy. Kidney biopsy would be unlikely to change the long-term management in this patient.

KEY POINT
In patients with proteinuria and chronic kidney disease, angiotensin-converting enzyme inhibitors or angiotensin receptor blockers should be used to lower blood pressure, decrease proteinuria, and slow disease progression.

Bibliography
Defarrari G, Ravera M, Berruti V, Leoncini G, Deferrari L. Optimizing therapy in the diabetic patient with renal disease: antihypertensive treatment. J Am Soc Nephrol. 2004;15(suppl 1):S6-S11. [PMID: 14684664]

Item 11   Answer: D
Educational Objective: *Know the indications for initiating dialysis in a patient with chronic kidney disease.*

At this time, no change in the management of this patient's disease is required. Patients with stage 5 chronic kidney disease (glomerular filtration rate [GRF] <15 mL/min/1.73 m^2 or receiving dialysis) often develop signs of uremia and require kidney replacement therapy. Absolute indications include uncontrollable hyperkalemia, uncontrollable hypervolemia, altered mental status or excess somnolence, pericarditis, or bleeding-diathesis secondary to uremic platelet dysfunction. Relative indications include nausea, vomiting, and poor nutrition caused by decreased appetite; severe metabolic acidosis; mild changes in mental status such as lethargy and malaise; asterixis; and worsening of kidney function with GFR less than 15 mL/min/1.73 m^2. However, the timing of hemodialysis in patients without fluid overload, hyperkalemia, metabolic acidosis, or uremic symptoms, such as this patient, is unclear. A recent study suggests early initiation of hemodialysis does not improve patient outcomes. Kidney transplantation is the treatment of choice for uremia. Transplantation in patients who have not yet been treated with hemodialysis is associated with better patient and allograft outcomes. This patient has several family members who are willing kidney donors, and it is possible that he could receive a transplant in the near future; therefore, the best course of action would be to follow the patient closely to ensure he does not develop uremic signs or symptoms or other indications for dialysis and strive for transplantation rather than dialysis.

No indication exists for increasing the lisinopril, especially with controlled blood pressure and a borderline high serum potassium level. Likewise, no reason exists to perform an abdominal ultrasound, because the bilateral flank masses are expected physical findings in a patient with enlarged kidneys secondary to polycystic kidney disease and are currently asymptomatic.

KEY POINT
Kidney replacement therapy for patients with stage 5 chronic kidney disease who are not hypervolemic, hyperkalemic, acidotic, or uremic may be delayed.

Bibliography
Cooper BA, Branley P, Bulfone L, et al; IDEAL Study. A randomized, controlled trial of early versus late initiation of dialysis. N Engl J Med. 2010;363(7):609-19. [PMID: 20581422]

Item 12   Answer: B
Educational Objective: *Evaluate a patient with non-diabetic kidney disease with a kidney biopsy.*

Kidney biopsy would be appropriate for this patient. This study is recommended in patients with features of nondiabetic kidney disease in order to establish a diagnosis and determine the most appropriate treatment. Diabetic nephropathy is characterized by proteinuria, hypertension, and a decline in the glomerular filtration rate in patients with a long-standing history of type 1 diabetes or a 5- to 10-year history of type 2 diabetes. This condition usually progresses from microalbuminuria to macroalbuminuria to an elevated serum creatinine level over a number of years. Although this patient's long-standing history of diabetes and proteinuria is suggestive of diabetic nephropathy, the presence of glomerular hematuria (dysmorphic erythrocytes and erythrocyte casts) and the rapid onset of symptomatic nephrotic syndrome are not consistent with diabetic nephropathy. These findings raise suspicion for primary glomerular disease. Furthermore, patients with diabetic nephropathy often have diabetic retinopathy, which is absent in this patient.

Cystoscopy would be considered in an adult with hematuria of uncertain origin in order to exclude bladder cancer. Similarly, imaging studies may help to evaluate urinary tract obstruction, kidney stones, kidney cysts or masses, renal vascular diseases, and vesicoureteral reflux. However, cystoscopy or a spiral CT would not be warranted in a patient with erythrocyte casts seen on urinalysis and dysmorphic erythrocytes, which suggests glomerular hematuria.

Observation alone would place this patient at risk for progressive kidney injury if her condition remains undiagnosed and untreated.

KEY POINT

Kidney biopsy is recommended in patients with diabetes mellitus who have features of nondiabetic kidney disease.

Bibliography

Lin YL, Peng SJ, Ferng SH, Tzen CY, Yang CS. Clinical indicators which necessitate renal biopsy in type 2 diabetes mellitus patients with renal disease. Int J Clin Pract. 2009;63(8):1167-1176. [PMID:18422591]

Item 13   Answer: D

Educational Objective: *Diagnose bone disease due to secondary hyperparathyroidism in a patient with end-stage kidney disease.*

The most likely cause of this patient's bone disease is secondary hyperparathyroidism. Chronic kidney disease (CKD) is associated with progressive alterations in mineral and bone metabolism that can cause bone disease. In patients with end-stage kidney disease (ESKD), the kidney's inability to excrete phosphorus leads to hyperphosphatemia. Loss of kidney function also is associated with 1,25-dihydroxyvitamin D deficiency. Hyperphosphatemia along with decreased 1,25 dihydroxyvitamin D levels result in hypocalcemia, which leads to direct stimulation of parathyroid hormone secretion. Furthermore, decreased 1,25 dihydroxyvitamin D levels cause increased production of parathyroid hormone. Therefore, bone disease due to secondary hyperparathyroidism, the most common bone pathologic finding seen in patients with ESKD, develops. This patient's hyperphosphatemia, hypocalcemia, and elevated serum parathyroid hormone and alkaline phosphatase levels are consistent with secondary hyperparathyroidism.

Adynamic bone disease commonly occurs in patients with ESKD and may cause fractures. However, unlike bone disease associated with secondary hyperparathyroidism, adynamic bone disease is often associated with hypoparathyroidism caused by excess vitamin D intake and/or calcium loading. This condition usually manifests as bone pain accompanied by

a serum parathyroid hormone level below 100 pg/mL (100 ng/L) and a normal alkaline phosphatase level.

Osteoporosis is defined by low bone mass, which is associated with reduced bone strength and an increased risk of fractures. Osteoporosis occurs most commonly in postmenopausal women but may develop secondary to drugs such as corticosteroids and anticonvulsants. Osteoporosis does not affect the concentrations of serum calcium, phosphorus, parathyroid hormone, or alkaline phosphatase.

Osteonecrosis is caused by transient or permanent lack of blood supply to bone, which causes death of bone and bone marrow infarction that results in mechanical failure. Patients typically present with chronic bone pain, not fracture, and normal concentrations of calcium, phosphorus, and parathyroid hormone.

KEY POINT

Bone disease due to secondary hyperparathyroidism commonly occurs in patients with end-stage kidney disease and may be associated with elevated serum parathyroid hormone and alkaline phosphatase levels, hyperphosphatemia, and hypocalcemia.

Bibliography

Abboud H, Henrich WL. Clinical practice. Stage IV chronic kidney disease. N Engl J Med. 2010;362(1):56-65. [PMID: 20054047]

Item 14   Answer: A

Educational Objective: *Diagnose a mixed acid-base disorder.*

The most likely acid-base disorder is metabolic acidosis, metabolic alkalosis, and respiratory acidosis. The low pH defines acidosis; the finding of a low carbon dioxide level further defines the acidosis as metabolic acidosis. The increased anion gap categorizes the metabolic acidosis as an increased anion-gap acidosis. The P_{CO_2} measurement determines if respiratory compensation is appropriate for the degree of metabolic acidosis. The adequacy of respiratory compensation can be checked using Winter formula:

$$\text{Expected } P_{CO_2} = (1.5 \times [HCO_3^-] + 8) \pm 2 = 24 \pm 2$$

This formula confirms the measured P_{CO_2} is elevated for the degree of metabolic acidosis, establishing the diagnosis of respiratory acidosis. Finally, the corrected carbon dioxide level is calculated to determine if a complicating metabolic disturbance is present:

$$\text{Corrected } [HCO_3^-] = \text{measured } [HCO_3^-] + (\text{measured anion gap} - 12)$$

Using this formula, the corrected carbon dioxide level (the expected carbon dioxide concentration if no other acid-base disturbances were present) is 31 meq/L (31 mmol/L), establishing the diagnosis of a complicating metabolic alkalosis.

To diagnose a mixed acid-base disorder, it is necessary to evaluate the pH, anion gap, expected P_{CO_2}, bicarbonate and corrected bicarbonate levels.

Bibliography

Kraut JA, Madias NE. Approach to patients with acid-base disorders. Respir Care. 2001;46(4):392-403. [PMID: 11262558]

Item 15   Answer: B

Educational Objective: *Diagnose renal tubular acidosis.*

The patient's low pH indicates an acidosis. The low carbon dioxide level confirms that it is a metabolic acidosis. The normal anion-gap calculation further classifies the acidosis as normal anion-gap acidosis. Normal anion-gap metabolic acidosis can be of kidney or extrarenal origin. Metabolic acidosis of kidney origin, such as renal tubular acidosis (RTA), is caused by abnormalities in tubular hydrogen transport. Metabolic acidosis of extrarenal origin is most commonly caused by gastrointestinal losses of carbon dioxide; other extrarenal causes include the external loss of biliary and pancreatic secretions and ureteral diversion procedures. The clinical history usually helps to distinguish between kidney and extrarenal causes of metabolic acidosis, but measuring the urine ammonium excretion can confirm the cause of this condition. Extrarenal causes of metabolic acidosis are associated with an appropriate increase in net acid excretion primarily reflected by high levels of urine ammonium excretion, whereas kidney causes of this condition are associated with low net acid excretion and decreased urine ammonium levels.

Urine ammonium measurement is not a commonly available study, but this value can be indirectly assessed by calculating the urine anion gap (UAG) using the following formula:

$$\text{Urine anion gap} = ([\text{urine sodium}] + [\text{urine potassium}]) - [\text{urine chloride}]$$

The UAG is normally between 30 and 50 meq/L (30 to 50 mmol/L). Metabolic acidosis of extrarenal origin is suggested by a large, negative UAG caused by significantly increased urine ammonium excretion. Conversely, metabolic acidosis of kidney origin is suggested by a positive UAG related to minimal urine ammonium excretion. This patient's UAG is 20 meq/L (20 mmol/L); although it is within the normal range, it is inappropriately low for the degree of the patient's acidosis. This type of acidosis is compatible with renal tubular acidosis. It is not compatible with gastroenteritis or laxative abuse, both causes of extrarenal normal anion-gap acidosis. Diabetic ketoacidosis causes an increased anion-gap acidosis and is not compatible with this patient's laboratory findings.

Normal anion-gap metabolic acidosis of extrarenal origin is suggested by a large, negative urine anion gap, whereas a positive urine anion gap suggests metabolic acidosis of kidney origin.

Bibliography

Kraut JA, Madias NE. Approach to patients with acid-base disorders. Respir Care. 2001;46(4):392-403. [PMID: 11262558]

Item 16   Answer: B

Educational Objective: *Diagnose respiratory acidosis due to chronic obstructive pulmonary disease.*

This patient's acid-base disorder is respiratory acidosis. Respiratory acidosis is produced by any process associated with primary retention of carbon dioxide. In this patient, the pH is less than 7.38 and the P_{CO_2} is >40 mm Hg (5.3 kPa), indicating the presence of a respiratory acidosis. Renal compensatory response occurs in respiratory acidosis. Persistent hypercapnia stimulates the secretion of protons at the level of the distal nephron. The urinary pH decreases, and excretion of urinary ammonium, titratable acid, and chloride is enhanced. Consequently, the reabsorption of bicarbonate throughout the nephron is enhanced. The predicted increase in serum bicarbonate is calculated as 1 meq/L (1 mmol/L) for each 10 mm Hg (1.3 kPa) increase in P_{CO_2} (acute) or 4 meq/L (4 mmol/L) for each 10 mm Hg (1.3 kPa) increase in P_{CO_2} (chronic). Because this patient with chronic obstructive pulmonary disease probably has chronic retention of carbon dioxide, an increase in the serum bicarbonate by at least 8 meq/L (8 mmol/L) is expected. This is consistent with the measured serum bicarbonate level. Therefore, there is appropriate compensation for the respiratory acidosis and no evidence for a coexisting metabolic acidosis. Respiratory alkalosis is not consistent with the observed decrease in the serum pH.

In respiratory acidosis, the predicted increase in serum bicarbonate is calculated as 1 meq/L (1 mmol/L) for each 10 mm Hg (1.3 kPa) increase in P_{CO_2} (acute) or 4 meq/L (4 mmol/L) for each 10 mm Hg (1.3 kPa) increase in P_{CO_2} (chronic).

Bibliography

Palmer BF. Approach to fluid and electrolyte disorders and acid-base problems. Prim Care. 2008;35:195-213, v. [PMID: 18486713]

Item 17   Answer: D

Educational Objective: *Diagnose respiratory alkalosis.*

This patient has a pure respiratory alkalosis. The presence of an alkaline pH with a low P_{CO_2} is compatible with respiratory alkalosis. Furthermore, there is appropriate metabolic compensation for the respiratory alkalosis. In acute respiratory alkalosis, for each 10 mm Hg (1.3 kPa) decline in P_{CO_2} the expected decline in serum bicarbonate is 2 meq/L (2 mmol/L). Since his P_{CO_2} declined by 10 mm Hg (1.3 kPa) to 30 mm Hg (4.0 kPa), the expected decline in the serum bicarbonate is 2 meq/L (2 mmol/L); this matches the measured serum bicarbonate concentration exactly. Because the decline in the serum bicarbonate level is appropriate for the degree of respiratory alkalosis the patient cannot have a metabolic acidosis or metabolic alkalosis. And since his anion gap is normal, there is no possibility that the acid-base disturbance is an anion-gap metabolic acidosis. The anion gap is 8, calculated as $[Na^+] - ([Cl^-] + [HCO_3^-])$. Normal anion gap is 12 ± 2.

Because the Pco_2 is depressed rather than elevated, the diagnosis cannot be respiratory acidosis.

There are many potential causes of respiratory alkalosis, and the physical examination is often helpful in identifying the correct diagnosis. Common causes of respiratory alkalosis include psychogenic (for example, hyperventilation associated with anxiety), normal pregnancy, pulmonary vascular disease (for example, pulmonary hypertension or pulmonary embolism), pulmonary parenchymal disease (for example, pneumonia and pulmonary fibrosis), heart failure, sepsis, and cirrhosis.

KEY POINT

In acute respiratory alkalosis, for each 10 mm Hg (1.33 kPa) decline in Pco_2, the expected decline in serum bicarbonate is 2 meq/L (2 mmol/L).

Bibliography

Palmer BF. Approach to fluid and electrolyte disorders and acid-base problems. Prim Care. 2008;35:195-213, v. [PMID: 18486713]

Item 18   Answer: C
Educational Objective: *Diagnose ethylene glycol poisoning.*

This patient has ethylene glycol poisoning, which may manifest as acute kidney injury associated with an increased anion gap metabolic acidosis and an increased osmolal gap. The osmolal gap is the difference between the calculated plasma osmolality and measured plasma osmolality. In this patient, the osmolality is calculated using the following formula:

$$2 \times [Sodium] + [Glucose]/18 + [Blood\ Urea\ Nitrogen]$$
$$/2.8 = 296\ mosm/kg\ (296\ \mu mol/kg)$$
Where sodium is meq/L and glucose and
blood urea nitrogen are mg/dL.

The difference between the measured and calculated osmolality is 40 mosm/kg (40 μmol/kg). The normal osmolal gap is approximately 10 mosm/kg (10 μmol/kg). An elevated osmolal gap suggests the presence of an unmeasured osmole that is most commonly ethanol but can be ethylene glycol or methanol. However, only ethylene glycol is associated with kidney injury and calcium oxalate crystals in the urine.

Although alcoholic and diabetic ketoacidosis and lactic acidosis can cause an anion gap metabolic acidosis, none of these conditions is associated with an osmolal gap.

KEY POINT

Ethylene glycol poisoning is associated with an anion gap metabolic acidosis, an increased osmolal gap, kidney injury, and calcium oxalate crystals in the urine.

Bibliography

Palmer BF. Approach to fluid and electrolyte disorders and acid-base problems. Prim Care. 2008;35:195-213, v. [PMID: 18486713]

Item 19   Answer: D
Educational Objective: *Diagnose a mixed metabolic and respiratory alkalosis disorder.*

Arterial blood gas values demonstrate a mixed metabolic and respiratory alkalosis. Metabolic alkalosis is indicated by the high serum bicarbonate level and a pH greater than 7.4. Respiratory compensation for the metabolic alkalosis is not appropriate; the Pco_2 would be expected to increase in compensation for the elevated serum bicarbonate level, but instead, the Pco_2 has decreased to 36 mm Hg (4.8 kPa), indicating the presence of a respiratory alkalosis. In most patients, for each 1 meq/L (1 mmol/L) increase in serum bicarbonate, the Pco_2 can be expected to increase by 0.7 mm Hg (0.09 kPa).

The anion gap is 7, calculated as $(141 - [100 + 34])$; thus, there is no hidden anion-gap metabolic acidosis (normal anion gap < 12 ± 2). The respiratory alkalosis is most likely due to pain-induced hyperventilation from the kidney stone, and metabolic alkalosis is probably a result of vomiting.

KEY POINT

A mixed metabolic and respiratory alkalosis is suggested by an elevated pH and serum bicarbonate concentration and a Pco_2 concentration that is lower than expected for the degree of alkalosis.

Bibliography

Palmer BF. Approach to fluid and electrolyte disorders and acid-base problems. Prim Care. 2008;35:195-213, v. [PMID: 18486713]

Item 20   Answer: B
Educational Objective: *Diagnose hyposmolar hyponatremia in a patient with heart failure.*

This patient has hyposmolar hyponatremia. Osmolality is defined as the number of solute particles per kilogram of solution. Plasma osmolality can be directly measured by an osmometer or calculated using the following equation:

$$Plasma\ osmolality\ (mosm/kg = 2\ serum\ [Na^+]\ (meq/L)$$
$$+ blood\ urea\ nitrogen\ (mg/dL)/2.8 + plasma\ glucose$$
$$(mg/dL)/18$$

Using this formula, the calculated plasma osmolality is 252 mosm/kg (normal, 275-295 mosm/kg [275-295 μmol/kg]). Therefore, the patient is hyposmolar and hyponatremic.

Hyponatremia can be caused by a decrease in effective arterial blood volume, which results in baroreceptor stimulation of antidiuretic hormone (ADH) secretion, which impairs water excretion. Consequently, distal delivery of filtrate to the tip of the loop of Henle decreases. A decrease in effective arterial blood volume may be associated with low extracellular fluid volume (hypovolemic hyponatremia) or high extracellular fluid volume in edematous patients (hypervolemic hyponatremia), including heart failure, cirrhosis, and nephrotic syndrome.

True hyponatremia may be associated with an elevation in the plasma concentration of an effective osmole, such as glucose. This elevation results in an increase in plasma osmolality (hyperosmolar hyponatremia), which causes water to leave the cells and results in a diluted serum sodium concentration. Hyponatremia that occurs in the absence of a hyposmolar state (pseudohyponatremia) is generally caused by an increased serum concentration of an effective osmole. Common causes of pseudohyponatremia include hyperglobulinemia and hypertriglyceridemia. Because these conditions are associated with a decrease of plasma water relative to plasma solids in the blood, the amount of sodium in a given volume of blood also decreases.

KEY POINT

Hyponatremia can be caused by a decrease in effective arterial blood volume, which results in baroreceptor stimulation of antidiuretic hormone (ADH) secretion.

Bibliography

Kazory A. Hyponatremia in heart failure: revisiting pathophysiology and therapeutic strategies. Clin Cardiol. 2010;33(6):322-9. [PMID: 20556801]

Item 21   Answer: C
Educational Objective: *Diagnose hydrochlorothiazide-induced hyponatremia.*

Hydrochlorothiazide is a common cause of hyponatremia in the outpatient setting. It is especially common in the elderly. Early signs of symptomatic hyposmolality may be very nonspecific, such as nausea, vomiting, and headaches (hyponatremic encephalopathy). Worsening of brain swelling then causes decreased mental status and seizures. Diuretic-induced hyponatremia most commonly occurs in patients taking thiazide diuretics. Elderly women with low body mass indices who tend to increase fluid intake after initiation of therapy with these agents are often affected. Thiazide diuretics work at the level of the convoluted tubule and collecting segment. Therefore, these agents maintain urinary concentrating capacity but not diluting capacity, which makes them prone to cause hyponatremic encephalopathy. By inducing relative volume depletion, antidiuretic hormone secretion is stimulated, which leads to urine concentration and water retention. Treatment includes stopping the diuretic and infusing normal saline (for mildly symptomatic patients) or 3% saline (for significantly symptomatic patients).

Acetazolamide acts in the proximal tubule as a carbonic anhydrase IV inhibitor. Blocking this enzyme in the proximal tubule impairs bicarbonate reabsorption but not diluting capacity and is most often associated with hypokalemia and metabolic acidosis. Acetazolamide is not associated with the development of hyponatremia. Metformin and glyburide do not affect fluid and electrolyte balance.

KEY POINT

Hydrochlorothiazide can cause severe hyponatremia.

Bibliography

Mann SJ. The silent epidemic of thiazide-induced hyponatremia. J Clin Hypertens (Greenwich). 2008;10:477-484. [PMID: 18550938]

Item 22   Answer: C
Educational Objective: *Manage hyperkalemia in a patient with chronic kidney disease.*

Discontinuation of ibuprofen and initiation of furosemide are the most appropriate next steps in the initial management of this patient's chronic kidney disease. This patient's long-standing history of diabetes mellitus, hypertension, proteinuria, and elevated serum creatinine level are consistent with diabetic nephropathy. Aggressive blood pressure control, particularly with pharmacologic modulators of the renin-angiotensin-aldosterone system, would help to slow the progression of this patient's disease but will likely worsen his hyperkalemia.

Until the glomerular filtration rate decreases to less than 15 mL/min/1.73 m^2, chronic kidney disease usually does not cause hyperkalemia without other mitigating factors. These factors include use of medications that interfere with the renin-angiotensin-aldosterone system and NSAIDs. Use of the NSAID ibuprofen is most likely contributing to this patient's hyperkalemia and reduced glomerular filtration rate and should be discontinued.

However, discontinuing ibuprofen alone would most likely not help to lower this patient's blood pressure, control volume overload, or fully correct his hyperkalemia; the addition of a loop diuretic is therefore warranted. If needed, additional interventions to help decrease the risk of hyperkalemia include adherence to a low-potassium diet and use of sodium bicarbonate.

Thiazide diuretics are largely ineffective in individuals with an estimated glomerular filtration rate below 30 mL/min/1.73 m^2.

The addition of losartan would worsen this patient's hyperkalemia and would not be recommended.

Spironolactone has been shown to further decrease urine protein excretion when added to either angiotensin-converting enzyme inhibitors or angiotensin receptor blockers in patients with diabetic nephropathy. However, this agent impairs kidney potassium excretion and also would further exacerbate this patient's hyperkalemia.

KEY POINT

Discontinuation of medications that interfere with the renin-angiotensin-aldosterone system, including NSAIDs and, if needed, angiotensin-converting enzyme inhibitors and angiotensin receptor blockers, is warranted to help correct significant hyperkalemia in the setting of chronic kidney disease.

Bibliography

Palmer BF. Managing hyperkalemia caused by inhibitors of the renin-angiotensin-aldosterone system. N Engl J Med. 2004;351(6):585-592. [PMID:15295051]

Item 23   Answer: A
Educational Objective: *Treat hyperkalemia with intravenous calcium gluconate.*

The best immediate treatment option is intravenous calcium gluconate. The electrocardiogram shows spiking of the T waves and widening of the QRS complexes, findings that indicate hyperkalemic cardiotoxicity in this patient with chronic kidney disease. The choice of treatment for hyperkalemia and the aggressiveness of its implementation depend largely on the severity of the hyperkalemia as well as on electrocardiographic and neuromuscular manifestations. The approximate relationship between electrocardiographic changes and the serum potassium concentration is substantially modified by changes of other cations in the serum and the acid–base status. (For example, with the simultaneous presence of hyponatremia, hypocalcemia, and acidemia, even modest degrees of hyperkalemia may result in serious and potentially fatal electrical disturbances.)

Urgent therapy of hyperkalemia consists of antagonism of the membrane effects of hyperkalemia and induction of intracellular potassium shift. Removing potassium from the body (for example, by sodium polystyrene sulfonate, hemodialysis, peritoneal dialysis) is important, but the effects cannot be accomplished with the necessary urgency. Therefore, the first step in treating urgent hyperkalemia is to administer calcium gluconate to antagonize hyperkalemic cardiac toxicity, an effect that usually begins within 2 to 3 minutes of administration of intravenous calcium gluconate. Sodium bicarbonate and β-antagonists such as albuterol and glucose (with or without insulin) would facilitate intracellular potassium shift. However, their effect is slower (10 minutes for sodium bicarbonate, 15 to 30 minutes for albuterol, and 30 minutes for glucose and insulin). Hypertonic glucose should not be administered without insulin when treating a patient with diabetes.

Dialysis, 50% glucose, and sodium polystyrene sulfonate are all helpful therapeutic steps in managing urgent hyperkalemia, but none is the ideal first step.

KEY POINT
The first step in treating urgent hyperkalemia is to administer calcium gluconate to antagonize hyperkalemic cardiac toxicity.

Bibliography
Alfonzo AV, Isles C, Geddes C, Deighan C. Potassium disorders: clinical spectrum and emergency management. Resuscitation. 2006;70(1):10-25. [PMID: 16600469]

Item 24   Answer: A
Educational Objective: *Diagnose laxative abuse in a patient with hypokalemia.*

This patient likely has been abusing laxatives. This is supported by the serum electrolyte pattern suggesting hypokalemia and a metabolic acidosis. In the absence of a cellular shift, a low serum potassium concentration can be caused by losses via the gastrointestinal tract, skin or kidney, or due to inadequate dietary intake of potassium. A urine potassium concentration of less than 20 meq/L (20 mmol/L) is suggestive of extrarenal losses, whereas a concentration higher than this value is suggestive of kidney losses. Therefore, this patient has a hypokalemic disorder associated nonrenal potassium loss. Gastrointestinal disorders are the most common clinical cause of extrarenal potassium losses. Diarrhea leads to fecal potassium wastage and is associated with a normal anion gap acidosis due to increased gastrointestinal loss of bicarbonate. Her low serum bicarbonate is consistent with metabolic acidosis but without an arterial blood gas, the acid-base disorder cannot be determined. Villous adenoma and laxative abuse are two such conditions that can cause gastrointestinal potassium losses. The fact that the patient is an underweight adolescent female, in whom eating disorders are common, suggests the possibility of surreptitious laxative abuse in an effort to control weight.

Although primary hyperaldosteronism may result hypokalemia, it is typically associated with hypertension and high urinary potassium concentration, both of which is absent in this patient. Hypoaldosteronism is associated with hyponatremia and hyperkalemia, which are not compatible with this patient's findings. Surreptitious diuretic abuse can cause of hypokalemia; however, it is associated with metabolic alkalosis and high urinary potassium concentration, findings not seen in this patient.

KEY POINT
In a patient with hypokalemia, a urine potassium concentration of less than 20 meq/L (20 mmol/L) is suggestive of extrarenal losses, whereas a concentration higher than this value is suggestive of kidney losses.

Bibliography
Alfonzo AV, Isles C, Geddes C, Deighan C. Potassium disorders: clinical spectrum and emergency management. Resuscitation. 2006;70(1):10-25. [PMID: 16600469]

Item 25   Answer: A
Educational Objective: *Diagnose central diabetes insipidus.*

The most likely cause of this patient's hypernatremia is central diabetes insipidus. This patient is clearly hyperosmolar, as estimated by multiplying the serum sodium level by 2 (310 mosm/kg [310 μmol/kg]; normal, 275-295 mosm/kg [275-295 μmol/kg]). The appropriate renal response to hyperosmolality is to maximally concentrate the urine (generally to greater than 800 mosm/kg [800 μmol/kg]). This response is not seen in this patient. Thus, he has either diabetes insipidus or a solute diuresis. A solute diuresis is most often caused by hyperglycemia. This patient does have a plasma glucose level of 150 mg/dL (8.3 mmol/L); however, this degree of elevation is unlikely to cause significant solute diuresis because the renal threshold for glucose reabsorption in most persons is 200 to 225 mg/dL (11.1 to 12.5 mmol/L). Furthermore, solute diuresis is usually characterized by isotonicity of the urine, whereas this patient has a markedly hypotonic urine. Consequently, diabetes mellitus is unlikely.

Hyperosmolar patients without glucosuria who have submaximally concentrated urine have diabetes insipidus by definition. Distinguishing between central and nephrogenic diabetes insipidus in a patient who is already hyperosmolar can be done by measuring plasma arginine vasopressin (AVP) (patients with central diabetes insipidus have an inappropriately low level, whereas patients with nephrogenic diabetes insipidus have a normal to elevated level); or by evaluating the response to administered AVP (5 U subcutaneously) or, preferably, the selective AVP V_2 receptor agonist desmopressin (arginine vasopressin, 1 to 2 μg subcutaneously or intravenously). A significant increase in urine osmolality (greater than 50%) within 1 to 2 hours after injection indicates insufficient endogenous AVP secretion, and, therefore, central diabetes insipidus, whereas a lack of response indicates renal resistance to the effects of AVP and, therefore, nephrogenic diabetes insipidus.

Patients with primary polydipsia also manifest polyuria and polydipsia but do not become hypernatremic and hyperosmolar. These patients may develop hyponatremia and typically have clearly identifiable psychiatric illness.

KEY POINT

Hyperosmolar patients without glucosuria who have submaximally concentrated urine have diabetes insipidus by definition.

Bibliography

Loh JA, Verbalis JG. Disorders of water and salt metabolism associated with pituitary disease. Endocrinol Metab Clin North Am. 2008;37:213-234, x. [PMID: 18226738]

Item 26   Answer: C

Educational Objective: *Diagnose acute pancreatitis as a cause for hypocalcemia.*

The most likely cause of the patient's hypocalcemia is calcium chelation with free fatty acids liberated by pancreatic enzymes during an episode of acute gallstone pancreatitis. When the pancreas is injured, the secretion of pancreatic enzymes is blocked, which leads to an autodigestive injury to the gland. The pancreatic enzymes are then released within the peritoneum and digest fat; the generated free fatty acids avidly chelate insoluble calcium salts, resulting in hypocalcemia and deposition of calcium salts in the pancreatic bed. This process is known as saponification and can lead to symptomatic hypocalcemia and calcium deposits identifiable on plain films of the abdomen. Pancreatic calcification identified by imaging studies is a diagnostic sign of chronic pancreatitis.

1,25-hydroxy vitamin D deficiency is most commonly seen in chronic kidney disease and is due to decreased activity of the 1α-hydroxylase enzyme responsible for converting 25-hydroxy vitamin D to the active form. This patient does not have a history of chronic kidney disease.

This patient has no history of previous thyroid surgery, which is the most common reason for parathyroid injury and hypoparathyroidism and is related to incidental removal or vascular injury to the parathyroid glands. Autoimmune destruction of the parathyroid gland usually occurs in the setting of other autoimmune disorders (polyglandular autoimmune syndrome) including adrenal insufficiency and mucocutaneous candidiasis, which are not present in this patient.

KEY POINT

Acute pancreatitis can generate free fatty acids that avidly chelate insoluble calcium salts in the pancreatic bed, resulting in hypocalcemia.

Bibliography

Juan D. Hypocalcemia. Differential diagnosis and mechanisms. Arch Intern Med. 1979;139(10):1166-71. [PMID: 226022]

Item 27   Answer: D

Educational Objective: *Treat hypercalcemia due to sarcoidosis with corticosteroids.*

This man presents with severe constipation due to hypercalcemia in the setting of sarcoidosis. Sarcoidosis is a multisystem, granulomatous, inflammatory condition of unknown cause that occurs in young adults of both sexes. The temporal pattern of disease progression ranges from asymptomatic to acute systemic presentations with fever, erythema nodosum, polyarthralgia, and hilar lymphadenopathy (Löfgren syndrome). Approximately 90% of patients have pulmonary involvement at the time of presentation. Hypercalcemia and hypercalciuria in sarcoidosis are caused by unregulated production of 1α-hydroxylase by activated macrophages in the granuloma tissue. Increased 1α-hydroxylase activity increases the production of 1,25 [OH]$_2$ vitamin D. Increased amounts of vitamin D$_3$ result in increased gastrointestinal absorption of calcium, resulting in hypercalcemia. Corticosteroid therapy decreases vitamin D$_3$ production by decreasing the number of activated macrophages.

Cinacalcet binds to the parathyroid calcium-sensing receptor, leading to decreased release of parathyroid hormone. This therapy is indicated only in refractory secondary hyperparathyroidism of chronic kidney disease (low serum calcium and elevated parathyroid hormone levels) or tertiary hyperparathyroidism (elevated serum calcium and elevated serum parathyroid hormone levels), neither of which applies to this patient.

Hydrochlorothiazide indirectly inhibits calcium excretion by the kidney, leading to calcium retention, and may cause hypercalcemia. Although this patient's blood pressure is elevated, it should be remeasured after his constipation is relieved and hypercalcemia is resolved; regardless, hydrochlorothiazide would be an inappropriate medication because of its propensity to cause hypercalcemia.

Measures taken to treat acute symptomatic hypercalcemia include increasing urinary excretion of calcium. Urine calcium excretion can be attained by inhibition of proximal tubular and loop sodium resorption, which is best achieved by volume expansion using intravenous normal saline infusion (1-2 L for 1 hour). This therapy is generally reserved for symptomatic patients with moderate calcium elevation (>12 mg/dL [3.0 mmol/L]) and is unnecessary in this patient.

KEY POINT

Sarcoidosis causes hypercalcemia through increased production of 1α-hydroxylase and can be treated with prednisone.

Bibliography

Iannuzzi MC, Fontana JR. Sarcoidosis: clinical presentation, immunopathogenesis, and therapeutics. JAMA. 2011;305(4):391-9. [PMID:21266686]

Item 28   Answer: C

Educational Objective: *Diagnose hyperparathyroidism by measuring the parathyroid hormone level.*

This patient's parathyroid hormone (PTH) level should be determined next. Primary hyperparathyroidism is the most common cause of hypercalcemia in the outpatient setting. The first step in the diagnosis of hypercalcemia is determination of the PTH level with an assay for intact PTH. If the PTH level is high or "inappropriately" normal, primary hyperparathyroidism is the diagnosis. If the PTH level is suppressed, a search for other entities that cause hypercalcemia must be conducted.

Calcitonin is secreted by thyroid parafollicular C cells. This serum level is elevated in patients with medullary thyroid cancer or C-cell hyperplasia. Calcitonin tends to lower the calcium level by enhancing cellular uptake, renal excretion, and bone formation. The effect of calcitonin on bone metabolism is weak and only relevant in pharmacologic amounts. Measurement of serum calcitonin is not indicated in a patient with hypercalcemia.

One of the ways in which PTH increases the serum calcium level is by up-regulation of the 1α-hydroxylase enzyme, which stimulates conversion of vitamin D to its most active form, 1,25-dihydroxy vitamin D. This form of vitamin D increases the percentage of dietary calcium absorbed by the intestine. Body stores of vitamin D are assessed by measuring the 25-hydroxy vitamin D level, which has a long half-life. Measurement of this patient's 25-hydroxy vitamin D and 1,25-dihydroxy vitamin D levels may be appropriate if the parathyroid hormone level is suppressed. At this time, however, such measurement is not indicated.

Humoral hypercalcemia of malignancy results from the systemic effect of a circulating factor produced by neoplastic cells. The hormone most commonly responsible for this syndrome is parathyroid hormone–related protein (PTHrP). This peptide's *N*-terminal shares many homologic features with PTH and most, if not all, of the metabolic effects of PTH. Tumors that elaborate PTHrP are most commonly squamous cell carcinomas, such as those of the lung, esophagus, and head and neck. This patient has no evidence of cancer. The diagnosis of humoral hypercalcemia of malignancy can often be made in the absence of PTHrP measurements if a compatible malignancy, hypercalcemia, and suppressed PTH level are present.

KEY POINT

The most common cause of hypercalcemia in the outpatient setting is hyperparathyroidism.

Bibliography

Moe SM. Disorders involving calcium, phosphorus, and magnesium. Prim Care. 2008;35(2):215-237, v-vi. [PMID:18486714]

Item 29   Answer: D

Educational Objective: *Diagnose hypophosphatemia in a patient with chronic alcoholism.*

This patient most likely has hypophosphatemia. Severe hypophosphatemia most often develops in patients with chronic alcoholism who have poor oral intake, decreased intestinal absorption due to frequent vomiting and diarrhea, and increased kidney excretion due to the direct effect of ethanol on the tubule. Despite total body phosphorus depletion, these patients may have normal serum phosphorus levels on admission to the hospital. Severe hypophosphatemia often develops over the first 12 to 24 hours after admission, usually because of intravenous glucose administration, which stimulates insulin release and causes phosphate to shift into cells. The sudden development of hypophosphatemia may cause confusion, rhabdomyolysis, hemolytic anemia, and severe muscle weakness that can lead to respiratory failure. Oral phosphate is the preferred treatment in this setting, but intravenous administration may be needed if oral therapy cannot be tolerated.

Hypercalcemia may manifest as decreased neuromuscular excitability that causes decreased muscular tone. Hypercalcemia is most commonly caused by alterations in calcium absorption from the gut and bone resorption due to primary hyperparathyroidism, malignancy, and granulomatous diseases. Primary hyperparathyroidism and thiazide diuretic use also may cause this condition. The sudden development of hypercalcemia in this patient is unlikely.

Hypokalemia can cause diffuse muscle weakness, gastrointestinal tract atony, respiratory failure, and cardiac arrhythmias. In chronic hypokalemia, muscle weakness is unusual in patients with a serum potassium level above 2.5 meq/L (2.5 mmol/L) and the risk of profound hypokalemia is low in a patient receiving potassium supplementation.

Early signs of hyponatremia typically include nausea, vomiting, and headaches; progressive manifestations include impaired mental status and seizures. These symptoms are not compatible with this patient's presentation. Finally, the development of acute hyponatremia would be unlikely in a patient receiving intravenous normal saline.

KEY POINT

Patients with chronic alcoholism may have normal serum phosphorus levels on admission to the hospital but may develop severe hypophosphatemia over the first 12 to 24 hours.

Bibliography

Moe S. Disorders involving calcium, phosphorus, and magnesium. Prim Care. 2008;35(2):215-237. [PMID:18486714]

Section 8

Neurology
Questions

Item 1 [Basic]

An 80-year old woman living in a nursing home with history of dementia is admitted to the hospital with pneumonia. In the emergency department, a peripheral intravenous line was inserted, appropriate antibiotics were initiated, she was given oxygen by nasal cannula, and a urinary catheter was placed.

On physical examination, temperature is 38.3°C (101.0°F), blood pressure is 140/88 mm Hg, pulse rate is 100/min, and respiration rate is 16/min. Pulmonary auscultation reveals left lower lobe crackles. Cardiac examination is normal. Moderate cognitive impairment is noted but no inattention or focal neurologic deficits.

She is provided access to her glasses and hearing aid, and a large clock and night light are in place in her room.

Which of the following additional steps should be taken to prevent delirium in this patient?

(A) Administer benzodiazepine, as needed
(B) Administer diphenhydramine for sleep
(C) Administer haloperidol twice daily
(D) Check vital signs every 4 hours through the night
(E) Remove her urinary catheter

Item 2 [Basic]

A 79-year-old woman was hospitalized 4 days ago after sustaining a right hip fracture in a fall. She underwent surgical repair with right hip replacement 3 days ago and did not fully awake from general anesthesia until 12 hours after extubation. As her alertness has increased, she has become increasingly agitated. The patient has a 4-year history of Alzheimer dementia. She has no other pertinent personal or family medical history. Current medications are donepezil, memantine, and low-molecular-weight heparin.

On physical examination today, temperature is 37.2°C (99.0°F), blood pressure is 100/68 mm Hg, pulse rate is 100/min and regular, and respiration rate is 18/min. The patient can move all four limbs with guarding of the right lower limb. She is inattentive and disoriented to time and place and exhibits combativeness alternating with hypersomnolence. The remainder of the neurologic examination is unremarkable, without evidence of focal findings or meningismus.

Which of the following is the most likely diagnosis?

(A) Acute stroke
(B) Acute worsening of Alzheimer dementia
(C) Meningitis
(D) Postoperative delirium

Item 3 [Advanced]

A 75-year-old woman with a history of chronic obstructive pulmonary disease is evaluated in the intensive care unit for delirium. She had a median sternotomy and repair of an aortic dissection and was extubated uneventfully on postoperative day 4. Two days later she developed fluctuations in her mental status and inattention. While still in the intensive care unit, she became agitated, pulling at her lines, attempting to climb out of bed, and asking to leave the hospital. Her arterial blood gas values are normal. The patient has no history of alcohol abuse or other substance abuse. The use of frequent orientation cues, calm reassurance, and presence of family members has done little to reduce the patient's agitated behavior. Medical evaluation identifies no focal neurologic deficits and no evidence of infection or metabolic abnormality.

Which of the following is the most appropriate therapy?

(A) Diphenhydramine
(B) Haloperidol
(C) Lorazepam
(D) Propofol

Item 4 [Basic]

A 36-year-old woman is evaluated in the emergency department for a 3-day history of confusion and falls. The patient lives alone and is accompanied by her neighbor who says that the patient's symptoms seem to be getting worse. The patient has a 10-year history of chronic alcoholism and has had recent weight loss due to diarrhea. She takes no medications.

On physical examination, temperature is 35.6°C (96.0°F), blood pressure is 142/76 mm Hg, pulse rate is 90/min, respiration rate is 14/min; BMI is 17. Temporal muscle wasting, sunken supraclavicular fossae, and absent adipose stores are noted. Abdominal examination findings are normal. On neurologic examination, the patient is confused; she is unable to state the date and does not know the name of the hospital. Marked horizontal nystagmus is noted. There is no nuchal rigidity or obvious motor weakness. Deep tendon reflexes are reduced, and plantar responses are flexor. The patient has a markedly ataxic gait.

Which of the following is the best initial management?

(A) Electroencephalography
(B) Haloperidol
(C) Thiamine
(D) Vancomycin, ampicillin, and ceftriaxone

Item 5 [Advanced]

A 73-year-old man is evaluated for confusion that began 2 weeks ago. He wanders aimlessly in the house, sometimes not recognizing his wife and mistaking the newspaper for his hat. He has visual hallucinations and believes he sees mice in the refrigerator. His medical history includes type 2 diabetes mellitus with painful peripheral neuropathy, coronary artery disease, depression, and heart failure. Medications are glyburide, nortriptyline, digoxin, lorazepam, metoprolol, lisinopril, aspirin, and pravastatin. He does not remember how long he has been taking these medications and if there have been any recent dosage changes. The patient drinks alcohol only occasionally, usually wine with a weekend meal.

On physical examination, the patient has asterixis. Vital signs are normal; oxygen saturation is normal with the patient breathing ambient air. He is inattentive and not oriented to time or place. His score on the Mini–Mental State Examination is 13/30 (28/30 6 months ago). Results of laboratory studies, including electrolyte levels and liver chemistry and renal function studies, are normal. An MRI of the brain is normal.

Which of the following is the most likely diagnosis?

(A) Alcohol hallucinosis
(B) Alzheimer dementia
(C) Depression
(D) Toxic encephalopathy (delirium)

Item 6 [Basic]

A 33-year-old woman is evaluated in the emergency department for paresthesia that began in the left face and spread over 30 minutes to the left arm and leg, clumsiness of the left hand that began 30 minutes ago, and a subsequent right-sided throbbing headache and nausea. This is the first time she has ever had such symptoms. She is otherwise healthy but has a family history of migraine. Her only medication is a daily oral contraceptive pill.

On physical examination, temperature is normal, blood pressure is 140/82 mm Hg, pulse rate is 110/min, and respiration rate is 20/min. All other examination findings are normal.

Results of laboratory studies and a CT scan of the head are also normal.

Which of the following is the most likely diagnosis?

(A) Migraine with aura
(B) Multiple sclerosis
(C) Partial complex seizure
(D) Transient ischemic attack
(E) Trigeminal neuralgia

Item 7 [Basic]

A 24-year-old woman is evaluated in the office for headache that occurs once or twice a week. The pain is a constant pressure in the back of the head. She has no nausea and can continue to work during the headaches. She has had these headaches since age 13 years and notes that they now seem to be more frequent and associated with less sleep and increased stress. When treated with ibuprofen or aceta-

minophen, the headaches abate in 30 minutes; untreated, they last several hours. She typically uses headache medication four to six times per month.

On physical examination, vital signs are normal. All other findings from the general physical examination findings, including those from a neurologic evaluation, are normal.

Which of the following is the most likely diagnosis?

(A) Chronic daily headache
(B) Cluster headache
(C) Migraine headache without aura
(D) Tension-type headache

Item 8 [Advanced]

A previously healthy 42-year-old woman is evaluated in the emergency department for the sudden onset of a severe occipital headache during defecation 8 hours ago, followed by two episodes of vomiting. The headache reached maximum intensity within seconds. She has never had a headache like this before. She reports no neck stiffness or neurologic symptoms. Her mother and two sisters have a history of migraine.

On physical examination, temperature is 36.8°C (98.2°F), blood pressure is 148/88 mm Hg, pulse rate is 90/min, and respiration rate is 20/min. The patient is in significant distress as a result of the pain. There is no evidence of meningismus, papilledema, or focal neurologic signs.

Which of the following is the most appropriate next step in management?

(A) CT angiography of the head and neck
(B) Lumbar puncture
(C) Noncontrast CT of the head
(D) Subcutaneous administration of sumatriptan

Item 9 [Basic]

A 32-year-old woman is evaluated for a gradual increase in migraine frequency and severity over the past 6 months. Migraine attacks, which formerly occurred two or three times each month, are now occurring approximately three times each week, with each attack lasting at least 12 hours. She has no other medial problems and takes only almotriptan as needed for acute migraine.

On physical examination, vital signs and results of a general physical examination, including a neurologic examination, are normal.

An MRI of the brain shows no abnormalities.

Which of the following is the most appropriate treatment for this patient?

(A) Botulinum toxin
(B) Propranolol
(C) Nortriptyline
(D) Sertraline

Item 10 [Basic]

A 75-year-old woman is evaluated in the emergency department after she was witnessed driving erratically on a city street. Initially, the patient was unable to answer any questions and had difficulty with her speech. Twenty minutes later, her speech was fluid, and, although she did not have any recollection of the past few hours' events, she was able to provide some details of her life, including her husband's name. When her husband arrived, the patient was able to recognize him, but 10 minutes later she did not recognize him. No evidence of hallucinations or delusions exists.

The husband reports that the patient has had a gradual and progressive cognitive impairment over the previous 5 years for which she takes donepezil. She often awakens at night and roams about the house. She has chronic problems with her memory and managing activities of daily living.

Which of the following is the most likely diagnosis?

(A) Delirium
(B) Delirium superimposed on dementia
(C) Dementia
(D) Psychosis

Item 11 [Basic]

A 68-year-old man is evaluated for memory difficulty that, according to his wife, began insidiously 3 or 4 years earlier. He has difficulty remembering recent events. For example, he forgets appointments and recent conversations and forgot that a close relative had recently died. He is no longer able to manage his own checkbook or operate his car without getting lost. Medical history is otherwise unremarkable.

Physical examination findings, including vital signs, are normal. Mental status examination shows prominent memory loss and difficulty drawing a complex figure.

Laboratory studies show that a complete blood count and routine chemistries are normal. An MRI of the brain shows only mild cerebral atrophy.

Which of the following is the most likely diagnosis?

(A) Alzheimer dementia
(B) Creutzfeldt-Jakob disease
(C) Dementia with Lewy bodies
(D) Frontotemporal dementia

Item 12 [Advanced]

An 84-year-old man is evaluated for the gradual onset of progressive memory loss over the past 2 years. In the past 4 months, he has twice been unable to find his way home after going to the local supermarket. His wife has assumed responsibility for the household finances after the patient overdrew their checking account for the third time. His mother had onset of Alzheimer dementia at age 79 years and died at age 86 years. His only medication is a daily multivitamin.

On physical examination, vital signs are normal. His level of alertness, speech, and gait are normal. His score on the Folstein Mini–Mental State Examination is 24/30, including

0/3 on the recall portion, which corresponds with a diagnosis of mild dementia.

Results of laboratory studies, including a complete blood count, serum vitamin B_{12} measurement, thyroid function tests, and a basic metabolic panel, are normal.

An unenhanced MRI of the brain shows no abnormalities.

Which of the following is the most appropriate treatment at this time?

(A) Donepezil
(B) Ginkgo biloba
(C) Quetiapine
(D) Sertraline

Item 13 [Advanced]

An 81-year-old woman is evaluated in the office for increasing difficulty with activities of daily living, including dressing and feeding herself, over the past 6 months. She has had gradually progressive cognitive decline for the past 5 years and now needs 24-hour help from a caregiver; Alzheimer dementia was previously diagnosed. Current medications are donepezil and a daily multivitamin.

On physical examination, vital signs are normal. Her level of alertness, speech, and gait are normal. The patient scores only 12/30 on the Folstein Mini–Mental State Examination.

Results of a complete blood count, a basic metabolic panel, a serum vitamin B_{12} measurement, and thyroid function tests are normal.

A CT scan of the head without contrast shows no evidence of tumor, hemorrhage, or infarction.

Which of the following is the most appropriate next step in treatment?

(A) Add memantine
(B) Add quetiapine
(C) Add sertraline
(D) Stop donepezil

Item 14 [Basic]

A 23-year-old man is evaluated in the emergency department because of the acute onset of uncontrolled head turning to one side and tongue protrusion. He was recently diagnosed with schizophrenia and had haloperidol treatment started 3 days ago. He has no other medical problems and takes no additional medications.

On examination, he appears anxious; temperature is normal, blood pressure is 140/80 mm Hg, pulse rate is 100/min, and respiration rate is 14/min. His head is turned 40 degrees to the right, and he has sustained tongue protrusion. He is unable to turn his head back to midline or retract his tongue back into his mouth. The remainder of his neurologic examination is normal.

Which of the following is the most likely diagnosis?

(A) Drug-induced dystonia
(B) Huntington disease
(C) Idiopathic cervical dystonia
(D) Neuroleptic malignant syndrome

Item 15 [Advanced]

A 66-year-old man is evaluated in the office for a 6-month history of a resting right arm tremor. He says that his writing has gotten smaller during this time and that he has had difficulty buttoning his dress shirts. The patient reports no prior medical problems and is not aware of any neurologic problems in his family. He takes no medications.

Results of a general medical examination are normal. Neurologic examination shows a paucity of facial expression (hypomimia). Cranial nerve function is normal. Motor examination shows normal strength but mild left upper limb rigidity and a 5-Hz resting tremor of the right upper limb. Deep tendon reflexes are normal, as are results of sensory examination. There is no truncal or appendicular ataxia. Diminished arm swing is noted bilaterally but is worse on the right. A tremor in the right upper limb is noted during ambulation. Left upper limb alternating motion rates are diminished.

Which of the following is the most likely diagnosis?

(A) Cervical dystonia
(B) Essential tremor
(C) Huntington disease
(D) Parkinson disease

Item 16 [Basic]

A 62-year-old woman is evaluated for a 1-year history of tremor that affects both upper extremities. She says that her handwriting has become sloppier since she first noticed the tremor and that she occasionally spills her morning coffee because of it. The patient is otherwise healthy. Her mother, who died at age 79 years, had a similar tremor. Her only medication is a daily multivitamin.

On examination, she has a mild tremor in the upper extremities that is present with the arms extended and during finger-to-nose testing. No resting tremor is apparent. Muscle tone and gait and limb coordination are normal.

Administration of which of the following drugs is the most appropriate treatment of this patient?

(A) Carbidopa-levodopa
(B) Pramipexole
(C) Propranolol
(D) Ropinirole

Item 17 [Advanced]

A 45-year-old woman with a history of heavy alcohol use is evaluated in the emergency department for a headache and altered mental status of 2-day's duration. One week earlier she had a diarrheal illness that quickly resolved.

On physical examination, she is lethargic and unable to follow commands. Temperature is 38.8°C (101.9°F), blood pressure is 110/70 mm Hg, pulse rate is 105/min, and respiration rate is 22/min. Jolt accentuation of her headache is present.

The leukocyte count is 14,500/µL (14.5×10^9/L) with 44% neutrophils, 42% bands, and 13% lymphocytes; platelet count is 146,000/µL (146×10^9/L). The serum albumin is 2.6 mg/dL (26 g/L), the INR is 1.5, and the partial thromboplastin time is 44.1 seconds.

A noncontrast head CT scan is normal. Cerebrospinal fluid (CSF) leukocyte count is 1500/µL (1500×10^6/L), with 60% neutrophils and 40% lymphocytes; glucose level is 5 mg/dL (0.3 mmol/L); and protein level is 328 mg/dL (3280 mg/L). The CSF Gram stain reveals intracellular gram-positive bacilli.

Which of the following is the most likely diagnosis?

(A) *Listeria monocytogenes* meningitis
(B) *Neisseria meningitidis* meningitis
(C) *Streptococcus pneumoniae* meningitis
(D) Viral meningitis

Item 18 [Advanced]

A 19-year-old-woman who is a sophomore in college is evaluated in December for a 24-hour history of fever and headache. She lives in a dormitory on campus. Her medical history is unremarkable. She takes no medications and is up to date with all of her immunizations, including the meningococcal vaccine, which she received before entering college. Two cases of meningococcal serogroup B-associated meningitis have been reported on campus.

On physical examination, the patient appears ill. Temperature is 39.1°C (102.4°F), blood pressure is 95/50 mm Hg, pulse rate is 125/min, and respiration rate is 25/min. A purpuric rash is appreciated over both lower extremities. Neck stiffness is present and jolt accentuation of the headache is elicited.

A noncontrast CT scan of the head is normal. The leukocyte count is 19,500/µL (19.5×10^9/L) with 87% neutrophils and 13% lymphocytes; platelet count is 110,000/µL (110×10^9/L). Cerebrospinal fluid (CSF) leukocyte count is 2000/µL (2000×10^6/L), with 95% neutrophils and 5% lymphocytes; glucose level is 20 mg/dL (1.1 mmol/L); and protein level is 100 mg/dL (1000 mg/L). The CSF Gram stain reveals gram-negative diplococci.

Which of the following is the most likely diagnosis?

(A) *Neisseria meningitidis* meningitis
(B) Rocky Mountain spotted fever
(C) *Streptococcus pneumoniae* meningitis
(D) *Vibrio vulnificus* meningitis

Item 19 [Advanced]

A 20-year-old female college student is evaluated in December because of a 12-hour history of fever, myalgia, headache, and a rash. She takes no medications.

On physical examination, the patient appears ill. Temperature is 38.8°C (101.8°F), blood pressure is 90/45 mm Hg, pulse rate is 112/min, and respiration rate is 24/min. A petechial rash, most prominent on the lower extremities, is present. Passive neck flexion causes discomfort.

Leukocyte count	10,500/μL (10.5 × 10⁹/L)
Platelet count	105,000/μL (105 × 10⁹/L)
Blood urea nitrogen	30 mg/dL (10.7 mmol/L)
Creatinine	2.5 mg/dL (221 μmol/L)
Bicarbonate	15 meq/L (15 mmol/L)

Leukocyte count 10,500/μL (10.5 × 10^9/L)
Platelet count 105,000/μL (105 × 10^9/L)
Blood urea nitrogen 30 mg/dL (10.7 mmol/L)
Creatinine 2.5 mg/dL (221 μmol/L)
Bicarbonate 15 meq/L (15 mmol/L)

Lumbar puncture is performed. Opening pressure is 300 mm H$_2$O. Cerebrospinal fluid leukocyte count is 1250/μL (1250 × 10^6/L) with 95% polymorphonuclear cells. Protein level is 100 mg/dL (1000 mg/L) and glucose level is 40 mg/dL (2.2 mmol/L). No organisms are seen Gram stain.

Which of the following is the most likely diagnosis?

(A) *Listeria monocytogenes* meningitis
(B) *Neisseria meningitidis* meningitis
(C) Rocky Mountain spotted fever
(D) Viral meningitis

Item 20 [Advanced]

A 65-year-old woman is evaluated for a 1-day history of fever, headache, and altered mental status. Medical history includes type 2 diabetes mellitus and hypertension treated with glipizide and hydrochlorothiazide. She has no allergies.

On physical examination, the patient is confused. Temperature is 38.9°C (102.0°F), blood pressure is 104/66 mm Hg, pulse rate is 100/min, and respiration rate is 20/min. Her neck is supple, and she has no rashes.

The leukocyte count is 19,000/μL (19 × 10^9/L); platelet count, 90,000/μL (90 × 10^9/L); and plasma glucose level, 120 mg/dL (6.7 mmol/L). A non–contrast-enhanced CT scan of the head is normal. Cerebrospinal fluid (CSF) analysis shows a leukocyte count of 1300/μL (1300 × 10^6/L) with 98% neutrophils, a glucose level of 20 mg/dL (1.1 mmol/L), and a protein level of 200 mg/dL (2000 mg/L). CSF Gram stain results are negative for any organisms.

Dexamethasone is begun.

Which of the following antimicrobial regimens should now be initiated?

(A) Ceftriaxone
(B) Penicillin G
(C) Vancomycin, ampicillin, and ceftriaxone
(D) Vancomycin plus ceftriaxone
(E) Vancomycin plus trimethoprim-sulfamethoxazole

Item 21 [Advanced]

A 75-year-old woman with an 8-hour history of aphasia and right-sided weakness is admitted to the hospital. She has a 35-year history of hypertension treated with chlorthalidone and a 10-year history of hyperlipidemia treated with simvastatin. Her medical history is otherwise unremarkable, and she takes no other medications.

On physical examination she is afebrile, blood pressure is 150/90 mm Hg, pulse rate is 88/min, and respiration rate is 12/min. Oxygen saturation on pulse oximetry is 96%. She is alert but has expressive aphasia and dense right hemiplegia. No carotid bruits are heard, and the cardiopulmonary examination is normal.

Coagulation studies, serum electrolytes, and comprehensive metabolic panel are normal. The electrocardiogram shows sinus rhythm without evidence of ischemia. The CT scan shows no signs of hemorrhage. Echocardiography is normal with an estimated ejection fraction of 54%.

Which of the following is the most appropriate next step in this patient's hospital management?

(A) Bed rest for the next 48 hours
(B) Bed rest for the next week
(C) Begin a mechanical soft diet
(D) Begin physical and occupational therapy

Item 22 [Basic]

A 74-year-old man is brought to the emergency department by ambulance 1 hour after he had an acute witnessed onset of aphasia and right hemiparesis. He has a history of hypertension. His current medications are hydrochlorothiazide and metoprolol.

On physical examination, blood pressure is 178/94 mm Hg and pulse rate is 80/min and regular. Neurologic examination confirms nonfluent aphasia, a right pronator drift, a right leg drift, and an extensor plantar response on the right.

An electrocardiogram obtained on the patient's arrival at the emergency department documents sinus rhythm. A CT scan of the head obtained within 1 hour of his arrival reveals early ischemic changes.

Which of the following is the best treatment?

(A) Aspirin
(B) Continuous intravenous heparin
(C) Intravenous labetalol
(D) Intravenous recombinant tissue plasminogen activator

Item 23 [Advanced]

A 74-year-old woman is admitted to the hospital after sustaining a severe left hemispheric ischemic stroke while alone at home. She was last known to be normal 8 hours ago. The patient has hypertension for which she takes enalapril but no history of ischemic heart disease or heart failure.

On physical examination, blood pressure is 190/105 mm Hg, pulse rate is 80/min, and respiration rate is 16/min. The patient has right hemiparesis, right facial droop, aphasia, and dysarthria. The remainder of the physical examination, including the cardiovascular examination, is normal.

Results of laboratory studies, including serum creatinine level, are normal.

A CT scan shows ischemic changes that occupy most of the left middle cerebral artery territory. An electrocardiogram and chest radiograph show normal findings.

Which of the following is the most appropriate treatment of her hypertension at this time?

(A) Intravenous labetalol
(B) Intravenous nicardipine
(C) Oral nifedipine
(D) No treatment at this time

Item 24 [Basic]

A 73-year-old retired woman is evaluated in the emergency department 6 hours after experiencing the sudden, explosive onset of a severe headache. The patient has hypertension controlled by diet and exercise. There is no relevant family history. She has no allergies and takes no over-the-counter medications.

On physical examination, she is in obvious distress from the headache. Temperature is normal, blood pressure is 179/108 mm Hg, pulse rate is 119/min, and respiration rate is 14/min. There is no meningismus. Neurologic examination shows a normal level of consciousness and no focal abnormalities.

Results of laboratory studies and a CT scan of the head without contrast are normal.

Which of the following is the most appropriate next management step?

(A) Lumbar puncture
(B) MRI of the brain
(C) Observation
(D) Sumatriptan, orally

Item 25 [Basic]

A 34-year-old woman is evaluated in the office for right-sided facial paralysis that she noticed on awakening 1 hour ago. She has a 10-pack-year smoking history. Personal and family medical history is noncontributory. Her only medication is a daily oral contraceptive.

On physical examination, vital signs are normal. Limb strength, reflexes, and tone are normal bilaterally. Findings from a sensory examination, which included her face, are also normal. When asked to raise her eyebrows, the patient does not elevate the right side. When asked to shut her eyes, she cannot close the right one but the globe rotates upward, partially covering the iris. When asked to smile, the patient does not move the right side of her face.

Which of the following is the most likely diagnosis?

(A) Graves ophthalmopathy
(B) Left cerebral infarction
(C) Right facial nerve (Bell) palsy
(D) Right trigeminal neuralgia

Item 26 [Advanced]

A 53-year-old woman is evaluated in the office for a 1-week history of paresthesias that began symmetrically in the feet and progressed to involve the distal legs and, more recently, the hands. She is unsteady when walking, has lower limb weakness, and has difficulty going upstairs. The patient has no history of pain or bowel or bladder impairment. Personal and family medical history is noncontributory, and she takes no medications.

On physical examination, vital signs are normal. Weakness of distal lower extremity muscles is noted, with stocking-glove sensory loss and areflexia. Deep tendon reflexes are absent. Plantar responses are normal, and gait is unsteady. No sensory level is present across the thorax. Mental status, language, and cranial nerve function are normal.

Complete blood count results, erythrocyte sedimentation rate, serum creatinine and creatine kinase levels, and liver chemistry test results are normal.

A chest radiograph shows no abnormalities.

Which of the following is the most likely diagnosis?

(A) Amyotrophic lateral sclerosis
(B) Diabetic neuropathy
(C) Guillain-Barré syndrome
(D) Myelopathy

Item 27 [Basic]

A 35-year-old woman is evaluated in the office for a 5-month history of right-hand numbness and tingling. She says that these symptoms involve the entire hand, seem to be worse when she drives or holds a book or newspaper, and have been awakening her at night. She reports no history of neck pain or hand weakness. Personal and family medical histories are noncontributory, and she takes no medication.

General physical examination reveals no abnormalities. Neurologic examination shows normal strength but sensory loss in the first three digits and the radial half of the fourth digit in the right hand.

Which of the following is the most likely diagnosis?

(A) Carpal tunnel syndrome
(B) de Quervain tenosynovitis
(C) Ganglion cysts
(D) Ulnar nerve compression (Guyon tunnel syndrome)

Item 28 [Basic]

An obese 66-year-old man has had increasing pain and tingling in his feet for more than 8 months. The patient has not seen a physician in more than 20 years. His only other symptoms are fatigue, blurry vision, and nocturia. He takes no medications.

On examination, vital signs are normal; BMI is 30. Results of skin, ophthalmoscopic, cardiopulmonary, and abdominal examinations are normal. On neurologic examination, he has sensory loss in the feet and distal legs. Muscle strength and reflexes are normal.

Which of the following tests will most likely diagnose the cause of the neurologic findings?

(A) Creatine kinase level
(B) Fasting blood glucose level
(C) Lumbar puncture and cerebrospinal fluid analysis
(D) Sural nerve biopsy

Item 1   **Answer: E**

Educational Objective: *Prevent delirium in patients at high risk.*

Elderly patients with a history of dementia are at very high risk for developing delirium during a hospitalization. Delirium is an acute state of confusion that may manifest as a reduced level of consciousness, cognitive abnormalities, perceptual disturbances, or emotional disturbances. Prevention involves addressing medical and environmental issues. Urinary catheters are associated with increased risk of delirium. In the absence of a medical indication for a catheter (e.g., relieve urinary retention, monitor fluid status in acutely ill patients when this directly impacts medical treatment, manage patients with stage 3 or 4 pressure ulcers on the buttocks), it should be removed.

Benzodiazepines and diphenhydramine have sedating effects but can cause delirium in the elderly. They should generally be avoided, unless a specific indication is presented, such as benzodiazepines for alcohol withdrawal or diphenhydramine for an allergic reaction. Alternative nonpharmacologic methods for relaxation include music, massage, and meditation.

In appropriate selected patients with severe delirium, low-dose haloperidol may lessen the severity and duration of delirium, but it is not indicated for the prevention of delirium. The use of antipsychotic medications in elderly patients with dementia is associated with an increased risk of death, primarily due to infection, such as pneumonia. A normal sleep-wake cycle should be maintained as much as possible, minimizing interruptions or unnecessary testing during the night, and keeping a light on and increasing stimulation during the day.

KEY POINT

Access to hearing aids, glasses, and canes and removal of unnecessary restraints and urinary catheters are basic procedures to reduce the risk of delirium in persons at risk.

Bibliography

Inouye SK. Delirium in older persons. N Engl J Med. 2006;354(11):1157-65. [PMID: 16540616]

Item 2   **Answer: D**

Educational Objective: *Diagnose postoperative delirium in a patient with dementia.*

The most likely diagnosis is postoperative delirium. Patients with delirium have acute, fluctuating mental status changes, with difficulty in focusing or maintaining attention and disorganized thinking. Based on psychomotor activity, there are four types of delirium: 1) hypoactive, 2) hyperactive, 3) mixed delirium with hypo- and hyperactivity, and 4) delirium without changes in psychomotor activity. Delirium in elderly patients with chronic dementia usually results from an acute medical problem. In addition, patients with chronic dementia from almost any cause are at greater risk for delirium after surgery with general anesthesia. This patient with a hip fracture who underwent right hip surgery with general anesthesia and did not recover from the anesthesia until 12 hours after extubation most likely has postoperative delirium. Such delirium is highly predictable and often easily managed by identification and correction of any underlying disorders and the removal or reduction of contributing factors.

The possibility of acute stroke must be considered in a patient with a change in mental status. However, this patient has no clinical evidence of such an event, which makes this diagnosis extremely unlikely.

Surgery does not exacerbate Alzheimer dementia (or dementia of any other cause) but rather produces a superimposed delirium. Finally, dementia does not acutely worsen over several hours; the decline is steadily progressive.

This patient has had dementia for 4 years that has abruptly gotten worse after surgery. Although not impossible, meningitis is highly unlikely in this setting, especially given the absence of any supporting physical examination findings, including meningeal irritation.

KEY POINT

Patients with chronic dementia are at greater risk for delirium after surgery with general anesthesia.

Bibliography

Rudolph JL, Jones RN, Rasmussen LS, Silverstein JH, Inouye SK, Marcantonio ER. Independent vascular and cognitive risk factors for postoperative delirium. Am J Med. 2007;120(9):807-813. [PMID: 17765051]

Item 3   Answer: B

Educational Objective: *Treat delirium in the intensive care unit with an antipsychotic agent (haloperidol).*

The appropriate treatment for this patient is haloperidol. When supportive care is insufficient for prevention or treatment of delirium, symptom control with medication is occasionally necessary to prevent harm or to allow evaluation and treatment in the intensive care unit. The recommended therapy for delirium is antipsychotic agents, although no drugs are approved by the U.S. Food and Drug Administration for this indication. Ongoing randomized, placebo-controlled trials are investigating different management strategies for intensive care unit delirium. A recent systematic evidence review found no evidence of superiority for second-generation antipsychotics compared with haloperidol for delirium. Haloperidol does not cause respiratory suppression, which is one reason that it is often used in patients with hypoventilatory respiratory failure who require sedation. All antipsychotic agents, and especially "typical" agents such as haloperidol, pose a risk of torsades de pointes, extrapyramidal side effects, and the neuroleptic malignant syndrome.

Diphenhydramine and other antihistamines are a major risk factor for delirium, especially in older patients. Lorazepam is actually deliriogenic, and its use in a delirious patient should be carefully re-evaluated, except perhaps in patients experiencing benzodiazepine withdrawal or delirium tremens. There is no evidence that propofol has any role in treating delirium.

KEY POINT

No drug is approved by the U.S. Food and Drug Administration for the treatment of delirium, but clinical practice guidelines recommend antipsychotic agents, such as haloperidol.

Bibliography

Campbell N, Boustani MA, Ayub A, et al. Pharmacological management of delirium in hospitalized adults—a systematic evidence review. J Gen Intern Med. 2009;24(7):848-853. [PMID: 19424763]

Item 4   Answer: C

Educational Objective: *Diagnose and treat Wernicke encephalopathy due to thiamine deficiency.*

This patient should receive thiamine now as the best initial management. She has Wernicke encephalopathy, a syndrome that results from deficiency of vitamin B_1, an important coenzyme in several biochemical pathways of the brain. Typical clinical manifestations of the disorder include mental status changes, nystagmus, ophthalmoplegia, and unsteady gait, all varying in intensity from minor to severe. When there is additional loss of memory with a confabulatory psychosis, the condition is described as Wernicke-Korsakoff syndrome. The classical clinical triad of gait ataxia, encephalopathy, and ophthalmoplegia is seen in only 19% of affected patients. Conditions associated with Wernicke encephalopathy include AIDS, alcohol abuse, cancer, hyperemesis gravidarum, pro-

longed total parenteral nutrition, postsurgical status (particularly bariatric surgeries), and glucose loading (in a predisposed patient).

Because Wernicke encephalopathy remains a clinical diagnosis, other neurologic disorders should be considered in this patient after thiamine has been administered. Electroencephalography can help exclude a seizure disorder, such as nonconvulsive status epilepticus. Infections, including encephalitis and meningitis, for which intravenous administration of broad-spectrum antibiotic drugs (such as vancomycin, ampicillin, and ceftriaxone) may be appropriate also should be part of the differential diagnosis and can be excluded with cerebrospinal fluid analysis.

Haloperidol is not indicated in this patient, who is confused but has no apparent history of psychosis or agitation. Some patients with Wernicke encephalopathy do have agitation, hallucinations, and behavioral disturbances that can mimic an acute psychosis.

KEY POINT

Wernicke encephalopathy is caused by thiamine deficiency and may result in mental status changes, ophthalmoplegia, nystagmus, and unsteady gait; it is best treated with thiamine.

Bibliography

Sechi G, Serra A. Wernicke's encephalopathy: new clinical settings and recent advances in diagnosis and management. Lancet Neurol. 2007;6(5):442-455. [PMID: 17434099]

Item 5   Answer: D

Educational Objective: *Diagnose medication-induced delirium.*

The most likely diagnosis is toxic encephalopathy presenting as delirium. Delirium is an acute state of confusion that may manifest as a reduced level of consciousness, cognitive abnormalities, perceptual disturbances, or emotional disturbances. The presence of asterixis suggests a toxic/metabolic cause of this patient's symptoms. The patient is taking several medications that might impair cognition. A prime suspect is nortriptyline; this drug has anticholinergic properties and is likely to cause impairment in patients with latent cholinergic deficiency (the elderly or patients with mild cognitive impairment, early dementia, or Parkinson disease). Digoxin and the sedative-hypnotic lorazepam may also contribute to cognitive impairment.

Symptoms of alcohol withdrawal most typically occur after cessation of prolonged, sustained alcohol intake. However, most people drink in an episodic fashion, as illustrated by this patient, and this pattern of drinking is not associated with sustained high blood alcohol levels that are requisite for withdrawal symptoms on abrupt cessation. Alcoholic hallucinosis develops 12 to 24 hours after the last drink and resolve within 24 to 48 hours, a symptomatic period much shorter than that experienced by this patient. Hallucinations are usually visual and are not associated with clouding of the sensorium and are not associated with asterixis.

In patients with early Alzheimer dementia, delirium is produced more readily by anticholinergic medications. Alzheimer dementia cannot be ruled out in this patient, but establishing the diagnosis would require removal of the causative agent and re-evaluation after recovery. However, asterixis, a sign of metabolic encephalopathy, would be unusual in this setting and points strongly to a metabolic encephalopathy and not dementia.

Depression may cause chronic cognitive impairment (pseudodementia) and difficulty concentrating, but not asterixis and an altered level of consciousness.

KEY POINT

Cognitive impairment accompanied by fluctuating lethargy and inattention, hallucinations, and asterixis most likely results from a toxic encephalopathy.

Bibliography

Inouye SK. Delirium in older persons [erratum in N Engl J Med. 2006;354:1655]. N Engl J Med. 2006;354(11):1157-1165. [PMID: 16540616]

Item 6   Answer: A

Educational Objective: *Diagnose migraine headache with aura.*

This patient is most likely experiencing a migraine with aura. Approximately 15% to 20% of patients with migraine experience aura within 1 hour of or during headache. Aura constitutes neurologic abnormalities, including visual loss, hallucinations, numbness, tingling, weakness, or confusion. Aura is caused by spreading cortical depression—a wave of abnormal electrical discharges that travel slowly across the brain's surface and essentially short-circuit the brain. Typically, aura lasts a few minutes but may last up to 1 hour per symptom. Additional clinical clues supporting a diagnosis of migraine are the patient's young age, the absence of vascular risk factors, and the family history of migraine. In addition, the diffuseness of this patient's symptoms and their progression are more compatible with migraine than a focal vascular process, such as a transient ischemic attack.

Although multiple sclerosis (MS) should be in the differential diagnosis of neurological symptoms in a young woman, this patient is less likely to have MS than a migraine or stroke because her presentation was more acute than would be typical in MS, and MS is not typically associated with a throbbing headache.

Partial seizures in which the patient maintains full awareness are classified as simple partial, whereas those involving an alteration of consciousness are classified as partial complex. Partial seizures that originate in the temporal lobe often begin with an aura, which may consist of a feeling of déjà vu, a rising epigastric sensation, or autonomic disturbances. Automatisms, such as lip smacking, are also suggestive of partial complex seizures, but a throbbing headache with nausea is not.

Trigeminal neuralgia is associated with pain occurring in paroxysms that involves one or more divisions of the trigeminal nerve. Each episode may persist between a few seconds and 2 minutes, and pain may be intensely sharp or stabbing. Behavior such as face washing or touching, tooth brushing, or chewing may trigger an event. The patient's symptoms are not consistent with trigeminal neuralgia.

KEY POINT

Between 15% and 20% of patients with migraine experience aura within 1 hour of or during headache characterized by a variety of neurologic symptoms, including visual loss, hallucinations, numbness, tingling, weakness, or confusion.

Bibliography

Wilson JF. In the clinic. Migraine [erratum in Ann Intern Med. 2008;148(5):408]. Ann Intern Med. 2007;147(9):ITC11-1-ITC11-16. [PMID: 17975180]

Item 7   Answer: D

Educational Objective: *Diagnose tension-type headache.*

This patient has tension-type headache, the most prevalent of all headache types. Tension-type headache is a dull, bilateral, or diffuse headache, often described as a pressure or squeezing sensation of mild to moderate intensity. There are no accompanying migraine features (nausea, emesis, photophobia, phonophobia), and the pain neither worsens with movement nor prohibits activity. The key feature that establishes a diagnosis of tension-type headache is the lack of disabling pain.

Chronic daily headache is a nonspecific term that refers to both primary (including migraine) and secondary headache disorders in which headache is present on more than 15 days per month for at least 3 months. Risk factors for chronic daily headache include obesity, a history of frequent headache (more than 1 per week), caffeine consumption, and overuse (>10 days per month) of acute headache medications, including analgesics, ergots, triptans, and opioids. In addition, more than half of all patients with chronic daily headache have sleep disturbance and mood disorders, such as depression and anxiety. Chronic migraine and medication overuse headache overwhelmingly represent the most common and challenging of the chronic daily headache disorders in clinical practice.

Cluster headache is a painful, disabling headache that may be associated with autonomic symptoms such as tearing or rhinorrhea. Cluster headaches are typically unilateral and periorbital/temporal and are associated with at least one of the following features on the same side as the headache: conjunctival irritation/lacrimation, rhinorrhea/nasal congestion, eyelid edema, facial/forehead sweating, and miosis/ptosis. Cluster episodes usually last 6 to 8 weeks and remission periods usually last 2 to 6 months.

Migraine headache is a recurrent headache disorder that manifests in attacks lasting 4 to 72 hours. Typical characteristics of migraine are its unilateral location, pulsating quality, moderate or severe intensity, aggravation by routine physical activity, and association with nausea and/or photophobia and phonophobia. This patient does not describe disability or any other features of migraine headache. A neurologic aura occurs in only one third of patients with migraine. The aura consists of such visual symptoms as perceptions of flashes of light, arcs of flashing light that often form a zigzag pattern, and an area of loss of vision surrounded by a normal field of vision.

KEY POINT

Tension-type headache is distinguished from migraine by the fact that patients with tension-type headache are not disabled and can carry out activities of daily living in a normal, expedient manner.

Bibliography

Sacco S. Diagnostic issues in tension-type headache. Curr Pain Headache Rep. 2008;12(6):437-441. [PMID: 18973737]

Item 8   Answer: C

Educational Objective: *Manage a thunderclap headache.*

This patient should undergo noncontrast CT of the head. She has experienced a thunderclap headache, which is a severe and explosive headache that is maximal in intensity at or within 60 seconds of onset. Every thunderclap headache must be immediately evaluated to detect potentially catastrophic conditions, especially subarachnoid hemorrhage. A negative CT scan of the head should be followed by a lumbar puncture to assess for blood in the cerebrospinal fluid not detected on the CT scan.

If both the CT scan of the head and lumbar puncture are negative, most of the other causes of thunderclap headache, such as an unruptured cerebral aneurysm, a carotid or vertebral artery dissection, cerebral venous sinus thrombosis, and reversible cerebral vasoconstriction syndrome, can be excluded by noninvasive angiography. CT angiography of the head and neck can detect unruptured aneurysms as small as 3 mm in diameter and thus is adequate to exclude this diagnosis. Magnetic resonance angiography (MRA) would also be appropriate in this setting. Both CT angiography and MRA can be performed with a venous phase to exclude cerebral venous sinus thrombosis. Given that most causes of thunderclap headache can be excluded by such noninvasive angiography, if prior cerebrospinal fluid analysis has shown no evidence of a subarachnoid hemorrhage, conventional cerebral angiography, in which a catheter is inserted into a large artery and advanced through the carotid artery, is unnecessary.

Because the patient may have intracerebral bleeding with mass effect, the performance of a lumbar puncture could result in brainstem herniation. This is why the lumbar puncture is performed only after a CT scan is performed. If the CT scan reveals intracerebral bleeding, a lumbar puncture is unnecessary.

Treatment with a vasoconstrictive drug, such as sumatriptan, would not be appropriate until the other causes of thunderclap headache have been excluded. Drugs with the potential to constrict extracranial and intracranial cerebral vessels can precipitate or exacerbate the cerebral ischemia that may be associated with arterial dissection and reversible cerebral vasoconstriction syndromes.

KEY POINT

A thunderclap headache is a potential neurologic emergency that must be immediately evaluated to detect potentially catastrophic conditions, especially subarachnoid hemorrhage.

Bibliography

Schwedt TJ, Matharu MS, Dodick DW. Thunderclap headache. Lancet Neurol. 2006;5(7):621-631. [PMID: 16781992]

Item 9   Answer: B

Educational Objective: *Treat a patient prophylactically for migraine with propranolol.*

The most appropriate treatment for this patient is propranolol. Prophylactic treatment should be considered in patients who experience 2 or more days of headache per week. Nearly 40% of patients with migraine need preventive treatment. There is evidence from at least two randomized, double-blind, placebo-controlled studies to support the use of eight drugs available in the United States (topiramate, valproic acid, amitriptyline, metoprolol, propranolol, timolol, and extract of the plant Butterbur root *Petasites hybridus*) and two nonpharmacologic approaches (relaxation therapy and biofeedback).

Several randomized placebo-controlled trials have found no consistent, statistically significant benefits for botulinum toxin injection in the treatment of episodic migraine headache. Similarly, there is no evidence of efficacy for nortriptyline or sertraline in the preventive treatment of migraine.

KEY POINT

Prophylactic medication should be initiated in patients with two or more migraine attacks per week.

Bibliography

Wilson JF. In the clinic. Migraine [erratum in Ann Intern Med. 2008;148(5):408]. Ann Intern Med. 2007;147(9):ITC11-1-ITC11-16. [PMID: 17975180]

Item 10   Answer: B

Educational Objective: *Diagnose delirium superimposed on dementia.*

This patient has delirium superimposed on dementia. Delirium is an altered level of alertness, often in connection with globally impaired cognition. It is typically characterized by abrupt onset and may be associated with rapid fluctuations of alertness, attention, memory, and psychomotor activity (for example, lethargy or agitation). Dementia is an acquired and persistent impairment of intellectual ability that compromises at least three areas of mental functioning: language, memory, visuospatial skills, emotion or personality, or cognition. Dementia typically has an insidious onset and is usually stable from day to day. Over the protracted course of dementia, many patients may experience an acute delirium, with confused and slurred speech, somnolence, agitation, tremulousness, unsteadiness, falls, and worsened incontinence. Often, the delirium is from a superimposed illness (most commonly, a urinary tract infection or pneumonia), a medication error, an injury, or some other cause that must be sought and managed.

Psychosis encompasses delusions, hallucinations, disorganized speech, and disorganized or catatonic behavior. Impaired cognition, including decrements in short-term memory and attention, is also characteristic. This patient's sudden decline in the setting of dementia and absence of hallucinations and delusions is more likely to represent an acute delirium rather than an acute psychosis.

KEY POINT

Over the course of dementia, many patients may experience an acute delirium, with confused and slurred speech, somnolence, agitation, tremulousness, unsteadiness, falls, and worsened incontinence.

Bibliography
Han JH, Wilson A, Ely EW. Delirium in the older emergency department patient: a quiet epidemic. Emerg Med Clin North Am. 2010;28(3):611-31. [PMID: 20709246]

Item 11   Answer: A
Educational Objective: *Diagnose Alzheimer dementia.*

The most likely diagnosis is Alzheimer dementia. Dementia is a clinical syndrome in which multiple cognitive domains—including memory, language, spatial skills, judgment, and problem solving—are impaired to a disabling degree. Some dementing illnesses can also affect noncognitive neurologic functions, such as gait. Diseases that cause dementia often produce characteristic patterns of cognitive (and sometimes noncognitive) impairment that can aid diagnosis. Alzheimer dementia is characterized by prominent memory loss, anomia, constructional apraxia, anosognosia (impaired recognition of illness), and variable degrees of personality change.

Creutzfeldt-Jakob disease (CJD) is the most common of the human prion diseases, with an annual incidence of less than 1 in 1,000,000 persons. The main clinical features of CJD are dementia that progresses over months (rather than years, as in this case) and startle myoclonus, although the latter may not be present early in the illness. Other prominent features include visual or cerebellar disturbance, pyramidal/extrapyramidal dysfunction, and akinetic mutism.

Dementia with Lewy bodies is accompanied by parkinsonism, visual hallucinations, and fluctuating symptoms, none of which this patient has. The characteristic cognitive profile of dementia in patients with dementia with Lewy bodies includes impaired learning and attention, psychomotor slowing, con-

structional apraxia, and more profound visuospatial impairment but less memory impairment than in similarly staged patients with Alzheimer dementia.

Frontotemporal dementia is a progressive neuropsychiatric condition. Patients initially have behavioral and personality changes that range from apathy to social disinhibition. They fail to change their clothes, brush their teeth, pursue their former interests, or initiate many of their previous activities that constituted a normal day. They may fixate, in a seemingly idiosyncratic fashion, on a particular activity, such as going to the bathroom, sorting through a wallet, hoarding magazines, or watching television. Some patients have greater disinhibition and emotional lability (crying or laughing inappropriately).

KEY POINT

Alzheimer dementia is characterized by prominent memory loss, anomia, constructional apraxia, anosognosia (impaired recognition of illness), and variable degrees of personality change.

Bibliography
Blass DM, Rabins PV. In the clinic. Dementia. Ann Intern Med. 2008;148(7):ITC4-1-ITC4-16. [PMID: 18378944]

Item 12   Answer: A
Educational Objective: *Treat Alzheimer dementia with an acetylcholinesterase inhibitor (donepezil).*

This patient should receive donepezil. The Folstein Mini–Mental State Examination (MMSE) discriminates well between the major stages of dementia used for prognosis and management purposes. The MMSE score range of 21 to 25 corresponds to mild dementia, 11 to 20 to moderate dementia, and 0 to 10 to severe dementia. This patient has Alzheimer dementia and is at a mild stage of impairment. The most appropriate medication with which to begin treatment is an acetylcholinesterase inhibitor of which there are currently three: donepezil, rivastigmine, and galantamine. In patients with mild, moderate, or severe Alzheimer dementia the use of acetylcholinesterase inhibitors are associated with a small but statistically significant improvement in performance of instrumental and functional activities of daily living and caregiver stress and may be associated with improved cognitive function compared with patients treated with placebo. Treatment effects are small and not always apparent in practice. Cholinesterase inhibitors are generally safe but have significantly more side effects than placebo, including diarrhea, nausea, vomiting, and symptomatic bradycardia. The gastrointestinal side effects are usually transient and mild.

Ginkgo biloba, although safe, has inconsistent and unconvincing evidence of benefit in the treatment of Alzheimer dementia. Also, there is no regulation regarding the contents of herbal extracts, which allows for variability in dose strength and quality.

Quetiapine is an antipsychotic drug, and sertraline is an antidepressant agent. Although both can be used in patients with

Alzheimer dementia, their use is limited to treatment of behavioral symptoms of psychosis and depression, respectively, neither of which this patient has exhibited. However, if these medications are to be used in such patients, the risks must first be carefully weighed against the benefits. Antipsychotics have limited effectiveness in treating behavioral problems and are associated with increased risk of death in patients with dementia.

KEY POINT

First-line pharmacotherapy for mild Alzheimer dementia is an acetylcholinesterase inhibitor.

Bibliography
Mayeux R. Early Alzheimer's disease. N Engl J Med. 2010;362(23): 2194-2201. [PMID: 20558370]

Item 13   Answer: A
Educational Objective: *Treat functional decline in a patient with advanced Alzheimer dementia with memantine.*

The most appropriate next step in treatment is the addition of memantine. This patient has Alzheimer dementia that is moderately advanced and now has difficulties with basic activities of daily living. The N-methyl-D-aspartate receptor antagonist memantine is the only drug approved by the U.S. Food and Drug Administration as first-line treatment of moderate to advanced Alzheimer dementia. Memantine has been shown to improve cognition and global assessment of dementia, but while the changes have been statistically significant, the clinical effect is not always evident. Memantine may improve quality-of-life measures, but these findings are not robust. Although evidence is limited, there is some suggestion that the stepped approach of adding memantine to a regimen that includes a cholinesterase inhibitor (such as donepezil) results in a modest additional benefit over substituting memantine for the cholinesterase inhibitor.

Quetiapine is an antipsychotic medication and sertraline is an antidepressant agent. Although both drugs can be used in patients with Alzheimer dementia, their use is limited to the treatment of the behavioral symptoms of psychosis and depression, respectively, neither of which this patient has at this time. The effectiveness of antipsychotic medications is on behavioral problems is limited and their use is associated with an increased risk of death in patients with dementia.

Discontinuing the donepezil taken by this patient without substituting another drug to manage her functional decline would not help slow or otherwise improve the course of her disease.

KEY POINT

Memantine is a first-line agent for treatment of moderate to advanced Alzheimer dementia.

Bibliography
Mayeux R. Early Alzheimer's disease. N Engl J Med. 2010;362(23): 2194-201. [PMID: 20558370]

Item 14   Answer: A
Educational Objective: *Diagnose drug-induced dystonia.*

The most likely diagnosis is drug-induced dystonia. All medications that block D_2 dopamine receptors can cause acute dystonic reactions. Dystonic movements are due to sustained contraction of agonist and antagonist muscles, which results in twisting and repetitive movements or sustained abnormal postures. These movements most frequently affect the ocular muscles (oculogyric crisis) and the face, jaw, tongue, neck, and trunk. The limbs are rarely affected. Neuroleptic, antiemetic, and serotoninergic agents have been implicated, and symptoms usually occur within 5 days of initiation of the drug. Treatment consists of parenteral diphenhydramine, benztropine mesylate, or biperiden.

Cervical dystonia, formerly known as torticollis, is a focal dystonia that involves the cervical musculature and causes abnormal postures of the head, neck, and shoulders. Quick, nonrhythmic, repetitive movements can also occur and can be mistaken for tremor. Cervical dystonia generally does not present so acutely and does not explain the sustained tongue protrusion.

Huntington disease is a hereditary, progressive, neurodegenerative disorder characterized by increasingly severe motor impairment, cognitive decline, and psychiatric symptoms. The associated movement disorder is chorea. Chorea refers to brief, irregular, nonstereotypical, nonrhythmic movements and can involve the extremities, head, trunk, and face. In addition to chorea, other motor symptoms include ataxia, dystonia, slurred speech, swallowing impairment, and myoclonus. Symptoms typically begin in the fourth and fifth decade. Huntington disease does not present acutely, as occurred in this patient.

The neuroleptic malignant syndrome is a life-threatening disorder caused by an idiosyncratic reaction to neuroleptic tranquilizers (dopamine D_2-receptor antagonists) and some antipsychotic drugs, of which haloperidol is the most common. Most patients with the syndrome develop muscle rigidity, hyperthermia, cognitive changes, autonomic instability, diaphoresis, sialorrhea, seizures, arrhythmias, and rhabdomyolysis within 2 weeks of initiating the drug. The lack of fever and generalized muscle rigidity argue strongly against this diagnosis.

KEY POINT

Neuroleptic, antiemetic, and serotoninergic agents have been implicated in acute dystonic reactions, which usually occur within 5 days of initiating the offending drug.

Bibliography
Tarsy D, Simon DK. Dystonia. N Engl J Med. 2006;355(8):818-29. [PMID: 16928997]

Item 15   Answer: D
Educational Objective: *Diagnose Parkinson disease.*

The most likely diagnosis is Parkinson disease. Parkinson disease remains a clinical diagnosis that is based on a cardinal set of clinical features, including resting tremor, bradykinesia, rigidity, and postural instability; the tremor, bradykinesia, and rigidity are asymmetric. Sustained levodopa responsiveness is expected in Parkinson disease and helps confirm the clinical diagnosis. Signs suggesting an alternative condition include symmetric symptoms or signs, early falls, rapid progression, poor or waning response to levodopa, dementia, early autonomic failure, and ataxia.

The patient's findings are not compatible with cervical dystonia, essential tremor, or Huntington disease. Cervical dystonia, formerly known as torticollis, is a focal dystonia that involves the cervical musculature and causes abnormal postures of the head, neck, and shoulders. Quick, nonrhythmic, repetitive movements can also occur and can be mistaken for tremor.

Essential tremor is characterized by an upper extremity high-frequency tremor, which is present with both limb movement and sustained posture of the involved extremities and is absent at rest. The tremor is characteristically bilateral, but there can be mild to moderate asymmetry. Essential tremors typically improve with alcohol and worsen with stress. Tremor amplitude over time generally increases and can be so severe as to interfere with writing, drinking, and other activities requiring smooth, coordinated upper limb movements.

Huntington disease is a hereditary, progressive, neurodegenerative disorder characterized by increasingly severe motor impairment, cognitive decline, and psychiatric symptoms. In addition to chorea, other motor symptoms include ataxia, dystonia, slurred speech, swallowing impairment, and myoclonus. Various psychiatric symptoms, such as dysphoria, agitation, irritability, anxiety, apathy, disinhibition, delusions, and hallucinations, are commonly seen.

KEY POINT

The diagnosis of Parkinson disease is based on a cardinal set of clinical features, including resting tremor, bradykinesia, rigidity, and postural instability.

Bibliography
Nutt JG, Wooten GF. Clinical practice. Diagnosis and initial management of Parkinson's disease. N Engl J Med. 2005;353(10):1021-1027. [PMID: 16148287]

Item 16   Answer: C
Educational Objective: *Treat essential tremor with propranolol.*

This patient should be treated with propranolol. She has a history and examination findings consistent with the presence of essential tremor. Essential tremor primarily occurs when a patient maintains a posture, such as when the hands are outstretched. Essential tremor also may be present during movement, particularly postural adjustments. Autosomal dominant transmission occurs in approximately half of patients with this condition. Essential tremor most commonly affects the upper extremities; however, the legs, head, trunk, face, and vocal cords may be involved. Up to 15% of patients with essential tremor have major disability associated with this condition. Progression of essential tremor is typically slow, with intermittent lengthy periods of stable symptoms. Features that may be predictive of a more severe essential tremor include a positive family history of tremor, longer tremor duration, voice tremor, and unilateral tremor onset. Alcoholic beverage consumption suppresses symptoms in most patients with this condition.

Treatment options for essential tremor are often limited and frequently only partially effective. It has been estimated that 50% of patients with essential tremor have no response to medical treatment. First-line medications used to treat essential tremor include propranolol, primidone, gabapentin, and topiramate. Propranolol is typically the drug of choice in most patients with essential tremor because of its effectiveness, which has been established in multiple well-designed randomized clinical trials.

Essential tremor is distinguished from Parkinson disease by its lack of parkinsonian features, such as rigidity, bradykinesia, postural instability, and resting tremor. Carbidopa-levodopa can be an appropriate choice to treat Parkinson disease but is not useful in the treatment of essential tremor. Parkinsonian tremor is typically postural and kinetic (occurring with movement). Ropinirole and pramipexole are dopamine agonist medications used to treat Parkinson disease. Given the absence of any other signs of Parkinson disease, these medications are not indicated in this patient.

KEY POINT

Propranolol is a first-line medication for essential tremor.

Bibliography
Lorenz D, Deuschl G. Update on pathogenesis and treatment of essential tremor. Curr Opin Neurol. 2007;20(4):447-452. [PMID: 17620881]

Item 17   Answer: A
Educational Objective: *Diagnose* Listeria monocytogenes *meningitis.*

The most likely diagnosis is *Listeria monocytogenes* meningitis. *Listeria monocytogenes* is a gram-positive bacillus that can cause invasive disease in immunocompromised states, including alcoholism, extremes of age (neonates and those >50 years of age), malignancy, immunosuppression, diabetes mellitus, pregnancy, hepatic failure, chronic kidney disease, iron overload, collagen vascular disorders, use of antitumor necrosis factor-α agents, and HIV infection. The gastrointestinal tract is the usual portal of entry with symptoms typically developing after consumption of contaminated cole slaw, raw vegetables, milk, cheese, processed meats, smoked seafood, and hot dogs, potentially resulting in a febrile gastroenteritis syndrome including diarrhea. The organism can continue to multiply at refrigerator-level temperatures.

Neisseria meningitidis meningitis occurs primarily in children and young adults. This illness is characterized by abrupt onset of flu-like illness including fever, headache, neck stiffness, altered mental status, intense myalgias, and rash. The rash is often petechial, purpuric, or maculopapular. The evolution of this infection can be rapid and fulminant, potentially resulting in septic shock and death. Invasive infections can be established by the growth of these gram-negative diplococci from CSF and blood cultures. Biopsy and culture of skin lesions may also reveal the organism.

Streptococcus pneumoniae is the most common cause of bacterial meningitis in adults. The clinical presentation of pneumococcal meningitis is not specific, but CSF and possibly blood cultures will reveal growth of gram-positive diplococci.

Patients with viral meningitis can present with a syndrome similar to bacterial meningitis. However, CSF findings typically reveal a lymphocytic pleocytosis, a glucose level greater than 45 mg/dL (2.5 mmol/L), protein level less than 200 mg/dL (2000 mg/L), and a negative Gram stain. In the evaluation of patients with acute bacterial or viral meningitis, a CSF protein concentration greater than 220 mg/dL (2200 mg/L), CSF glucose less than 34 mg/dL (1.9 mmol/L), CSF blood-glucose ratio less than 0.2, CSF leukocytes greater than 2000/μL (2000 × 10⁶/L), or CSF neutrophils greater than 1180/μL (1180 × 10⁶/L) are individual predictors of bacterial etiology with a 99% or greater certainty.

KEY POINT

Listeria monocytogenes is a gram-positive bacillus that can cause invasive disease in immunocompromised patients, particularly those with cell-mediated immunodeficiency.

Bibliography
Nudelman Y, Tunkel AR. Bacterial meningitis: epidemiology, pathogenesis and management update. Drugs. 2009;69(18):2577-96. [PMID: 19943708]

Item 18   Answer: A
Educational Objective: *Diagnose* N. meningitidis *serogroup B meningitis.*

This patient's illness, physical examination, and CSF profile are consistent with *N. meningitidis* meningitis. This infection most commonly occurs in children and young adults. The Centers for Disease Control and Prevention (CDC) recommends routine immunization with the meningococcal vaccine, which protects against serogroups A, C, Y, and W-135, but not serogroup B, the causative agent in as many as one third of U.S. cases and the recent cause of other cases of meningitis on campus.

Rocky Mountain spotted fever (RMSF) can manifest as headache, fever, myalgia, abdominal pain, and rash. The purpuric rash typically develops 3 to 4 days after the onset of constitutional symptoms and begins on the wrists and ankles before spreading centripetally. Thrombocytopenia, a relative leukopenia, and elevated transaminases may provide clues to the diagnosis, particularly if the patient resides or has traveled to areas where RMSF-associated American dog ticks are present. These ticks transmit infection in spring and early summer but not in December, which is when this patient became ill.

Streptococcus pneumoniae is the most common cause of bacterial meningitis in adults. The clinical presentation of pneumococcal meningitis is not specific, but CSF and, possibly, blood cultures will reveal gram-positive (not gram-negative) diplococci.

Vibrio vulnificus is a gram-negative bacillus that can cause septicemia, wound infection, and, rarely, gastroenteritis. Wound infection typically occurs by inoculation through the skin, and septicemia and gastroenteritis occurs after ingestion of raw or undercooked shellfish. Invasive disease typically occurs in immunocompromised hosts, particularly those with liver disease. These infections are more common in summer months when warmer sea water temperatures support the growth of this organism. Meningitis is not characteristic of infection with this organism.

KEY POINT

The *N. meningitidis* vaccine does not provide protection against *N. meningitidis* serogroup B meningitis.

Bibliography
Nudelman Y, Tunkel AR. Bacterial meningitis: epidemiology, pathogenesis and management update. Drugs. 2009;69(18):2577-2596. [PMID: 19943708]

Item 19   Answer: B
Educational Objective: *Diagnose meningococcal meningitis.*

This patient's illness is most consistent with *Neisseria meningitidis* (meningococcal) infection, which is characterized by the sudden onset of fever, myalgia, headache, and rash in a previously healthy patient. Early in its course, meningococcal disease may be indistinguishable from other common viral illnesses; however, the rapidity with which the disease worsens (often over hours) and progresses to septic shock differentiates it from these other illnesses. A petechial rash is most common and may coalesce to form purpuric lesions. The diagnosis is established on the basis of clinical presentation and confirmed with blood and cerebrospinal fluid (CSF) cultures.

Meningitis caused by *Listeria monocytogenes* is associated with extremes of age (neonates and persons age >50 years), alcoholism, malignancy, immunosuppression, diabetes mellitus, hepatic failure, renal failure, iron overload, collagen vascular disorders, and HIV infection. The clinical presentation of *Lis-*

teria meningoencephalitis ranges from a mild illness with fever and mental status changes to a fulminant course with coma. It is not associated with a rash.

The classic presentation of Rocky Mountain spotted fever is a severe headache, fever, myalgia, and arthralgia. Thrombocytopenia and acute kidney injury can occur. A maculopapular rash develops 3 to 5 days later, beginning on the wrists and ankles and potentially involving the palms and soles. Rocky Mountain spotted fever is transmitted by the American dog tick in the spring and early summer, which is inconsistent with the timing of this patient's presentation.

Viral meningitis can present with fever, headache, stiff neck, and photophobia and may be associated with a maculopapular eruption. However, acute viral meningitis is rarely associated with thrombocytopenia, metabolic acidosis, and acute kidney injury. Finally, CSF findings typically show a lymphocyte-predominant leukocytosis (leukocyte count <1000/µL [1000×10^6/L]), a glucose level greater than 45 mg/dL (2.5 mmol/L), a protein level less than 200 mg/dL (2000 mg/L), and a Gram stain negative for organisms.

KEY POINT

Meningococcal infection should be considered in the differential diagnosis of any previously healthy patient who presents with acute-onset fever, headache, rash, and myalgia.

Bibliography

van de Beek D, de Gans J, Tunkel AR, Wijdicks EF. Community-acquired bacterial meningitis in adults. N Engl J Med. 2006;354(1):44-53. [PMID:16394301]

Item 20   Answer: C

Educational Objective: *Treat bacterial meningitis empirically with vancomycin, ampicillin, and ceftriaxone.*

This patient most likely has bacterial meningitis and requires therapy with vancomycin, ampicillin, and ceftriaxone. Bacterial meningitis in adults is characterized by fever, headache, nuchal rigidity, and signs of cerebral dysfunction. In elderly patients, such as this one, insidious onset with lethargy or obtundation and variable signs of meningeal irritation may be present, particularly in the setting of diabetes mellitus. This patient's symptoms and cerebrospinal fluid results are consistent with acute bacterial meningitis. The most likely etiologic agents are *Streptococcus pneumoniae*, *Listeria monocytogenes*, *Neisseria meningitidis*, and aerobic gram-negative bacilli. Pending culture results and results of in vitro susceptibility testing, empiric treatment with antimicrobial therapy consisting of vancomycin, ampicillin, and ceftriaxone for infection caused by penicillin-resistant pneumococci and *L. monocytogenes* is necessary. Administration of adjunctive dexamethasone should be strongly considered in patients with acute bacterial meningitis because clinical trials have established the benefit of adjunctive dexamethasone on adverse outcomes and

death in adults with suspected or proven *S. pneumoniae* meningitis.

Intravenous ceftriaxone or intravenous penicillin G alone might not provide adequate cerebrospinal fluid levels for treatment of penicillin-resistant *S. pneumoniae*. Most infectious disease experts would recommend vancomycin plus ceftriaxone for the treatment of penicillin-resistant *S. pneumoniae*; however, this combination would not adequately treat meningitis caused by *L. monocytogenes*, which requires the addition of ampicillin. Trimethoprim-sulfamethoxazole does treat *Listeria* meningitis, but the combination of vancomycin plus trimethoprim-sulfamethoxazole would be potentially inadequate treatment for *S. pneumoniae* meningitis.

KEY POINT

Empiric therapy of acute bacterial meningitis in an older adult should include a third-generation cephalosporin, vancomycin, and ampicillin.

Bibliography

Tunkel AR, Hartman BJ, Kaplan SL, et al. Practice guidelines for the management of bacterial meningitis. Clin Infect Dis. 2004;39(9):1267-1284. [PMID:15494903]

Item 21   Answer: D

Educational Objective: *Treat acute stroke with early mobilization.*

The patient should begin physical and occupational therapy. A total of 40% of patients who have a stroke retain moderate functional impairment, and 15% to 30% have severe disability. Current evidence points to the benefits of early mobilization and graded exercise in promoting more complete recovery from stroke and in preventing complications such as decubitus ulcers, deconditioning, and loss of function. For this reason, early mobilization with physical and occupational therapy and a variety of approaches is recommended. Confining the patient to bed for 48 hours or longer is associated with a greater incidence of preventable complications and less than optimal functional recovery.

On admission to a hospital ward, a patient with stroke should be given nothing by mouth until a swallowing assessment is conducted. In a patient with significant language disturbance, there is concern for the possibility of aspiration and complications from it; the patient should not be prescribed a diet until a swallowing assessment has been conducted to determine safety in swallowing. The American Heart Association/American Stroke Association recommends a water swallow test performed at the bedside by a trained observer as the best bedside predictor of aspiration. A prospective study of the water swallow test demonstrated a significantly decreased risk of aspiration pneumonia of 2.4% versus 5.4% in patients who were not screened.

Early mobilization of stroke patients is recommended as a strategy for reducing complications.

Bibliography

Smith LN, James R, Barber M, Ramsay S, Gillespie D, Chung C; Guideline Development Group. Rehabilitation of patients with stroke: summary of SIGN guidance. BMJ. 2010;340:c2845. [PMID: 20551122]

Item 22   Answer: D

Educational Objective: *Treat an acute hemispheric stroke with thrombolytic therapy (intravenous recombinant tissue plasminogen activator).*

This patient should receive intravenous recombinant tissue plasminogen activator (rtPA). He has clinical symptoms and signs and radiologic evidence of an acute left hemispheric stroke. The probable mechanism of stroke is ischemic infarction, given the results of the head CT scan. He was brought to the emergency department within 1 hour of the witnessed onset of stroke symptoms, and his evaluation is completed 1 hour later. He does not appear to have any clinical, radiologic, or laboratory contraindication to receiving the preferred treatment of intravenous rtPA, and he can receive it within the recommended window of 3 hours from stroke onset.

Aspirin is indicated for acute ischemic stroke in patients who are not eligible for rtPA. For patients with acute stroke who are eligible for thrombolysis, aspirin should be withheld in the emergency department and for 24 hours after rtPA administration.

Although long-term anticoagulation is an effective treatment for prevention of cardioembolic stroke in patients with atrial fibrillation, acute anticoagulation with heparin has not been shown to be beneficial in patients with acute ischemic stroke.

Elevated blood pressure is common at the time of initial stroke presentation, even among patients without chronic hypertension. Rapid lowering of blood pressure may further impair cerebral blood flow and worsen the ischemic injury. Elevated blood pressure often will resolve spontaneously or improve gradually during the first few days after a stroke. The threshold for acute blood pressure lowering in patients with acute stroke who are eligible for thrombolysis is 185/110 mm Hg. In such a setting, preferred agents include intravenous infusions of labetalol or nicardipine. Because this patient's blood pressure is already below that threshold, there is no indication for intravenous use of labetalol at this time.

The preferred treatment of ischemic stroke is intravenous recombinant tissue plasminogen activator if it can be administered within 3 hours from stroke onset.

Bibliography

van der Worp HB, van Gijn J. Clinical practice. Acute ischemic stroke. N Engl J Med. 2007;357(6):572-579. [PMID: 17687132]

Item 23   Answer: D

Educational Objective: *Manage hypertension in a patient with an acute ischemic stroke.*

There is no urgent need to treat hypertension in an uncomplicated ischemic stroke. For uncomplicated ischemic strokes in patients without concurrent acute coronary artery disease or heart failure, consensus exists that antihypertensive medications, such as intravenous labetalol or nicardipine, should be withheld if the systolic blood pressure is less than 220 mm Hg or the diastolic blood pressure is less than 120 mm Hg, unless there are other manifestations of end-organ damage. This patient's systolic and diastolic blood pressure levels are below these limits and there is no urgent need to treat hypertension, such as aortic dissection, myocardial infarction, or heart failure. Many such patients have spontaneous declines in blood pressure during the first 24 hours after stroke onset.

Oral nifedipine is an inappropriate treatment for this patient not only because of its antihypertensive qualities, but also because of its route of administration. Given the severity of her stroke deficits, in particular the dysarthria, she should receive nothing by mouth until a swallowing evaluation is carried out because of the high risk of aspiration.

Notably, the patient is not eligible for recombinant tissue plasminogen activator therapy because the time interval between now and her previous symptom-free state is more than 3 hours. Aspirin (160 to 325 mg/d) administered within 48 hours of stroke onset results in a small but significant reduction in the risk for recurrent stroke during the first 2 weeks after the stroke and improves outcome at 6 months. Therefore, aspirin is recommended as initial therapy for most patients with acute stroke. However, aspirin should not be administered for at least 24 hours after administration of thrombolytics.

For uncomplicated ischemic strokes in patients without concurrent acute coronary artery disease, aortic dissection, or heart failure, antihypertensive medications should be withheld if the systolic blood pressure is less than 220 mm Hg or the diastolic blood pressure is less than 120 mm Hg.

Bibliography

Urrutia VC, Wityk RJ. Blood pressure management in acute stroke. Neurol Clin. 2008;26(2):565-583, x-xi. [PMID: 18514827]

Item 24   Answer: A

Educational Objective: *Evaluate a subarachnoid hemorrhage with a lumbar puncture and cerebrospinal fluid analysis.*

This patient should have a lumbar puncture. A thunderclap headache is a severe and explosive headache that is maximal in intensity at or within 60 seconds of onset. CT scanning is the first test to be conducted in a patient with thunderclap headache in whom a subarachnoid hemorrhage is suspected;

a ruptured intracranial aneurysm is the most serious cause of such headaches. The ability to detect subarachnoid hemorrhage is dependent on the amount of subarachnoid blood, the interval after symptom onset, the resolution of the scanner, and the skills of the radiologist. On the day of the hemorrhage, extravasated blood will be present in more than 95% of patients, but in the following days, this proportion falls sharply. If an initial CT scan of the head reveals nothing, a lumbar puncture should be performed next in patients with this presentation. The finding of xanthochromia or gross hemorrhage is diagnostic for subarachnoid hemorrhage. Subsequent angiography (CT or MRI) can confirm the presence of a ruptured aneurysm in patients with a positive lumbar puncture.

Early in the diagnosis of subarachnoid hemorrhage, brain MRI is no more accurate than head CT. There is nothing to be gained by performing brain MRI in this patient with negative findings on a head CT scan.

In patients with an initial subarachnoid hemorrhage, there is substantial risk of rebleeding (2% per day for the first month). Rebleeding is associated with high mortality. The treatment of subarachnoid hemorrhage involves localizing the aneurysm with cerebral angiography and securing it to prevent subsequent bleeding. Traditionally, surgical clipping within 72 hours of onset has been recommended. Aneurysms also may be treated endovascularly by filling them with metallic coils and promoting localized thrombosis within the aneurysm to obliterate it from the cerebral circulation. Hospital observation as the sole management option for this patient places her at increased risk for rebleeding and death.

Treatment with sumatriptan is indicated for migraine headache. All of the triptans promote vasoconstriction and block pain pathways in the brainstem. They are contraindicated in patients with stroke and uncontrolled hypertension. The use of sumatriptan in this patient who has a high likelihood of subarachnoid hemorrhage is contraindicated.

KEY POINT

A lumbar puncture with subsequent cerebrospinal fluid analysis is necessary in any patient with thunderclap headache and normal findings on a CT scan to fully evaluate a possible subarachnoid hemorrhage.

Bibliography
van Gijn J, Kerr RS, Rinkel GJ. Subarachnoid haemorrhage. Lancet. 2007;369(9558):306-318. [PMID: 17258671]

Item 25   Answer: C
Educational Objective: *Diagnose Bell palsy.*

This patient's physical examination findings most strongly suggest right facial nerve (Bell) palsy. The precise cause of Bell palsy is not known, and it is still considered an idiopathic disorder. Research strongly suggests it may be the result of herpes simplex virus infection of the facial nerve. Bell palsy is not considered contagious. The seventh cranial nerve innervates

all muscles of facial expression (the mimetic muscles). Any cause of a complete facial neuropathy will therefore impair the entire hemiface, including the forehead corrugators typically spared by cerebral lesions. Bell phenomenon describes the reflexive rolling upwards of the globe during eye closure. When a normal patient is asked to close the eyes, forced eyelid opening will reveal this phenomenon, as will the selective paralysis of the orbicularis oculi due to a facial neuropathy. Facial neuropathies will otherwise spare the extraocular muscles that govern globe movement. Because Bell palsy is a diagnosis of exclusion, clinicians need to make every effort to exclude other identifiable causes of facial paralysis, such as Lyme disease, HIV disease, acute and chronic otitis media, cholesteatoma, and multiple sclerosis. Other common causes of acute peripheral facial paralysis will often have findings on history or physical examination that suggest the correct diagnosis.

Graves ophthalmopathy can cause proptosis or extraocular muscle edema with consequent eye movement abnormalities but is not associated with the facial hemiparalysis typical of facial nerve (Bell) palsy.

Cerebral infarction, brain hemorrhage, or any structural brain lesion can cause weakness of the lower face but not of the forehead because the bilateral cortical representation of the midline forehead spares the forehead corrugators. Some limb or sensory abnormality is also often, but not universally, observed in the setting of cerebral infarction; no such abnormality was observed in this patient. Therefore, despite her cerebrovascular risk factors of oral contraception and cigarette smoking, this patient is unlikely to have had a cerebral infarction.

The trigeminal nerve provides sensation, not movement, to the muscles of facial expression, so trigeminal neuralgia is not a likely diagnosis in this patient with normal sensation.

KEY POINT

Any cause of a complete facial neuropathy will impair the entire hemiface, including the forehead muscles.

Bibliography
Tiemstra JD, Khatkhate N. Bell's palsy: diagnosis and management. Am Fam Physician. 2007;76(7):997-1002. [PMID: 17956069]

Item 26   Answer: C
Educational Objective: *Diagnose Guillain-Barré syndrome.*

This patient has a rapidly progressive disorder affecting the peripheral nervous system, most compatible with a clinical diagnosis of Guillain-Barré syndrome. Patients with Guillain-Barré syndrome typically develop paresthesias distally in the lower extremities that are followed by limb weakness and gait unsteadiness. In addition to sensory loss and limb weakness, deep tendon reflexes are characteristically absent or markedly reduced. The diagnosis is confirmed by electromyography, which usually shows a demyelinating polyradiculoneuropathy.

Cerebrospinal fluid (CSF) analysis characteristically shows albuminocytologic dissociation, whereby the spinal fluid cell count is normal but the spinal fluid protein level is elevated. CSF analysis may also yield normal results early in the course of the disease. However, a normal CSF cell count is useful in excluding other infectious conditions, such as polyradiculoneuropathies associated with HIV and cytomegalovirus infection, infection due to West Nile virus, and carcinomatous or lymphomatous nerve root infiltration. By definition, symptoms in patients with Guillain-Barré syndrome peak within 4 weeks of onset. Intravenous immune globulin and plasma exchange are equally efficacious in the treatment of Guillain-Barré syndrome.

Amyotrophic lateral sclerosis (ALS) is a degenerative disease of the anterior horn cells of the spinal cord and presents with both upper and lower motor neuron signs, including hyperreflexia, spasticity, and an extensor plantar response (upper motor neuron signs) and weakness, muscle atrophy, and fasciculations (lower motor neuron signs). The patient's findings are not compatible with ALS.

Diabetes mellitus most commonly causes a slowly progressive, distal, symmetric sensorimotor polyneuropathy. Autonomic dysfunction frequently is associated with diabetic neuropathy and is characterized by symptoms of impotence, orthostatic hypotension, and gastroparesis. The symptoms of a distal symmetric sensorimotor neuropathy may be the first clinical manifestation, but the rapidly progressive course of this patient's neuropathy rules out diabetic neuropathy.

A spinal cord lesion (myelopathy) would be an unlikely cause of the symptoms noted on clinical examination. The absence of bowel or bladder impairment, the lack of a sensory level across the thorax, and the upper and lower limb areflexia argue against a central nervous system disorder affecting the spinal cord.

KEY POINT

Guillain-Barré syndrome is a disorder associated with rapidly progressive extremity weakness, paresthesias, and areflexia.

Bibliography

Burns TM. Guillain-Barré syndrome. Semin Neurol. 2008;28(2):152-167. [PMID: 18351518]

Item 27   Answer: A
Educational Objective: *Diagnose carpal tunnel syndrome.*

This patient most likely has carpal tunnel syndrome. Carpal tunnel syndrome refers to median nerve compression at the wrist in the carpal tunnel. Symptoms include aching wrist pain with sparing of the palm, numbness and tingling in the median nerve sensory distribution of the fingers, and weakness of the thenar muscles. The paresthesias are often worse at night or when holding a book or steering a car.

de Quervain tenosynovitis is an exercise-related injury associated with knitting and sports involving extensive wrist action. Tenderness may be elicited in the anatomic snuffbox (the extensor pollicis brevis and abductor pollicis longus tendons). Pain elicited by flexing the thumb into the palm, closing the fingers over the thumb, and then bending the wrist in the ulnar direction (Finkelstein test) is confirmatory.

Ganglion cysts are synovia-filled cysts arising from joints or tendon sheaths that typically appear on the dorsal hand or ventral wrist. They can cause pain and compress other structures. The absence of cystic structures on the dorsal and ventral wrist and the distribution of the patient's pain eliminate this diagnosis.

Ulnar nerve compression at the wrist is also called Guyon tunnel syndrome, because the entrapment occurs where the ulnar nerve transverses the Guyon tunnel between the pisiform and hamate bones on the anterolateral side of the wrist, and cyclist's palsy, because the compression of the ulnar nerve often occurs as the hand rests on the handlebars. However, the ulnar nerve can be compressed by muscles, tumors (lipomas), scar tissue, synovial cysts, or any other internal structure that passes close to the tunnel. The presentation is similar to that of carpal tunnel syndrome, but with symptoms and signs on the ulnar distribution of the hand.

KEY POINT

Symptoms of carpal tunnel syndrome include aching wrist pain with sparing of the palm, numbness and tingling in the median nerve sensory distribution of the fingers, and weakness of the thenar muscles.

Bibliography

Keith MW, Masear V, Chung K, et al. Diagnosis of carpal tunnel syndrome. J Am Acad Orthop Surg. 2009;17(6):389-396. [PMID: 19474448]

Item 28   Answer: B
Educational Objective: *Diagnose diabetic polyneuropathy.*

The fasting blood glucose level will most likely provide a diagnosis for the patient's neurologic findings. Diabetic neuropathy involves injury to sensory, motor, and autonomic nerves. Loss of sensation in a "stocking-glove" distribution that is associated with paresthesias or painful dysesthesias is the most common presentation of this condition. Loss of sensation in the lower extremities is typical and plays a major part in the development of foot ulcerations, which can lead to limb loss. No direct treatment for diabetic neuropathy exists, other than to improve glycemic control. Pharmacologic therapy, however, may help symptoms. Partial serotonin and norepinephrine reuptake inhibitors (duloxetine), tricyclic antidepressants (amitriptyline), and various antiseizure medications (gabapentin, phenytoin, carbamazepine) are frequently used to treat the pain associated with this condition.

Obtaining a creatine kinase level would be appropriate in someone with suspected primary muscle disease, but this diagnosis is not likely in this patient, given the presence of neuropathic pain and sensory loss without muscle weakness. Lumbar puncture and cerebrospinal fluid examination should be considered in patients with acute, severe, or rapidly progressive neuropathy and in those with a demyelinating neuropathy; in these situations, lumbar puncture may help to confirm the presence of an inflammatory process in the cerebrospinal fluid but would not result in a specific diagnosis. Multiple sclerosis, the most common example of a demyelinating disorder, is characterized by discrete subacute episodes of neurologic dysfunction that progress over days to weeks, plateau, and then improve partially or completely over subsequent days to months. Sural nerve biopsy is most typically performed in patients with suspected vasculitis or amyloidosis. Patients with vasculitic neuropathy typically have a systemic illness with manifestations in other organs, including the skin, lungs, and kidneys; vasculitic neuropathy as the sole presenting feature of a systemic illness would be very unusual. Like vasculitis, amyloidosis is a systemic disease with manifestations involving many organ systems and would not likely present with symptoms confined to the peripheral nervous system of the lower extremities.

KEY POINT

Loss of sensation in a "stocking-glove" distribution that is associated with paresthesias or painful dysesthesias is the most common presentation of diabetic neuropathy.

Bibliography

Kanji JN, Anglin RE, Hunt DL, Panju A. Does this patient with diabetes have large-fiber peripheral neuropathy? JAMA. 2010;303(15):1526-1532. [PMID: 20407062]

Section 9

Oncology
Questions

Item 1 [Advanced]

A 45-year-old woman is evaluated for a lump in the right breast that has been present for 3 months. The patient is gravida 1, para 1. She has menses every 28 days. She is otherwise healthy. No family history of breast cancer exists. Her mother died of endometrial cancer at the age of 63 years.

On physical examination, vital signs are normal. A firm and nontender 2-cm mass in the upper outer quadrant of the right breast is palpated. No other masses or axillary adenopathy are noted.

A mammogram is BI-RADS 2 (benign findings).

Which of the following is the most appropriate next step in the management of this patient?

(A) Obtain a fine needle aspirate
(B) Obtain an ultrasound of the right breast
(C) Repeat mammogram in 1 year
(D) Test for *BRCA-1* and *BRCA-2* genes

Item 2 [Advanced]

A 55-year-old woman undergoes follow-up evaluation for a mildly pruritic eruption on and surrounding her right nipple, which developed about 5 months ago. Triamcinolone acetonide cream was begun 1 month ago with no improvement in the lesion. She has no personal or family history of eczema or psoriasis, and she is otherwise healthy. Her only medication is triamcinolone.

Breast findings are shown (Plate 23).

Which of the following is the most likely diagnosis?

(A) Chronic cutaneous lupus erythematosus
(B) Lichen simplex chronicus
(C) Paget disease of the breast
(D) Psoriasis

Item 3 [Basic]

A 49-year-old woman is evaluated after noticing a small lump in her right breast 3 weeks ago. It is painless and has not changed in size. She has no other pertinent medical history. Her last menstrual period was 2 weeks ago. Her mother had breast cancer at age 55 years; there is no other family history of cancer.

On physical examination, vital signs are normal. There is a 1.0 × 1.5-cm firm, discrete, mobile mass in the upper outer quadrant of the right breast. There is no lymphadenopathy or other abnormalities on examination.

A bilateral mammogram does not reveal any suspicious lesion in either breast.

Which of the following is the most appropriate management option for this patient?

(A) Aspiration or biopsy
(B) Clinical reevaluation in 1 month
(C) MRI of both breasts
(D) Repeat mammography in 6 months

Item 4 [Basic]

A 52-year-old woman undergoes evaluation after a recent diagnosis of invasive ductal adenocarcinoma of the right breast. Her aunt died of breast cancer at age 85 years, but there is no other family history of breast or ovarian cancer. The patient is otherwise healthy. Her physical examination is normal.

The patient undergoes tumor resection and a sentinel lymph node biopsy of the right axilla. On pathologic examination, a 1.2-cm invasive ductal adenocarcinoma with free margins is confirmed, and the lymph node reveals no metastases. Complete blood count, metabolic profile, and liver chemistry tests are normal as are diagnostic mammography and chest radiography.

Which of the following will be most helpful in directing the approach to management of this patient?

(A) Full right axillary lymph node dissection
(B) Genetic testing for the *BRCA1/2* mutation
(C) Tumor estrogen and progesterone receptor assay
(D) Whole-body positron emission tomography

Item 5 [Basic]

A 48-year-old postmenopausal woman is evaluated after a recent diagnosis of breast cancer. Her annual screening mammogram revealed a new 1.5-cm area of microcalcification in the left breast without any associated mass. Stereotactic biopsy revealed grade 2, estrogen receptor–progesterone receptor–negative and *HER2*-negative infiltrating ductal carcinoma. She is otherwise healthy.

Her physical examination is normal except for ecchymosis at the biopsy site.

Which of the following is the most appropriate next step in management?

(A) Left lumpectomy and tamoxifen
(B) Left lumpectomy followed by breast irradiation
(C) Left lumpectomy with sentinel lymph node biopsy and tamoxifen
(D) Left lumpectomy with sentinel lymph node biopsy followed by breast irradiation

Item 6 [Advanced]

A 51-year-old woman is evaluated during a routine health maintenance examination. She is healthy and takes no medications. She does not smoke or drink alcohol. She is up to date on all of her immunizations and cancer screening tests. Her most recent screening colonoscopy was performed at age 50 years. The only new addition to her history is a recent diagnosis of colorectal cancer in her 55-year-old brother.

What is the best colorectal cancer screening strategy for this patient?

(A) *APC* gene mutations screening
(B) Colonoscopy at age 55 years and then every 3 to 5 years
(C) Colonoscopy at age 60 years and then every 10 years
(D) Colonoscopy now and then every 2 years

Item 7 [Advanced]

A 59-year-old man is evaluated for a change in his bowel habits over the past 2 months. Typically, he has a soft, formed bowel movement every other day, but he now passes hard, pellet-like stools alternating with loose stools associated with a sense of bloating and abdominal fullness; there is no blood. He has not lost weight. He has never undergone colon cancer screening.

On physical examination, vital signs are normal. Abdominal examination reveals normal bowel sounds and no evidence of tenderness or masses. Rectal examination is normal, and the stool is negative for occult blood. Routine screening chemistry tests are normal.

Which of the following is the most appropriate next step in the management of this patient?

(A) Colonoscopy
(B) Contrast-enhanced abdominal CT scan
(C) Flexible sigmoidoscopy
(D) Testing three stools for occult blood

Item 8 [Basic]

A 58-year-old woman undergoes a general physical examination. She is asymptomatic and takes no medications or over-the-counter drugs. Family history is unremarkable. Her preferred method of colorectal cancer screening has been annual fecal occult blood testing (FOBT). Annual testing for the past 8 years has been negative for fecal occult blood.

Physical examination is normal. Results of routine laboratory studies are also normal, including a hemoglobin level of 14.8 g/dL (148 g/L). One of three stool samples submitted by the patient for FOBT is positive.

Which of the following is the most appropriate next step in evaluating this patient?

(A) Colonoscopy
(B) Flexible sigmoidoscopy
(C) Repeat FOBT now
(D) Repeat FOBT in 1 year

Item 9 [Advanced]

A 27-year-old woman with an 8-year history of ulcerative colitis is evaluated during a follow-up examination. The initial colonoscopy after diagnosis showed pancolitis. She has been treated with mesalamine since diagnosis and has had episodes of bloody diarrhea two or three times a year but has otherwise been well. Her most recent colonoscopy 1 year ago when she had increased diarrhea and bleeding showed no progression of disease. Since then, she has been clinically stable. The patient's medical history is otherwise unremarkable, and her only medications are low-dose mesalamine and a multivitamin. There is no family history of colorectal cancer.

On physical examination, vital signs are normal. There is mild abdominal tenderness in the right lower quadrant without rebound or guarding. The rest of the physical examination is normal.

Laboratory studies reveal a normal complete blood count, including leukocyte differential, and a normal serum C-reactive protein level.

Which of the following is the most appropriate management for this patient?

(A) Annual colonoscopy
(B) Annual fecal occult blood testing
(C) Annual flexible sigmoidoscopy
(D) Annual wireless capsule endoscopy

Item 10 [Basic]

A 66-year-old man is evaluated during a routine examination. The patient has a 25-pack-year cigarette-smoking history. He has tried to quit smoking with nicotine gum and varenicline with no success. He has mild airway obstruction but good exercise tolerance and no cough, sputum production, or hemoptysis. The importance of smoking cessation is reviewed with the patient.

Which of the following is the recommended screening strategy for lung cancer in this patient?

(A) 18F-fluorodeoxyglucose and positron emission tomography scan (FDG-PET)
(B) Chest radiography
(C) Spiral CT scan of the chest
(D) Sputum cytology
(E) No screening

Item 11 [Advanced]

A 52-year-old woman is evaluated after an abdominal CT scan detected a 3-mm nodule in the right lower pulmonary lobe. The CT scan was obtained to evaluate abdominal pain, which has since completely resolved. The patient has never smoked. She works in the home and has not been exposed to potential carcinogens. She has not had a chest radiograph or other imaging procedure, except mammography. Her medical history is unremarkable, and she takes no medication. Her family history is unremarkable.

The physical examination is normal.

Which of the following is the most appropriate next step in the management of this patient?

(A) Chest radiograph in 3 months
(B) CT scan of the chest in 3 months
(C) CT scan of the chest in 6 months
(D) No follow-up

Item 12 [Basic]

A 78-year-old woman is evaluated for a 6-month history of fatigue and an unintentional 9.0-kg (20-lb) weight loss.

On physical examination, vital signs are normal. There is a palpable 1.5-cm left supraclavicular lymph node. The skin is normal, the lungs are clear, and the abdomen is soft and without organomegaly.

Complete blood count, liver enzymes, and serum calcium level are normal. Chest radiograph shows a 5-cm left lung mass with left hilar lymphadenopathy. CT scan shows a 5-cm left upper lobe mass with left hilar lymphadenopathy and normal-sized mediastinal lymph nodes.

Which of the following is the most appropriate management?

(A) Bronchoscopy with biopsy of the mass
(B) CT-guided transthoracic needle biopsy of the mass
(C) Positron emission tomography–CT (PET–CT)
(D) Supraclavicular lymph node biopsy

Item 13 [Advanced]

A 62-year-old man is evaluated for a recent diagnosis of biopsy-proven, limited-stage small cell lung cancer involving the right upper lobe. The patient has excellent performance status and has recently stopped smoking cigarettes. He has no other medical problems and takes no medications.

On physical examination, vital signs are normal; BMI is 24. Pulmonary examination discloses decreased breath sounds throughout all lung fields and a few early wheezes in the right upper chest. Neurologic examination results are normal.

Which of the following is the most appropriate treatment for this patient?

(A) Chemotherapy and radiation therapy
(B) Chemotherapy followed by autologous stem cell transplantation
(C) Radiation therapy
(D) Right upper lobectomy
(E) Small cell lung cancer vaccination

Item 14 [Basic]

A 60-year-old man is evaluated during a routine visit. He has no chronic medical problems or genitourinary symptoms. His physical examination is normal, including a digital rectal examination that reveals a slightly enlarged, nontender, smooth prostate gland.

He has previously decided to undergo annual prostate-specific antigen (PSA) cancer screening. One year ago, his PSA was 2.5 ng/mL (2.5 µg/L). A PSA measured yesterday was 5.4 ng/mL (5.4 µg/L).

Which of the following is the most appropriate next management step?

(A) CT scan of the pelvis
(B) Transrectal prostate biopsy
(C) Radical prostatectomy
(D) Repeat PSA measurement in 6 months

Item 15 [Advanced]

A 57-year-old man is evaluated during a routine examination. He asks if he should undergo prostate-specific antigen (PSA) testing. Medical history is otherwise unremarkable. There is no family history of cancer. Results of the physical examination are unremarkable.

Which of the following is the best prostate cancer screening option for this patient?

(A) Discuss the risks and benefits of screening for prostate cancer
(B) Order PSA testing
(C) Order PSA testing and perform digital rectal examination (DRE)
(D) Perform DRE

Item 16 [Basic]

An 80-year-old man is evaluated after an elevated serum prostate-specific antigen (PSA) level of 5.7 ng/mL (5.7 µg/L) was noted during a community screening program. He has no symptoms related to the genitourinary system and denies bone pain, weight loss, or any change in his health status. The patient has hypertension and hypercholesterolemia. He also underwent four-vessel coronary artery bypass graft surgery 5 years ago and has chronic stable angina. His current medications are hydrochlorothiazide, atenolol, lisinopril, pravastatin, nitroglycerin, and low-dose aspirin.

On physical examination, the patient is afebrile, blood pressure is 140/80 mm Hg, and the pulse rate is 72/min and regular. The lungs are clear, and the abdomen is soft and nontender. There is trace pedal edema in the lower extremities.

Which of the following is the most appropriate next step in management?

(A) Bone scan
(B) Repeat PSA
(C) Transrectal prostate biopsy
(D) Observation

Item 17 [Advanced]

A 66-year-old man is evaluated because of an increasingly elevated serum prostate-specific antigen (PSA) level. The patient received a prostate cancer diagnosis 4 years ago and underwent definitive radiation therapy, following which his PSA level became undetectable. He is currently asymptomatic.

A bone scan now shows multiple metastatic lesions.

Which of the following is the most appropriate management?

(A) Docetaxel plus prednisone
(B) Hospice care
(C) Leuprolide
(D) Samarium-153
(E) Observation

Item 18 [Basic]

A 27-year-old woman with a history of multiple sex partners is evaluated during a routine office visit. She feels well and has no symptoms. She has never had an abnormal Pap smear. She has been sexually active for 10 years and has not had any sexually transmitted diseases, although she has not usually used condoms. Safe sex counseling is provided.

Results of a pelvic examination are normal, and a Pap smear is obtained. HIV testing is performed. Results of the Pap smear are positive for atypical squamous cells of undetermined significance (ASCUS). Subsequent human papillomavirus testing is positive for subtype 16.

Which of the following is the best next management step?

(A) Colposcopy
(B) Repeat human papillomavirus testing in 1 year
(C) Repeat Pap testing in 1 year
(D) Treatment with interferon

Item 19 [Basic]

A 19-year-old asymptomatic woman is evaluated during a routine annual physical examination. The patient states she is not sexually active and has not engaged in prior sexual activity. She has a boyfriend whom she has dated for the past year. The patient completed her menstrual cycle 3 days ago. She has no pertinent family history or known drug allergies and takes no medications. She has not received a human papillomavirus vaccine.

Results of the physical examination, including a breast and pelvic examination, are normal.

Which of the following is the most appropriate management option for this patient?

(A) Human papillomavirus (HPV) vaccine at age 21 years
(B) HPV vaccine at onset of sexual activity
(C) HPV vaccine at time of HPV seroconversion
(D) HPV vaccine now

Item 20 [Basic]

A 38-year-old woman comes to the office for a routine physical examination and Pap smear. Her husband has been her only sexual partner for the past 14 years, and they are both human immunodeficiency virus–negative. She has received annual Pap tests since the onset of sexual activity at age 21 years and has never had an abnormal Pap smear.

If her current Pap smear is normal, when does she need to have her next Pap test?

(A) Today
(B) In 6 months
(C) In 3 years
(D) In 5 years
(E) Never, unless she has a new sexual partner

Item 21 [Basic]

A 47-year-old woman undergoes her annual physical examination. She has no medical problems and takes no medications. She had a complete vaginal hysterectomy for abnormal uterine bleeding caused by leiomyoma 2 years ago. She has had a monogamous sexual relationship with her husband since her marriage 24 years ago. She has had cervical Pap tests every 3 years since the age of 30 years until 2 years ago, all of which have been normal.

Which of the following is the most appropriate frequency of Pap tests for this patient?

(A) Annually, indefinitely
(B) Every 3 years, indefinitely
(C) Every 3 years until age 65 years
(D) Discontinue Pap smear

Item 22 [Advanced]

A 72-year-old man is evaluated for an asymptomatic lesion on his forearm. It is firm to palpation and has been gradually enlarging over the past year. It does not itch. No other similar skin lesions are present.

Skin findings are shown (Plate 24).

Which of the following is the most likely diagnosis?

(A) Nummular eczema
(B) Psoriasis
(C) Squamous cell carcinoma in situ
(D) Superficial basal cell carcinoma
(E) Superficial spreading melanoma

Item 23 [Basic]

A 62-year-old man is evaluated for a dark blue "berry-like" lesion that has been enlarging over the past 6 months. It is bothersome, because it now tends to catch on his clothing.

Skin findings are shown (Plate 25).

Which of the following is the most likely diagnosis?

(A) Basal cell carcinoma
(B) Keratoacanthoma
(C) Nodular melanoma
(D) Seborrheic keratosis
(E) Spitz nevus

Item 24 [Advanced]

A 70-year-old man comes to the office to ask about the skin changes on his hands, as shown (Plate 26).

The skin changes have been present for years, but he is concerned now about the possibility of skin cancer.

Which of the following is the most likely diagnosis?

(A) Actinic keratoses
(B) Basal cell carcinoma
(C) Malignant melanoma
(D) Seborrheic keratoses

Item 25 [Basic]

A 62-year-old man is evaluated for an asymptomatic nodule on his shoulder that has been present for more than 1 year.

Skin findings are shown (Plate 27).

Which of the following is the most likely diagnosis?

(A) Basal cell carcinoma
(B) Pyogenic granuloma
(C) Seborrheic keratosis
(D) Squamous cell carcinoma

Item 26 [Advanced]

A 62-year-old man is evaluated for a rapidly growing nodule on his face. The lesion has arisen within the past 4 to 6 weeks and is painless. He does not recall a history of trauma.

The lesion is shown (Plate 28). It is not tender, warm to the touch, or fluctuant. There is no associated lymphadenopathy.

Which of the following is the most likely diagnosis?

(A) Abscess
(B) Keloid
(C) Keratoacanthoma
(D) Nodular basal cell carcinoma

Item 27 [Basic]

A 69-year-old man is evaluated for low back discomfort. He has a history of metastatic prostate cancer to the spine without evidence of spinal cord compression. He is ambulatory and functional in all activities of daily living. He recently received palliative radiation therapy to treat metastatic disease in L1 and L3. The patient takes at least two naproxen 250-mg tablets daily. The pain medication reduces, but does not eliminate, his back discomfort.

On physical examination, vital signs are normal as are results of neurologic and mental status examinations. There is no point tenderness over the lumbar vertebrae.

Which of the following is the most appropriate next therapeutic step?

(A) Add a fentanyl patch
(B) Add an extended-release opioid
(C) Add a short-acting opioid
(D) Discontinue naproxen and substitute ibuprofen

Item 28 [Basic]

A 74-year-old man with metastatic lung cancer to the liver and pelvis is evaluated for low back pain. The pain is localized to the right ischial region and has progressively worsened over the past month despite the use of immediate-release morphine (15 mg) every 6 hours. He states the pain returns about 4 hours after taking his medication. He has no symptoms of spinal cord compression. He has declined radiation therapy for his bony lesions.

On physical examination, vital signs are normal as are results of neurologic and mental status examinations.

Which of the following is the most appropriate maintenance pain management strategy?

(A) Add gabapentin three times daily
(B) Increase frequency of immediate-release morphine to every 4 hours
(C) Switch to immediate-release oxycodone every 4 hours
(D) Switch to sustained-release morphine twice daily

Item 29 [Advanced]

A 67-year-old man with newly diagnosed, widely metastatic prostate cancer is hospitalized for severe hip, chest wall, and shoulder pain. Adequate dosages of acetaminophen, ibuprofen, and hydrocodone have not relieved his pain. Several boluses of intravenous morphine sulfate are administered followed by a continuous infusion. After 24 hours, his pain is adequately controlled, and he is not experiencing any adverse effects related to the morphine administration.

Which of the following is the most appropriate oral drug regimen after hospital discharge?

(A) Hydrocodone as needed
(B) Long-acting morphine sulfate twice daily and immediate-release morphine sulfate as needed
(C) Long-acting morphine sulfate twice daily and oxycodone as needed
(D) Oxycodone as needed

Item 30 [Advanced]

A 79-year-old woman is evaluated at home by a visiting hospice nurse for dyspnea that began 4 days ago and has worsened in the past 24 hours. The patient has metastatic breast cancer. She has executed a do-not-resuscitate order and has discontinued cancer treatment. Over the past 6 weeks, her oral intake has worsened, and she cannot walk without assistance because of weakness. Her pain is well controlled with extended-release morphine and immediate-release morphine as needed for breakthrough pain.

The hospice nurse reports that the patient is alert and oriented. Vital signs are normal. Oxygen saturation is 97% with the patient breathing ambient air. She has crackles and early inspiratory wheezing over both lung fields and a reduced cough effort. She has mild dullness to percussion and reduced breath sounds over the right base. There is no S_3, jugular venous distention, or peripheral edema. Her last dose of extended-release morphine was 6 hours ago, and her last dose of immediate-release morphine was yesterday.

Which of the following is the best management option for her dyspnea?

(A) A supplemental dose of immediate-release morphine
(B) Emergency department evaluation
(C) Furosemide
(D) Home oxygen therapy

Section 9

Oncology
Answers and Critiques

Item 1   **Answer: B**
Educational Objective: *Evaluate a breast mass.*

The next management step for this patient is to obtain an ultrasound of the right breast. The Breast Imaging Reporting and Data System (BI-RADS) is a standardized reporting system for mammography findings and a source of recommendations for further management. Category assignments are either incomplete (category 0) or final assessment (categories 1 through 6). Category 2 findings correspond to findings compatible with benign nodules or cysts or benign calcifications. But because this patient's mass has persisted through several menstrual cycles, she needs further evaluation despite the normal mammogram. Because she is older than 30 years and the mammogram is classified as BI-RADS 2, the ultrasound is the next appropriate test. This is true for mammograms rated BI-RADS 1-3. Ultrasound serves to distinguish cystic from solid masses. A cystic mass should be aspirated and the fluid sent for cytologic evaluation if bloody or recurrent. A solid mass requires biopsy by fine-needle aspiration, core needle, or excision. If the mammogram is classified as BI-RADS 4 or 5, malignancy is much more likely and a tissue diagnosis with fine needle aspirate or biopsy is the most appropriate management.

Inherited germline abnormalities in *BRCA-1* and *BRCA-2* genes confer very high risk for breast and ovarian cancer (absolute risk of breast cancer greater than 60% by age 50 years). Fewer than 5% of all cases of breast cancer are attributed to germline abnormalities in these genes, however, and the prevalence of these abnormalities in the general population is approximately 1/800. Testing for *BRCA-1* and *BRCA-2* genes should be performed only in women who appear to have a genetic risk (multiple relatives with breast or ovarian cancer, especially with early-onset of disease). These women and their families should be referred to a genetic counselor for discussion and consideration of these complex issues. This patient does not have an increased genetic risk for breast cancer and testing for *BRCA-1* and *BRCA-2* genes is not indicated.

KEY POINT

Breast ultrasonography serves to distinguish cystic from solid masses.

Bibliography
Stein L, Chellman-Jeffers M. The radiologic workup of a palpable breast mass. Cleve Clin J Med. 2009;76(3):175-80. [PMID: 19258464]

Item 2   **Answer: C**
Educational Objective: *Diagnose Paget disease of the breast.*

This patient has Paget disease of the breast, defined as a persistent, scaling, eczematous, or ulcerated lesion involving the nipple/areolar complex. Histologically, the hallmark of Paget disease of the breast is the presence of malignant, intraepithelial adenocarcinoma cells (Paget cells) within the epidermis of the nipple associated with an underlying invasive or intraductal cancer. It is often misdiagnosed on the first presentation as either eczema or psoriasis, but when there is a lack of response to appropriate therapy, a biopsy should be performed.

The most characteristic lesions of chronic cutaneous lupus erythematosus are discoid lesions appearing as erythematous, infiltrated plaques that are covered with scale and are associated with follicular plugging. These lesions are most often found on the face, neck, and scalp. As they expand, they develop depressed central scars. This patient's lesion, location, and appearance are not clinically compatible with chronic cutaneous lupus.

Lichen simplex chronicus is a localized disorder characterized by intense pruritus, which leads to a localized area of lichenified skin (thickened skin with increased and exaggerated skin markings due to scratching). This patient has no evidence of lichenification.

The most common form of psoriasis is plaque psoriasis. The skin lesions of this disorder are sharply demarcated, erythematous plaques covered by silvery-white scales that affect the scalp and extensor surfaces (elbows and knees) as well as the nails. A single patch of psoriasis located on the nipple would be a very rare presentation.

KEY POINT

Paget disease of the breast is a ductal carcinoma that presents as a persistent, scaling, eczematous, or ulcerated lesion involving the nipple/areolar complex and may be mistaken for more benign conditions such as eczema.

Bibliography
Caliskan M, Gatti G, Sosnovskikh I, et al. Paget's disease of the breast: the experience of the European Institute of Oncology and review of the literature. Breast Cancer Res Treat. 2008;112(3):513-521. [PMID: 18240020]

Item 3   Answer: A

Educational Objective: *Manage a breast mass with aspiration or biopsy.*

The most appropriate management option is fine-needle aspiration or biopsy of the breast mass. A patient with a breast mass requires triple assessment: palpation, mammography with or without ultrasonography, and surgical evaluation for biopsy. Mammograms may be normal in 10% to 15% of patients with breast lumps, some of which may be cancerous. After performance of bilateral diagnostic mammography, the initial focus of the workup of a dominant breast mass is to distinguish a simple cyst from a solid mass by fine-needle aspiration (FNA) or ultrasonography. If the fluid from FNA is bloody, the fluid should undergo cytologic evaluation. Women with simple cysts should undergo a breast examination 4 to 6 weeks after cyst aspiration to evaluate for cyst recurrence or a residual lump. A solid mass requires a tissue diagnosis by fine-needle aspiration biopsy (FNAB), core-needle biopsy, or excisional biopsy. Patients with benign FNAB or core-needle biopsy results and negative mammogram require close clinical follow-up of the breast abnormality.

It is inappropriate to observe the patient without further workup or to just repeat mammography later, because she has a discrete mass that may represent breast cancer despite the normal mammographic findings. Even if an ultrasound is negative, the patient requires tissue sampling.

The role of breast MRI for screening high-risk patients is currently being evaluated. In patients with an established diagnosis of breast cancer, it may be of value in determining the extent of disease. In this patient, a breast MRI would not obviate the need for fine-needle aspiration or biopsy and is much more expensive than ultrasonography.

KEY POINT

A patient with a breast mass requires aspiration or biopsy regardless of mammography results.

Bibliography

Kerlikowske K, Smith-Bindman R, Ljung BM, Grady D. Evaluation of abnormal mammography results and palpable breast abnormalities. Ann Intern Med 2003;139(4):274-284. [PMID:12965983]

Item 4   Answer: C

Educational Objective: *Evaluate a patient with early-stage breast cancer for tumor estrogen- and progesterone-receptor status.*

The next step is a tumor estrogen-receptor (ER) and progesterone-receptor (PR) assay. This patient has early-stage breast cancer (stage I) based on the tumor size (<2 cm); absent lymph node involvement; and no apparent metastases based on her symptoms, physical examination findings, and routine blood tests. The step that would be most helpful in directing the approach to management of this patient is to perform an assay for expression of ER and PR to determine the optimal sys-

temic treatment, and this evaluative step should be performed in all cases of primary breast cancer. Endocrine therapy (for example, tamoxifen, aromatase inhibitors, fulvestrant, and megestrol acetate) is beneficial only in patients with ER–positive or PR–positive tumors. Patients whose tumors are hormone receptor–negative are refractory to endocrine treatment and should receive chemotherapy instead.

In patients with early-stage breast cancer, the routine evaluation is limited to a thorough history and physical examination, diagnostic mammography, chest radiography, and routine blood tests (including liver chemistry tests). The use of additional imaging studies or blood tests is not warranted in the absence of specific symptoms because they may lead to the detection of abnormalities of no significance (a false-positive test result).

In early-stage disease, the positive predictive value of abnormal findings of whole-body positron emission tomography is approximately 1%; therefore, this type of imaging modality is not recommended. The absence of metastases in a sentinel axillary lymph node has a high negative predictive value, obviating the need for a complete axillary lymph node dissection with its associated morbidity.

About 5% of breast cancer cases are attributable to rare, high-penetrance mutations in a few specific genes; mutations in *BRCA1* and *BRCA2* account for up to 50% of all cases of hereditary and familial breast cancer. This proportion is higher in patients with breast cancer at a younger age of onset and in families with multiple breast or ovarian cancer cases. Testing for the *BRCA1* or *BRCA2* gene in this patient would not be indicated without a more compelling family history of disease.

KEY POINT

Assay for expression of estrogen and progesterone receptors is crucial in determining the optimal systemic treatment for breast cancer and should be performed in all patients with primary breast cancer.

Bibliography

Carlson RW, Allred DC, Anderson BO, Burstein HJ, Carter WB, Edge SB, Erban JK, Farrar WB, Goldstein LJ, Gradishar WJ, Hayes DF, Hudis CA, Jahanzeb M, Kiel K, Ljung BM, Marcom PK, Mayer IA, McCormick B, Nabell LM, Pierce LJ, Reed EC, Smith ML, Somlo G, Theriault RL, Topham NS, Ward JH, Winer EP, Wolff AC; NCCN Breast Cancer Clinical Practice Guidelines Panel. Breast cancer. Clinical practice guidelines in oncology. J Natl Compr Canc Netw. 2009;7(2):122-92. [PMID: 19200416]

Item 5   Answer: D

Educational Objective: *Treat a patient with breast cancer and a small focal tumor with lumpectomy, sentinel node dissection, and radiation.*

This patient should undergo breast lumpectomy plus sentinel lymph node biopsy followed by radiation therapy. Breast lumpectomy plus radiation therapy is known as "breast-conserving therapy." Breast-conserving therapy consists of excision of the primary tumor followed by radiation to the remaining ipsilateral breast tissue and is generally indicated for patients with focal disease and small tumors for which conservation will offer a good cosmetic result. However, patient preferences must be considered in the surgical decision-making process. The survival rate for women undergoing breast-conserving therapy is equivalent to that of those who undergo mastectomy, with breast-conserving therapy resulting in improved cosmetic outcomes and less morbidity than mastectomy. Most patients treated with lumpectomy without radiation therapy have a high risk for local recurrence; therefore, this treatment modality cannot be recommended. In addition, sentinel lymph node biopsy is a safe and accurate method for screening the axillary lymph nodes for metastases in women with small breast tumors. Sentinel lymph node biopsy has replaced full axillary lymph node dissection for the staging of disease in many women with early-stage, clinically lymph node–negative breast cancer. The first draining (or sentinel) lymph node is identified by injecting blue dye and radioactive colloid into the tumor site. If the sentinel lymph node does not contain metastases, it is unlikely that more distal axillary lymph nodes will contain metastases; consequently, no further surgery is indicated in this setting, and the toxicity from a full axillary lymph node dissection is avoided. However, if the sentinel lymph node shows metastatic involvement, then axillary lymph node dissection is performed to determine the number of involved lymph nodes.

Selective estrogen receptor modulators such as tamoxifen are not indicated in patients with estrogen receptor–negative tumors.

KEY POINT

Lumpectomy with sentinel lymph node biopsy followed by breast irradiation is the appropriate management of women with small, focal breast cancer.

Bibliography

Buchholz TA. Radiation therapy for early-stage breast cancer after breast-conserving surgery. N Engl J Med. 2009;360(1):63-70. [PMID: 19118305]

Item 6   Answer: B

Educational Objective: *Screen a patient at high risk for colorectal cancer.*

The best colorectal cancer screening strategy for this patient is colonoscopy at age 55 years and then every 3 to 5 years. A family history of colorectal cancer or adenomatous polyps significantly increases a person's risk for colorectal cancer. The presence of colorectal cancer in a first-degree relative carries a twofold to threefold increased lifetime risk over the general population; that risk is doubled again if the affected relative was diagnosed before age 45 years. If two first-degree relatives have colorectal cancer, the colorectal cancer risk approaches 20%. For persons with a family history of colorectal cancer in a first-degree relative, screening is initiated either at age 40

years or beginning 10 years earlier than the diagnosis of the youngest affected family member. If normal, colonoscopy is repeated every 3 to 5 years. Because this patient had colonoscopy screening at the age of 50 years, colonoscopy should be offered at some time between ages 53 and 55 years.

Familial adenomatous polyposis and attenuated familial adenomatous polyposis are most commonly diagnosed after polyposis is detected on endoscopy. In these patients, testing for mutations in the *APC* gene is reasonable. However, this patient does not have a personal history of polyposis.

Performing colonoscopy at age 50 years and then every 10 years is the recommendation for patients at average risk for colorectal cancer. Persons at average risk for colorectal cancer include those with no personal or family history of colon adenoma or cancer and who do not have a condition that predisposes them to cancer.

Patients with inflammatory bowel disease have an increased risk for colorectal cancer. The most reliable estimates suggest an annual colorectal cancer rate in extensive colitis of at least 0.5% per year after the first decade of colitis. Screening recommendations include colonoscopy every 1 to 2 years beginning 8 years after diagnosis. This screening interval is not appropriate for this patient who does not have inflammatory bowel disease.

KEY POINT

For persons with a family history of colorectal cancer in a first-degree relative, screening is initiated either at age 40 years or beginning 10 years earlier than the diagnosis of the youngest affected family member.

Bibliography

Geiger TM, Ricciardi R. Screening options and recommendations for colorectal cancer. Clin Colon Rectal Surg. 2009;22(4):209-17. [PMID: 21037811]

Item 7   Answer: A

Educational Objective: *Evaluate a symptomatic patient for colon cancer with colonoscopy.*

This patient requires a colonoscopy. Common signs and symptoms of colorectal cancer are influenced by the site of the primary tumor and may include a change in bowel habits, diarrhea, constipation, a feeling that the bowel does not empty completely, bright red blood in the stool or melanotic stools, and stools that are narrower in caliber than usual. Other signs include general abdominal discomfort (frequent gas pains, bloating, fullness, or cramps), weight loss for no known reason, fatigue, and vomiting. Findings that should prompt investigation for colon cancer include a rectal or abdominal mass, hepatomegaly, abdominal tenderness, or iron deficiency anemia. If one or more such findings are present, a full colorectal examination with colonoscopy should be done. However, the examination may be limited to sigmoidoscopy for rectal bleeding in most persons younger than 40 years of age because colorectal cancer is uncommon in such patients (except those with hereditary colorectal cancer syndromes), and in most young patients with hematochezia, a rectosigmoid lesion, usually hemorrhoids, is the cause of rectal bleeding. This patient is older than 40 years, has concerning symptoms, and therefore requires an immediate colonoscopy.

A contrast-enhanced CT scan of the abdomen is not sensitive for diagnosing colon cancer. Options for colorectal cancer screening include colonoscopy, fecal occult blood testing, flexible sigmoidoscopy, or barium enema used alone or in combination for screening. However, these screening modalities are reserved for asymptomatic patients. This patient is not asymptomatic and screening modalities, such as fecal occult blood testing, are not adequate owing to lack of sensitivity in a patient with a higher than average probability of disease. Even if the test results were positive, additional diagnostic studies would be needed to clarify the diagnosis. Direct visualization of the colonic mucosa with colonoscopy is needed for this patient with symptoms suggestive of colon cancer.

KEY POINT

Patients with suspected colon cancer should be evaluated with colonoscopy.

Bibliography

Kahi CJ, Rex DK, Imperiale TF. Screening, surveillance, and primary prevention for colorectal cancer: a review of the recent literature. Gastroenterology. 2008;135(2):380-99. Epub 2008 Jun 26. [PMID: 18582467]

Item 8   Answer: A

Educational Objective: *Evaluate a patient with a positive fecal occult blood test result with colonoscopy.*

This patient has a positive result on a screening test for colorectal neoplasia and should be evaluated next with colonoscopy. Fecal occult blood testing (FOBT) is associated with a 15% to 33% reduction in mortality rates from colorectal cancer when annual or biennial testing is done. Six-window FOBT is performed by taking two separate samples from each of three spontaneously passed stools (six samples). Even though only one of three of this patient's samples submitted for fecal occult blood testing was positive, she requires appropriate follow-up with a diagnostic test such as colonoscopy.

Repeating the FOBT is inappropriate because one test result was already positive. Since bleeding from colorectal neoplasia can occur intermittently, a subsequent negative FOBT would not rule out colon cancer or an adenomatous polyp. Flexible sigmoidoscopy, because of its limited ability to examine the entire colon, is inadequate for determining whether this patient has colorectal neoplasia. Waiting a year to repeat the FOBT potentially places this patient at risk for missing a curable colon cancer and cannot be recommended.

KEY POINT

An asymptomatic patient with a single positive fecal occult blood test on routine screening requires follow-up with colonoscopy.

Bibliography

Weinberg DS. In the clinic. Colorectal cancer screening. Ann Intern Med. 2008;148:ITC2-1-ITC2-16. [PMID: 18252680]

Item 9   Answer: A

Educational Objective: *Screen for colon cancer in a patient with inflammatory bowel disease.*

The most appropriate management for this patient is annual colonoscopy beginning now. This patient has pancolitis of 8 years' duration. The inflammation involves the ileum and proximal colon. The colon cancer risk in patients with ulcerative colitis or Crohn disease reaches a significant level (estimate annual cancer risk of 1% to 2% per year) after 8 years of inflammation. The cancer risk is slightly delayed for patients with inflammation limited to the distal colon. The recommendation is to initiate a surveillance program with colonoscopy 8 years after onset of disease, with follow-up colonoscopy every 1 to 2 years thereafter. Random biopsies are performed in four-quadrant fashion throughout the entire colon. Colectomy is recommended for patients with dysplastic findings on biopsy.

In wireless capsule endoscopy, a patient swallows a video capsule that by intestinal motility passes through the stomach and into the small intestine. The video capsule transmits images to a recording device worn by the patient. The images are downloaded onto a computer where they can be reviewed. With capsule endoscopy, the small bowel can be visualized in its entirety. There is no recommendation for standard screening for small-bowel carcinoma in the setting of ulcerative colitis or Crohn disease, and therefore, capsule endoscopy is not indicated. Furthermore, capsule endoscopy has no ability to biopsy the bowel wall and assess for dysplasia. Flexible sigmoidoscopy would not reach the at-risk colonic mucosa in the proximal colon beyond the reach of the sigmoidoscope, and annual fecal occult blood testing is insensitive to the diagnosis of colonic dysplasia, the earliest precursor of colon cancer.

KEY POINT

Patients with inflammatory bowel disease should initiate screening for colorectal cancer after 8 years' disease duration.

Bibliography

Weinberg DS. In the clinic. Colorectal cancer screening. Ann Intern Med. 2008;148:ITC2-1-ITC2-16. [PMID: 18252680]

Item 10   Answer: E

Educational Objective: *Do not screen for lung cancer.*

Screening for early-stage lung cancer is not now recommended with the use of any methodology, including spiral CT scan, chest radiography, sputum cytology, or 18F-fluorodeoxyglucose (FDG)-PET scan. No method has been shown to reduce death from lung cancer. Lung cancer screening with spiral CT scanning detects 60% or more of incident Stage I cancers. However, the false-positive rate (number of benign nodules detected) with spiral CT lung cancer screening is high and may result in patient anxiety and unnecessary invasive testing. Recent large, single-arm observational studies of spiral CT screening show that about 60% to 85% of incident cancers (detected after the baseline scan) are stage I and that the survival rate is better than that of historical unscreened cohorts. However, this finding alone does not prove that lung cancer screening is effective. Proof of efficacy for a lung cancer screening test would be a reduction in the mortality rate among those screened compared with a comparable group at risk who were not screened. Although survival results may be provocative in an observational study, they are subject to bias. The survival rate may be dramatically improved without actually resulting in a reduction in deaths from lung cancer because of lead-time bias, length-time bias, and overdiagnosis. A randomized, controlled trial is generally accepted as the definitive means of establishing efficacy for a screening test. Various screening studies now under way are randomized trials that might answer the question of the efficacy of screening for lung cancer.

KEY POINT

Screening for early-stage lung cancer is not now recommended with the use of any methodology.

Bibliography

Smith RA, Cokkinides V, Brawley OW. Cancer screening in the United States, 2008: a review of current American Cancer Society guidelines and cancer screening issues. CA Cancer J Clin. 2008;58(3):161-179. [PMID: 18443206]

Item 11   Answer: D

Educational Objective: *Evaluate a patient at low-risk for lung cancer with a very small pulmonary nodule.*

This patient requires no further follow up. Studies of chest CT screening have shown that 25% to 50% of patients have one or more pulmonary nodules detected on the initial CT scan. Even in patients at relatively high risk for lung cancer, the likelihood that a small nodule is malignant is low. For example, the risk of malignancy is about 0.2% for nodules smaller than 3 mm in diameter and 0.9% for nodules measuring 4 to 7 mm in diameter. The Fleischner Society recommendations include no follow-up for low-risk patients with nodules 4 mm or smaller and follow-up CT at 12 months for patients with such nodules who are at risk for lung cancer. This small nodule is not likely to be visible on chest radiograph, and, therefore, such imaging would not be helpful.

KEY POINT

In a patient at low risk for malignancy, no follow-up is required for an incidentally noted pulmonary nodule of 4 mm or smaller in diameter.

Bibliography

MacMahon H, Austin JH, Gamsu G, et al; Fleischner Society. Guidelines for management of small pulmonary nodules detected on CT scans: a statement from the Fleischner Society. Radiology. 2005;237(2):395-400. [PMID: 16244247]

Item 12   Answer: D

Educational Objective: *Diagnose and stage advanced lung cancer with a peripheral lymph node biopsy.*

The most appropriate management for this patient is supraclavicular lymph node biopsy. In the evaluation of a patient with suspected lung cancer, obtaining a tissue diagnosis is critical for treatment planning and determining prognosis. Staging the cancer and determining whether the patient is a candidate for resection are also important parts of the evaluation. In this patient, determining whether the supraclavicular lymph node contains non–small cell cancer should be done, and the next step in the evaluation would be to sample the lymph node; this would likely establish both a diagnosis and that the patient has advanced unresectable disease.

Because the clinical stage is already suggesting an advanced stage of disease, positron emission tomography (PET)–CT would not be needed for staging if the supraclavicular lymph node is positive, and a positive PET-CT result of the supraclavicular lymph nodes would not obviate the need for lymph node sampling. Biopsy of the mass or hilar lymph nodes by CT guidance or bronchoscopy would establish the diagnosis but not the stage and would not determine resectability.

KEY POINT

In the evaluation of possible lung cancer, obtaining a tissue diagnosis and staging for lung cancer should be done simultaneously whenever possible.

Bibliography

Silvestri GA, Gould MK, Margolis ML, et al; American College of Chest Physicians. Noninvasive staging of non-small cell lung cancer: ACCP evidenced-based clinical practice guidelines (2nd edition). Chest. 2007;132(3 Suppl):178S-201S. [PMID: 17873168]

Item 13   Answer: A

Educational Objective: *Manage a patient with limited-stage, small cell lung cancer.*

This patient has limited-stage small-cell lung cancer (SCLC) and should receive chemotherapy and radiation therapy. SCLC is considered a systemic disease; patients who present with seemingly localized disease almost always have concurrent micrometastases and consequently the more complicated staging system of non–small cell lung cancer does not apply. Patients with visibly localized disease that can be encompassed within a radiation therapy port are designated as having limited-stage disease. Patients with tumor beyond the confines of a radiation port are considered to have extensive-stage disease. Chemotherapy plus radiation therapy is considered first-line treatment for patients with limited-stage SCLC. Typical regimens consist of a combination of a platinum agent (carboplatin or cisplatin) and etoposide or irinotecan. Combination chemotherapy and radiation therapy is associated with a substantially improved median survival compared with chemotherapy, surgery, or radiotherapy alone, although cure remains rare.

High-dose chemotherapy with autologous hematopoietic stem cell transplantation is not recommended for patients with SCLC because the substantial morbidity associated with this therapy negates any benefit. Local treatment consisting of surgery or radiation as single-modality therapies does not have the potential for cure. SCLC vaccination is not an effective therapy for SCLC.

KEY POINT

Chemotherapy and radiation therapy is considered the first-line treatment for patients with limited-stage small cell lung cancer.

Bibliography

Simon GR, Turrisi A; American College of Chest Physicians. Management of small cell lung cancer: ACCP evidence-based clinical practice guidelines (2nd edition). Chest. 2007;132(3 Suppl):324S-339S. [PMID: 17873178]

Item 14   Answer: B

Educational Objective: *Manage a rising PSA level with prostate biopsy.*

Prostate cancer is most often diagnosed following prostate-specific antigen (PSA) screening in asymptomatic men. Patients with an elevated or rising serum PSA level noted during routine screening should also undergo prostate biopsy, even if they are asymptomatic. Specifically, these patients need ultrasound-guided biopsies of their prostate (typically in 6 random areas) to assess for the presence of prostate cancer. After prostate cancer is diagnosed, additional studies such as a bone scan or CT scan of the abdomen and pelvis should be considered in patients with signs or symptoms suggestive of distant spread of the malignancy.

Pathologic proof of prostate cancer is needed before embarking on definitive therapy such as radical prostatectomy. A PSA greater than 4.0 ng/mL (4.0 µg/L) is only 25% sensitive for prostate cancer. In the absence of a histologic diagnosis for prostate cancer, surgical intervention is not appropriate.

Patients with "borderline" PSA measurements might be appropriately managed by repeating the measurement in 6 months; however, this patient has had a rapid rise in the PSA level. Any rise greater than 0.75 ng/mL/year (0.75 µg/L/year) is considered abnormal and should be evaluated.

KEY POINT

Patients with a prostate-specific antigen (PSA) level greater than 4.0 ng/dL (4.0 µg/L) should have further evaluation for prostate cancer.

Bibliography

Lin K, Lipsitz R, Miller T, Janakiraman S; U.S. Preventive Services Task Force. Benefits and harms of prostate-specific antigen screening for prostate cancer: an evidence update for the U.S. Preventive Services Task Force. Ann Intern Med. 2008;149(3):192-9. [PMID: 18678846]

Item 15   Answer: A

Educational Objective: *Manage prostate cancer screening by discussing risks and benefits.*

This 57-year-old asymptomatic man should participate in a discussion with his doctor about the risks and benefits of prostate cancer screening. The U.S. Preventive Services Task Force (USPSTF) concluded that the evidence was insufficient to recommend for or against prostate cancer screening using prostate-specific antigen (PSA) testing or digital rectal examination (DRE) and recommended that physicians discuss potential, but uncertain, benefits and possible harms (complications of future diagnostic testing and therapies, including incontinence; erectile dysfunction; and bowel dysfunction) before ordering PSA testing. The USPSTF also recommended against prostate cancer screening in men aged 75 years or older. They noted that if screening were to be performed, men ages 50 to 70 years would benefit most. The USPSTF stated that men should be informed of the gaps and conflicting results in the evidence and should be assisted in considering their personal preferences before deciding whether to be tested. The American Cancer Society recommends that PSA testing be offered to men at age 50 years (age 45 years for men at high risk owing to a positive family history of prostate cancer or who are black) and that information about limitations and benefits be provided.

Two large randomized screening trials studied the effect of screening on rate of death from prostate cancer. There was no difference in the rate of death from prostate cancer between screened and control groups in one study. In the second study, the prostate cancer death rate per 1000 person-years was 0.35 in the screened group versus 0.41 in the control group ($P =$ 0.04). The number needed to screen was 1410 and the number needed to treat to prevent one prostate cancer-related death over a 10-year period was 48. About 50% to 75% of those 48 men would be expected to have some complication of treatment. In evaluating the limited benefit demonstrated in this trial, one must consider the increased number of false diagnoses (false-positive rate of 75.9% of those undergoing biopsy) and unnecessary treatments.

KEY POINT

Physicians should discuss potential, but uncertain, benefits and possible harms before ordering prostate-specific antigen testing.

Bibliography
U.S. Preventive Services Task Force. Screening for prostate cancer: U.S. Preventive Services Task Force recommendation statement. Ann Intern Med. 2008;149(3):185-91. [PMID: 18678845]

Item 16   Answer: D
Educational Objective: *Manage an elderly patient with prostate cancer and medical comorbidities.*

The most appropriate next step in the management of this patient is observation. Although screening by prostate-specific antigen (PSA) measurement does result in detection of some cases of cancer, no definitive benefits resulting from such detection have been reported. In this older patient, observation or watchful waiting is the most appropriate management.

According to the U.S. Preventive Services Task Force (USPSTF), there is inadequate evidence to suggest that treatment of patients younger than 75 years with screening-detected prostate cancer results in improved outcomes compared with treatment of patients with clinically detected (symptomatic) prostate cancer. Adequate evidence indicates that the incremental benefits of treatment of patients 75 years of age or older with screening-detected prostate cancer are small to none. Moderate to substantial harms, including erectile dysfunction, urinary incontinence, bowel dysfunction, and death, in addition to small harms, including prostate biopsy-induced pain and discomfort and psychological effects of false-positive test results, are associated with prostate cancer screening. Because prostate cancer symptoms may not develop in many older patients who receive treatment for screening-detected prostate cancer during their lifetime, consideration of these harms is important.

In view of the recommendations from the USPSTF and the evidence supporting those recommendations, repeating the PSA, bone scan, and transrectal prostate biopsy are all inappropriate choices for this 80-year-old man with significant comorbidities.

KEY POINT
In men age 75 years or older there is little to no benefit associated with prostate cancer screening.

Bibliography
U.S. Preventive Services Task Force. Screening for prostate cancer: U.S. Preventive Services Task Force recommendation statement. Ann Intern Med. 2008;149(3):185-I91. [PMID:18678845]

Item 17   Answer: C
Educational Objective: *Treat asymptomatic metastatic prostate cancer with androgen deprivation therapy.*

The most appropriate management of this patient is androgen deprivation therapy with leuprolide. This patient has metastatic prostate cancer involving the bones. Prostate cancer is a hormone-responsive tumor, and his disease will most likely respond to hormone deprivation therapy with surgical castra-

tion or gonadotropin hormone–releasing hormone (GnRH) agonists such as leuprolide. GnRH therapy causes impotence, hot flushes, gynecomastia, and loss of libido, as does orchiectomy. Patients may experience tumor-flare reactions with the use of GnRH agonists, which initially cause an increase in luteinizing and follicle-stimulating hormones. These hormones lead to a transient increase in testosterone, which can exacerbate prostate cancer symptoms. This reaction can be prevented by a brief course of concomitant antiandrogen therapy with agents such as bicalutamide, nilutamide, or flutamide.

Although docetaxel-based chemotherapy has been shown to improve survival, this agent is generally indicated only for patients with hormone-refractory cancer. Several studies have demonstrated an improvement in overall survival with docetaxel-based chemotherapy in this setting.

Hospice care is premature because multiple sequential medical interventions are likely to improve this patient's overall and progression-free survival. Observation is inappropriate because his disease is likely to progress without any intervention.

Samarium-153 is a radionuclide that is taken up by bone. It may be useful in treating prostate cancer with painful bone metastases but may cause bone marrow suppression and should be used only in patients whose cancer is no longer responsive to other therapies.

KEY POINT
Androgen deprivation therapy with surgical castration or gonadotropin hormone–releasing hormone agonists is first-line therapy for asymptomatic patients with metastatic prostate cancer.

Bibliography
Ramirez ML, Keane TE, Evans CP. Managing prostate cancer: the role of hormone therapy. Can J Urol. 2007;14 Suppl 1:10-8. [PMID: 18163939]

Item 18   Answer: A
Educational Objective: *Manage an adult patient with an abnormal Pap smear and high-risk human papillomavirus serology with colposcopy.*

The most appropriate next management step is colposcopy. The most common abnormal finding following cervical cancer screening is atypical squamous cells (ASC), which is reported in approximately 5% of test results. Most ASC abnormalities resolve spontaneously, but approximately 15% of patients harbor a precancerous lesion discovered on biopsy. Adult women with ASC should be tested for human papillomavirus infection. If the patient with ASC tests positive for high-risk human papillomavirus subtypes (for example, 16 or 18), colposcopy with biopsy is performed. Colposcopy provides an illuminated, magnified view of the cervix, vagina, and vulva and enhances the ability of the operator to detect premalignant and malignant lesions that can biopsied.

In a patient with ASC and high-risk human papillomavirus infection, delaying investigation for the presence of possible premalignant or malignant lesions for 1 year is excessively long and inappropriate. There is no effective treatment for cervical human papillomavirus infection, including interferon.

KEY POINT

Colposcopy with biopsy is indicated for patients with atypical squamous cells on cervical cytologic screening and who test positive for high-risk human papillomavirus subtypes.

Bibliography

Apgar BS, Kittendorf AL, Bettcher CM, Wong J, Kaufman AJ. Update on ASCCP consensus guidelines for abnormal cervical screening tests and cervical histology. Am Fam Physician. 2009;80(2):147-55. [PMID: 19621855]

Item 19   Answer: D
Educational Objective: *Prevent human papillomavirus infection with human papillomavirus immunization.*

The Advisory Committee on Immunization Practices of the Centers for Disease Control and Prevention recommends the quadrivalent human papillomavirus (HPV) vaccine for cervical cancer prevention for all girls and women between the ages of 9 and 26 years regardless of sexual activity. The vaccine has a high success rate in preventing infections with HPV strains 6, 11, 16, and 18, which cause most cases of genital warts and cervical cancer.

HPV infection is predominantly spread by sexual contact. This patient states she is not sexually active; however, the vaccine should be recommended now because it is of low risk, and vaccine efficacy lasts for at least several years. The vaccine does not protect against all types of HPV, and roughly 30% of cervical cancers will not be prevented by the vaccine; therefore, women should continue to receive regular Pap smears even after completing the vaccination series.

The HPV quadrivalent vaccine is not effective in preventing HPV-related diseases in women who have an established infection at the time of vaccination; therefore, waiting for HPV seroconversion prior to vaccination is inappropriate.

Although the HPV vaccine is well tolerated in men, and high rates of seroconversion against pathologic HPV have been demonstrated, efficacy of male vaccination in preventing clinical disease in men and women remains uncertain, and cost-effectiveness is unproved. The Centers for Disease Control and Prevention does not recommend routine HPV immunization for boys.

KEY POINT

A human papillomavirus quadrivalent vaccination series should be offered to all girls and women ages 9 through 26 years, and women should continue to get regular Pap smears even after completing the vaccination series.

Bibliography

Barr E, Sings HL. Prophylactic HPV vaccines: new interventions for cancer control. Vaccine. 2008;26:6244-57. Epub 2008 Aug 9. [PMID: 18694795]

Item 20   Answer: C
Educational Objective: *Screen for cervical cancer every 3 years in low-risk women.*

This patient is at low risk for cervical cancer. She is in a long-term, monogamous relationship and has had many normal Pap smears, so it is appropriate to lengthen the screening interval for Pap tests to every 3 years. The United States Preventive Services Task Force recommends cervical cancer screening for women who are sexually active and have a cervix. Screening should begin within 3 years of onset of sexual activity but no later than age 21 years. After age 65 years, the effectiveness of screening is low in women who have had recent negative Pap smears. Women at normal risk can be screened every 3 years, although the American Cancer Society recommends waiting until age 30 years before lengthening the screening interval from an annual basis. Annual Pap tests do not identify more invasive cancer than tests performed every 2 or 3 years in low-risk women who have had several normal tests.

Women who have human immunodeficiency virus infection should be screened for cervical cancer more frequently, because human papillomavirus can grow faster and lesions can progress more quickly in significantly immunosuppressed patients. Women who have multiple sex partners, have a history of abnormal Pap smears, or have recently been diagnosed with a sexually transmitted disease are at higher risk for cervical cancer, and current guidelines suggest screening such women annually.

KEY POINT

In women older than 30 years with three previous normal annual Pap smears, the screening interval can be lengthened to every 3 years.

Bibliography

Safaeian M, Solomon D, Castle PE. Cervical cancer prevention—cervical screening: science in evolution. Obstet Gynecol Clin North Am. 2007;34:739-60, ix. [PMID: 18061867]

Item 21   Answer: D
Educational Objective: *Discontinue screening for cervical cancer in patients who have had a hysterectomy for benign disease.*

In asymptomatic women who have had a vaginal hysterectomy for benign disease, there is no proven benefit to routine Pap testing to detect cancer. The United States Preventive Service Task Force recommends cervical cancer screening only for women who are sexually active and have a cervix. Vaginal hysterectomy for benign disease is not associated with an increased incidence of vaginal malignancy. Estimates of the positive predictive value of an abnormal vaginal smear in this setting approach zero.

KEY POINT

In asymptomatic women who have had a vaginal hysterectomy for benign disease, there is no proven benefit to routine Pap testing to detect cancer.

Bibliography

Stokes-Lampard H, Wilson S, Waddell C, Ryan A, Holder R, Kehoe S. Vaginal vault smears after hysterectomy for reasons other than malignancy: a systematic review of the literature. BJOG. 2006;113:1354-65. [PMID: 17081187]

Item 22   Answer: C
Educational Objective: *Diagnose squamous cell carcinoma in situ (Bowen disease).*

This lesion is most consistent with squamous cell carcinoma in situ (Bowen disease). It is a form of intraepidermal carcinoma, a malignant tumor of keratinocytes. It presents as a single lesion in two thirds of cases. The head, neck, and extremities are the most commonly affected sites in men. The cheeks and lower extremities are the most commonly affected sites in women. Lesions vary from a few millimeters to several centimeters in diameter. Lesions can arise de novo or from a pre-existing actinic keratosis. Etiology is most likely multifactorial and includes chronic ultraviolet radiation, arsenic exposure, human papillomavirus, immunosuppression, genetic factors, trauma, x-ray radiation, and chemical carcinogens.

Nummular eczema presents as circular, erythematous, well-demarcated, intensely pruritic, patches 2 to 10 cm in diameter, usually found on the trunk and lower extremities. Onset is usually spontaneous with no inciting event.

Psoriasis is a chronic skin condition that usually presents in young adults. Lesions are characterized as 1 to 10 cm in diameter erythematous papules and plaques with silver scales, having sharply defined margins raised above the normal surrounding skin. These plaques are symmetrically distributed and usually involve the scalp, extensor elbows, knees, and back.

Superficial basal cell carcinoma is recognized as a solitary, well-defined, pink, pearly translucent, dome-shaped papule with telangiectasias. With time, the center may umbilicate and ulcerate to produce the characteristic rolled borders. Eighty percent of these occur on the head and neck.

Superficial spreading melanoma presents as a variably pigmented plaque with an irregular border, ranging from a few to several centimeters. It is not scaly. It can occur anywhere, but is commonly seen on the back in men and the legs in women.

KEY POINT

Bowen disease is recognized as a gradually enlarging, well-demarcated, erythematous scaly plaque that can resemble superficial basal cell carcinoma, psoriasis, or eczema.

Bibliography

Madan V, Lear JT, Szeimies RM. Non-melanoma skin cancer. Lancet. 2010;375(9715):673-85. [PMID: 20171403]

Item 23   Answer: C
Educational Objective: *Diagnose nodular melanoma.*

The most likely diagnosis is nodular melanoma. Nodular melanoma often presents as uniformly dark blue or black "berry-like" lesions that most commonly originate from normal skin. It is most often found in people aged 60 years or older. Nodular melanomas often do not fulfill the ABCDE (*a*symmetry, irregular *b*orders, *c*olor variegation, expanding *d*iameter, *e*volution over time) criteria for melanoma and tend to expand vertically rather than horizontally. Nodular melanomas are mostly symmetric, elevated, and one color.

Basal cell carcinoma presents classically as a solitary, well-defined, pink, pearly translucent, dome-shaped papule with telangiectasias. With time, the center may umbilicate and ulcerate to produce the characteristic rolled borders. Eighty percent of these occur on the head and neck.

Keratocanthoma is a rapidly growing skin cancer thought to be a form of squamous cell cancer. Early lesions present as solitary, round nodules that grow rapidly. As the lesions mature, a central keratotic plug becomes visible and the lesion becomes crater-like. It rarely progresses to invasive or metastatic cancer and often involutes within months.

Seborrheic keratosis is a benign common epidermal tumor, usually tan, brown, or black in color with discrete borders most commonly found on the trunk, face, and upper extremities. It is elevated from the surface of the skin and has a "stuck-on" warty or waxy appearance. It is most commonly found in persons older than 50 years. The number of lesions can vary from one to hundreds in a person.

Spitz nevus is a clinically benign mole usually found in children or young adults that presents as a dome-shaped uniformly pink, red, or pigmented nodule. Its surface can be smooth or verrucous and is most commonly found on the face and lower extremities. It can have histopathologic features that overlap with those of melanoma.

KEY POINT

Nodular melanomas often present as uniformly dark blue or black "berry-like" lesions that are mostly symmetric, elevated, and one color.

Bibliography

Chamberlain AJ, Fritschi L, Kelly JW. Nodular melanoma: patients' perceptions of presenting features and implications for earlier detection. J Am Acad Dermatol. 2003:48(5):694-701. [PMID: 12734497]

Item 24   Answer: A
Educational Objective: *Diagnose actinic keratoses.*

This patient has actinic keratoses, common lesions that occur on sun-exposed skin of older white-skinned persons. Actinic keratoses are believed to be the earliest clinically recognized step in a biologic continuum that may result in invasive squamous cell carcinoma. Actinic keratoses are 1- to 3-mm, elevated, flesh-colored or red papules, surrounded by a whitish scale. They are often easier to feel as "rough spots" on the skin than they are to see. Most patients will have, on average, 6 to 8 lesions. Most remain stable and some regress, but others enlarge to become invasive squamous cell carcinomas. The appearance of the patient's lesion is not consistent with basal cell carcinoma, melanoma, or seborrheic keratosis.

A basal cell carcinoma classically presents as a pink, pearly or translucent, dome-shaped papule with telangiectasias. The papule may have central umbilication.

A melanoma is classically a pigmented macule or plaque that is asymmetric and has irregular, scalloped, notched, or indistinct borders. It is black or dark brown or has variegated (multiple) coloration, including shades of black, red, and blue. Melanomas may also have depigmented or white areas, which represent regression of the lesion. Rarely, melanomas are not pigmented and can resemble basal cell carcinomas.

Seborrheic keratoses can be brown or black but have discrete borders, are elevated above the surface of the skin, and have a "stuck-on" warty or waxy appearance.

KEY POINT

Actinic keratoses are precancerous lesions that can develop into invasive squamous cell carcinoma and that typically appear as erythematous lesions with overlying hyperkeratosis.

Bibliography
Schwartz RA, Bridges TM, Butani AK, Ehrlich A. Actinic keratosis: an occupational and environmental disorder. J Eur Acad Dermatol Venereol. 2008;22(5):606-615. [PMID:18410618]

Item 25   Answer: A
Educational Objective: *Diagnose basal cell carcinoma.*

The most likely diagnosis is basal cell carcinoma. Basal cell carcinoma (BCC) typically presents as a pearly, pink papule or nodule with telangiectatic vessels. As BCC grows, the central area often ulcerates, resulting in its characteristic rolled edge. Flecks of melanin pigment are commonly present. A biopsy is necessary, as amelanotic melanoma may have a similar appearance. Common biopsy techniques include shave or punch. Most nodular BCCs are treated with excision, whereas ill-defined lesions, high-risk histologic types, and tumors on the face and hands are treated with Mohs micrographic surgery. Selected superficial lesions can be treated with curettage, imiquimod, cryotherapy, or excision.

Pyogenic granulomas are typically bright red and friable, are commonly crusted, and develop over a few days to weeks. Removal is necessary only if the lesion is cosmetically unacceptable, painful, causes unwanted bleeding, or is otherwise bothersome.

Seborrheic keratosis is a painless, nonmalignant growth appearing as a waxy brownish patch or plaque. Seborrheic keratoses lack a pearly appearance and typically exhibit horn cysts (epidermal cysts filled with keratin) on the surface that can best be visualized with a magnifying lens. Treatment is necessary only if lesions are symptomatic or interfere with function.

Squamous cell carcinomas are rapidly growing, hyperkeratotic, flesh-colored, pink or red ulcerated macules, papules, or nodules that commonly appear on the scalp, neck, and pinnae. A shave or punch biopsy is used to confirm the diagnosis of suspicious lesions.

KEY POINT

Basal cell carcinomas present as pink, pearly nodules with telangiectases and, commonly, flecks of melanin pigment.

Bibliography
Mogensen M, Jemec GB. Diagnosis of nonmelanoma skin cancer/keratinocyte carcinoma: a review of diagnostic accuracy of nonmelanoma skin cancer diagnostic tests and technologies. Dermatol Surg. 2007;33(10):1158-1174. [PMID:17903149]

Item 26   Answer: C
Educational Objective: *Diagnose keratoacanthoma.*

The most likely diagnosis is keratoacanthoma. Keratoacanthoma is an epithelial neoplasm that is characterized by rapid growth over 2 to 6 weeks and by a crater-like configuration. Early lesions are frequently misdiagnosed as skin infections. The typical early lesion is a hard, erythematous nodule with a keratotic (horny) center. Keratoacanthomas typically occur on heavily sun-damaged skin, usually in older persons, with a peak age of 60 years. As the lesion enlarges, the center of the crater becomes more prominent. Unlike typical squamous cell carcinomas, keratoacanthomas are capable of spontaneous resolution by terminal differentiation, in which the tumor "keratinizes itself to death." The clinical presentation and characteristic histologic features establish the diagnosis.

Because keratoacanthomas may cause significant local tissue destruction, simple observation is generally not recommended despite the tendency for spontaneous involution. Prompt surgical excision is recommended for solitary lesions on the trunk or extremities. Intralesional 5-fluorouracil or methotrexate, topical imiquimod, and radiation therapy have also been used to treat large lesions or those in areas where surgical excision would be anatomically difficult.

An abscess is warm, red, and tender and may be fluctuant if palpated. This is not consistent with the patient's findings.

Keloids present as slow-growing, hard nodules, often with a dumbbell shape. They occur at sites of prior trauma.

Nodular basal cell carcinoma is often found on the face and is characterized by slow growth and the presence of a skin-toned to pink, pearly, translucent papule with telangiectasia, rolled borders, and central depression, often with ulceration. The rapid growth and appearance of the patient's lesion is not consistent with nodular basal cell carcinoma.

KEY POINT

Keratoacanthomas are rapidly growing, nontender, firm nodules with depressed keratotic centers.

Bibliography

Sarabi K, Selim A, Khachemoune A. Sporadic and syndromic keratoacanthomas: diagnosis and management. Dermatol Nurs. 2007;19(2):166-170. [PMID:17526304]

Item 27   Answer: C

Educational Objective: *Use short-acting opioid medications for mild to moderate cancer-related pain.*

The most appropriate next therapeutic step is to add a short-acting opioid. The pain in patients with advanced malignancy often outpaces the ability of non-narcotic analgesics to control the pain. In patients with cancer who have mild to moderate pain such as this one, an effective strategy is moving to step 2 on the World Health Organization three-step pain relief ladder by prescribing an intermittent low-dose narcotic in addition to adjuvant, non-narcotic pain medicine. Appropriate choices include immediate-release formulations of oxycodone, morphine, or oxymorphone.

Initiating a long-acting narcotic such as a fentanyl transdermal patch or extended-release oxycodone would not be indicated until the patient's pain is adequately controlled with short-acting narcotics, which can be rapidly titrated to achieve adequate pain control. Once pain control is established, the cumulative dose of the short-acting opioid can be used to calculate an effective dose of a long-acting opioid, with the dose reduced by 30% to 50% and access to a short-acting opioid maintained for break-through pain. If the short-acting opioid is needed more than three times daily, the amount of long-acting opioid is increased.

Changing to a different NSAID is much less likely to control this patient's pain than is adding a short-acting opioid analgesic.

KEY POINT

For mild to moderate cancer-associated pain, a short-acting opioid is indicated when non-opioid drugs fail to adequately control pain.

Bibliography

Bruera E, Kim HN. Cancer Pain. JAMA. 2003;290(18):2476-2479. [PMID:14612485]

Item 28   Answer: D

Educational Objective: *Use sustained-release morphine to treat moderate to severe cancer-related pain.*

The most appropriate pain management strategy for this patient is switching to sustained-release morphine. Pain control is a common management issue in terminally ill patients. The use of as-needed doses of opioid analgesics combined with non-opioid adjunctive therapy is an effective management strategy for mild to moderate cancer pain. When this strategy no longer suffices, however, additional pain relief must be given. This patient has discomfort from pain that returns before he is scheduled to take his next dose of analgesic therapy, and he is taking the medication on a continual basis. This patient would benefit most from the addition of a longer-acting narcotic to treat his pain. An appropriate solution would be to give him sustained-release morphine twice daily. A breakthrough pain strategy should be continued so the patient has options if the longer-acting pain medication does not provide complete relief. When adding a long-acting opioid, a strategy to avoid overmedication is to give a starting dose of 30% to 50% of the patient's average 24-hour dosage of narcotic. The dose of the opioid for breakthrough pain is calculated as 10% of the total daily opioid dose given as an immediate-release opioid.

Gabapentin can be useful in treating neuropathic pain but would likely not be useful for reducing pain from bony metastases. Increasing the frequency of the immediate-release medication is not the best answer because of the patient's need to re-dose frequently owing to multiple recurrent bouts of pain. The goal of palliative therapy for pain is to relieve the patient of significant pain for most of the day, which will result in the infrequent need for additional doses of immediate-release pain medication. Switching the medication from one immediate-release formulation to another is also unlikely to make the patient more comfortable.

KEY POINT

Long-acting narcotics are useful in pain control for patients with recurrent pain while on short-acting, as-needed narcotic therapy.

Bibliography

Bruera E, Kim HN. Cancer Pain. JAMA. 2003;290(18):2476-2479. [PMID:14612485]

Item 29   Answer: B

Educational Objective: *Treat cancer pain with long-acting and immediate-release morphine sulfate.*

Because of the severity of this patient's pain, long-acting morphine sulfate (or other strong opioids such as hydromorphone or fentanyl) and immediate-acting morphine sulfate for breakthrough pain is the therapy of choice. The transition from parenteral to oral morphine is straightforward: 10 mg of intravenous morphine is equivalent to 30 mg of oral morphine. In this case, the patient's total daily dose of morphine sulfate should be calculated (including total doses of bolus and continuous infusion) and is multiplied by 3 to obtain the equivalent oral dose. Because long-acting morphine is dosed every 12 hours, half of the calculated oral dose is given twice daily. Ten percent of the total oral dose is made available as immediate-acting morphine to use as needed for breakthrough pain (the "rescue dose"). If the immediate-acting opioid is needed more than three times per day, the dose of long-acting opioid can be increased.

Hydrocodone is a weak opiate and is not indicated in the treatment of severe pain. Furthermore, hydrocodone has proven ineffective for this patient in the past. Although long-acting morphine sulfate and oxycodone as needed may provide adequate pain relief, it is appropriate to use the same drug whenever possible for both breakthrough and basal dosing in order to simplify future dose titrations as well as minimize drug-related side effects. In addition, in treating severe pain, analgesics provided on an as-needed basis are less effective than regularly dosed, long-acting opioids supplemented with immediate-acting agents for breakthrough pain.

KEY POINT

Moderate to severe pain requires treatment with a strong opioid analgesic, usually in both long-acting and immediate-acting formulations.

Bibliography

Jost L, Roila F; ESMO Guidelines Working Group. Management of cancer pain: ESMO clinical recommendations. Ann Oncol. 2009;20 Suppl 4:170-3. [PMID: 19454446]

Item 30   Answer: A

Educational Objective: *Treat dyspnea in a palliative care setting with an opioid.*

The home hospice nurse of this patient should be advised to administer the immediate-release morphine to treat the dyspnea. In terminally ill patients with malignancy or cardiopulmonary disease, narcotics can be an effective treatment for dyspnea. In a randomized trial that evaluated narcotics for dyspnea in patients already on these medications for pain, the intensity of dyspnea and the respiration rate improved with administration of a supplemental dose of opioid. In a study of patients with cancer who were not oxygen dependent, cautious titration of parenteral opioids was not associated with respiratory depression. Similar studies have not been performed with oral agents.

An emergency department visit would be unlikely to provide long-term improvements in comfort or prognosis and would be generally inappropriate for a hospice patient.

The results of the patient's physical examination are consistent with a right pleural effusion, which could be a sign of heart failure. However, the patient has no other signs suggestive of heart failure, and a diuretic such as furosemide is therefore not indicated.

Although supplemental oxygen is often used in the palliative care setting to relieve dyspnea in nonhypoxemic patients with malignancy, this approach is not effective. A meta-analysis demonstrated no improvement in patients' perception of dyspnea at activity or at rest after receiving 4 to 10 L/min of oxygen.

KEY POINT

Morphine is effective in treating cancer-related dyspnea as well as dyspnea related to end-stage cardiopulmonary disorders.

Bibliography

Estfan B, Mahmoud F, Shaheen P, et al. Respiratory function during parenteral opioid titration for cancer pain. Palliat Med. 2007;21(2):81-86. [PMID:17344255]

Section 10

Pulmonary Medicine
Questions

Item 1 [Basic]

A 60-year-old man is evaluated for progressive exertional dyspnea. For the past year, he has been unable to walk three blocks without stopping twice because of shortness of breath. He has a daily cough productive of a small amount of white sputum. He has smoked 1 pack per day since the age of 20 years.

On physical examination, he is comfortable at rest. Vital signs are normal. Oxygen saturation by pulse oximetry is 90% on ambient air. Estimated central venous pressure is normal and no murmurs or extra cardiac sounds are heard. His lung examination reveals decreased air movement without wheezes or crackles. The remainder of the examination is normal.

Chest x-ray shows increased radiolucency and low-lying diaphragms.

Pulmonary function studies following administration of a bronchodilator:

FEV_1	65% of predicted
FVC	75% of predicted
FEV_1/FVC ratio	0.60
Total lung capacity (TLC)	105% of predicted
Diffusing capacity of lung for carbon dioxide (D_{LCO})	44% of predicted

Which of the following is the most likely diagnosis?

(A) Asthma
(B) Chronic obstructive pulmonary disease
(C) Heart failure
(D) Interstitial lung disease

Item 2 [Basic]

A 25-year-old woman is evaluated for a 3-month history of progressive breathlessness and decreased exercise capacity. She reports no recent illness, fever, cough, or previous history of breathing problems. She has a 1-year history of pain and stiffness in the joints of her hands and wrists.

On physical examination, her vital signs are normal. She has a normal cardiopulmonary examination. She has active synovitis involving her wrists and second and third metacarpophalangeal joints bilaterally.

The chest x-ray is normal.

Pulmonary function studies following administration of a bronchodilator:

FEV_1	60% of predicted
FVC	63% of predicted
FEV_1/FVC ratio	0.85
Total lung capacity(TLC)	65% of predicted
Diffusing capacity of lung for carbon dioxide (D_{LCO})	45% of predicted

Which of the following is the most likely diagnosis in this patient?

(A) Chronic obstructive lung disease
(B) Asthma
(C) Pulmonary embolism
(D) Interstitial lung disease

Item 3 [Basic]

A 56-year-old woman is evaluated for a 2 year history of episodic cough and chest tightness. Her symptoms began after a severe respiratory tract infection. Since then, she has had cough and chest discomfort after similar infections, typically lasting several weeks before resolving. She feels well between episodes. She is otherwise healthy and takes no medications. Physical examination reveals no abnormalities. Chest radiograph and spirometry are normal.

Which of the following is the most appropriate next diagnostic test?

(A) Bronchoscopy
(B) CT scan of the sinuses
(C) Exercise echocardiography
(D) Methacholine challenge test

Item 4 [Advanced]

A 60-year-old man is hospitalized because of progressive dyspnea during the past month. He has a 45-pack-year smoking history, but he has no other medical problems.

On physical examination, he is cyanotic and has paradoxical respiratory movements of his rib cage and abdomen. Blood pressure is 140/78 mm Hg, pulse rate is 105/min, and respiration rate is 28/min. Jugular venous distention is present. The lungs are clear. The remainder of the examination is normal.

Pulmonary function studies:

Total lung capacity	85% of predicted
Residual volume	72% of predicted
FVC	60% of predicted
FEV_1	63% of predicted
FEV_1/FVC ratio	105%
Residual volume/total lung capacity	163%
Maximum inspiratory pressure	36% of predicted
Maximum expiratory pressure	45% of predicted
D_{LCO}	82% of predicted

Arterial blood gases studies show a pH of 7.3, a PO_2 of 42 mm Hg (5.6 kPa), a PCO_2 of 55 mm Hg (7.3 kPa), and a bicarbonate level of 27 meq/L (27 mmol/L).

Which of the following is the most likely cause of his respiratory failure?

(A) Chronic obstructive pulmonary disease
(B) Idiopathic pulmonary fibrosis
(C) Neuromuscular weakness
(D) Pulmonary arterial hypertension

Item 5 [Advanced]

A 63-year-old man is evaluated for a 1-year history of dyspnea that has gradually worsened during the past 6 months. He has dyspnea at rest, but has no orthopnea. The patient reports his breathing is better when lying flat and is worse when sitting upright. He previously abused alcohol and intravenous drugs. Medical history is significant for cirrhosis and portal hypertension.

On physical examination, the patient is afebrile. Blood pressure is 110/68 mm Hg, pulse rate is 80/min, and respiration rate is 24/min. Oxygen saturation by pulse oximetry is 85% on ambient air. The cardiac examination is normal. Lungs are clear. Ascites is present as are clubbing, peripheral cyanosis, and spider nevi. Lower extremities show 1+ pitting edema.

The chest x-ray is normal.

Which of the following is the most likely cause of this patient's dyspnea?

(A) Bronchogenic carcinoma
(B) Constrictive pericarditis
(C) Emphysema
(D) Hepatopulmonary syndrome

Item 6 [Basic]

A 60-year-old woman is evaluated for an 18–month history of progressive dyspnea on exertion and a 3–month history of orthopnea. She is otherwise well and takes no medications.

On examination, she is afebrile, blood pressure is 110/85 mm Hg, pulse rate is 100/min, and respiration rate is 24/min. The carotid upstroke is diminished and delayed compared with the apical pulsation. Cardiac examination shows a sustained cardiac apex impulse, grade 3/6 late-peaking systolic ejection murmur at the right upper sternal border radiating to the carotid arteries, and an S_4. Lungs are clear to auscultation. The remainder of the examination is normal.

Which of the following is the most likely diagnosis?

(A) Aortic stenosis
(B) Atrial septal defect
(C) Pulmonary arterial hypertension
(D) Pulmonary valvular stenosis

Item 7 [Basic]

A previously healthy 30-year-old man who is a lifelong non-smoker is evaluated in the emergency department for sudden onset of right-sided chest pain and shortness of breath.

On physical examination, vital signs are normal. There are decreased breath sounds over the posterior right thorax. The cardiac examination is normal.

A chest radiograph is obtained and is shown.

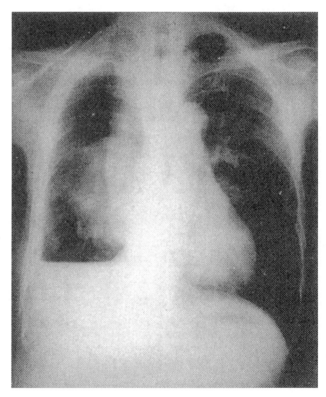

Which of the following is the most likely diagnosis?

(A) Heart failure
(B) Hydropneumothorax
(C) Pneumonia
(D) Pulmonary embolism

Item 8 [Advanced]

A 20-year-old woman is evaluated in the emergency department for an acute episode of wheezing and dyspnea without cough or sputum production. She has had frequent evaluations in emergency departments for similar episodes. In between these episodes, findings on physical examination and pulmonary function testing, including methacholine challenge, have been normal. She is otherwise healthy and takes no medications.

On physical examination, the patient has inspiratory and expiratory wheezing and is in moderate discomfort. The temperature is 37.1°C (98.8°F), pulse rate is 100/min, and respiration rate is 24/min; oxygen saturation on ambient air is 96%. After receiving albuterol and intravenous corticosteroids, she continues to wheeze and is in moderate respiratory distress. Oxygen saturation on ambient air remains at 96%. Chest radiograph shows decreased lung volumes.

Which of the following is the most appropriate management for this patient?

(A) Chest CT scan
(B) Intravenous aminophylline
(C) Intravenous azithromycin
(D) Laryngoscopy

Item 9 [Advanced]

A 60-year-old woman is evaluated for a 4-month history of progressive fatigue and dyspnea on exertion. She does not smoke cigarettes and denies chest pain, palpitations, dizziness, or syncope. She has a 12-year history of limited cutaneous systemic sclerosis. A screening cardiopulmonary evaluation 3 years ago was normal. She also has gastroesophageal reflux disease and Raynaud phenomenon. She intermittently develops ulcers on the fingertips. Current medications are amlodipine, omeprazole, and nitroglycerin ointment.

On physical examination, temperature is 37.0°F (98.6°F), blood pressure is 120/80 mm Hg, pulse rate is 84/min, and respiration rate is 16/min. Cardiac examination reveals a loud pulmonic component of S_2 with fixed splitting and a 2/6 early systolic murmur at the lower left sternal border that increases with inspiration. The lungs are clear to auscultation. The abdominal examination is unremarkable. Sclerodactyly is present, and pitting scars are visible over several fingertips. There is no peripheral edema.

Complete blood count and erythrocyte sedimentation rate are normal. Electrocardiogram shows evidence of right ventricular hypertrophy. Chest radiograph shows no infiltrates.

Pulmonary function studies:

FVC	84% of predicted
FEV_1/FVC	80%
DLCO	44% of predicted

Which of the following is the most likely diagnosis?

(A) Chronic obstructive pulmonary disease
(B) Interstitial lung disease
(C) Left ventricular failure
(D) Pulmonary arterial hypertension

Item 10 [Advanced]

A 55-year-old man is found to have a pleural effusion after a 2-week history of cough, sputum production, dyspnea, chills, and pleuritic chest pain. Upright and lateral decubitus chest x-rays confirm that the effusion is free flowing (without evidence of loculation). He has otherwise been in good health and takes no medications.

A thoracentesis is performed and 1.2 L of fluid is removed. Analysis of the pleural fluid is performed.

Leukocytes	3000/μL (3×10^9/L) with 82% neutrophils
Glucose	25 mg/dL (1.4 mmol/L)
Lactate dehydrogenase	2500 U/L
pH	6.95

Gram stain and culture are pending. Blood cultures are obtained. Empiric broad-spectrum antibiotics are begun.

Which of the following is the most appropriate next step in the management of this patient?

(A) Chest CT
(B) Chest tube drainage of the effusion
(C) Video-assisted thorascopic surgery (VATS)
(D) No additional treatment

Item 11 [Basic]

A 24-year-old man is evaluated in the emergency department for a 10-day history of increasing shortness of breath and dry cough. Before this time, the patient was healthy and took no medications.

On physical examination, temperature is 37.9°C (100.3°F), blood pressure is 105/70 mm Hg, pulse is 106/min, and respirations are 32/min. A lung examination reveals dullness to percussion, decreased tactile fremitus, and decreased breath sounds at the right base. The remainder of his physical examination is unremarkable.

Which of the following is the most likely diagnosis?

(A) Heart failure
(B) Lobar consolidation
(C) Pleural effusion
(D) Pneumothorax

Item 12 [Advanced]

A 30-year-old medical resident is evaluated for cough, right-sided chest pain, and fever of 3 weeks' duration. He has no significant medical history, and he takes no medications.

Hemoglobin is 14 g/dL (140 g/L), and the leukocyte count is 8000/μL (8.0×10^9/L). Chest radiograph shows a right pleural effusion occupying approximately 50% of the hemithorax without other abnormalities. Thoracentesis yields turbid, yellow fluid, and analysis shows the following:

Erythrocyte count	500/μL (500 x 10^6/L)
Nucleated cell count	3500/μL (3.5×10^9/L) with 20% neutrophils, 60% lymphocytes, 10% macrophages, 4% mesothelial cells, and 6% eosinophils
Total protein	4.2 g/dL (42 g/L)
Lactate dehydrogenase	240 U/L
pH	7.35
Glucose	68 mg/dL (3.8 mmol/L)

Serum total protein is 7.0 g/dL (70 g/L) and serum lactate dehydrogenase is 100 U/L. Gram stain shows no organisms and culture is pending.

Which of the following is the most appropriate next step in management?

(A) Azithromycin for 5 days
(B) Chest CT scan
(C) Flexible bronchoscopy
(D) Pleural biopsy

Item 13 [Advanced]

A 40-year-old man is evaluated for shortness of breath and left-sided chest discomfort without cough, fever, or hemoptysis. The patient has a history of lymphoma that is now in remission.

Examination of the chest shows dullness to percussion and decreased breath sounds on the left side. Chest radiograph shows a moderate-sized, left-sided pleural effusion without a pneumothorax. Serum protein is 5.8 g/dL (58 g/L), cholesterol is 200 mg/dL (5.2 mmol/L), and triglycerides are 100 mg/dL (1.1 mmol/L). Thoracentesis yields 500 mL of milky-appearing pleural fluid, and analysis shows the following:

Cell count	Erythrocytes 300/µL (300 × 106/L); leukocytes 890/µL (890 × 10⁹/L) with 65% lymphocytes, 22% neutrophils, 8% mesothelial cells, and 4% eosinophils
Total protein	3.5 g/dL (35 g/L)
Lactate dehydrogenase	250 U/L
pH	7.50
Amylase	25 U/L
Triglycerides	145 mg/dL (1.6 mmol/L)
Cholesterol	38 mg/dL (1.0 mmol/L)

Cytology, Gram stain, acid-fast bacilli stain, and bacterial culture are negative.

Which of the following is the most likely diagnosis?

(A) Chylothorax
(B) Heart failure
(C) Parapneumonic effusion
(D) Tuberculous pleural effusion

Item 14 [Advanced]

A 33-year-old woman is evaluated in the emergency department for a 6-hour history of worsening asthma symptoms. Her medications include albuterol and an inhaled corticosteroid. She is treated with intravenous corticosteroids and albuterol. After 4 hours of treatment, she remains symptomatic and can speak only one to two words between breaths.

On physical examination, she appears uncomfortable and tired. Temperature is 36.8°C (98.2°F), blood pressure is 150/90 mm Hg, heart rate is 124/min, and respiration rate is 32/min. Oxygen saturation by pulse oximetry is 92% with oxygen 2 L/min by nasal cannula. Lung examination reveals poor air movement and diffuse expiratory wheezes.

Results of arterial blood gas studies: pH, 7.2; PCO_2, 45 mm Hg (6.0 kPa); PO_2, 70 mm Hg (9.3 kPa). Peak flow is 30% of best performance.

Which of the following the most appropriate management for this patient?

(A) Admission to the hospital ward
(B) Intubation and mechanical ventilation
(C) Continued therapy in the emergency department
(D) Discharge home

Item 15 [Basic]

A 40-year-old woman is evaluated for worsening asthma symptoms after resolution of an acute respiratory tract infection that was treated with supportive measures. The patient has a 15-year history of asthma that has been well controlled on moderate-dose inhaled corticosteroids plus as-needed inhaled albuterol. Since her respiratory tract infection 10 days ago, her asthma symptoms have worsened; she has had frequent nighttime episodes of wheezing and has used her albuterol inhaler six to eight times a day.

On physical examination, the patient is afebrile and has no chest pain or significant sputum production. Her peak flow is more than 40% below her baseline value.

Which of the following is the most appropriate management for this patient?

(A) 7-Day course of a fluoroquinolone
(B) Leukotriene-modifying agent
(C) Long-acting β-agonist
(D) Nebulized albuterol at home
(E) Short course of an oral corticosteroid

Item 16 [Basic]

A 24-year-old woman with persistent asthma, which is well controlled on low-dose fluticasone and albuterol as needed, became pregnant 2 months ago and asks for advice about asthma therapy during her pregnancy. Before she started fluticasone therapy, she had frequent asthma symptoms and occasional exacerbations requiring emergency department treatment. Since she became pregnant, her asthma has remained under good control. The physical examination is unremarkable, and spirometry is normal.

Which of the following is the most appropriate management for this patient?

(A) Continue the current regimen
(B) Stop fluticasone; add inhaled cromolyn
(C) Stop fluticasone; add salmeterol
(D) Stop fluticasone; add theophylline

Item 17 [Basic]

A 75-year-old woman with long-standing asthma is evaluated for a 1-month history of nocturnal asthma symptoms at least weekly and the need to use an albuterol inhaler daily. Her asthma therapy is a moderate-dose inhaled corticosteroid. The patient is otherwise healthy.

On physical examination, she has occasional wheezing, but the rest of the examination is unremarkable. On office spirometry, the FEV_1 is 70% of predicted and FVC is 85% of predicted.

Which of the following is the most appropriate management?

(A) Adding a leukotriene-modifying agent
(B) Adding a long-acting anticholinergic agent
(C) Adding a long-acting β-agonist
(D) Adding theophylline
(E) Doubling the corticosteroid dose

Item 18 [Advanced]

A 37-year-old man with asthma is evaluated for frequent episodes of wheezing and dyspnea unrelieved by short-acting β-agonist therapy. He uses his controller medications regularly, including an inhaled long-acting β-agonist and inhaled high-dose corticosteroids. He has symptoms daily and frequent nocturnal symptoms.

On physical examination, the patient is in mild respiratory distress. The temperature is 37.0°C (98.6°F), blood pressure is 140/85 mm Hg, pulse rate is 90/min, and respiration rate is 18/min. He has bilateral wheezing. Spirometry shows an FEV_1 of 65% of predicted. After the supervised use of a bronchodilator in the office, there was relief of symptoms, and repeat spirometry 10 minutes after the administration of the bronchodilator showed that the FEV_1 increased to 85% of predicted.

Which of the following is the most appropriate next step in this patient's management?

(A) Add a leukotriene-modifying drug
(B) Have the patient demonstrate his inhaler technique
(C) Have the patient keep a symptom and treatment log
(D) Start oral prednisone therapy

Item 19 [Advanced]

A 65-year-old man with chronic obstructive pulmonary disease is evaluated in the emergency department for a 4-day history of worsening dyspnea, cough, and increased production of purulent sputum. His albuterol inhaler has been ineffective in relieving his symptoms.

On physical examination, the patient is in respiratory distress using pursed-lip breathing. Temperature is 36.7°C (98.0°F), blood pressure is 145/84 mm Hg, pulse rate is 102/min, and respiration rate is 20/min. He has audible polyphonic wheezes but no crackles. Heart sounds are distant but otherwise normal. The remainder of his physical examination is normal.

Arterial blood gases performed on 2 L/min nasal cannula: pH, 7.31; PCO_2, 50 mm Hg (6.7 kPa); PO_2, 65 mm Hg (8.6 kPa). Chest radiograph displays hyperinflation but no infiltrates.

Intravenous corticosteroids and inhaled albuterol are begun.

Which of the following treatments should also be initiated?

(A) Amoxicillin
(B) Inhaled corticosteroids
(C) Levofloxacin
(D) Theophylline

Item 20 [Basic]

A 58-year-old man with chronic obstructive pulmonary disease (COPD) is evaluated for slowly progressive dyspnea beginning 6 months ago. He now has dyspnea with minimal exertion, such as walking two blocks, and he can no longer climb a flight of stairs. He has a 42-pack-year smoking history, quitting 2 years ago. His medications are albuterol and tiotropium inhalers.

On physical examination, temperature is 36.6°C (97.8°F), blood pressure is 140/86 mm Hg, pulse rate is 90/min, and respiration rate is 16/min. Oxygen saturation by pulse oximetry is 87% on ambient air. Breath sounds are decreased, but no audible wheezes are present.

Arterial blood gas analysis, on ambient air, reveals: pH, 7.38; PO_2, 54 mm Hg (7.2 kPa); PCO_2, 45 mm Hg (6.0 kPa). Chest radiograph shows hyperinflation. Spirometry shows an FEV_1 of 30% of predicted and an FEV_1/FVC ratio of 50%.

Which of the following interventions is most likely to improve this patient's survival?

(A) Continuous oxygen therapy
(B) Inhaled corticosteroid
(C) Inhaled salmeterol
(D) Theophylline

Item 21 [Basic]

A 55-year-old man with a 7-year history of severe chronic obstructive pulmonary disease is evaluated after being discharged from the hospital following an acute exacerbation; he has had three exacerbations over the previous 18 months. He is a long-term smoker who stopped smoking 1 year ago. His medications are albuterol as needed and inhaled tiotropium and salmeterol.

On physical examination, vital signs are normal. Breath sounds are decreased bilaterally; there is no edema or cyanosis. Oxygen saturation after exertion is 92% on ambient air. Spirometry shows an FEV_1 of 32% of predicted and an FEV_1/FVC ratio of 40%. Chest radiograph done in the hospital 3 weeks ago showed no active disease.

Which of the following medications should now be initiated?

(A) An inhaled corticosteroid
(B) Ipratropium
(C) N-acetylcysteine
(D) Oral prednisone

Item 22 [Advanced]

A 64-year-old man with a history of chronic obstructive pulmonary disease is evaluated in the emergency department for increased dyspnea over the past 48 hours. There is no change in his baseline production of white sputum, but he has increased nasal congestion and sore throat. His medications are inhaled tiotropium, fluticasone, salmeterol, and albuterol. Therapy with methylprednisolone, inhaled albuterol, and ipratropium bromide is started.

The patient is alert but in mild respiratory distress. The temperature is 38.6°C (101.5°F), the blood pressure is 150/90 mm Hg, the pulse rate is 108/min, and the respiration rate is 30/min. Breath sounds are diffusely decreased with bilateral expiratory wheezes; he is using accessory muscles to breathe. With the patient breathing oxygen, 2 L/min by nasal cannula, arterial blood gases are pH 7.27, P_{CO_2} 60 mm Hg (8.0 kPa), and P_{O_2} 62 mm Hg (8.2 kPa); oxygen saturation is 91%.

Which of the following is the most appropriate next step?

(A) Increase oxygen to 5 L/min
(B) Intubation and mechanical ventilation
(C) Start aminophylline infusion
(D) Start noninvasive positive-pressure ventilation

Item 23 [Advanced]

A 72-year-old woman is evaluated for fatigue and decreased exercise capacity. She has severe chronic obstructive pulmonary disease, which was first diagnosed 10 years ago. She was hospitalized 1 month ago for her second exacerbation this year. She stopped smoking 5 years ago. She has no other significant medical problems. Her medications are albuterol as needed, an inhaled corticosteroid, a long-acting bronchodilator, and oxygen, 2 L/min by nasal cannula.

On physical examination, vital signs are normal. Breath sounds are decreased. Spirometry done 1 month ago showed an FEV_1 of 28% of predicted, and blood gases measured at that time (on supplemental oxygen) showed a pH of 7.41, P_{CO_2} of 43 mm Hg (5.7 kPa), and P_{O_2} of 64 mm Hg (8.4 kPa); D_{LCO} is 30% of predicted. There is no nocturnal oxygen desaturation. Chest radiograph at this time shows hyperinflation. CT scan of the chest shows homogeneous distribution of emphysema.

Which of the following is the most appropriate management for this patient?

(A) Lung transplantation
(B) Lung volume reduction surgery
(C) Nocturnal assisted ventilation
(D) Pulmonary rehabilitation

Item 24 [Basic]

A 40-year-old man who is a new patient is evaluated for a 6-month history of mild shortness of breath, which occurs primarily with exertion, and also occasional wheezing. He has smoked a half pack of cigarettes daily since the age of 18 years. He is otherwise healthy and takes no medications. He works in an automobile repair shop. His father, a cigarette smoker, died of emphysema at the age of 55 years.

On physical examination, vital signs are normal. Breath sounds are diminished bilaterally, and there is occasional wheezing posteriorly. Spirometry shows an FEV_1 of 58% of predicted and an FEV_1/FVC ratio of 65%. Chest radiograph shows bilateral basilar lucency (lung bullae).

Which of the following is the most appropriate next step in management?

(A) Measure plasma α_1-antitrypsin
(B) Measure sweat chloride
(C) Obtain a flow-volume loop
(D) Obtain high-resolution CT scan of the chest

Item 25 [Basic]

A 45-year-old man is evaluated at the insistence of his wife because of his loud snoring. On questioning, the patient admits to morning headaches, nasal congestion, and falling asleep once while driving. He does not smoke cigarettes. He has no other medical problems and takes no medications.

On physical examination, temperature is 36.6°C (97.8°F), blood pressure is 148/90 mm Hg, pulse rate is 80/min, and respiration rate is 12/min. BMI is 34. Oxygen saturation by pulse oximetry is 90% on ambient air. The cardiopulmonary examination is normal. No peripheral edema is present.

Which of the following should be done next to evaluate this patient's symptoms?

(A) Brain natriuretic peptide (BNP) measurement
(B) Coronary artery calcium (CAC) score
(C) CT pulmonary angiography
(D) Polysomnography and arterial blood gas measurement

Item 26 [Advanced]

A 55-year-old man is evaluated for fatigue that has been present for more than 1 year. He feels tired on awakening and requires at least one nap daily to accomplish his work tasks. He reports no other changes in his sleep pattern or symptoms of depression. He does not smoke cigarettes, drink alcohol, or take illicit drugs. His only other medical problem is a 2-year history of difficult-to-control hypertension. Medications are lisinopril, hydrochlorothiazide, and amlodipine.

On physical examination, temperature is normal, blood pressure is 140/92 mm Hg, pulse rate is 78/min, and respiration rate is 14/min. BMI is 36. The cardiopulmonary examination is normal. The vascular examination is normal without evidence of carotid, abdominal, or femoral bruits. The remainder of the physical examination is unremarkable.

Routine laboratory testing, including fasting blood glucose, serum electrolytes, and kidney function tests are normal.

Which of the following diagnostic tests should be done next?

(A) 24-Hour urine free cortisol measurement
(B) Percutaneous renal artery angiography
(C) Plasma aldosterone–renin activity ratio
(D) Polysomnography

Item 27 [Advanced]

A 64-year-old woman is evaluated for a 6-week history of dyspnea, dry cough, fever, chills, night sweats, and fatigue, which have not responded to treatment with azithromycin and levofloxacin; she has lost 2.2 kg (5 lb) during that time. The patient had an examination 6 months ago while she was asymptomatic that included routine laboratory studies, age- and sex-appropriate cancer screening, and a chest radiograph; all results were normal. The patient has never smoked, has had no known environmental exposures, and has not traveled recently or been exposed to anyone with a similar illness. Her only medications are aspirin and a multivitamin.

On physical examination, temperature is 37.8°C (100.0°F); other vital signs are normal. Cardiac examination is normal. There are scattered crackles in the mid-lung zones with associated rare expiratory wheezes. There is no digital clubbing. Musculoskeletal and skin examinations are normal. Chest radiograph is shown.

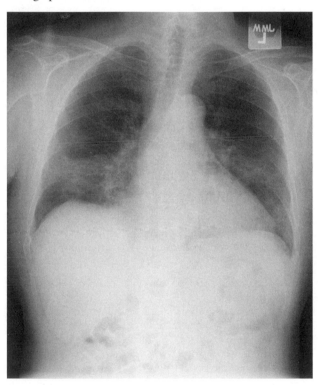

Which of the following is the most likely diagnosis?

(A) Asbestosis
(B) Community-acquired pneumonia
(C) Cryptogenic organizing pneumonia
(D) Idiopathic pulmonary fibrosis

Item 28 [Advanced]

A 74-year-old man is evaluated for a 5-year history of gradually progressive dyspnea and dry cough without wheezing or hemoptysis. He has not had fever or lost weight. He smoked one pack of cigarettes per day between the ages of 18 and 60 years. He worked as an insulator for 40 years.

Physical examination shows no digital clubbing or cyanosis. Auscultation of the lungs reveals bilateral end-inspiratory crackles. Pulmonary function testing shows the following:

Total lung capacity	67% of predicted
Residual volume	72% of predicted
FVC	65% of predicted
FEV_1	75% of predicted
FEV_1/FVC ratio	89%
D_{LCO}	52% of predicted

His chest radiograph is shown.

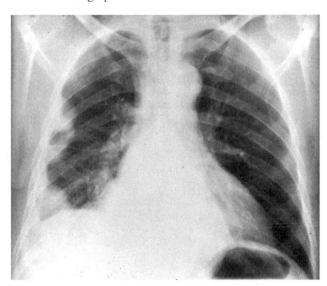

Which of the following is the most likely diagnosis?

(A) Asbestosis
(B) Idiopathic pulmonary fibrosis
(C) Pulmonary sarcoidosis
(D) Rheumatoid interstitial lung disease

Item 29 [Basic]

A 55-year-old man has a 1-year history of fatigue, chronic morning headache, daytime hypersomnolence, and frequent nighttime awakenings. The patient has hypertension and a 48-pack-year smoking history. His only medication is lisinopril. His family history is noncontributory.

On physical examination, temperature is normal, blood pressure is 135/85 mm Hg, pulse rate is 88/min, and respiration rate is 28/min. BMI is 35. The examination is otherwise unremarkable.

Hematocrit	53% (normal 5 years ago)
Leukocyte count	5700/µL (5.7 × 10⁹/L)
Platelet count	345,000/µL (345 × 10⁹/L)
Erythropoietin	Elevated
Arterial oxygen saturation (on ambient air)	98%

Cytogenetic studies are negative for the *JAK2* gene mutation.

Which of the following is the most likely cause of the patient's elevated hematocrit?

(A) High-oxygen–affinity hemoglobin
(B) Polycythemia vera
(C) Sleep apnea
(D) Volume contraction

Item 30 [Advanced]

A 38-year-old woman with a 4-year history of systemic sclerosis is evaluated for a 6-month history of dry cough and shortness of breath. She has no fever, sputum production, or orthopnea. The clinical manifestations of her systemic sclerosis include arthralgia, gastroesophageal reflux disease, and Raynaud phenomenon.

On physical examination, temperature is 36.9°C (98.5°F), blood pressure is 120/76 mm Hg, pulse rate is 88/min, and respiration rate is 18/min. Oxygen saturation by pulse oximetry is 90% on ambient air. Fine bibasilar late inspiratory crackles are heard. Cardiac examination is normal without murmurs or extra sounds.

Complete blood count, serum electrolytes, and metabolic panel are normal. Chest x-ray is normal. Results of pulmonary function testing: FEV_1, 75% of predicted; FVC, 71% of predicted; FEV_1/FVC ratio, 100% of predicted; and diffusing capacity of lung for carbon monoxide (D_{LCO}), 64% of predicted. Antitopoisomerase I antibody testing is positive.

Which of the following is the most appropriate next diagnostic test?

(A) Bronchoalveolar lavage
(B) High resolution chest CT
(C) Lung biopsy
(D) Pulmonary artery angiogram

Item 31 [Advanced]

A 60-year-old woman is evaluated for a 2-month history of progressive exertional dyspnea, low-grade fever, and cough. She has never smoked and has worked all her life as a homemaker. Medical history includes 10-year history of hypertension and a 3-month history of atrial fibrillation. Her medications are hydrochlorothiazide, atenolol, amiodarone, and warfarin.

On physical examination, temperature is 37.8°C (100.0°F), blood pressure is 138/78 mm Hg, pulse rate is 92/min, respiration rate is 24/min. Oxygen saturation on pulse oximetry is 94% on ambient air. No evidence of jugular venous distention is seen. Heart sounds are normal without extra cardiac sounds or murmur. Bilateral crackles at the lung bases are noted. No clubbing is noted.

Hemoglobin is 11 mg/dL (110 g/L), leukocyte count is 12,800/μL (12.8×10^9/L) with 9% eosinophils. Chest x-ray shows diffuse interstitial infiltrates with basilar predominance.

Which of the following is the most likely diagnosis?

(A) Acute eosinophilic pneumonitis
(B) Asbestosis
(C) Drug-induced lung toxicity
(D) Heart failure

Item 32 [Basic]

A 75-year-old woman is admitted to the hospital from her home for treatment of community-acquired pneumonia because of extreme weakness and nausea. She has a history of hypertension and compensated heart failure. Medications are metoprolol, lisinopril, and hydrochlorothiazide.

On physical examination, temperature is 38.9°C (102.0°F), blood pressure is 110/74 mm Hg, pulse rate is 100/min, and respiration rate is 20/min. Oxygen saturation by pulse oximetry is 92% on ambient air. Crackles are heard at the left lower lung base. Cardiopulmonary examination is otherwise normal.

Hemoglobin	15 g/dL (150 g/L)
Leukocyte count	18,500/μL (18.5×10^9/L)
Platelet count	150,000/μL (150×10^9/L)
Creatinine	1.2 mg/dL (106.1 mmol/L)
Electrolytes	Normal

Which of the following venous thrombosis prophylactic interventions is most appropriate for this patient?

(A) Aspirin
(B) Knee-high compression stockings
(C) Lepirudin
(D) Unfractionated heparin
(E) Prophylaxis not indicated

Item 33 [Advanced]

A 54-year-old man is evaluated in the emergency department for a 1-hour history of chest pain and dyspnea. The patient had been hospitalized 1 week ago for a colectomy for colon cancer. His medical history also includes hypertension and nephrotic syndrome secondary to membranous glomerulonephritis. His medications are furosemide, ramipril, and pravastatin.

On physical examination, the temperature is 37.5°C (99.5°F), the blood pressure is 110/60 mm Hg, the pulse rate is 120/min, the respiration rate is 24/min, and the BMI is 30. Oxygen saturation is 89% with the patient breathing ambient air and 97% on oxygen, 4 L/min. Cardiac examination shows tachycardia and an S_4. Breath sounds are normal. Serum creatinine concentration is 2.1 mg/dL (185.6 μmol/L). Chest radiograph is normal. Empiric unfractionated heparin therapy is begun.

Which of the following tests should be done next?

(A) Assay for plasma D-dimer
(B) CT pulmonary angiography
(C) Lower extremity ultrasonography
(D) Measurement of antithrombin III
(E) Ventilation/perfusion scan

Item 34 [Advanced]

A 50-year-old woman is evaluated in the emergency department for a 4-day history of pain, swelling, and erythema of the left leg. There is no history of recent immobilization, cancer, surgery, or deep venous thrombosis.

On physical examination, temperature is 37.7°C (100.0°F), blood pressure is 132/82 mm Hg, pulse rate is 65/min, and respiration rate is 16/min. Examination of the left leg discloses warmth and circumscribed erythema and tenderness limited to the posterior tibial portion of the leg. The circumference of the left leg is 1 cm greater than the right when measured 10 cm below the tibial tuberosity. Localized tenderness along the distribution of the deep venous system and pitting edema are absent, as are venous varicosities.

Which of the following is the most appropriate next step in diagnosis?

(A) CT of the leg
(B) D-dimer assay
(C) MRI of the leg
(D) Venography

Item 35 [Advanced]

A 57-year-old woman is evaluated in the emergency department for a 1-week history of swelling and pain in the left leg. She has had two normal pregnancies and no miscarriages. There is no family or personal history of thromboembolic disease. The patient is otherwise healthy.

A proximal deep venous thrombosis is confirmed on ultrasound. Unfractionated heparin is given as an initial bolus followed by a continuous infusion at a dose to prolong the activated partial thromboplastin time to two times the control value. Warfarin, 5 mg/d, is also initiated.

Which of the following is the most appropriate duration of heparin therapy for this patient?

(A) Minimum of 3 days
(B) Minimum of 3 days, with one INR measurement of >2
(C) Minimum of 5 days
(D) Minimum of 5 days, with two INR measurements of >2, 24 h apart

Section 10

Pulmonary Medicine
Answers and Critiques

Item 1   **Answer: B**

Educational Objective: *Diagnose chronic obstructive pulmonary disease.*

The most likely diagnosis is chronic obstructive pulmonary disease (COPD). A clinical diagnosis of COPD should be considered in any patient who has dyspnea, chronic cough or sputum production, or a history of risk factors for the disease. The diagnosis of COPD is confirmed and staged by spirometry. Spirometry should be performed after the administration of an adequate dose of an inhaled bronchodilator (for example, salbutamol 400 μg) to minimize variability. Although measurements of postbronchodilator FEV_1/FVC ratio and FEV_1 are recommended for the diagnosis and assessment of severity of COPD, respectively, determining the degree of reversibility of airflow limitation (change in FEV_1 after administration of bronchodilators or corticosteroids) is no longer recommended for diagnosis, for distinguishing COPD from asthma, or for predicting the response to long-term treatment with bronchodilators or corticosteroids. A postbronchodilator FEV_1 less than 80% of predicted and FEV_1/FVC ratio less than 0.70 confirm the presence of airflow limitation that is not fully reversible, establishes the diagnosis of COPD, and excludes the diagnosis of asthma. Finally, this patient has a low DLCO, which is not compatible with asthma. DLCO measures the ability of the lungs to transfer gas from alveoli to the red blood cells in pulmonary capillaries. It is low in conditions characterized by barriers to diffusion (interstitial edema, interstitial infiltrates, tissue fibrosis) or loss of lung tissue (for example, emphysema).

Heart failure is usually associated with increased central venous pressure, an S_3 on cardiac examination, and crackles on lung auscultation. Patients with heart failure typically have normal pulmonary function testing, except for the possibility of decreased DLCO due to interstitial edema. In interstitial lung disease, the patient may have dry crackles on examination. Additionally, pulmonary function testing typically shows a proportionate decrease in FEV1 and FVC resulting in a normal FEV1/FVC ratio, a decreased TLC, and decreased DLCO.

KEY POINT

A postbronchodilator FEV_1 less than 80% of predicted and FEV_1/FVC ratio less than 0.70 confirm the presence of airflow limitation that is not fully reversible and establishes the diagnosis of chronic obstructive pulmonary disease.

Bibliography

Sweitzer BJ, Smetana GW. Identification and evaluation of the patient with lung disease. Med Clin North Am. 2009;93(5):1017-30. [PMID: 19665617]

Item 2   **Answer: D**

Educational Objective: *Diagnose interstitial lung disease.*

The most likely diagnosis is rheumatoid arthritis-interstitial lung disease. The diagnosis of rheumatoid arthritis is suggested by the symmetrical synovitis of the wrists and metacarpophalangeal joints. The chest x-ray is often normal in patients with rheumatoid arthritis-interstitial lung disease, particularly in the early course of the disease. However, the pulmonary function tests show proportionate reduction in FEV_1 and FVC resulting in a normal FEV_1/FVC ratio. This finding is consistent with a restrictive pattern, which is supported by the finding of reduced TLC. Additionally, the decreased DLCO is compatible with interstitial lung disease. DLCO measures the ability of the lungs to transfer gas from alveoli to the red blood cells in pulmonary capillaries. It is low in conditions characterized by loss of lung tissue or barriers to gas diffusion (for example, interstitial edema, interstitial infiltrates, tissue fibrosis) or loss of lung tissue (emphysema).

Chronic obstructive lung disease and asthma would have shown an obstructive pattern, with reduced FEV_1/FVC ratio; the TLC may be normal or increased. In COPD, the DLCO is often low but it is normal in patients with asthma. A pulmonary embolism would not affect the spirometry or lung volumes, but may show a decrease in DLCO.

KEY POINT

Interstitial lung disease is characterized by pulmonary function tests showing proportionate reduction in FEV_1 and FVC, resulting in a normal FEV_1/FVC ratio, reduced TLC and *decreased DLCO*.

Bibliography

Dempsey OJ, Kerr KM, Remmen H, Denison AR. How to investigate a patient with suspected interstitial lung disease. BMJ. 2010;340:c2843. [PMID: 20534676]

Item 3   Answer: D

Educational Objective: *Diagnose asthma with a methacholine challenge test.*

The most appropriate next diagnostic test is a methacholine challenge. This patient's history is consistent with, but not typical of, asthma. This presentation is sometimes referred to as cough-variant asthma. Asthma is often an episodic disease, with normal examination findings and spirometry between episodes. In such cases, a bronchial challenge test, such as with methacholine, can induce bronchoconstriction even when the patient is asymptomatic and spirometry is normal. Methacholine challenge testing is done by giving the patient increasing concentrations of methacholine by nebulization and performing spirometry after each dose until there is a greater than 20% decrease in FEV_1 from baseline. The methacholine dose that leads to a 20% decrease in the FEV_1 is known as the provocative concentration 20 (PC_{20}) and is calculated from a dose-response curve. In general, a PC_{20} of less than 4 mg/mL is consistent with asthma. A PC_{20} between 4 and 16 mg/mL suggests some bronchial hyperreactivity and is less specific for asthma. A PC_{20} above 16 mg/mL is considered normal. The sensitivity of a positive methacholine challenge test in asthma is in the range of 85% to 95%. False-positive results can occur in patients with allergic rhinitis, chronic obstructive pulmonary disease, heart failure, cystic fibrosis, or bronchitis.

Bronchoscopy to evaluate the trachea could be helpful if an anatomic lesion is suspected. However, the symptoms in patients with such lesions are persistent or progressive rather than intermittent. Since this patient has intermittent symptoms, bronchoscopy is not indicated. Exercise echocardiography could help determine the presence of cardiac ischemia or myocardial dysfunction, the typical symptoms of which are dyspnea on exertion, chest tightness, or pain. Cough and wheezing can occur in coronary artery disease, particularly when associated with acute decompensation of the left ventricle, but this patient's intermittent episodes of cough and wheezing are provoked by an upper respiratory tract infection, making the diagnosis of coronary artery disease unlikely. Patients with rhinosinusitis have symptoms consisting of nasal congestion, purulent nasal secretions, sinus tenderness, and facial pain. Radiography, including sinus CT scan, is not indicated in the initial evaluation of acute sinusitis.

KEY POINT

Methacholine challenge testing is most useful in evaluating patients with suspected asthma who have episodic symptoms and normal baseline spirometry.

Bibliography

Panettieri RA Jr. In the clinic. Asthma. Ann Intern Med. 2007;146(11): ITC6-1-ITC6-16. [PMID: 17548407]

Item 4   Answer: C

Educational Objective: *Diagnose respiratory failure caused by neuromuscular weakness.*

This patient most likely has severe muscle weakness due to a subacute or chronic neuromuscular disorder such as amyotrophic lateral sclerosis or myasthenia gravis. Either condition can present with respiratory failure. An increased residual volume/total lung capacity (RV/TLC) ratio is commonly seen in obstructive disorders, but it may also be caused by a neuromuscular restrictive disorder. In such cases, the normal FEV_1/FVC ratio and the low maximum respiratory pressures indicate neuromuscular weakness rather than an obstructive lung disease.

Interstitial lung diseases, such as idiopathic pulmonary fibrosis (IPF), cause restriction but would not explain the increased RV/TLC ratio, normal D_{LCO}, and reduced maximum respiratory pressures. When respiratory failure develops with IPF, it is usually characterized by hypoxemia. Hypercapnic respiratory failure is rare in IPF.

Similarly, pulmonary hypertension presents with hypoxia and hypocapnia; hypercapnia would be unusual. In some patients, pulmonary arterial hypertension may be associated with a mild decrease FEV_1 or FVC but the RV/TLC and maximal inspiratory pressure are normal. Finally, the D_{LCO} is usually decreased in pulmonary arterial hypertension, and this is not compatible with this patient's findings.

KEY POINT

In patients with neuromuscular respiratory failure, an increased residual volume/total lung capacity ratio, normal FEV_1/FVC ratio, low maximum respiratory pressures, and normal D_{LCO} are typical.

Bibliography

Vazquez-Sandoval A, Huang EJ, Jones SF. Hypoventilation in neuromuscular disease. Semin Respir Crit Care Med. 2009;30(3):348-358. [PMID: 19452395]

Item 5   Answer: D

Educational Objective: *Diagnose hepatopulmonary syndrome.*

This patient most likely has hepatopulmonary syndrome, which manifests as dyspnea at rest or on exertion, platypnea, and hypoxemia in the setting of chronic liver disease. In the context of chronic liver disease, clubbing, cyanosis, and hypoxemia are characteristic of hepatopulmonary syndrome. The hypoxemia results from pulmonary vascular dilatation with intrapulmonary shunt and ventilation-perfusion mismatch, which may worsen when the individual is in an upright position. These can cause orthodeoxia (fall in partial pressure of oxygen with upright posture) and platypnea (dyspnea worse when sitting upright). The chest x-ray in patients with hepatopulmonary syndrome is typically normal; occasionally, subtle bibasilar infiltrates may be seen.

Bronchogenic carcinoma may be associated with clubbing, but the patient has no cough, hemoptysis, or focal pulmonary findings on physical examination to suggest this diagnosis, and the chest x-ray is normal.

Emphysema can cause dyspnea, hypoxemia, and diminished breath sounds. However, no features, such as cough, or physical examination findings, such as hyperresonance to percussion, wheezes, or prolonged expiration, are present. Finally, emphysema would not explain the platypnea.

Constrictive pericarditis may present with two types of symptom complexes: fluid overload causing ascites, jugular venous distention, hepatic congestion, and lower extremity edema; and diminished cardiac output causing fatigue and dyspnea on exertion. The patient has no suggestive findings of constrictive pericarditis such as elevated jugular venous pressure, pulsus paradoxus, or pericardial knock.

KEY POINT

The main features of hepatopulmonary syndrome include signs of portal hypertension, dyspnea, platypnea, hypoxemia with orthodeoxia, cyanosis, and clubbing.

Bibliography

Rodríguez-Roisin R, Krowka MJ. Hepatopulmonary syndrome—a liver-induced lung vascular disorder. N Engl J Med. 2008;358(22):2378-87. [PMID: 18509123]

Item 6   Answer: A
Educational Objective: *Diagnose severe aortic stenosis.*

Heart failure due to aortic stenosis is the most likely cause of this patient's dyspnea on exertion and orthopnea. Classic manifestations of severe aortic stenosis are angina, syncope, and heart failure. In early stages, aortic stenosis may present subtly, with dyspnea or a decrease in exercise tolerance. About one half of patients with aortic stenosis are diagnosed when heart failure develops. This patient has characteristic findings of severe aortic stenosis, including narrow pulse pressure; delayed, diminished carotid upstroke; sustained apical impulse; late-peaking systolic ejection murmur radiating to the carotids; and S_4.

Adults with unrepaired atrial septal defects may be asymptomatic or may present with symptoms related to excess pulmonary blood flow, including fatigue, dyspnea, palpitations, or right-sided heart failure. Atrial arrhythmias, including atrial fibrillation or flutter and sick sinus syndrome, are common. The characteristic physical examination findings in atrial septal defect are fixed splitting of the S_2 and a right ventricular heave. A pulmonary midsystolic flow murmur and a tricuspid diastolic flow rumble caused by increased flow through the right-sided valves from a large left-to-right shunt may be heard. The patient is quite old to be diagnosed with congenital heart disease and she has no findings to support this diagnosis.

The symptoms of pulmonary arterial hypertension tend to be nonspecific, including progressively worsening dyspnea and dizziness, although these symptoms usually occur in the absence of (or out of proportion to) pulmonary disease or left-sided heart disease. Physical examination may disclose signs of elevated pulmonary artery pressure and right ventricular strain (loud P_2, fixed split S_2, tricuspid regurgitation, elevated jugular venous distention), which are not present in this patient.

Valvular pulmonary stenosis is usually an isolated congenital abnormality and causes obstruction to the right ventricular outflow. Severe valvular obstruction may be tolerated for many years before development of symptoms. In severe pulmonary stenosis, the jugular venous pressure demonstrates a prominent *a* wave. A right ventricular lift is common. An ejection click is common, and a systolic murmur is present, with the pulmonic component of the S_2 delayed.

KEY POINT

Classic manifestations of severe aortic stenosis are angina, syncope, and heart failure.

Bibliography

Cheitlin MD. Pathophysiology of valvular aortic stenosis in the elderly. Am J Geriatr Cardiol. 2003;12(3):173-7. [PMID: 12732812]

Item 7   Answer: B
Educational Objective: *Diagnose hydropneumothorax on a chest radiograph.*

This patient has a hydropneumothorax. Spontaneous pneumothorax is a relatively common event in healthy young persons. The radiographic abnormality is characterized by the loss of normal lung markings in the periphery of the hemithorax and the presence of a well-defined, visceral pleural line at some point between the chest wall and the hilum. Spontaneous pneumothorax occurs when a subpleural bleb ruptures into the pleural space, an event that commonly occurs during exertion. The presence of air within the pleural space allows the lung to collapse toward the hilum. Frequently, a small amount of bleeding accompanies rupture of the bleb and produces the characteristic appearance of a flat-line junction between the air and the fluid that collects at the base of the hemithorax; this is known as a hydropneumothorax. Large pneumothoraces require insertion of a chest tube to drain the pleural space and reexpand the lung. An initial chest radiograph showing shift of the mediastinum away from the side of the pneumothorax indicates the development of a tension pneumothorax and requires immediate chest tube insertion.

Typical radiographic findings of heart failure include cardiomegaly, pulmonary vascular congestion, Kerley B-lines, and pleural effusions; pulmonary edema may be recognized as perihilar interstitial infiltrates. Pneumonia may have various radiographic presentations, including lobar consolidation, interstitial infiltrates, and cavitation. Radiographic abnormalities are commonly associated with pulmonary embolism but are not specific. Findings such as atelectasis, infiltrates, and pleural effusions are found as frequently in patients with pulmonary embolism as in patients without pulmonary embolism. Slightly over 10% of patients with pulmonary embolism will have a normal chest radiograph.

KEY POINT

The radiographic abnormality that defines pneumothorax is the loss of normal lung markings in the periphery of the hemithorax and the presence of a well-defined, visceral pleural line at some point between the chest wall and the hilum.

Bibliography

Currie GP, Alluri R, Christie GL, Legge JS. Pneumothorax: an update. Postgrad Med J. 2007;83:461-465. Erratum in: Postgrad Med J. 2007;83:722. [PMID: 17621614]

Item 8   Answer: D
Educational Objective: *Diagnose vocal cord dysfunction with laryngoscopy.*

The most appropriate management for this patient is laryngoscopy. She likely has vocal cord dysfunction (VCD). Patients with VCD can have throat or neck discomfort, wheezing, stridor, and anxiety. The disorder can be difficult to differentiate from asthma; however, affected patients do not respond to the usual asthma therapy. Diagnosing VCD is made more difficult by the fact that many of these patients also have asthma. The chest radiograph in this patient showed decreased lung volumes, which is in contrast to hyperinflation that would be expected in acute asthma. Oxygen saturation is typically normal in patients with VCD.

Laryngoscopy, especially when done while the patient is symptomatic, can reveal characteristic adduction of the vocal cords during inspiration. Another test that helps make the diagnosis is flow volume loops, in which the inspiratory and expiratory flow rates are recorded while a patient is asked to take a deep breath and then to exhale. In patients with VCD, the inspiratory limb of the flow volume loop is "flattened" owing to narrowing of the extrathoracic airway (at the level of the vocal cords) during inspiration. Recognition of VCD is essential to prevent lengthy courses of corticosteroids and to initiate therapies targeted at VCD, which include speech therapy, relaxation techniques, and treating underlying causes such as anxiety.

The chest CT scan can be used to exclude parenchymal lung disease or evaluate the possibility of a pulmonary embolism; however, these disorders are unlikely in this patient with previous normal pulmonary examinations and radiographs and excellent oxygenation.

Intravenous aminophylline is not recommended for treating either acute asthma or VCD.

Azithromycin is a reasonable choice for acute bronchitis in patients with underlying lung disease, but there is little evidence that this patient has acute bronchitis, which would manifest with cough, sputum production, and fever.

KEY POINT

Laryngoscopy during an exacerbation of vocal cord dysfunction shows adduction of the vocal cords during inspiration.

Bibliography

King CS, Moores LK. Clinical asthma syndromes and important asthma mimics. Respir Care. 2008;53(5):568-580. [PMID: 18426611]

Item 9   Answer: D
Educational Objective: *Diagnose pulmonary arterial hypertension associated with systemic sclerosis.*

This patient most likely has pulmonary arterial hypertension (PAH) associated with collagen vascular disease related to systemic sclerosis. Pulmonary disease is the primary cause of morbidity in patients with systemic sclerosis; PAH is among the most common manifestations of lung involvement in these patients, particularly in those with limited cutaneous disease. This patient's worsening fatigue and dyspnea on exertion in the presence of clear lung fields are consistent with PAH.

Physical signs of elevated pulmonary artery pressure include a loud P_2, fixed split S_2, pulmonic flow murmur, and tricuspid regurgitation. Chest radiographs are usually normal in early disease but may show enlargement of the pulmonary arteries, the right atrium, and the right ventricle. Electrocardiograms in these patients may show right ventricular strain or hypertrophy.

Pulmonary function studies in patients with PAH usually reveal an isolated decreased D_{LCO} in the setting of normal airflow and lung volumes (excluding restrictive lung disease). Echocardiography is an early diagnostic test for patients with signs and symptoms of PAH. This study is used to exclude congenital heart disease, such as atrial septal defect, and valvular heart disease, such as mitral stenosis, that may manifest as pulmonary hypertension. Echocardiography may be used to estimate peak right ventricular systolic pressure if tricuspid regurgitation is noted on examination.

A clinical diagnosis of chronic obstructive pulmonary disease (COPD) should be considered in any patient who has dyspnea, chronic cough or sputum production, and/or a history of risk factors for the disease. The diagnosis of COPD is confirmed and staged by spirometry. This patient has no risk factors, symptoms, or physical examination findings (barrel chest, decreased breath sounds, wheezing) to support the diagnosis of COPD. Patients with COPD have $FEV_1/FVC < 70\%$.

Interstitial lung disease (ILD) is a common pulmonary manifestation in patients with systemic sclerosis who also have dyspnea and fatigue, and patients with ILD also usually have dry cough. The absence of late inspiratory crackles on pulmonary examination and the presence of normal lung volumes on pulmonary function testing further argue against this condition. In patients with ILD, the lung volumes are less than 80% of predicted.

Left ventricular failure may manifest as dyspnea and fatigue and may be associated with cardiac murmurs. However, this condition is unlikely in the absence of additional abnormal cardiopulmonary examination findings, such as an S_3 or S_4 gallop and pulmonary crackles. In addition, chest radiographs in patients with left ventricular heart failure usually demonstrate pulmonary vascular congestion.

Physical signs of elevated pulmonary artery pressure include a loud P_2, fixed split S_2, pulmonic flow murmur, and tricuspid regurgitation.

Bibliography

Highland KB, Garin MC, Brown KK. The spectrum of scleroderma lung disease. Semin Respir Crit Care Med. 2007;28(4):418-429. [PMID: 17764059]

Item 10   Answer: B
Educational Objective: *Treat a complicated pleural effusion with chest tube drainage.*

The next step in the management of this patient is chest tube drainage of the pleural effusion. In pleural effusions associated with pneumonia, the presence of loculated pleural fluid, pleural fluid with a pH less than 7.20, pleural fluid with a glucose level less than 60 mg/dL (3.3 mmol/L), lactate dehydrogenase level greater than 1000 U/L, positive pleural fluid Gram stain or culture, or the presence of gross pus in the pleural space predicts a poor response to antibiotics alone; such effusions are treated with drainage of the fluid through a catheter or chest tube.

This patient's history is compatible with community-acquired pneumonia (cough, sputum, fever, chills), and the radiographic findings are consistent with a free-flowing pleural effusion. Because this patient's pleural fluid findings predict a poor response to antibiotics alone, his effusion is called a *complicated parapneumonic effusion*. A CT scan may be helpful to detect very small effusions, to determine thickness of the pleural lining, to distinguish empyema (pus in the pleural space) from a lung abscess, or to detect an underlying malignancy obscured by the pleural fluid; however, none of these indications apply to this patient and a CT scan is not needed.

Most pleural effusions resolve with treatment of the underlying disease. The only effusions that usually require invasive treatment are complicated parapneumonic effusions (such as this one), empyema, and malignancy. In patients with pneumonia, thoracic empyema develops when antibiotics are not given (or delayed) and the pleural space is not drained in a timely manner. In this case, video-assisted thoracoscopic surgery (VATS) is indicated to break down loculations and drain pus from the pleural cavity. Therefore, not intervening with chest tube placement is inappropriate for this patient, and VATS surgery is overly aggressive therapy at this point in time.

In parapneumonic effusion, the presence of loculated pleural fluid, pleural fluid with a pH less than 7.20, pleural fluid with a glucose level less than 60 mg/dL (3.3 mmol/L), lactate dehydrogenase greater than 1000 U//L, positive pleural fluid Gram stain or culture, or the presence of gross pus in the pleural space predicts the need for chest tube drainage.

Bibliography

Sahn SA. Diagnosis and management of parapneumonic effusions and empyema. Clin Infect Dis. 2007;45(11):1480-6. [PMID: 17990232]

Item 11   Answer: C
Educational Objective: *Diagnose pleural effusion.*

The most likely diagnosis is parapneumonic pleural effusion. Large fluid accumulation in the pleural space blocks transmission of sound between the lung and the chest wall; percussion over an effusion is dull, and tactile (vocal) fremitus is diminished or absent. On auscultation, the most common findings are decreased to absent breath sounds over the effusion. Fever and pleural effusion suggests an underlying infection, malignancy, or associated collagen vascular disease. The patient's history of recent onset of fever and cough makes a pneumonia-related parapneumonic effusion most likely.

Heart failure can be associated with a pleural effusion, but other symptoms and signs of heart failure such as orthopnea, elevated central venous pressure, S_3, and peripheral edema are likely to be present. Furthermore, heart failure in a 24-year-old person who was previously well is very unusual.

Patients with lobar pneumonia typically have tachypnea, fever, crackles, bronchial breath sounds, and dullness to percussion with reduced breath sounds. Because consolidated lung tissue is an excellent transmitter of sound and vibration, tactile fremitus is increased, not decreased as in pleural effusion

Pneumothorax should be considered in any patient with sudden onset of pleuritic chest pain and dyspnea. The physical examination may show decreased breath sounds and hyperresonance to percussion on the affected side rather than dullness to percussion.

Large pleural effusion is associated with dullness to percussion and absent or decreased tactile (vocal) fremitus and breath sounds over the affected area.

Bibliography

Wong CL, Holroyd-Leduc J, Straus SE. Does this patient have a pleural effusion? JAMA. 2009;301(3):309-17. [PMID: 19155458]

Item 12   Answer: D
Educational Objective: *Evaluate a tuberculous pleural effusion with a pleural biopsy.*

The most appropriate next step is a pleural biopsy. He likely has a tuberculous pleural effusion based on the subacute (3-week) duration of symptoms and the characteristics of the pleural effusion. Because of the patient's age and the presentation with an isolated pleural effusion, primary tuberculosis is most likely. A tuberculous effusion is typically exudative by both protein (pleural fluid to serum protein ratio greater than 0.5) and lactate dehydrogenase (LDH) criteria (pleural fluid to serum LDH ratio greater than 0.6 and pleural fluid to serum upper limits of normal LDH ratio greater than 0.6). The cellular response in the pleural fluid is classically lymphocytic (greater than 80% mature lymphocytes). However, it can be neutrophilic within the first 2 weeks, after which it typically evolves into the classic lymphocyte-predominant exudate. Whereas pleural fluid cultures for *Mycobacterium* are positive in less than one third of cases, the combination of pleural biopsy for histologic evaluation and culture is typically positive in more than two thirds of cases.

The 3-week history of symptoms is too long for a typical bacterial pneumonia, no definite infiltrate was present on the chest radiograph, and the cellular response in the pleural fluid was primarily lymphocytic rather than neutrophilic. Therefore, a bacterial pneumonia with a parapneumonic effusion is unlikely, and an empiric course of azithromycin would not be appropriate.

Chest CT scan might be helpful to assess whether there is an underlying parenchymal infiltrate that was not visible on plain chest radiograph, but it would not help in determining the underlying cause of the pleural effusion.

Flexible bronchoscopy, with collection of samples for histology and culture, is useful for diagnosing pulmonary tuberculosis in the setting of pulmonary parenchymal disease. However, the yield from culture of bronchopulmonary secretions (obtained either as sputum or bronchoscopic samples) is low, especially in the absence of pulmonary parenchymal abnormalities on chest radiograph.

KEY POINT
A patient with tuberculous pleural effusion typically presents with a lymphocyte-predominant exudative effusion.

Bibliography
Escalante P. In the clinic. Tuberculosis [erratum in Ann Intern Med. 2009;151(4):292.]. Ann Intern Med. 2009;150(11):ITC61-614; quiz ITV616. [PMID: 19487708]

Item 13   Answer: A
Educational Objective: *Diagnose chylothorax.*

The most likely diagnosis is chylothorax. Chylothorax is drainage of lymphatic fluid into the pleural space secondary to disruption or blockage of the thoracic duct or one of its lymphatic tributaries. Malignancy is the most common cause of chylothorax, but trauma is the second most common cause. Chylothorax can also occur in association with pulmonary tuberculosis and chronic mediastinal infections, sarcoidosis, lymphangioleiomyomatosis, and radiation fibrosis. The pleural fluid in chylothorax is usually milky but may also be serous or serosanguineous in malnourished patients with little fat intake. The pleural fluid triglyceride concentration in a chylothorax is typically greater than 110 mg/dL (1.24 mmol/L) and occurs in association with a low pleural fluid cholesterol concentration. If the pleural fluid triglyceride level is less than 50 mg/dL (0.6 mmol/L), chylothorax is unlikely.

Heart failure is associated with a transudative pleural effusion. The pleural fluid protein to serum protein ratio is >0.5 and milky appearance of the effusion excludes heart failure as a possible diagnosis. Parapneumonic effusion is usually associated with a neutrophilic pleocytosis. Tuberculosis is the most common cause of lymphocyte-predominant exudate worldwide, typically as high as 90% to 95% lymphocytes. Patients with tuberculous pleural effusion usually present with a nonproductive cough, chest pain, and fever, and the effusion is usually pale yellow in color. This patient's presentation and history of lymphoma do not support tuberculosis as the cause of the effusion.

KEY POINT
The most common causes of chylothorax are cancer and trauma; other causes are pulmonary tuberculosis, chronic mediastinal infections, sarcoidosis, lymphangioleiomyomatosis, and radiation fibrosis.

Bibliography
Agrawal V, Doelken P, Sahn SA. Pleural fluid analysis in chylothorax. Chest. 2008;133(6):1436-1441. [PMID: 18339791]

Item 14   Answer: B
Educational Objective: *Treat respiratory failure with mechanical ventilation.*

The most appropriate management for this patient is intubation and mechanical ventilation and admission to the intensive care unit. The cause of acute ventilatory failure in patients with exacerbations of asthma is increased airway resistance and also dynamic hyperinflation that reduces chest-wall compliance. Both contribute to excessive work of breathing. Bronchospasm, airway edema, and secretions, as well as excessive expiratory airway collapse, can severely reduce airway diameter, resulting in markedly prolonged expiration. Increased respiratory drive and high metabolic demands increase minute ventilation, and expiration between breaths is incomplete. Progressive stacking of breaths leads to an equilibration at a higher lung volume with higher positive end-expiratory alveolar pressure (auto-PEEP or intrinsic PEEP), associated with dynamic air trapping and hyperinflation. The associated flattening of the diaphragm decreases its function and forces greater reliance on accessory muscles, further increasing carbon dioxide production and oxygen consumption as a result of the inefficiency of these muscles compared with a properly functioning diaphragm. Severe air trapping can also cause alveolar rupture and marked reductions in venous return to the right heart, resulting in pneumothorax and hypotension, respectively. Typically, patients with an asthma exacerbation initially present with respiratory alkalosis. Slightly elevated or even normal $PaCO_2$ levels often indicate impending respiratory failure rather than recovery, and clinical correlation is critical for interpreting arterial blood gas findings in this setting. Additional features that suggest respiratory failure in this patient include pulse oximetry less than 95%, PO_2 less than 75 mm Hg (10.0 kPa), respiration rate greater than 30/min, and heart rate greater than 120/min.

KEY POINT

Respiratory acidosis, hypoxemia, and fatigue are indications for intubation and mechanical ventilation in patients with an acute exacerbation of asthma.

Bibliography

Lazarus SC. Clinical practice. Emergency treatment of asthma. N Engl J Med. 2010;363(8):755-64. [PMID: 20818877]

Item 15   Answer: E
Educational Objective: *Begin step-up therapy for asthma with systemic corticosteroids.*

The most appropriate management for this patient is a short course of oral corticosteroids. This patient with previously well-controlled asthma has had "loss of control" after a respiratory tract infection. A short course of an oral corticosteroid (for example, prednisone, 0.5 mg/kg daily, for 5 to 7 days) can resolve the asthma symptoms and enable the patient to regain control of her disease. It is unclear whether doubling (or even quadrupling) the dose of inhaled corticosteroids is an effective strategy in place of oral corticosteroids.

Antibiotics are generally not recommended for acute respiratory infections in asthma because most of these infections are viral and the routine use of antibiotics in patients with an asthma exacerbation is not recommended.

Nebulized therapy at home should be reserved for patients who cannot use a metered-dose inhaler appropriately. Although nebulized bronchodilator therapy can be more effective in reversing bronchoconstriction than metered-dose inhaled bronchodilators, nebulized therapy should not be used as a substitute for oral corticosteroid therapy in patients with asthma exacerbations. Adding a leukotriene-modifying agent can be considered in patients who cannot or will not take oral

corticosteroids; however, leukotriene receptor antagonists are less potent anti-inflammatory agents than corticosteroids and are not effective in patients with significant exacerbations. Adding a long-acting β-agonist would be reasonable in this patient if her symptoms persist after the oral corticosteroid therapy, but the persistence and severity of the patient's current symptoms suggest that there is ongoing airway inflammation and that a systemic corticosteroid is warranted.

KEY POINT

A short course of oral corticosteroids may help restore asthma control in previously well-controlled patients who have developed unstable disease as a result of a respiratory tract infection.

Bibliography

Panettieri RA Jr. In the clinic. Asthma. Ann Intern Med. 2007;146(11): ITC6-1-ITC6-16. [PMID: 17548407]

Item 16   Answer: A
Educational Objective: *Manage persistent asthma during pregnancy with inhaled corticosteroids.*

The best management for this patient is to continue her current asthma regimen. Asthma during pregnancy follows the rule of thirds: the condition improves in one third of patients, worsens in one third, and remains unchanged in one third. Uncontrolled asthma has a significantly worse impact on pregnancy outcome than the potential risk of medications during pregnancy. Short-acting β-agonists are regarded as safe during pregnancy. Budesonide has been studied in pregnancy and has been shown to be safe. There are fewer data on other inhaled corticosteroids, such as fluticasone, which is a U.S. Food and Drug Administration pregnancy risk category C drug (studies of safety in pregnancy are lacking but the potential benefit of the drug may justify the potential risk). The inhaled corticosteroids are, however, believed from clinical experience to be safe during pregnancy; therefore, it is generally recommended to keep the patient on the regimen that has been effective for control of asthma.

Theophylline and aminophylline are pregnancy risk category C drugs also, but extensive clinical experience suggests that they are safe during pregnancy. However, the metabolism of these agents may be altered in pregnancy, requiring increased drug level monitoring. Also, inhaled corticosteroids are as effective as theophylline with fewer side effects in pregnant patients.

The National Asthma Education and Prevention Program expert panel guidelines in 2007 affirmed the recommendation of adding long-acting β-agonists to patients whose asthma is not controlled with an inhaled corticosteroid but advised against using long-acting β-agonists as a single controller therapy. There is no need to add a long-acting β-agonist to this patient's asthma regimen because her symptoms are well controlled, and substituting the long-acting β-agonist for inhaled fluticasone may result in loss of symptom control and possible increased risk of asthma-related death. Cromolyn is also considered safe in pregnancy but no safer than inhaled corticosteroids and less effective in persistent asthma.

KEY POINT

Clinical experience has shown that inhaled corticosteroids are safe and effective in pregnant patients with asthma.

Bibliography

Schatz M, Dombrowski MP. Clinical practice. Asthma in pregnancy. N Engl J Med. 2009;360(18):1862-1869. [PMID: 19403904]

Item 17   Answer: C

Educational Objective: *Treat inadequately controlled persistent asthma by adding a long-acting β-agonist.*

The most appropriate management for this patient is the addition of a long-acting β-agonist. She has persistent asthma, which is defined as asthma symptoms occurring 2 or more days per week or 2 or more nights per month. Patients with persistent asthma should be treated with daily inhaled corticosteroid therapy. When asthma is not adequately controlled on low- or moderate-dose inhaled corticosteroid therapy, adding a long-acting β-agonist (salmeterol or formoterol) has been shown to be superior to doubling the dose of the corticosteroid for improving asthma control and quality of life. The concerns about increased asthma-related deaths in patients using a long-acting β-agonist led the U.S. Food and Drug Administration to include a black box warning in the package insert for these drugs. The National Asthma Education and Prevention Program expert panel guidelines in 2007 affirmed the recommendation of adding a long-acting β-agonist in patients whose disease is not controlled with an inhaled corticosteroid but advised against using a long-acting β-agonist as a single controller therapy.

Theophylline and leukotriene-modifying drugs are third-line agents that should be considered in patients who remain symptomatic despite the addition of a long-acting β-agonist to the corticosteroid therapy. Long-acting anticholinergic drugs are beneficial in patients with chronic obstructive pulmonary disease; however, their role in management of asthma is not defined.

KEY POINT

In patients with persistent asthma not adequately controlled with daily low- or moderate-dose inhaled corticosteroids, adding a long-acting β-agonist improves asthma control and quality of life.

Bibliography

Panettieri RA Jr. In the clinic. Asthma. Ann Intern Med. 2007;146(11): ITC6-1-ITC6-16. [PMID: 17548407]

Item 18   Answer: B

Educational Objective: *Recognize poor inhaler technique as a possible cause of medication failure in asthma.*

The best initial management approach for this patient is to have him demonstrate his inhaler technique. Patient education is a key component in asthma care. Studies have shown that patient education by the physician decreases the number of visits to the emergency department and improves asthma control. Improper technique in the use of inhalers is a major reason that patients do not respond well to medications. A clue suggesting poor inhaler technique is the patient's rapid improvement in FEV_1 after the supervised use of a bronchodilator. Although there used to be one type of inhalation device (the metered-dose inhaler) with one technique that could be taught to the patient, there are now several new and different devices with significant differences in the technique needed for their use. Physicians should learn the proper technique for use of these inhalers before prescribing them to patients in order to ensure proper technique to optimize drug delivery and effectiveness and to reduce side effects.

Adding a leukotriene-modifying agent would be appropriate if the patient is effectively using the current medications. Oral prednisone would be appropriate for an exacerbation of poorly controlled severe persistent asthma. It would improve asthma control, but without proper education in the use of the inhaler, symptoms would most likely return when the corticosteroid dosage is tapered. Furthermore, oral corticosteroids have increased adverse effects. Simply having the patient return with a symptom and treatment log would not be expected to identify poor inhaler technique, although it would be helpful to assess compliance and symptom pattern.

KEY POINT

Poor inhaler technique is a major reason why patients with asthma do not respond well to specific asthma therapy.

Bibliography

Panettieri RA Jr. In the clinic. Asthma. Ann Intern Med. 2007;146(11): ITC6-1-ITC6-16. [PMID: 17548407]

Item 19   Answer: C

Educational Objective: *Treat an exacerbation of chronic obstructive pulmonary disease (COPD) with antibiotics.*

Levofloxacin should be initiated at this time. Oral or intravenous corticosteroids, short-acting bronchodilators (such as albuterol or ipratropium), and supplemental oxygen are the principle treatments for acute exacerbations of COPD; however, many patients will also benefit from the addition antibiotics. In select populations, antibiotics have improved several clinical outcomes, including resolution of symptoms, shorter hospital stay, and mortality. Antibiotics are recommended for patients with severe COPD exacerbations and those on mechanical ventilation. Patients with moderate to severe exacerbations characterized by increased dyspnea, increased sputum volume, increased sputum purulence, or need for hospitalization also benefit from antibiotics.

The optimal antibiotic regimen for the treatment of exacerbations is based on the most commonly isolated bacterial pathogens, including *Haemophilus influenzae*, *Streptococcus pneumoniae*, and *Moraxella catarrhalis*. Generally, antibiotic regimens for community-acquired infection include coverage with a third-generation cephalosporin in combination with a macrolide or monotherapy with a fluoroquinolone. Because of the high incidence of *H. influenzae* and *M. catarrhalis* resistance, amoxicillin is no longer considered a first-line agent for patients with moderate to severe COPD exacerbations.

The addition of inhaled corticosteroids would not likely add any benefit to a patient already receiving intravenous (or oral) corticosteroids. Theophylline is not recommended for the treatment of acute exacerbations of COPD because it provides no additional benefit beyond that of inhaled bronchodilators and oral or inhaled corticosteroids but is associated with significant side effects, including nausea, vomiting, palpitations, and arrhythmias.

KEY POINT

Recommended antibiotics for moderate to severe exacerbations of COPD include a third-generation cephalosporin combined with a macrolide or monotherapy with a fluoroquinolone.

Bibliography

Littner MR. Chronic obstructive pulmonary disease. Ann Intern Med. 2011;154(7):ITC41. [PMID: 21464346]

Item 20   Answer: A
Educational Objective: *Treat hypoxic COPD with oxygen.*

The use of long-term oxygen therapy in patients with chronic respiratory failure improves survival and has a beneficial effect on hemodynamics, exercise capacity, and mental status. Oxygen is usually prescribed for patients who have arterial P_{O_2} less than 55 mm Hg (7.3 kPa) or oxygen saturation less than 88% with or without hypercapnia or who exhibit arterial P_{O_2} of 56 to 59 mm Hg (7.4 to 7.8 kPa) or oxygen saturation less than 89% with one or more of the following: pulmonary hypertension, evidence of cor pulmonale or edema as a result of right heart failure, or hematocrit greater than 56%. The duration of treatment should be at least 15 hours a day. Oxygen as needed or oxygen with activity has no proven mortality benefit.

Inhaled corticosteroids and a long-acting β-agonist, such as salmeterol, may be indicated in this patient and likely would reduce the frequency of exacerbations, reduce hospitalizations, and improve lung function, but these medications do not increase survival. Methylxanthines, such as theophylline, are usually used only after other long-acting bronchodilators have been tried. They have a narrow therapeutic window, and most patients are effectively treated with plasma levels of 5 to 12 µg/mL (27.8 to 66.6 µmol/L). Toxicity is dose-related, and common side effects include headache, insomnia, nausea, and heartburn, as well as a potential for development of arrhythmias and tremor. Methylxanthines are metabolized by cytochrome P450, and drug interactions are common. Methylxanthines decrease dyspnea and improve lung function, but do not impact survival.

KEY POINT

Continuous oxygen improves mortality in patients with hypoxic COPD.

Bibliography

Littner MR. Chronic obstructive pulmonary disease. Ann Intern Med. 2011;154(7):ITC41. [PMID: 21464346]

Item 21   Answer: A
Educational Objective: *Treat severe chronic obstructive pulmonary disease by adding an inhaled corticosteroid.*

This patient should be started on an inhaled corticosteroid. Regular use of inhaled corticosteroids in patients with chronic obstructive pulmonary disease (COPD) is associated with a reduction in the rate of exacerbations, and patients who have frequent exacerbations benefit most. The Global Initiative for Chronic Obstructive Lung Disease guidelines recommend consideration of inhaled corticosteroids in patients whose lung function is less than 50% and those who have exacerbations. When inhaled corticosteroids are combined with a long-acting β₂-agonist, the rate of decline in quality of life and health status is significantly reduced; lung function is also improved and dyspnea is alleviated. The effects of combination therapy on mortality are uncertain.

Anticholinergic agents in COPD are especially useful when combined with short-acting or long-acting β₂-agonists. Tiotropium is effective in patients with stable COPD for up to 24 hours and should not be combined with short-acting anticholinergic agents, such as ipratropium. Mucolytic agents have little effect on lung function. The antioxidant *N*-acetylcysteine, a drug with both mucolytic and antioxidant action, did not reduce the number of exacerbations of COPD in a large prospective 3-year trial. Oral corticosteroids are not recommended for regular use in a long-term maintenance program because their use is not associated with superior outcomes compared with standard therapy and is associated with increased side effects.

KEY POINT

Inhaled corticosteroids may offer significant benefit in patients with severe chronic obstructive pulmonary disease.

Bibliography

Littner MR. In the clinic. Chronic obstructive pulmonary disease. Ann Intern Med. 2008;148(5):ITC3-1-ITC3-16. [PMID: 18316750]

Item 22   Answer: D

Educational Objective: *Manage chronic obstructive pulmonary disease exacerbation with noninvasive positive-pressure ventilation.*

The patient is having a moderate to severe exacerbation of chronic obstructive pulmonary disease (COPD) and should be placed on noninvasive positive-pressure ventilation (NPPV). A landmark study found that NPPV reduced the need for intubation, the length of hospital stay, and the mortality rate in such patients. Suitable candidates for NPPV include patients with moderate to severe dyspnea, use of accessory respiratory muscles, respiration rate greater than 25/min, and pH less than 7.35 with P_{CO_2} greater than 45 mm Hg (6.0 kPa). Contraindications to NPPV include impending respiratory arrest, cardiovascular instability, altered mental status, high aspiration risk, production of copious secretions, and extreme obesity, as well as surgery, trauma, or deformity of the face or upper airway.

Intubation is inappropriate because the patient is not in respiratory arrest and is a suitable candidate for NPPV. However, if the patient's condition deteriorates or does not improve after 1 to 2 hours of NPPV, intubation should be considered. Most patients with exacerbations of COPD are usually easily oxygenated on low levels of inspired oxygen, as was the patient in this case. Excessive oxygen supplementation can worsen carbon dioxide retention during a COPD exacerbation. Therefore, oxygen should be titrated to maintain a saturation of approximately 90%; increasing the nasal oxygen to 5 L/min is not indicated at this time.

Methylxanthines are generally not recommended for the treatment of acute exacerbations of COPD because they are not more effective than inhaled bronchodilators and corticosteroid therapy but can cause nausea and vomiting.

KEY POINT

Noninvasive positive-pressure ventilation should be initiated early in the course of moderate or severe exacerbations of chronic obstructive pulmonary disease.

Bibliography
Littner MR. In the clinic. Chronic obstructive pulmonary disease. Ann Intern Med. 2008;148(5):ITC3-1-ITC3-16. [PMID: 18316750]

Item 23   Answer: D

Educational Objective: *Prescribe pulmonary rehabilitation for a patient with severe chronic obstructive pulmonary disease.*

This patient, who is on maximum medical treatment for chronic obstructive pulmonary disease (COPD) and is still symptomatic, would benefit from pulmonary rehabilitation. Comprehensive pulmonary rehabilitation includes patient education, exercise training, psychosocial support, and nutritional intervention as well as the evaluation for oxygen supplementation. Referral should be considered for any patient with chronic respiratory disease who remains symptomatic or has decreased functional status despite otherwise optimal medical therapy. Pulmonary rehabilitation increases exercise capacity, reduces dyspnea, improves quality of life, and decreases health care utilization.

Lung transplantation should be considered in patients who are hospitalized with COPD exacerbation complicated by hypercapnia (P_{CO_2} greater than 50 mm Hg [6.7 kPa]) and patients with FEV_1 not exceeding 20% of predicted and either homogeneous disease on high-resolution CT scan or D_{LCO} less than 20% of predicted who are at high risk of death after lung volume reduction surgery. Lung transplantation is, therefore, not an option for this patient.

The effect of lung volume reduction surgery is larger in patients with predominantly upper-lobe disease and limited exercise performance after rehabilitation. The ideal candidate should have an FEV_1 between 20% and 35% of predicted, a D_{LCO} no lower than 20% of predicted, hyperinflation, and limited comorbidities.

There is no indication for nocturnal assisted ventilation in this patient because she does not have daytime hypercapnia and worsening oxygen desaturation during sleep.

KEY POINT

Pulmonary rehabilitation in patients with advanced lung disease can increase exercise capacity, decrease dyspnea, improve quality of life, and decrease health care utilization.

Bibliography
ZuWallack R, Hedges H. Primary care of the patient with chronic obstructive pulmonary disease – part 3: pulmonary rehabilitation and comprehensive care for the patient with chronic obstructive pulmonary disease. Am J Med. 2008;121(suppl 7):S25-S32. [PMID: 18558104]

Item 24   Answer: A

Educational Objective: *Diagnose α_1-antitrypsin deficiency.*

This patient may have α_1-antitrypsin (AAT) deficiency, a clinically underdiagnosed disorder that primarily affects the lungs but also the liver and, rarely, the skin. AAT protects against proteolytic degradation of elastin, a protein that promotes elasticity of connective tissue. The normal plasma concentration of AAT is 150 to 350 mg/dL (1.5 to 3.5 g/L). Patients with plasma levels lower than 50 to 80 mg/dL (0.5 to 0.8 g/L) have severe deficiency. In the lungs, severe deficiency of AAT predisposes to early-onset chronic obstructive pulmonary disease, especially panacinar emphysema, which involves the lung bases. This patient is younger than 45 years and has bilateral basilar emphysema, and, therefore, AAT deficiency must be ruled out.

The sweat chloride test is a screening test for cystic fibrosis. Nearly 10% of patients diagnosed with cystic fibrosis are older than 18 years. Of these patients, gastrointestinal symptoms and infertility are the most common presenting problems. In cystic fibrosis lung disease, chest radiography typically shows hyperinflation and accentuated bronchovascular markings, appearing first in the upper lobes, followed by bronchiectasis and cyst formation. This patient's age, presenting symptoms, and chest radiograph findings make cystic fibrosis unlikely.

A flow volume loop, which includes forced inspiratory and expiratory maneuvers, is indicated for patients with unexplained dyspnea and can detect upper airway obstruction that cannot be diagnosed with spirometry. However, this patient has no physical findings suggestive of upper airway obstruction (for example, stridor), and even if such findings were present, they would not explain the patient's findings on chest radiography.

High-resolution CT scan is not helpful in the diagnosis of AAT deficiency, although it may be useful in evaluating the extent of the disease.

KEY POINT

Patients with severe α_1-antitryspin deficiency are predisposed to early-onset chronic obstructive pulmonary disease, especially panacinar emphysema, which involves the lung bases.

Bibliography

American Thoracic Society; European Respiratory Society. American Thoracic Society/European Respiratory Society Standards for the diagnosis and management of individuals with alpha 1 antitryspin deficiency. Am J Respir Crit Care Med. 2003;168(7):818-900. [PMID: 14522813]

Item 25   Answer: D

Educational Objective: *Evaluate a patient with probable obstructive sleep apnea with polysomnography and arterial blood gases.*

Polysomnography and arterial blood gas measurement should be performed next to evaluate this patient. Although snoring, morning headaches, and daytime sleepiness are common symptoms of obstructive sleep apnea (OSA), clinical and physical examination features are neither sensitive nor specific enough for the diagnosis. Polysomnography is required to determine the presence and severity of OSA. However, this patient also has low oxygen saturation while awake as measured by pulse oximetry, suggesting the presence of obesity-hypoventilation syndrome. The symptoms of obesity-hypoventilation syndrome are the same as obstructive sleep apnea, and most patients with obesity-hypoventilation syndrome also have obstructive sleep apnea. The diagnosis is established by documenting alveolar hypoventilation (PCO_2 >45 mm Hg [6.0 kPa]) in the absence of other known causes. Additional studies to evaluate other causes of alveolar hypoventilation include chest x-ray and pulmonary function testing.

B-type natriuretic peptide (BNP) may be helpful for differentiating heart failure from noncardiac causes of shortness of breath in the acute setting. Patients presenting to the emergency department with acute dyspnea with a serum BNP concentration less than 100 pg/mL are unlikely to have acute

heart failure. However, this patient does not have acute dyspnea or any signs of heart failure, and BNP testing is not indicated. Additionally, factors other than ventricular wall stress that influence BNP levels include renal failure, older age, and female sex, all of which increase BNP, and obesity, which reduces BNP. Interpretation of BNP results should take these factors into account.

The CAC score correlates with cardiovascular risk but is not a direct measure of the severity of luminal coronary disease, and CAC scores are not indicated for routine screening. CAC measurement may be considered in asymptomatic patients with an intermediate risk of coronary artery disease (10%-20% 10-year risk), because a high CAC score is an indication for more intensive preventive medical treatment. This patient may have an increased risk of coronary artery disease, and a lipid profile and use of the Framingham risk calculator will estimate the patient's 10-year risk for a major cardiovascular event. However, an abnormal CAC cannot explain the patient's symptoms or waking hypoxemia and is, therefore, not the most appropriate next diagnostic test.

A CT pulmonary angiogram is a reasonable diagnostic test if pulmonary embolism is a consideration. However, the patient has no symptoms referable to possible pulmonary embolism such as dyspnea and chest pain. Pulmonary embolism should be considered in all patients with obstructive sleep apnea and compatible symptoms, because it is a frequent cause of death in this group of patients.

KEY POINT

The symptoms of obesity-hypoventilation syndrome are the same as obstructive sleep apnea, and most patients with obesity-hypoventilation syndrome also have obstructive sleep apnea.

Bibliography

Piper AJ, Grunstein RR. Obesity hypoventilation syndrome: mechanisms and management. Am J Respir Crit Care Med. 2011;183(3):292-98. [PMID: 21037018]

Item 26   Answer: D

Educational Objective: *Diagnose obstructive sleep apnea as a secondary cause of hypertension.*

The next diagnostic test should be polysomnography. Risk factors for obstructive sleep apnea (OSA) include excessive body weight, abnormalities of craniofacial anatomy, male sex, underlying medical or neurologic disorders (myxedema, acromegaly, and stroke), alcohol use, certain medications (muscle relaxants, sedatives, opioids, and anesthetics), and aging. Patients with untreated OSA have a greater likelihood of developing systemic and pulmonary arterial hypertension, coronary artery disease, acute myocardial infarction during sleep, heart failure, recurrent atrial fibrillation, stroke, insulin resistance, mood disorders, and parasomnias. OSA may also negatively affect quality of life and academic and occupational performance, may increase the risk of vehicular and work-related accidents, and may increase the overall mortality rate.

Polysomnography is required to determine the presence and severity of OSA. Therapy is recommended for all patients with OSA and excessive daytime sleepiness, insomnia, impaired cognition, mood disorder, hypertension, ischemic heart disease, or stroke. Treatment of OSA modestly reduces blood pressure in many, but not all, patients with hypertension.

A 24-hour urine free cortisol measurement is a screening test for Cushing syndrome. Although patients with hypercortisolism may develop obesity and hypertension, this patient has few other findings compatible with this disorder such as muscle weakness, ecchymosis, hypokalemia, unexplained osteoporosis, and diabetes mellitus. Percutaneous renal artery angiography is used to diagnose renal artery stenosis. Atherosclerotic renovascular disease is usually associated with widespread atherosclerosis, peripheral vascular disease, cardiovascular disease, and ischemic target organ damage, which is not evident in this patient. The ratio of plasma aldosterone to plasma renin activity is the preferred screening test for hyperaldosteronism. Hyperaldosteronism causes hypertension, hypokalemia, and metabolic alkalosis. Because these findings are not present in this patient, a plasma aldosterone–renin activity ratio is not indicated.

KEY POINT

Patients with untreated obstructive sleep apnea have a greater likelihood of developing systemic hypertension.

Bibliography
Bagai K. Obstructive sleep apnea, stroke, and cardiovascular diseases. Neurologist. 2010;16(6):329-39. [PMID: 21150380]

Item 27   Answer: C
Educational Objective: *Diagnose cryptogenic organizing pneumonia.*

The most likely diagnosis is cryptogenic organizing pneumonia (COP). This nonsmoker without any exposure history has acute to subacute development of nonspecific systemic and respiratory symptoms with a dominant alveolar (opacification) process on chest radiograph. The tempo of the disease process is the key to differentiating COP from other interstitial lung diseases. COP is often acute or subacute, with symptom onset occurring within 2 months of presentation in the majority of patients. The presentation is so suggestive of an acute or subacute lower respiratory tract infection that patients have almost always been treated with and failed to respond to one or more courses of antibiotics before diagnosis.

The diagnosis of asbestosis is based on a convincing history of asbestos exposure and definite evidence of interstitial fibrosis. The most specific finding on chest radiograph is bilateral partially calcified pleural plaques. This patient lacks an exposure history, an interstitial infiltrate and evidence of pleural disease, making asbestosis an unlikely diagnosis.

Community-acquired pneumonia is an acute infectious process that progresses over days, not weeks, and would have responded to levofloxacin.

Idiopathic pulmonary fibrosis (IPF) typically follows a prolonged course with evidence of respiratory symptoms and radiographic findings that progress slowly over months or years. Radiographic findings in COP are also distinct from those in IPF. A dominant alveolar opacification process is typically present in patients with COP. The opacities are almost always bilateral with varied distribution. One of the key radiographic features of COP is the tendency for COP opacities to "migrate" or involve different areas of the lung on serial examinations. Although the radiographic findings of IPF are varied, it has a dominant interstitial (reticular) pattern with or without opacities.

KEY POINT

Cryptogenic organizing pneumonia most often presents with subacute disease progression and bilateral alveolar-filling opacities on chest radiograph.

Bibliography
Ryu JH, Daniels CE, Hartman TE, et al. Diagnosis of interstitial lung diseases. Mayo Clin Proc. 2007;82(8):976-986. [PMID: 17673067]

Item 28   Answer: A
Educational Objective: *Diagnose asbestosis.*

The diagnosis of asbestosis is based on a convincing history of asbestos exposure with an appropriately long latent period (10 to 15 years) and definite evidence of interstitial fibrosis without other likely causes. This patient worked as an insulator when asbestos exposure was still widespread and is at risk for asbestos-related lung disease. The most specific finding on chest radiograph is bilateral partially calcified pleural plaques. Pleural plaques are focal, often partially calcified, fibrous tissue collections on the parietal pleura and are considered a marker of asbestos exposure.

Idiopathic pulmonary fibrosis presents with slowly progressive dyspnea and a chronic, nonproductive cough. The chest radiograph is almost always abnormal at the time of presentation, with decreased lung volumes and basal reticular opacities. Almost all patients have a physiologic restrictive process (decreased FVC, total lung capacity, functional residual capacity) as well as impaired gas exchange with a decreased D_{LCO}. However, asbestosis is a much more likely diagnosis in a patient with a positive exposure history and radiographic evidence of pleural plaques.

Sarcoidosis occurs most commonly in young and middle-aged adults, with a peak incidence in the third decade. More than 90% of patients with sarcoidosis have lung involvement. The chest radiograph may show hilar lymphadenopathy alone, hilar lymphadenopathy and reticular opacities predominantly in the upper lung zone, or reticular opacities without hilar lymphadenopathy. Pulmonary function tests may reveal a restrictive pattern and reduction in D$_{LCO}$ or may be normal. The patient's age, predominantly lower lobe involvement, occupational history, and pleural plaques argue against pulmonary sarcoidosis.

Rheumatoid lung disease has many manifestations, including an interstitial lung disease, which is most common in patients with severe rheumatoid arthritis. This patient does not have evidence of rheumatoid arthritis.

KEY POINT

Pleural plaques are focal, often partially calcified, fibrous tissue collections on the parietal pleura and are a marker of asbestos exposure.

Bibliography

Aberle DR, Balmes JR. Computed tomography of asbestos-related pulmonary parenchymal and pleural disease. Clin Chest Med. 1991;12(1): 115-131. [PMID: 2009740]

Item 29   Answer: C

Educational Objective: *Diagnose secondary polycythemia due to sleep apnea.*

This obese man most likely has sleep apnea with secondary polycythemia. Excessive daytime sleepiness is the hallmark of sleep apnea. Other clinical manifestations that should alert the clinician to the presence of sleep apnea include morning headaches, nocturia, and alterations in mood. Hypoxia is the main inducer of erythropoietin production by the proximal nephrons, and an elevated erythropoietin level strongly supports a diagnosis of secondary polycythemia. Some patients with cardiopulmonary disease or sleep apnea will not show reduced oxygen saturation at rest or during the daytime. In these cases, pulse oximetry should be obtained after exertion, and, depending on the clinical history, sleep studies may be indicated to confirm the diagnosis of sleep apnea and to detect nocturnal oxygen desaturation. In patients with sleep apnea, the secondary polycythemia will most likely resolve once the sleep apnea is corrected.

Congenital polycythemia due to a high-oxygen–affinity hemoglobin is suspected when polycythemia is discovered during childhood or when it is associated with a positive family history of polycythemia. In these cases, the serum erythropoietin level is normal. This patient lacks an appropriate childhood or family history, and his normal hematocrit 5 years ago and elevated erythropoietin level argue against a high-oxygen–affinity hemoglobin.

Polycythemia vera is characterized by a low serum erythropoietin level and an increased erythrocyte mass and may be accompanied by mild elevation in leukocyte and platelet counts. Hematocrit values greater than 60% for men and 56% for women in the absence of secondary causes of erythrocytosis and the presence of splenomegaly establish the diagnosis of polycythemia vera. A *JAK2* mutation is detected in 95% of patients with polycythemia vera, and a polymerase chain reaction assay for this mutation can aid in establishing the differential from secondary causes of erythrocytosis. This patient's history, which is strongly suggestive of sleep apnea, argues strongly against the diagnosis of polycythemia vera.

Relative polycythemia often accompanies plasma volume contraction as a result of excessive sweating, diarrhea, vomiting, capillary leak syndrome, and, occasionally, diuretic use. The hematocrit or hemoglobin appears increased because of a reduction in plasma volume. There is nothing in the history to suggest the presence of relative polycythemia, and relative polycythemia is not associated with an increase in the erythropoietin level as seen in this case.

KEY POINT

Sleep apnea with nocturnal hypoxemia may be associated with secondary polycythemia.

Bibliography

Lengfelder E, Merx K, Hehlmann R. Diagnosis and therapy of polycythemia vera. Semin Thromb Hemost. 2006;32(3):267-275. [PMID: 16673281]

Item 30   Answer: B

Educational Objective: *Diagnose scleroderma-related diffuse parenchymal lung disease.*

The most appropriate next diagnostic test is high resolution chest CT. Connective tissue diseases, along with drugs and environmental causes, are the most common known causes of diffuse parenchymal lung disease (DPLD). DPLD is most likely in patients with systemic sclerosis who develop anti-topoisomerase I (anti–Scl-70) antibody positivity. DPLD associated with systemic sclerosis usually manifests as dyspnea, dry cough, and decreased exercise tolerance. Fine bibasilar crackles that extend into late inspiration are heard on physical examination. On pulmonary function testing, these patients have a restrictive pattern with a decreased FVC and D$_{LCO}$ (and normal FEV$_1$/FVC ratio). High-resolution CT (HRCT) is more sensitive than chest x-ray for DPLD and reveals ground-glass and reticular linear opacities, subpleural cysts, and honeycombing in patients with advanced disease. Together, the clinical findings and HRCT can establish the diagnosis in this patient.

If the clinical context, temporal pattern of disease, and HRCT findings do not yield a diagnosis, it may be reasonable to obtain a bronchoscopic or surgical lung biopsy. The diagnostic yield of surgical lung biopsy is approximately 90%. However, a limited number of histopathologic patterns are recognized for a large number of DPLDs, and the specificity of lung biopsy depends on the pattern. Bronchoalveolar lavage can provide additional diagnostic information, including culture, cytology, and cell differential. Bronchoalveolar lavage is safe and simple to perform and may be helpful to diagnose infections and carcinoma, as well as eosinophilic pneumonia. Neither test is recommended before an HRCT.

In patients with systemic sclerosis, pulmonary vascular disease may manifest as isolated pulmonary arterial hypertension (PAH) or as a complication of vascular obliteration in patients with DPLD. Patients with PAH may present with fatigue, decreased exercise tolerance, dyspnea, or syncope. Physical examination findings include an increased P_2 and a persistently split S_2. Chest radiographs are usually normal. A decrease in DLCO in the setting of normal lung volumes is consistent with PAH. This patient has a restrictive physiology on pulmonary function testing and no physical examination findings to support PAH.

KEY POINT

Connective tissue diseases, along with drugs and environmental causes, are the most common known causes of diffuse parenchymal lung disease

Bibliography

Eickelberg O, Selman M. Update in diffuse parenchymal lung disease 2009. Am J Respir Crit Care Med. 2010;181(9):883-8. [PMID: 20430925]

Item 31   Answer: C

Educational Objective: *Diagnose drug-induced lung toxicity.*

The most likely diagnosis is drug-induced lung toxicity. A high index of suspicion for drug-induced lung disease is essential, because early identification and drug withdrawal can prevent morbidity and mortality. Establishment of a definitive diagnosis of drug-induced lung disease requires exclusion of other known causes and symptom improvement with drug withdrawal. Most offending drugs cause a hypersensitivity-type reaction, with presenting symptoms of fatigue, low-grade fever, and cough. Peripheral blood eosinophilia may be present. Amiodarone is a well-known cause of drug-induced lung toxicity, and this diagnosis is supported by the temporal relationship between starting amiodarone for atrial fibrillation and onset of symptoms.

The diagnosis of heart failure is unlikely in the absence of orthopnea, jugular venous distention, or an S_3. Additionally, heart failure cannot account for the patient's low-grade fever and eosinophilia.

Acute eosinophilic pneumonitis is a rapidly progressive illness occurring over days to 3 weeks associated with fever, sputum production, eosinophilia, and a peripherally distributed infiltrate. The patient's subacute illness that began 2 months ago is not consistent with this diagnosis nor is the pattern of infiltrates on her chest x-ray.

The term asbestosis refers to bilateral interstitial fibrosis of the lung parenchyma caused by inhalation of asbestos fibers. An exposure history of appropriate duration, latency (typically 20-30 years), and intensity and radiographic evidence of interstitial fibrosis on chest radiograph or chest CT scan are usually sufficient for diagnosis. Symptoms include breathlessness, bibasilar inspiratory crackles, and digital clubbing and pulmonary function testing showing a restrictive pattern. This patient has a subacute process and no history of asbestos exposure, making asbestosis an unlikely diagnosis.

KEY POINT

Drug-induced lung toxicity typically presents as a hypersensitivity-type reaction, with symptoms of fatigue, low-grade fever, cough, and peripheral eosinophilia.

Bibliography

Dempsey OJ, Kerr KM, Remmen H, Denison AR. How to investigate a patient with suspected interstitial lung disease. BMJ. 2010;340:c2843. [PMID: 20534676]

Item 32   Answer: D

Educational Objective: *Prevent deep venous thrombosis with prophylactic unfractionated heparin.*

The most appropriate venous thrombosis prophylactic intervention for this patient is unfractionated heparin. Preventing venous thromboembolism (VTE) was the highest ranked intervention for patient safety in a recent Agency for Healthcare Research and Quality report. Appropriate prophylaxis can reduce the rate of VTE by approximately two thirds; however, various studies have shown suboptimal use of prophylaxis in medical and surgical patients. The American College of Chest Physicians (ACCP) guidelines recommends the use of unfractionated heparin, low-molecular-weight heparin (LMWH), and fondaparinux for prevention of venous thromboembolism in hospitalized, medically ill patients. In patients with renal impairment (glomerular filtration rate <30 mL/min/ 1.73 m^2), dosing of LMWH must be adjusted and fondaparinux is contraindicated.

ACCP guidelines state that aspirin should not be used as the sole prophylaxis in any high-risk group because it is not as effective as equally safe alternatives. The evidence for graduated compression stockings in the prevention of venous thromboembolism is weak, and compression stockings are not recommended as primary prophylaxis in hospitalized patients.

Three direct thrombin inhibitors are in clinical use: lepirudin, the recombinant form of the leech enzyme hirudin; bivalirudin, an engineered form of hirudin that alters its thrombin-binding capacity and half-life; and argatroban, a small molecule that binds irreversibly to the active site of thrombin. Each of these is a parenterally administered drug with limited Food and Drug Administration–approved indications, and all require therapeutic monitoring. Lepirudin should be considered when a patient has heparin-induced thrombocytopenia, which is not present in this patient. Additionally, lepirudin is very expensive. Lepirudin is not indicated for routine prevention of venous thromboembolism in the hospitalized, medically-ill patient.

Unfractionated heparin, low-molecular-weight heparin (LMWH), and fondaparinux can be used for prevention of venous thromboembolism in hospitalized, medically ill patients.

Bibliography
Goodacre S. In the clinic. Deep venous thrombosis. Ann Intern Med. 2008;149(5):ITC3-1. [PMID: 18765697]

Item 33   Answer: E
Educational Objective: *Diagnose acute pulmonary embolism with a ventilation/perfusion scan.*

A ventilation/perfusion lung scan should be done next. This patient is at high risk for pulmonary embolism (PE) because of his recent hospitalization, cancer, and nephrotic syndrome. A positive ventilation/perfusion scan would confirm the diagnosis of PE in this patient with a high pretest probability for the condition, especially in the absence of parenchymal lung defects on chest radiograph.

The probability of PE is very high based on this patient's presentation that included chest pain, dyspnea, recent hospitalization and surgery, active cancer, and protein-losing nephropathy. A negative D-dimer test would not be sufficient evidence to rule out a PE under these circumstances, and a high D-dimer level would add little to the diagnostic evaluation.

CT angiography is an acceptable modality to diagnose acute PE but requires a significant amount of contrast infusion, which would be contraindicated in a patient with an elevated serum creatinine level.

Lower extremity ultrasonography can disclose asymptomatic deep venous thrombosis in a small percentage of patients presenting with symptoms of PE. However, the yield is relatively low and ventilation/perfusion scanning would have a much higher degree of accuracy.

Decreased antithrombin III levels may result from nephrotic syndrome, and levels are lowered during acute thrombosis, especially during treatment with heparin. Therefore, measuring antithrombin III would add little to the accuracy of the diagnosis of PE or have any implication for immediate management decisions.

KEY POINT
Ventilation/perfusion scanning is an appropriate noninvasive test to diagnose acute pulmonary embolism, especially in the presence of chronic kidney disease.

Bibliography
Agnelli G, Becattini C. Acute pulmonary embolism. N Engl J Med. 2010;363(3):266-74. [PMID: 20592294]

Item 34   Answer: B
Educational Objective: *Evaluate low-probability venous thrombosis with a D-dimer test.*

The most appropriate next diagnostic test is a D-dimer assay. Several imaging procedures can exclude deep venous thrombosis (DVT), but the diagnostic goal is to use the most efficient, least invasive, and least expensive method with the fewest side effects. A D-dimer assay is a simple, relatively noninvasive test that has been shown to have a high negative predictive value, especially if the suspicion for DVT is low. The Wells criteria have been established to help the clinician assess the likelihood of DVT, and studies have shown that with a low clinical suspicion (as in this patient) and a negative D-dimer assay, the presence of DVT can be reliably excluded without the need for more invasive or complex imaging.

In the Wells criteria, the following clinical variables each earn 1 point: active cancer; paralysis or recent plaster cast; recent immobilization or major surgery; tenderness along the deep veins; swelling of the entire leg; greater than a 3-cm difference in calf circumference compared with the other leg; pitting edema; and collateral superficial veins. The clinical suspicion that an alternative diagnosis is likely earns -2 points. Based on this system, the pretest probability of DVT is considered high in patients with scores of greater than or equal to 3, moderate in patients with scores of 1 to 2, and low in patients with scores less than or equal to 0. This patient's Wells score is -2, and the likelihood for DVT is therefore low. This patient's fever, circumscribed area of warmth, and tenderness localized to the posterior calf could represent cellulitis, a reasonable alternative to the diagnosis of venous thrombosis.

Venography, the traditional gold standard for diagnosis of DVT, is rarely performed today because of its invasiveness, discomfort, costs, and complexity. Neither an MRI nor CT of the leg has been substantially validated as a reliable diagnostic test for DVT.

KEY POINT
Negative D-dimer assay results and a low Wells criteria probability score reliably exclude a diagnosis of deep venous thrombosis.

Bibliography
Hargett CW, Tapson VF. Clinical probability and D-dimer testing: how should we use them in clinical practice? Semin Respir Crit Care Med. 2008;29(1):15-24. [PMID: 18302083]

Item 35   Answer: D
Educational Objective: *Treat a patient with an idiopathic deep venous thrombosis with heparin.*

The appropriate treatment for a patient with deep venous thrombosis that is either idiopathic or associated with a transient risk factor is an initial short course of an immediate-acting anticoagulant such as unfractionated heparin, low-molecular-weight heparin, or fondaparinux for at least 5 days. Warfarin should be started at approximately the same time that heparin is administered, and the two drugs should be overlapped until the INR reaches a therapeutic range (>2) measured on two occasions approximately 24 hours apart. This timing allows for further reduction of prothrombin, the vitamin K–dependent factor with the longest half-life (approximately 60 h), which is responsible for much of the antithrombotic effect of warfarin. Usually 5 to 7 days of therapy are required to achieve this therapeutic level. The initial recommended daily warfarin dose is 5 mg, but occasionally 7.5 to 10 mg may be used. Lower doses (2.5 mg) are recommended in the elderly, especially in the setting of malnourishment, liver disease, or recent major surgery.

KEY POINT

Treatment of deep venous thrombosis consists of an immediate-acting anticoagulant such as unfractionated heparin, low-molecular-weight heparin, or fondaparinux for at least 5 days.

Bibliography

Gage BF, Fihn SD, White RH. Management and dosing of warfarin therapy. Am J Med. 2000;109(6):481-488. [PMID: 11042238]

Rheumatology

Questions

Item 1 [Basic]

A 60-year-old woman has noted recurrent, right elbow pain. The pain occurs mainly with the use of the arm and hand, not with bending the elbow. She has noted no pain or tenderness in other joints.

Examination of the right arm shows marked tenderness over the lateral epicondyle. The elbow range of motion is normal, and there is no redness or swelling. Resisted wrist extension exacerbates the elbow pain.

Which one of the following is the most likely diagnosis?

(A) Cubital tunnel syndrome
(B) Lateral epicondylitis
(C) Olecranon bursitis
(D) Septic arthritis

Item 2 [Advanced]

A 45-year-old woman is evaluated in the office for a 3-month history of pain, stiffness, and swelling of the small joints of the hands and feet. She also has increasing fatigue that has caused her to miss work at least 1 day per week. She has no other medical problems.

On physical examination, the vital signs and general physical examination, including skin examination, are normal. A photograph of one of her hands is shown (Plate 29).

Complete blood count, serum chemistries, and urinalysis are all normal. Erythrocyte sedimentation rate is 44 mm/h.

Which of the following is the most likely diagnosis?

(A) Osteoarthritis
(B) Psoriatic arthritis
(C) Rheumatoid arthritis
(D) Systemic lupus erythematosus

Item 3 [Basic]

A 78-year-old obese woman is evaluated because right hip pain that worsens when she goes up and down stairs. She says that she cannot sleep on her right side because of pain over the hip and can localize the pain by pointing the lateral aspect of her hip. She has been active and in good health.

On physical examination, moving the hip through rotation, flexion, and extension does not elicit pain, but abduction reproduces the pain minimally. There is full, unrestricted range of motion. There is tenderness to pressure over the lateral aspect of the right hip.

Which of the following is the most likely diagnosis?

(A) Avascular necrosis of the femoral head
(B) Osteoarthritis
(C) Rheumatoid arthritis
(D) Trochanteric bursitis

Item 4 [Basic]

A 35-year-old woman is evaluated for a 5-day history of acute right knee pain that began when she hopped down from the bed of a truck, twisting her knee. She experienced a popping sensation and a gradual onset of knee joint swelling over the next several hours. Since then, she has continued to have moderate pain, particularly when walking up or down stairs. She reports no locking or giving way of the knee or any previous knee injury.

On physical examination, the right knee has a minimal effusion with full range of motion. The medial aspect of the joint line is tender to palpation. Maximally flexing the hip and knee and applying abduction (valgus) force to the knee while externally rotating the foot and passively extending the knee (McMurray test) result in a palpable snap but no crepitus.

Which of the following is the most likely diagnosis?

(A) Anserine bursitis
(B) Anterior cruciate ligament tear
(C) Meniscal tear
(D) Patellofemoral pain syndrome

Item 5 [Advanced]

A 66-year-old woman is evaluated because of right knee pain of 4 weeks' duration. Although the knee is stiff for 20 to 30 minutes in the morning, she does not have much pain at work. Walking up the stairs in her house, however, causes a good deal of pain, which is not relieved by ibuprofen or acetaminophen. Kneeling also causes pain. Knee radiographs done 6 weeks ago show mild medial compartment osteoarthritis bilaterally.

On physical examination, she is overweight. There is coarse crepitus with flexion and extension of the right knee. Both knees are in slight varus angulation ("bow-legged"). On palpation, there is tenderness along the joint margins of both knees and exquisite tenderness to digital pressure at the medial upper tibia on the right that reproduces her pain. In addition, with the patient's right knee semiflexed, palpation along the medial semimembranous tendinous (hamstring) edge of the thigh elicits pain when the examining fingers meet the tibia.

Which of the following is most likely responsible for the exacerbation of the right knee pain?

(A) Anserine bursitis
(B) Gout
(C) Osteoarthritis
(D) Rheumatoid arthritis

Item 6 [Basic]

A 47-year-old man is evaluated for right lateral shoulder pain. He has been pitching during batting practice for his son's baseball team for the past 2 months. He has shoulder pain when lifting his right arm overhead and also when lying on the shoulder while sleeping. Acetaminophen does not relieve the pain.

On physical examination, he has no shoulder deformities or swelling. Range of motion is normal. He has subacromial tenderness to palpation, with shoulder pain elicited at 60 degrees of passive abduction. He also has pain with resisted mid-arc abduction but no pain with resisted elbow flexion or forearm supination. He is able to lower his right arm smoothly from a fully abducted position, and his arm strength for abduction and external rotation against resistance is normal.

Which of the following is the most likely diagnosis?

(A) Adhesive capsulitis
(B) Bicipital tendinitis
(C) Glenohumeral arthritis
(D) Rotator cuff tear (complete)
(E) Rotator cuff tendinitis

Item 7 [Advanced]

A 59-year-old woman is evaluated for a 3-week history of pain in the right upper scapula and trapezius areas. There are no paresthesias.

On physical examination, the shoulder has full range of motion without eliciting worse pain or altering the character of the pain. There is no sign of rotator cuff pain or weakness with testing against resistance. There are no signs of impingement. The shoulder apprehension test is negative. Strength, deep tendon reflexes, and sensation are normal bilaterally.

What is the most appropriate next step in this patient's management?

(A) Chest radiograph
(B) Intra-articular corticosteroid injection
(C) Physical therapy
(D) Radiograph of the shoulder
(E) Skeletal muscle relaxant

Item 8 [Advanced]

An 82-year-old woman is evaluated for a flare of polymyalgia rheumatica manifested by aching in the shoulders and hips that began 2 weeks ago. She also has fatigue and malaise. She was diagnosed with polymyalgia rheumatica 8 months ago. At that time, she was prescribed prednisone, 20 mg/d; her symptoms promptly resolved; and her prednisone dosage was grad-

ually tapered. Four months ago, her prednisone dosage was decreased from 7.5 mg/d to 5 mg/d, and her symptoms returned. Her prednisone dosage was then increased to 10 mg/d followed by a slow taper of this agent. Her prednisone dosage was most recently decreased from 7 mg/d to 6 mg/d, which is her current dosage. She also takes calcium and vitamin D supplements and a bisphosphonate.

On physical examination, vital signs are normal. Range of motion of the shoulders, neck, and hips elicits mild pain. There is no temporal artery tenderness.

Which of the following is the most appropriate treatment for this patient?

(A) Increase prednisone to 20 mg/d
(B) Increase prednisone to 7.5 mg/d; add methotrexate
(C) Increase prednisone to 20 mg/d; add methotrexate
(D) Increase prednisone to 7.5 mg/d; add infliximab

Item 9 [Advanced]

A 62-year-old woman is evaluated for a 3-day history of fever and left knee pain and swelling. She has a 30-year history of rheumatoid arthritis treated with methotrexate and nonsteroidal anti-inflammatory drugs. She has no other medical problems.

On physical examination, temperature is 37.8°C (100.0°F), blood pressure is 140/78 mm Hg, pulse rate is 86/min, and respiration rate is 14/min. The left knee is swollen, red, warm, and tender to palpation. Range of motion is limited because of pain.

Arthrocentesis is performed, and the following results are reported: synovial fluid leukocyte count 75,000/µL (75 × 10^9/L) with 69% neutrophils. Gram stain is positive for gram-positive cocci.

Which would be the most appropriate initial antibiotic therapy pending culture results?

(A) Cefazolin
(B) Ceftriaxone
(C) Nafcillin
(D) Vancomycin

Item 10 [Basic]

A 32-year-old woman is evaluated in the emergency department for a 4-day history of pain and swelling of the right wrist and low-grade fever. She has a 7-year history of severe rheumatoid arthritis. She does not recall any specific trauma involving the wrist but has recently been very physically active. Medications are methotrexate, a folic acid supplement, etanercept, prednisone, and ibuprofen.

On physical examination, temperature is 37.8°C (100.0°F), blood pressure is 118/68 mm Hg, pulse rate is 90/min, and respiration rate is 18/min. BMI is 22. Cardiopulmonary examination is normal. There is no rash. The right wrist is swollen and tender and has a decreased range of motion. There are a subcutaneous nodule and small flexion deformity on the left elbow but no active synovitis. Mild synovitis is present on the second metacarpophalangeal joints bilaterally. The hips, knees, and feet are not tender or swollen and have full range of motion.

Which of the following diagnostic studies of the wrist will be most helpful in establishing this patient's diagnosis?

(A) Arthrocentesis
(B) Arthroscopy
(C) Bone scan
(D) MRI
(E) Radiography

Item 11 [Advanced]

A 67-year-old man is evaluated in the emergency department for a 2-week history of pain involving the left hip. He has had no fever. Four years ago, he underwent total arthroplasty of the left hip joint to treat osteoarthritis. One month ago, he underwent tooth extraction for an abscessed tooth.

On physical examination, temperature is 36.6°C (98.0°F), blood pressure is normal, and pulse rate is 90/min. Cardiopulmonary examination is normal. A well-healed surgical scar is present over the left hip, and there is no warmth or tenderness. External rotation of the left hip joint is markedly painful.

Laboratory studies reveal an erythrocyte sedimentation rate of 88 mm/h.

Radiograph of the left hip shows a normally seated left hip prosthesis. Fluoroscopic-guided arthrocentesis is performed. The synovial fluid leukocyte count is 38,000/µL (38 x 10⁹/L) (90% neutrophils). Polarized light microscopy of the fluid shows no crystals, and Gram stain is negative. Culture results are pending.

Which of the following is the most likely diagnosis?

(A) Aseptic loosening
(B) Gout
(C) Pigmented villonodular synovitis
(D) Prosthetic joint infection

Item 12 [Basic]

A 36-year-old man is evaluated for the acute onset of a warm swollen right ankle of 3 days' duration. He had a similar episode 2 years ago involving his left great toe that resolved in 5 days. He is otherwise healthy and takes no medications.

On physical examination, temperature is 36.7°C (98.0°F), blood pressure is 140/90 mm Hg, pulse rate is 80/min, and respiration rate is 12/min. Abnormal findings are limited to a warm swollen right ankle with painful range of motion.

An arthrocentesis is performed. Synovial fluid cell count is 30,000/µL (30 × 10⁹/L) with 95% polymorphonuclear cells and 5% lymphocytes. Gram stain is negative for bacteria.

Polarized microscopy demonstrates intracellular monosodium urate crystals.

Which of the following is the most appropriate treatment?

(A) Allopurinol
(B) Colchicine
(C) Febuxostat
(D) Indomethacin

Item 13 [Basic]

A 68-year-old man is evaluated for hyperuricemia. He has had multiple attacks of acute gout typically affecting the great toe, but 2 weeks ago he had an attack involving his right great toe and both ankles. Arthrocentesis confirmed the presence of monosodium urate crystals. He was successfully treated with ibuprofen.

Physical examination is normal except for a tophaceous deposit on the right forefoot.

Laboratory studies are normal except for a serum uric acid level of 11.2 mg/dL (0.7 mmol/L).

Which of the following is the most appropriate therapy for this patient?

(A) Allopurinol
(B) Low-dose colchicine
(C) Low-dose colchicine and allopurinol
(D) Low-dose indomethacin

Item 14 [Basic]

An 82-year-old woman with a 2-year history of osteoarthritis of the knees is evaluated for persistent swelling and pain in the right knee of 3 months' duration. She now uses a cane for ambulation and is unable to go grocery shopping. Medications are naproxen and hydrocodone-acetaminophen as needed.

On physical examination, vital signs are normal. The right knee has a large effusion and a valgus deformity. There is decreased flexion of the right knee secondary to pain and stiffness, and she is unable to fully extend this joint. Range of motion of both knees elicits coarse crepitus.

Laboratory studies reveal a serum creatinine level of 1.1 mg/dL (97.2 µmol/L) and a serum uric acid level of 8.2 mg/dL (0.5 mmol/L).

Radiograph of the right knee reveals a large effusion and changes consistent with end-stage osteoarthritis. Aspiration of the right knee is performed. Synovial fluid leukocyte count is 3200/µL (3.2 x 10⁹/L). Polarized light microscopy of the fluid demonstrates rhomboid-shaped weakly positively birefringent crystals. Results of Gram stain and cultures are pending.

Which of the following is the most likely diagnosis?

(A) Calcium pyrophosphate dihydrate deposition disease
(B) Chronic apatite deposition disease
(C) Gout
(D) Septic arthritis

Item 15 [Advanced]

A 70-year-old male dairy farmer is evaluated for a 1-year history of pain in the left knee that worsens with activity and is relieved with rest. On physical examination, vital signs are normal. A small effusion is present on the left knee, but there is no erythema or warmth. Range of motion of the left knee elicits pain and is slightly limited. Extension of this joint is limited to approximately 10 degrees, but flexion is nearly full. The remainder of the musculoskeletal examination is normal.

The erythrocyte sedimentation rate is 15 mm/h. A standing radiograph of the left knee is shown.

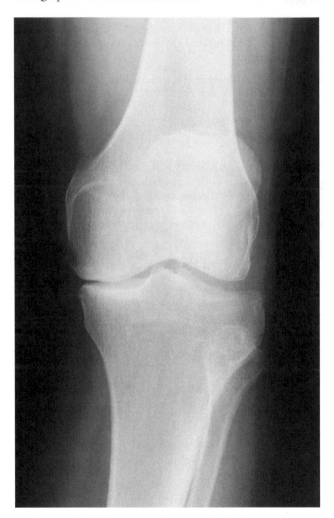

Which of the following is the most likely diagnosis?

(A) Avascular necrosis
(B) Osteoarthritis
(C) Rheumatoid arthritis
(D) Torn medial meniscus

Item 16 [Basic]

A 72-year-old woman is evaluated for a 1-year history of progressive pain in the right knee. The pain is most acute along the medial aspect of the joint, worsens with activity, and is relieved with rest. She has no stiffness in the morning and has had no swelling. She also has not experienced locking or giving away of this joint.

On physical examination, vital signs are normal. There is bony enlargement of the proximal and distal interphalangeal joints. There is no evidence of a right knee effusion. Passive flexion and extension of the right knee are painful.

Laboratory studies, including complete blood count, erythrocyte sedimentation rate, and C-reactive protein, are normal. Radiograph of the right knee also is normal.

In addition to acetaminophen as needed, which of the following is the most appropriate next step in this patient's management?

(A) Arthroscopy
(B) Aspiration of the knee
(C) MRI of the knee
(D) Physical therapy

Item 17 [Basic]

A 60-year-old woman is evaluated for wrist pain of 6 months' duration. The pain is located at the base of the right thumb at the wrist. She is a watercolor artist and a graphic designer and is right handed. The pain is described as a persistent ache for which she takes acetaminophen, which provides moderate relief. She has 20 minutes of morning stiffness in the right thumb that improves with a hot shower.

On physical examination, vital signs are normal. Examination of her hands shows no soft tissue swelling, warmth, or redness of any hand or wrist joints. Bilateral boney hypertrophy of the proximal interphalangeal joints is present bilaterally. Range of motion of the right thumb is limited by pain. Point tenderness is elicited at the base of the right thumb at the first carpometacarpal joint. Circular movement of her right thumb exacerbates the pain. Tapping the flexor retinaculum does not reproduce or aggravate the pain nor does passively stretching the tendons over the radial styloid.

Which of the following is the most likely diagnosis?

(A) Carpal tunnel syndrome
(B) Crystal-induced arthritis
(C) de Quervain tenosynovitis
(D) Osteoarthritis
(E) Rheumatoid arthritis

Item 18 [Basic]

A 67-year-old man is evaluated in the office for acute right knee pain that developed 6 days ago after working on his car. The pain is worse when he walks or climbs stairs and improves when he rests. He has no fever and denies knee stiffness. He has minimal pain relief with maximal dosage of acetaminophen and the application of ice. He has no other medical illness and takes no medications.

On examination, his temperature is 36.8°C (98.2°F), blood pressure is 132/75 mm Hg, heart rate is 92/min and respiratory rate is 14/min. BMI is 27. Moderate valgus deformity of both knees is present. The right knee has a moderate effusion without warmth or erythema. Pain is elicited with passive and active range of motion. The remainder of his examination is normal.

Plain radiographs of his left knee show severe medial joint space narrowing with subchondral sclerosis and osteophyte formation. Analysis of the synovial fluid reveals 1100 leukocytes/μL (1.1 x 10^9/L) (79% lymphocytes, 10 % macrophages).

Which of the following is the best management for this patient's knee pain?

(A) Begin a nonsteroidal anti-inflammatory drug
(B) Begin empiric antibiotics
(C) Inject intra-articular corticosteroids
(D) Obtain right knee magnetic resonance imaging (MRI)
(E) Refer for total knee arthroplasty

Item 19 [Advanced]

A 60-year-old woman is evaluated for bilateral joint pain and swelling in her hands. She has 2 hours of morning stiffness that improves slightly with activity. Acetaminophen and nonsteroidal anti-inflammatory drugs provide only minimal symptom relief. She has no other medical problems and takes no additional medications.

On physical exam, vital signs are normal. She has symmetric joint swelling and tenderness the second and third metacarpophalangeal joints and tenderness over the left fifth metatarsophalangeal joint.

Which of the following test results would most likely support a diagnosis of rheumatoid arthritis in this patient?

(A) Elevated erythrocyte sedimentation rate
(B) Normocytic, normochromic anemia
(C) Positive rheumatoid factor
(D) Radiographs showing marginal joint erosions

Item 20 [Advanced]

A 19-year-old woman with a 4-year history of rheumatoid arthritis is evaluated because of a 3-month history of worsening symptoms. She had previously good disease control with methotrexate. She is otherwise well and denies fevers, night sweats and weight loss.

On physical examination, vital signs are normal. There is active synovitis involving the left first and second metacarpophalangeal joints and right wrist. The remainder of the physical examination is normal.

Hand x-rays reveal a new erosion on the right ulnar styloid and the left second MCP joint.

Initiation of the tumor necrosis factor (TNF)-α inhibitor, adalimumab, is recommended.

Which of the following tests should be performed prior to initiating adalimumab therapy?

(A) Brain MRI
(B) Chest CT
(C) Thyroid stimulating hormone measurement
(D) Tuberculin skin test

Item 21 [Basic]

A 26-year-old woman is evaluated for a 2-month history of pain and swelling in the hands and daily morning stiffness that lasts for 3 to 4 hours. She is 4 months postpartum, and her pregnancy was without complications. She has no history of rash and is otherwise well. Her only medication is ibuprofen, which has not sufficiently relieved her symptoms.

On physical examination, temperature is normal, blood pressure is 110/68 mm Hg, pulse rate is 82/min, and respiration rate is 16/min. The second and third proximal interphalangeal and metacarpophalangeal joints and the wrists are tender and swollen bilaterally.

Laboratory studies show an erythrocyte sedimentation rate of 67 mm/h, and titers of IgM antibodies against parvovirus B19 are negative.

Which of the following is the most likely diagnosis?

(A) Gout
(B) Osteoarthritis
(C) Parvovirus B19 infection
(D) Rheumatoid arthritis

Item 22 [Basic]

A 55-year-old woman is evaluated for a 3-month history of fatigue, morning stiffness lasting for 1 hour, and decreased grip strength. She drinks two glasses of wine daily and is unwilling to stop. Her only medication is over-the-counter ibuprofen, 400 mg three times daily, which has helped to relieve her joint stiffness.

On physical examination, vital signs are normal. Musculoskeletal examination reveals swelling of the metacarpophalangeal and proximal interphalangeal joints of the hands and decreased grip strength. There are effusions on both knees. The remainder of the physical examination is normal.

Erythrocyte sedimentation rate	35 mm/h
C-reactive protein	Normal
Rheumatoid factor	Positive
Antinuclear antibodies	Positive
Anti–cyclic citrullinated peptide antibodies	Positive
Alanine aminotransferase	25 U/L
Aspartate aminotransferase	28 U/L

Radiographs of the hands show soft-tissue swelling but no erosions or joint-space narrowing. Radiographs of the feet are normal.

Which of the following is the most appropriate treatment for this patient?

(A) Add hydroxychloroquine
(B) Add methotrexate
(C) Add subcutaneous etanercept
(D) Increase ibuprofen dosage

Item 23 [Advanced]

A 23-year-old man is evaluated for arthritis of 6 weeks' duration involving his hands and right knee. He also reports a history of psoriasis that began abruptly 3 months ago and has spread rapidly. He has no history of trauma or preceding illness, including diarrhea, urethritis, or conjunctivitis. He has no other medical problems and takes no medications.

On physical examination, temperature is 37.2°C (99.0°F), blood pressure is 120/76 mm Hg, pulse rate is 78/min, and respiration rate is 12/min. A right knee effusion is present. The right knee is erythematous, warm, and tender to palpation with limited range of motion because of pain. The third right toe is swollen and red. Evidence of synovitis is present involving the distal interphalangeal joints of both hands. Typical psoriatic lesions are noted involving the elbows, knees, periumbilical area, sacrum, soles, and palms.

A right knee arthrocentesis is performed and results are compatible with an inflammatory arthritis. Synovial fluid Gram stain is negative and fluid is sent for culture.

Which of the following additional tests should be performed?

(A) Antinuclear antibody
(B) HIV testing
(C) HLA-B27 antigen
(D) Rheumatoid factor

Item 24 [Advanced]

A 28-year-old woman is evaluated for a 3-week history of pain and swelling of the right knee and ankle. For the past 6 weeks, she has had diffuse, crampy abdominal pain. For the past week, the pain has been accompanied by four to six daily episodes of bloody diarrhea and fecal urgency. She has lost approximately 1.5 kg (3.3 lb) since the onset of her symptoms. She has not noticed a rash or other joint or soft-tissue involvement. She has not traveled outside of her hometown and has a monogamous sexual relationship with her husband. She has no other medical problems and does not take any medications.

On physical examination, temperature is 37.7°C (99.9°F), blood pressure is 128/72 mm Hg, pulse rate is 98/min, and respiration rate is 18/min. The abdomen is soft and diffusely tender to palpation. Bowel sounds are normal, and there is no organomegaly. Rectal examination reveals tenderness of the rectal canal and stool associated with bright red blood. The right ankle and knee are swollen and slightly warm to the touch, and range of motion of these joints elicits pain. The remainder of the physical examination is normal.

Plain radiographs of the ankle and knee are normal. Arthrocentesis is performed. Synovial fluid analysis reveals a leukocyte count of 14,000/μL (14 x 10⁹/L) (92% polymorphonuclear cells, 8% macrophages).

Which of the following is the most likely cause of this patient's joint symptoms?

(A) Crystal-induced arthritis
(B) Enteropathic arthritis
(C) Gonococcal arthritis
(D) Whipple disease

Item 25 [Basic]

A 23-year-old man is evaluated in the emergency department for a 5-day history of headache, blurred vision, and right eye pain. His eye pain increases when he attempts to read or when exposed to light. He also has a 3-year history of back stiffness that is worse in the morning and tends to improve as he becomes more active. He does not have arthralgia, arthritis, or rash. He takes no medications and is monogamous.

On physical examination, temperature is 36.8°C (98.2°F), blood pressure is 130/76 mm Hg, pulse rate is 85/min, and respiration rate is 14/min. There are no skin lesions. The appearance of the right eye is shown (Plate 30).

Photophobia is present during the penlight examination of the pupil. Both pupils react to light. An emergency referral is made to an ophthalmologist.

Following resolution of the eye problem, this patient should be evaluated for which of the following systemic diseases?

(A) Ankylosing spondylitis
(B) Sarcoidosis
(C) Sjögren syndrome
(D) Systemic lupus erythematosus

Item 26 [Advanced]

A 26-year-old female electrical engineer is evaluated for a 2-year history of persistent pain and stiffness involving the low back. These symptoms are worse in the morning and are alleviated with exercise and hot showers. There are no radicular symptoms. Her only medication is ibuprofen, which has helped to relieve her symptoms. She has no other medical problems and takes no additional medications.

On physical examination, vital signs are normal. Cutaneous examination is normal. Palpation of the pelvis and low back elicits pain. There is loss of normal lumbar lordosis, and forward flexion of the lumbar spine is decreased. Reflexes and strength are intact.

Radiographs of the lumbar spine and pelvis are normal.

Which of the following studies is most likely to establish the diagnosis in this patient?

(A) Anti–cyclic citrullinated peptide antibodies
(B) Erythrocyte sedimentation rate
(C) HLA-B27
(D) MRI of the sacroiliac joints

Item 27 [Basic]

A 36-year-old woman is evaluated for a 5–month history of fever, joint swelling, and pleuritic chest pain. Her symptoms have not responded to daily naproxen.

On physical examination, temperature is 36.6°C (97.8°F), blood pressure is 140/85 mm Hg, pulse rate is 102/min, and respiration rate is 14/min. She has a shallow, nontender hard palate ulcer and central facial redness sparing the nasolabial folds. She has bilateral synovitis of her wrist and metacarpophalangeal joints.

Hemoglobin	10.7 mg/dL (107 g/L)
Leukocyte count	3000/μL (3 × 10⁹/L)
Antinuclear antibody (ANA)	Positive, 1:640
Urine protein	1.5 g/24 hours

Which of the following serologic tests is most likely to confirm the diagnosis?

(A) Anti–double-stranded DNA antibody
(B) Antiribonucleoprotein antibody
(C) Anti–SS-A (Ro) and anti–SS-B (La) antibodies
(D) Anti-topoisomerase I (anti–Scl-70) antibody
(E) Rheumatoid factor

Item 28 [Advanced]

A 55-year-old woman is evaluated for progressive polyarthralgia, photosensitive rash, and lower-extremity purpura of 7 weeks' duration. She also has daily low-grade fever and intermittent pleuritic chest pain. She has an 11-year history of rheumatoid arthritis treated with oral methotrexate and intravenous infliximab. Her disease has been mostly stable except for occasional flares treated with prednisone.

On physical examination, vital signs are normal except for a temperature of 38.0°C (100.4°F). Malar rash is present. Cardiopulmonary examination reveals normal breath sounds, and no rubs are heard. She is unable to take a deep breath because of pain. Several small 1-cm maculopapular eruptions are visible on the lower extremities bilaterally. Musculoskeletal examination reveals synovitis of the metacarpophalangeal and proximal interphalangeal joints and the wrists bilaterally. The left elbow has a nodule. Range of motion of the right wrist is decreased.

Rheumatoid factor	Positive
Antinuclear antibodies	Titer of 1:640
Anti–double-stranded DNA antibodies	Positive

Chest radiograph reveals small bilateral pleural effusions.

Which of the following is the most appropriate next step in this patient's treatment?

(A) Add sulfasalazine
(B) Discontinue infliximab; begin prednisone
(C) Discontinue methotrexate; begin hydroxychloroquine
(D) Discontinue methotrexate; begin sulfasalazine

Item 29 [Advanced]

A 25-year-old woman is evaluated during a routine follow-up visit. Four months ago, she was diagnosed with systemic lupus erythematosus that manifested as fatigue, malar rash, oral ulcers, pleuritis, and arthralgia. At that time, she began treatment with hydroxychloroquine and a 1-month course of low-dose prednisone.

On physical examination today, she states that her symptoms have resolved somewhat but that she still has slight fatigue and mild arthralgia in her hands, feet, and knees. Temperature is 36.4°C (97.6°F), blood pressure is 130/92 mm Hg, pulse rate is 84/min, and respiration rate is 18/min. She has a mild malar flush, a painless ulcer on the hard palate, and

trace bilateral ankle edema. The remainder of the examination is normal.

Hemoglobin	10 g/dL (100 g/L)
Leukocyte count	2300/μL (2.3 × 10⁹/L)
Platelet count	132,000/μL (132 × 10⁹/L)
Erythrocyte sedimentation rate	45 mm/h
Serum creatinine	1.0 mg/dL (88.4 μmol/L)
Albumin	3.1 g/dL (31 g/L)
Serum complement (C3 and C4)	Decreased
Urinalysis	2+ protein; 3+ blood; 5-10 leukocytes, 15-20 erythrocytes, and 1 erythrocyte cast/hpf

Which of the following is the next best step in this patient's treatment?

(A) Amlodipine
(B) High-dose prednisone
(C) Ibuprofen
(D) Low-dose prednisone

Item 30 [Basic]

A 22-year-old woman is evaluated because of a 3-week history of pain in her joints and a rash. Both the skin rash and arthralgia began after a 2-week sailing vacation in July on Lake Michigan. The joint pain involves primarily the wrists and hands bilaterally, and tends to be worse in the morning and improve as the day progresses. She originally thought that the rash was the result of sunburn, but it has not gone away, and is shown (Plate 31). It is not painful and does not itch.

Which of the following conditions is most likely responsible for this patient's rash?

(A) Dermatomyositis
(B) Rosacea
(C) Seborrheic dermatitis
(D) Systemic lupus erythematosus

Item 31 [Advanced]

A 63-year-old woman with dermatomyositis is evaluated for cough and dyspnea. She was diagnosed with polymyositis 6 months ago and has been treated with prednisone and methotrexate. She was doing very well until 6 weeks ago when she developed a dry cough and progressive dyspnea. She has no history of pulmonary disease and does not smoke.

On physical examination, temperature is 37.0°C (98.6°F), blood pressure is 110/60 mm Hg, pulse rate is 88/min, and respiration rate is 20/min. The cardiac examination is normal. No jugular venous distention or peripheral edema is evident. On pulmonary auscultation, bibasilar crackles are heard. Muscle strength is normal, and no skin rash is evident.

Laboratory evaluation shows a normal complete blood count, comprehensive chemistry panel, and serum creatine kinase level. Chest x-ray shows increased interstitial markings in both lung bases.

Which of the following is the most likely diagnosis?

(A) Community-acquired pneumonia
(B) Heart failure
(C) Interstitial lung disease
(D) Pneumocystis pneumonia

Item 32 [Advanced]

A 41-year-old woman is evaluated for intermittent pain and cyanosis of the fingers that is usually associated with exposure to cold temperatures or stress. She does not smoke, and her efforts to keep room temperatures warm and to wear gloves and layers of clothing to maintain her core temperature have not been successful in managing her symptoms.

She was diagnosed with limited cutaneous systemic sclerosis 1 year ago. She also has gastroesophageal reflux disease. Her only medication is omeprazole.

On physical examination, temperature is 37.0°C (98.6°F), blood pressure is 128/72 mm Hg, and pulse rate is 88/min. Cutaneous examination of the hands shows sclerodactyly. Radial and ulnar pulses are 2+ and equal bilaterally.

Which of the following is the most appropriate additional treatment for this patient?

(A) Amlodipine
(B) Isosorbide dinitrate
(C) Prednisone
(D) Propranolol

Item 33 [Basic]

A 25-year-old woman is evaluated during a follow-up visit for a 6-month history of diffuse muscle and joint pain above and below the waist, fatigue, and difficulty sleeping. She has a 2-year history of hypothyroidism treated with levothyroxine. Her only other medication is hydrocodone-acetaminophen, which has not relieved her pain.

On physical examination, temperature is 37.0°C (98.6°F), blood pressure is 125/78 mm Hg, pulse rate is 85/min, and respiration rate is 12/min. Cardiopulmonary examination is normal. Musculoskeletal examination reveals diffuse periarticular tenderness, including bilateral tenderness in the biceps brachii, thighs, and calves. Muscle strength testing cannot be completed because of pain. The joints are not swollen, and she does not have lower-extremity edema.

Complete blood count	Normal
Complete metabolic panel	Normal
Erythrocyte sedimentation rate	10 mm/h
Creatine kinase	100 U/L
Antinuclear antibodies	Titer of 1:640
Thyroid-stimulating hormone	1.5 µU/mL (1.5 mU/L)
Urinalysis	Normal

Which of following is the most likely diagnosis?

(A) Fibromyalgia
(B) Polymyositis
(C) Sjögren syndrome
(D) Systemic lupus erythematosus

Item 34 [Basic]

A 68-year-old woman is evaluated because of recent soft tissue swelling posterior to the mandible, and dryness of both eyes, dry mouth. Her medical history is otherwise unremarkable.

Physical examination reveals normal vital signs, bilateral parotid gland swelling, diffuse lymphadenopathy, and trace joint effusion in both knees. Schirmer's test shows 8 mm, right eye; 5 mm, left eye (normal, greater than 15 mm/5 min), consistent with decreased tear production.

Which of the following is the most likely diagnosis?

(A) Hodgkin disease
(B) Sarcoidosis
(C) Sjögren syndrome
(D) Systemic lupus erythematosus

Item 35 [Advanced]

A 69-year-old woman is evaluated for a progressive 6-month history of fatigue and weakness. She has had painful paresthesias on the dorsum of the right foot for the past 10 days and weakness in the right wrist for the past 2 days. She also has had fever and night sweats accompanied by arthralgia and myalgia. She has had a 4.1-kg (9-lb) weight loss during this time and over the past month has developed anorexia and nausea. Colonoscopy, mammography, and Pap smear performed 2 months ago were normal. Her medical history is otherwise unremarkable, and she takes no medications.

On physical examination, temperature is normal, blood pressure is 155/115 mm Hg, pulse rate is 102/min, and respiration rate is 18/min. BMI is 28. There is jugular venous distention. Cardiac examination reveals a summation gallop. Left and right renal bruits are heard during systole and diastole. The lungs are clear to auscultation. She is unable to dorsiflex the right foot, and extension of the right wrist is weak. There is 2+ ankle edema bilaterally. There are no skin lesions and no evidence of synovitis.

Hemoglobin	10 g/dL (100 g/L)
Erythrocyte sedimentation rate	98 mm/h
Blood urea nitrogen	30 mg/dL (10.7 mmol/L)
Serum creatinine	1.2 mg/dL (106.0 µmol/L)
Antinuclear antibodies	Negative
Rheumatoid factor	Negative
c-ANCA	Negative
p-ANCA	Negative
C3 and C4	Normal
Urinalysis	2+ protein; no casts
Urine protein-creatinine ratio	0.36 mg/mg

Serum and urine electrophoreses are negative. Blood cultures are pending. Echocardiography is negative for valvular disease, valvular vegetation, or tumor. On kidney ultrasound, the kidneys are 11 cm bilaterally. There is no hydronephrosis.

Which of the following studies is most likely to yield a definitive diagnosis?

(A) Abdominal fat pad aspiration
(B) Angiography of the renal arteries
(C) Kidney biopsy
(D) Skin biopsy

Item 36 [Advanced]

A 57-year-old man is evaluated in the emergency department for the acute onset of rapidly worsening dyspnea. For the past 10 weeks, he has had pain and swelling in the small joints of the hands and in the knees; he was diagnosed with seronegative symmetric inflammatory polyarthritis 2 weeks ago and was started on low-dose methotrexate, a folic acid supplement, low-dose prednisone, and naproxen at that time. He also has a history of refractory otitis media and underwent bilateral tympanostomy tube placement 6 months ago.

He is in respiratory failure and is intubated, mechanically ventilated, and admitted to the hospital. Blood is noted when he is intubated. On physical examination on admission, temperature is 38.5°C (101.3°F), blood pressure is 135/95 mm Hg, pulse rate is 125/min, and respiration rate is 24/min. There is no bleeding from the gums. Pulmonary examination reveals diffuse crackles throughout all lung fields. The metacarpophalangeal and proximal interphalangeal joints are swollen, and both knees have medium-sized effusions. Palpable purpura is present on the calves.

Hemoglobin	10 g/dL (100 g/L)
Leukocyte count	12,500/µL (12.5 × 10⁹/L) (80% neutrophils)
Serum creatinine	2.6 mg/dL (229.8 µmol/L)
Rheumatoid factor	Negative
Antinuclear antibodies	Negative
c-ANCA	Positive
Anti–cyclic citrullinated peptide antibodies	Negative
Antiproteinase-3 antibodies	Positive
Serologic test for HIV antibodies	Negative
Urinalysis	2+ protein; 1+ blood; 15 erythrocytes/hpf

A chest radiograph shows normal heart size and diffuse alveolar infiltrates in both lung fields.

Ceftriaxone, azithromycin, and hydrocortisone are started. His previous medications are discontinued.

Which of the following is the most likely diagnosis?

(A) Interstitial pneumonitis
(B) Methotrexate-induced pneumonitis
(C) *Pneumocystis* pneumonia
(D) Wegener granulomatosis

Item 37 [Basic]

A 75-year-old woman is evaluated for a sudden loss of vision in the left eye that began 30 minutes ago. She has a 2-week history of fatigue; malaise; and pain in the shoulders, neck, hips, and lower back. She also has a 5-day history of mild bitemporal headache.

On physical examination, temperature is 37.3°C (99.1°F), blood pressure is 140/85 mm Hg, pulse rate is 72/min, and respiration rate is 16/min. BMI is 31. The left temporal artery is tender. Funduscopic examination reveals a pale, swollen optic disc. Range of motion of the shoulders and hips elicits moderate pain.

Hemoglobin	9.9 g/dL (99 g/L)
Leukocyte count	7300/µL (7.3 × 10⁹/L)
Platelet count	456,000/µL (456 × 10⁹/L)
Erythrocyte sedimentation rate	116 mm/h

Which of the following is the most appropriate next step in this patient's management?

(A) Brain MRI
(B) High-dose intravenous methylprednisolone
(C) Low-dose oral prednisone
(D) Temporal artery biopsy

Section 11

Rheumatology
Answers and Critiques

Item 1   **Answer: B**

Educational Objective: *Diagnose lateral epicondylitis of the elbow ("tennis elbow").*

This woman has lateral epicondylitis of the elbow, commonly referred to as "tennis elbow." Epicondylitis is caused by microtearing of the tendons resulting from repetitive motions. Lateral epicondylitis is the most common cause of elbow pain. Symptoms are tenderness of the lateral epicondyle and pain on resisted wrist extension and hand gripping. Medial epicondylitis, or golfer's elbow, is less common. There is tenderness in the medial epicondyle and pain with wrist flexion. Only a minority of cases of lateral epicondylitis can be attributed to playing tennis. Treatment of the disorder consists of application of ice, nonsteroidal anti-inflammatory drugs, local steroid injection, and a forearm brace or isometric exercises to strengthen the forearm.

Cubital tunnel syndrome, or ulnar nerve entrapment, is a common cause for pain and sensory and motor loss in the ulnar region and for paresthesias in the ulnar aspect of the arm and hand. Systemic diseases such as end-stage renal disease may be involved; extrinsic causes such as ganglion cysts or external pressure are common as well.

Olecranon bursitis, or carpet-layers elbow, occurs when the olecranon bursa develops an effusion, either from trauma, an inflammatory process, or infection. On examination, an inflamed bursa does not cause restriction or pain with range of motion of the elbow, providing evidence that the joint is not involved. However, the bursa can be extremely tender to palpation.

A history of joint pain, joint swelling, and fever are the only findings associated with septic arthritis that occur in more than 50% of affected patients. Approximately 85% to 90% of patients have involvement of only one joint. Common sites of infection include the knee, wrists, ankles, and hips. The hallmark of a septic joint is pain on passive range of motion in the absence of trauma, and an infected joint typically appears swollen and warm with overlying erythema.

KEY POINT

Lateral epicondylitis is a clinical diagnosis based upon the presence of localized pain made worse by wrist extension, point tenderness, and an absence of signs of limitation of motion or inflammation of the elbow joint.

Bibliography

Calfee RP, Patel A, DaSilva MF, Akelman E. Management of lateral epicondylitis: current concepts. J Am Acad Orthop Surg. 2008;16(1):19-29. [PMID: 18180389]

Item 2   **Answer: C**

Educational Objective: *Diagnose rheumatoid arthritis.*

This patient has symptoms and signs consistent with rheumatoid arthritis. Different joints are variably affected by different disorders. Rheumatoid arthritis and osteoarthritis can both involve the proximal interphalangeal joints of the hands, but metacarpophalangeal joint involvement occurs in rheumatoid arthritis but not typically in osteoarthritis. Distal interphalangeal joint involvement is characteristic of osteoarthritis but not rheumatoid arthritis. Unless a secondary condition, such as trauma, metabolic disorder, or inflammatory arthritis, has already affected the joint, osteoarthritis does not occur in the metacarpophalangeal, wrist, elbow, shoulder, and ankle joints. This patient has erythema and swelling of the metacarpophalangeal joints and loss of function leading to absenteeism from work; these findings are most consistent with rheumatoid arthritis.

Psoriasis is associated with an underlying inflammatory arthritis in up to 30% of patients with skin disease; nail pitting suggests psoriatic arthritis, even in the absence of psoriatic skin lesions. These changes are not present in this patient.

More than 90% of patients with SLE develop joint involvement that can manifest as arthralgia or true arthritis. Joint pain is often migratory and can be oligoarticular or polyarticular and asymmetric or symmetric. Pain typically involves the large and small joints; the wrists and metacarpophalangeal and proximal interphalangeal joints in particular are most commonly affected. The absence of other manifestations of SLE (serositis, cytopenias, kidney disease, rash, photosensitivity) make this diagnosis unlikely.

KEY POINT

Rheumatoid arthritis and osteoarthritis can both involve the proximal interphalangeal joints of the hands, but metacarpophalangeal joint involvement occurs in rheumatoid arthritis and not osteoarthritis.

Bibliography

Majithia V, Geraci SA. Rheumatoid arthritis: diagnosis and management. Am J Med. 2007;120:936-9. [PMID: 17976416]

Item 3 Answer: D
Educational Objective: *Diagnose trochanteric bursitis.*

Many patients with pain over the greater trochanter describe it as hip pain. Often patients can point with one finger to the source of the pain on the lateral hip. Actively resisted abduction of the hip worsens the pain. The treatment of choice is a corticosteroid injection. Formal instruction in exercises to stretch the iliotibial band and strengthen the gluteus medius and minimus muscles may be helpful, as will nonsteroidal anti-inflammatory drugs or hot packs.

Patients with hip joint pathology typically have pain that is localized to the groin and have painful, often restricted range of hip motion. The patient's ability to precisely localize the pain to the lateral aspect of the hip is not consistent with hip joint pathology. Finally, findings on physical examination indicate that the source of pain is not the hip joint itself; therefore, osteoarthritis, rheumatoid arthritis, and avascular necrosis of the femoral head are unlikely causes of the pain.

KEY POINT

Patients with trochanteric bursitis can point with one finger to the source of the pain on the lateral hip and actively resisted abduction of the hip worsens the pain.

Bibliography
Shbeeb MI, Matteson EL. Trochanteric bursitis (greater trochanter pain syndrome). Mayo Clin Proc. 1996;71:565-9. [PMID: 8642885]

Item 4 Answer: C
Educational Objective: *Diagnose meniscal tear.*

The patient's history is suspicious for a meniscal tear. Patients typically describe a twisting injury with the foot in a weight-bearing position, in which a popping or tearing sensation is often felt, followed by severe pain. Swelling occurs over several hours, in contrast to ligamentous injuries, in which swelling is immediate. Patients with meniscal tears may report a clicking or locking of the knee secondary to loose cartilage in the knee but often have pain only on walking, particularly going up or down stairs. Pain along the joint line is 76% sensitive for a meniscal tear, and an audible pop or snap on the McMurray test is 97% specific for a meniscal tear.

Anserine bursitis is characterized by pain and tenderness over the anteromedial aspect of the lower leg below the joint line of the knee. The location of the patient's pain and her abnormal physical examination findings do not support the diagnosis of anserine bursitis.

Ligamentous damage usually occurs as a result of forceful stress or direct blows to the knee while the extremity is bearing weight. Excessive medial rotation with a planted foot stresses the anterior cruciate ligament. A popping or tearing sensation is frequently reported in patients with ligamentous damage. This patient's physical examination findings, particularly the result of the McMurray test, support a diagnosis of meniscal, rather than ligamentous, injury.

Patellofemoral pain syndrome is the most common cause of chronic knee pain in active adults, particularly women, younger than 45 years. The exacerbation of the pain by going down steps and the development of knee stiffness and pain at rest when the knee is flexed for an extended period of time are clues to the diagnosis. Reproducing the pain by firmly moving the patella along the femur confirms the diagnosis. This patient's history and physical examination findings are consistent with acute injury to the meniscus rather than the patellofemoral pain syndrome.

KEY POINT

Pain along the joint line is 76% sensitive for a meniscal tear, and a pop or snap on the McMurray test is 97% specific.

Bibliography
Jackson JL, O'Malley PG, Kroenke K. Evaluation of acute knee pain in primary care. Ann Intern Med. 2003;139(7):575-588. [PMID: 14530229]

Item 5 Answer: A
Educational Objective: *Diagnose anserine bursitis.*

The patient has anserine bursitis; the maneuver with the knee semiflexed helps to confirm the diagnosis. In anserine bursitis, the diagnosis rests on the finding of focal tenderness on the upper, inner tibia, about 5 cm distal to the medial articular line of the knee. Patients are usually middle-aged or older and often have knee osteoarthritis, but the problem can occur in active young people also. Usually, there is no redness, swelling, or increased warmth at the painful site. It may be that the underlying problem is strain of the pes anserinus tendon rather than true bursitis. Corticosteroid injection at the bursal site almost always provides relief of pain. Often, knee pain attributed to even severe osteoarthritis of the knee disappears after treatment of the anserine bursitis. Because the corticosteroid is injected into soft tissue, the risk of tendon rupture is minimal. In addition, patients should adhere to a regimen of isometric quadriceps exercises and, if applicable, weight reduction.

Osteoarthritis and gout would produce findings limited to the knee joint, and are not associated with focal tenderness of the upper, inner tibia. Rheumatoid arthritis of the knee is uncommon, particularly if it is asymmetrical, and would not produce focal tenderness along the upper tibia.

KEY POINT

In anserine bursitis, the diagnosis rests on the finding of focal tenderness on the upper, inner tibia, about 5 cm distal to the medial articular line of the knee.

Bibliography
Larsson LG, Baum J. The syndrome of anserine bursitis: An overlooked diagnosis. Arthritis Rheum. 1985;28:1062-5. [PMID: 4038358]

Item 6   Answer: E
Educational Objective: *Diagnose rotator cuff tendinitis.*

Rotator cuff tendinitis, an inflammation of the supraspinatus and/or infraspinatus tendon that can also involve the subacromial bursa, is a common overuse injury. This injury is characterized by subacromial tenderness and impingement—painful compression of the rotator cuff tendons and subacromial bursa between the humeral head and the acromion with arm elevation. Pain in patients with rotator cuff tendinitis often occurs with reaching overhead and when lying on the shoulder. The passive painful-arc maneuver assesses the degree of impingement. The examiner places one hand on the acromion and the other on the forearm and abducts the arm while preventing the patient from shrugging. Subacromial pain at 60 to 70 degrees of abduction suggests moderate impingement, while pain at 45 degrees or less suggests severe impingement. Pain with resisted mid-arc abduction is a specific finding for rotator cuff tendinitis. Appropriate treatments for acute tendinitis include NSAIDs, ice, and exercises; overhead reaching and lifting should be limited.

Adhesive capsulitis (frozen shoulder) is characterized by a decreased range of shoulder motion predominantly resulting from stiffness rather than from pain or weakness.

Bicipital tendinitis is also an overuse injury in which the bicipital groove may be tender, and anterior shoulder pain is elicited with resisted forearm supination or elbow flexion.

Glenohumeral arthritis is often related to trauma and the gradual onset of pain and stiffness over months to years.

A torn rotator cuff usually results in arm weakness, particularly with abduction and/or external rotation. A positive drop-arm test (inability to smoothly lower the affected arm from full abduction) is a very specific but relatively insensitive method for diagnosing rotator cuff tear.

KEY POINT
Rotator cuff tendinitis is characterized by subacromial tenderness and impingement; pain often occurs with reaching overhead and when lying on the shoulder.

Bibliography
Koester MC, George MS, Kuhn JE. Shoulder impingement syndrome. Am J Med. 2005;118(5):452-455. [PMID:15866244]

Item 7   Answer: A
Educational Objective: *Diagnose referred shoulder pain.*

The most appropriate next step in this patient's management is a chest radiograph to evaluate for a cause of referred pain to the shoulder. Referred shoulder pain, in contrast to intrinsic shoulder problems, is always associated with a normal shoulder examination that does not alter the severity or the character of the pain. This patient's examination is not specific for a process involving the shoulder apparatus. There are no physical examination signs that localize the pain to any shoulder structure. Radicular symptoms due to nerve entrapment at the level of the cervical spine might be poorly localized to the trapezius or arm; however, these symptoms are usually accompanied by paresthesias, muscle weakness, and abnormal reflexes, which are absent in this patient. Referred shoulder pain is often the result of an underlying intrathoracic process. A chest radiograph may help to identify an underlying intrathoracic process, such as an apical lung tumor, effusion, or pneumothorax.

Physical therapy would be a reasonable option if the shoulder pain were found to be musculoskeletal in nature; however, given her full range of motion and no localizing signs on examination, physical therapy is unlikely to be helpful and further evaluation for the cause of the shoulder pain is warranted. Likewise, without evidence of either a musculoskeletal or an intra-articular etiology, neither a skeletal muscle relaxant nor intra-articular corticosteroid injection would be appropriate.

Plain radiography has limited utility in the initial evaluation of shoulder pain in the absence of trauma or shoulder deformity. Imaging may be necessary in patients with severe or persistent pain and/or functional loss. In this patient, a radiograph would be unlikely to demonstrate changes, given that she has had no trauma and her physical examination shows no findings of shoulder pathology.

KEY POINT
Referred shoulder pain, in contrast to intrinsic shoulder problems, is always associated with a normal shoulder examination that does not alter the severity or the character of the pain.

Bibliography
Mitchell C, Adebajo A, Hay E, Carr A. Shoulder pain: diagnosis and management in primary care. BMJ. 2005;331(7525):1124-8. [PMID: 16282408]

Item 8   Answer: B
Educational Objective: *Treat polymyalgia rheumatica.*

The most appropriate management in this patient is to increase the prednisone dosage to 7.5 mg/d and add methotrexate, 10 mg weekly. Typically, patients with polymyalgia achieve resolution of their symptoms with low-dose prednisone (10 to 20 mg/d); once these symptoms are controlled, the prednisone dosage can then be tapered. However, polymyalgia rheumatica commonly recurs when the prednisone dosage is being tapered. During flares, the prednisone dosage should be increased to the minimum amount needed to provide symptomatic relief; once symptoms subside, slower tapering of the dosage is warranted.

Because two previous attempts to taper this patient's prednisone dosage below 7.5 mg/d have been unsuccessful, the addition of a steroid-sparing agent as well as an increase in her prednisone dosage is warranted. Methotrexate in particular has been shown to be an effective steroid-sparing agent in patients with polymyalgia rheumatica.

This patient's prednisone dosage should be increased to the minimum dosage needed to control her symptoms, which in this individual has been shown to be between 7 and 7.5 mg/d. Increasing this patient's prednisone dosage to 20 mg/d would unnecessarily place her at greater risk for corticosteroid toxicity. Infliximab has not been shown to be an effective steroid-sparing agent in patients with polymyalgia rheumatica and therefore would not be indicated for this patient.

KEY POINT

Methotrexate is an effective steroid-sparing agent in the treatment of polymyalgia rheumatica.

Bibliography

Caporali R, Cimmino MA, Feraccioli G, et al; Systemic Vasculitis Study Group of the Italian Society for Rheumatology. Prednisone plus methotrexate for polymyalgia rheumatica: a randomized, double-blind, placebo-controlled trial. Ann Intern Med. 2004;141(7):493-500. [PMID:15466766]

Item 9   Answer: D

Educational Objective: *Treat presumed methicillin-resistant* Staphylococcus aureus *septic arthritis with vancomycin.*

The most appropriate initial antibiotic selection for this patient is vancomycin. Septic arthritis is a medical emergency. Hematogenous spread is the most common mechanism of joint infection, because the synovium has no basement membrane and is, therefore, particularly vulnerable to infection. *Staphylococcus* is the most common gram-positive organism affecting native and prosthetic joints, and infection with the methicillin-resistant strain is becoming increasingly common. Joints that have been previously damaged are more likely to become infected than structurally normal joints. In particular, patients with rheumatoid arthritis have usually used intra-articular corticosteroids or immunosuppressive agents at some point in their disease course and are, therefore, particularly susceptible to infection. Septic arthritis also is more likely to have a polyarticular presentation in patients with pre-existing rheumatoid arthritis than in other patients. In general, vancomycin is the empiric therapy of choice for community-acquired septic arthritis and synovial fluid positive for gram-positive cocci or in patients at low risk for gram-negative infection and with a negative synovial fluid Gram stain. Because this patient's synovial fluid is positive for gram-positive cocci and because of increasing concern about methicillin-resistant *Staphylococcus aureus* (MRSA) infection in the community, vancomycin is the initial treatment of choice pending culture results. Modifications of the initial antibiotic regimen can be made to narrow coverage with cefazolin or nafcillin when culture results are available but are not generally recommended as initial empiric therapy because of the prevalence of MRSA in the community.

Ceftriaxone is the initial antibiotic of choice in patients at risk for gonococcal infection. Gonococcal arthritis is the most common form of bacterial arthritis in young, sexually active persons and should be considered in patients who present with migratory tenosynovitis and arthralgia.

KEY POINT

In general, vancomycin is the empiric therapy of choice for community-acquired septic arthritis with synovial fluid positive for gram-positive cocci and in patients at low risk for gram-negative infections and with a negative Gram stain result.

Bibliography

Mathews CJ, Weston VC, Jones A, Field M, Coakley G. Bacterial septic arthritis in adults. Lancet. 2010;375(9717):846-55. [PMID: 20206778]

Item 10   Answer: A

Educational Objective: *Diagnose septic arthritis in a patient with rheumatoid arthritis.*

This patient most likely has septic arthritis, which usually manifests as acute monoarthritis and is characterized by pain on passive range of motion in the absence of known trauma. Arthrocentesis of the wrist will most likely help to establish a diagnosis in this patient.

Septic arthritis should particularly be suspected in patients with underlying rheumatologic disorders such as rheumatoid arthritis who present with a sudden single joint flare that is not accompanied by other features of the pre-existing disorder. However, all patients who present with acute monoarthritis should be presumed to have septic arthritis until synovial fluid analysis via arthrocentesis excludes this condition. Synovial fluid analysis is the only definitive way to diagnose septic arthritis and is critical to guide antibiotic treatment. Patients with suspicion for this condition should begin empiric systemic antibiotic therapy until culture results are available.

Surgical drainage or débridement via arthroscopy may be warranted in patients with septic arthritis who do not respond to repeated percutaneous drainage and appropriate antibiotic therapy but would not be an appropriate initial intervention.

Joint and bone damage due to infection are relatively late radiographic findings. In acute septic arthritis, nonspecific soft-tissue fullness and joint effusions are often the only initial radiographic findings and do not establish the diagnosis of infection. Bone scans are more sensitive in detecting inflammatory lesions in bones and joints but also are not specific for infection.

MRI of the affected joint is especially useful in detecting avascular necrosis, soft-tissue masses, and collections of fluid not visualized by other imaging modalities but would not establish the diagnosis of infection.

KEY POINT

All patients who present with acute monoarthritis should be presumed to have septic arthritis until synovial fluid analysis via arthrocentesis excludes this condition.

Bibliography

Kherani RB, Shojania K. Septic arthritis in patients with pre-existing inflammatory arthritis. CMAJ. 2007;176(11):1605-1608. [PMID: 17515588]

Item 11   Answer: D
Educational Objective: *Diagnose prosthetic joint infection.*

This patient most likely has prosthetic joint infection, which may occur at any time in the postoperative period. Prosthetic joint infections that occur after the first postoperative year are most frequently caused by hematogenous spread of organisms to the prosthetic joint. The source of infection in this setting is often obvious and includes skin or genitourinary tract infection or, as in this patient, an abscessed tooth. Pain is the predominant or only symptom in patients with prosthetic joint infection, and fever and leukocytosis are frequently absent. Patients with prosthetic joint infection usually have an elevated erythrocyte sedimentation rate. Radiography may reveal prosthetic loosening, but hardware loosening may occur in patients without infection, as well.

The gold standard for diagnosing prosthetic joint infection is arthrocentesis or intraoperative tissue sampling with culture before antibiotic therapy is initiated. The synovial fluid leukocyte count in patients with prosthetic joint infection is usually lower compared with that in patients with other forms of septic arthritis.

Aseptic loosening refers to loss of fixation of the arthroplasty components, which is a major long-term complication of hip arthroplasty. The most striking manifestation of this condition is pain in the proximal and medial aspect of the thigh that is worse with weight bearing. Osteolysis is typically seen on radiographs of affected patients, which this patient does not have. Aseptic loosening also would not explain this patient's inflammatory synovial fluid.

This patient's elevated synovial fluid leukocyte count with a predominance of neutrophils is suggestive of gout, but this condition does not have a subacute onset and does not commonly affect the hips. An acute attack of gout also would be associated with crystals visible on polarized light microscopy of the synovial fluid.

Pigmented villonodular synovitis is a rare proliferative synovitis that most commonly involves the hip or knee. Radiographs in patients with this condition may reveal bone erosions or may be normal. Pigmented villonodular synovitis typically develops in young patients and is not associated with prosthetic joint placement.

KEY POINT

In patients with prosthetic joint infection, pain is the predominant or only symptom, and fever and leukocytosis are frequently absent.

Bibliography

Trampuz A, Zimmerli W. Diagnosis and treatment of implant-associated septic arthritis and osteomyelitis. Curr Infect Dis Rep. 2008;10(5):394-403. [PMID: 18687204]

Item 12   Answer: D
Educational Objective: *Treat acute gout with a non-steroidal anti-inflammatory drug (NSAID).*

The most appropriate treatment for this patient is administration of an NSAID such as indomethacin. Definitive diagnosis of gout requires the identification of monosodium urate crystals on arthrocentesis or aspiration of a tophus. During an attack of gout, needle-shaped monosodium urate crystals that typically appear engulfed by the neutrophils are visible on compensated polarized light microscopy. NSAIDs, corticosteroids, and colchicine are options in the treatment of an acute attack of gout. NSAIDs are highly effective when administered during an acute attack, but they should be used with caution in patients at risk for renal impairment, bleeding, or ulcer disorders, especially in the elderly. Oral, intra-articular, or intravenous corticosteroid therapy is also effective in acute gouty attacks. However, oral and intravenous therapy may be problematic in patients with diabetes mellitus. Colchicine is most effective in patients with monoarticular involvement and, when used within the first 24 hours of symptoms, can abort a severe attack. At the first sign of an attack in patients with normal renal function, this agent is usually administered two or three times daily until the patient experiences symptomatic relief, develops gastrointestinal toxicity, or reaches a maximum dose of 6 mg per attack.

Allopurinol and febuxostat are xanthine oxidase inhibitors useful in reducing uric acid levels in patients with recurrent attacks of acute gout and patients with uric acid tophi or renal stones. Rapid control of serum uric acid levels generally is not necessary during an acute attack, and acute increases and decreases in the uric acid level alter the steady state and may prolong the current attack or precipitate new attacks. Prophylactic colchicine, low-dose corticosteroids, or NSAIDs initiated at least 1 week before beginning or adjusting the dose of uric acid–lowering therapy help to prevent disease flares associated with changes in uric acid levels and may need to be continued until therapeutic serum uric acid levels have been achieved (<6 mg/dL [0.4 mmol/L]). Prolonged use of these agents may be indicated in patients with chronic tophaceous gout until the disease is controlled.

KEY POINT

NSAIDs, corticosteroids, and colchicine are options in the treatment of an acute attack of gout.

Bibliography

Wilson JF. In the clinic. Gout. Ann Intern Med. 2010;152(3):ITC2-1-ITC2-16. [PMID: 20124228]

Item 13   Answer: C

Educational Objective: *Treat hyperuricemia with uric acid–lowering therapy.*

The most appropriate therapy for this patient is low-dose colchicine and allopurinol. Criteria for initiating treatment of hyperuricemia in patients with symptomatic gout include the presence of tophi or renal stones, multiple attacks of acute gout, or a history of a decreasing period between attacks. Uric acid–lowering therapy typically is not initiated until a patient experiences two documented acute attacks. Dietary purine restriction, weight loss, and discontinuation of alcohol may help to decrease uric acid levels in patients with mild hyperuricemia and symptomatic gout. Medications that raise serum uric acid levels, such as thiazide diuretics and low-dose salicylates, should be discontinued if alternative therapy is available. However, most patients with recurrent gouty attacks, particularly those with tophaceous deposits, require pharmacologic therapy to lower serum levels of uric acid. The goal in uric acid–lowering therapy is to achieve a serum uric acid level less than 6.0 mg/dL (0.4 mmol/L), not just levels within the normal range. When the uric acid levels are below 6.0 mg/dL (0.4 mmol/L), monosodium urate crystals from within the joint and from soft-tissue tophaceous deposits are reabsorbed. Prophylactic colchicine, low-dose corticosteroids (10 mg/d or less), or nonsteroidal anti-inflammatory drugs (NSAIDs) initiated at least 1 week before beginning or adjusting the dose of uric acid–lowering therapy help to prevent disease flares associated with changes in uric acid levels and may need to be continued until therapeutic serum uric acid levels have been achieved.

Low-dose NSAIDs, such as indomethacin, or low-dose colchicine may prevent attacks of gout but do not lower uric acid levels and, therefore, cannot prevent the continued accumulation of uric acid in soft tissues (tophi), uric acid kidney stones, or destructive arthritis.

KEY POINT

Prophylactic colchicine, low-dose corticosteroids, or NSAIDs are initiated at least 1 week before beginning or adjusting the dose of uric acid–lowering therapy to prevent disease flares associated with changes in uric acid levels.

Bibliography

Wilson JF. In the clinic. Gout. Ann Intern Med. 2010;152(3):ITC2-1-ITC2-16. [PMID: 20124228]

Item 14   Answer: A

Educational Objective: *Diagnose calcium pyrophosphate dihydrate deposition disease.*

This patient has calcium pyrophosphate dihydrate (CPPD) deposition disease presenting as pseudogout. Pseudogout manifests as acute or subacute attacks of warmth and swelling in one to two joints that resemble acute gouty arthropathy. Pseudogout is associated with inflammatory synovial fluid and the presence of CPPD crystals that are weakly positively birefringent and rhomboid in shape seen on polarized light microscopy. Treatment of an acute pseudogout attack primarily involves NSAIDs, but a corticosteroid or colchicine would be appropriate alternative choices.

This patient's radiographic and physical examination findings also are suggestive of osteoarthritis. Osteoarthritis that manifests in patients with CPPD deposition or the presence of chondrocalcinosis on radiography is known as pseudo-osteoarthritis. This degenerative condition mimics osteoarthritis except that it may affect joints not typically involved in osteoarthritis, such as the wrists, metacarpophalangeal joints, shoulders, and ankles. The synovial fluid in patients with pseudo-osteoarthritis is noninflammatory. Both pseudo-osteoarthritis and pseudogout may be present in the same patient. The treatment of pseudo-osteoarthritis is no different than the treatment of osteoarthritis and includes adequate analgesia, physical and occupational therapy, and arthroplasty for symptomatic disease unresponsive to more conservative therapy.

Characteristic features of chronic apatite deposition disease include large, minimally inflammatory effusions that usually develop in the shoulder or knee, destruction of associated tendon structures, and chronic pain. Calcium apatite crystals may only appear as amorphous nonbirefringent crystalline clumps on synovial fluid analysis and therefore are not identified on routine examination. Identification of these crystals requires special staining or crystal analysis that is not routinely available. The absence of these crystals in this patient excludes this condition.

Gout is caused by the deposition of monosodium urate crystals in the tissues of and around the joints. Early attacks of gout are monoarticular and most commonly involve the first metatarsophalangeal joint, whereas chronic gout may manifest as symmetric involvement of the small joints of the hands and feet accompanied by tophi and subcortical erosions on radiography. Definitive diagnosis of gout is established by the presence of strongly negatively birefringent needle-shaped crystals on polarized light microscopy of synovial fluid or fluid from a tophus, which is not consistent with this patient's findings.

The diagnosis of septic arthritis should be considered in all patients with acute monoarthritis and a sudden increase in pain in a chronically damaged joint. This patient's joint fluid is inflammatory, but the leukocyte count is not sufficiently elevated to suggest septic arthritis.

KEY POINT

Pseudogout is associated with acute or subacute attacks of warmth and swelling in one to two joints that resemble acute gouty arthropathy and weakly positive birefringent crystals that are rhomboid in shape seen on polarized light microscopy of synovial fluid.

Bibliography

Rosenthal AK. Update in calcium deposition diseases. Curr Opin Rheumatol. 2007;19(2):158-162. [PMID: 17278931]

Item 15   Answer: B

Educational Objective: *Diagnose osteoarthritis of the knee.*

This patient most likely has osteoarthritis of the knee. He has two risk factors for this condition, advanced age and an occupation involving repetitive bending and physical labor. Osteoarthritis commonly affects weight-bearing joints such as the knees and is characterized by pain on activity that is relieved with rest. Swelling in patients with this condition is usually minimal, and range of motion may be limited. According to the American College of Rheumatology, osteoarthritis of the knee can be diagnosed if knee pain is accompanied by at least three of the following features: age greater than 50 years, morning stiffness lasting less than 30 minutes, crepitus, bony tenderness, bony enlargement, and an absence of palpable warmth. This patient's radiographic findings of osteophytes, joint-space narrowing, sclerosis, and cyst formation are typical of this condition. Arthrocentesis is not necessary to establish a diagnosis of osteoarthritis.

Patients with avascular necrosis of the knee typically experience pain on weight bearing and may have a painful, limited range of motion. However, this condition also is associated with pain on rest and most commonly occurs in patients who use corticosteroids, have systemic lupus erythematosus, or consume excessive amounts of alcoholic beverages. Radiographs in patients with avascular necrosis usually reveal density changes; subchondral radiolucency; cysts; sclerosis; and, eventually, joint-space narrowing.

Rheumatoid arthritis may be associated with a limited range of motion and joint-space narrowing visible on radiography. Patients with rheumatoid arthritis usually have symmetric arthritis that affects at least three joints as well as an elevated erythrocyte sedimentation rate and is associated with morning stiffness that persists for more than 30 minutes. In addition, rheumatoid arthritis also would not explain the presence of subchondral sclerosis and osteophytes on radiography.

A torn medial meniscus would cause pain in the knee and can occur in the elderly in association with osteoarthritis. Patients with acute meniscal damage often describe a twisting injury with the foot in a weight-bearing position in which a popping or tearing sensation is felt, followed by severe pain; in addition, this condition is characterized by the sensation that the knee "locks" or "gives out."

KEY POINT

Physical examination findings consistent with osteoarthritis of the knee include crepitus, bony tenderness, bony enlargement, and an absence of palpable warmth.

Bibliography

Felson DT. Clinical practice. Osteoarthritis of the knee [erratum in N Engl J Med. 2006;354(23):2520]. N Engl J Med. 2006;354(8):841-848. [PMID:16495396]

Item 16   Answer: D

Educational Objective: *Manage osteoarthritis of the knee.*

This patient has osteoarthritis of the knee. The most appropriate next step in her management is referral for physical therapy, which is an appropriate first-line management option for patients with this condition. Quadriceps muscle training in particular has been shown to reduce pain in this population group. Use of over-the-counter acetaminophen or an NSAID on an as-needed basis also may benefit this patient.

Arthroscopy and MRI of the knee would most likely reveal abnormalities of the articular cartilage not visible on plain radiography but are not needed to establish the diagnosis of osteoarthritis. Similarly, aspiration of the knee joint would be warranted in patients with an effusion to obtain a synovial fluid leukocyte count but is not needed to establish a diagnosis; furthermore, this patient does not have an effusion.

KEY POINT

Physical therapy is an appropriate first-line management option for patients with osteoarthritis of the knee, and quadriceps muscle training in particular has been shown to reduce pain in this setting.

Bibliography

Bennell KL, Hinman RS, Metcalf BR, et al. Efficacy of physiotherapy management of knee joint osteoarthritis: a randomised, double blind, placebo controlled trial. Ann Rheum Dis. 2005;64(6):906-912. [PMID: 15897310]

Item 17   Answer: D

Educational Objective: *Diagnose osteoarthritis of the first carpometacarpal joint.*

This patient most likely has osteoarthritis of the first carpometacarpal joint. Osteoarthritis in this location often presents with well localized tenderness to palpation. Movement of the thumb in a circular motion ("grind test") will often elicit the pain. Predisposing factors include repetitive use of the wrist or thumb. Patients may present with pain, swelling, or enlargement of the carpometacarpal joint recognized as squaring or boxing at the base of the thumb. Associated findings of osteoarthritis are common and may include boney enlargement of the distal interphalangeal joints (Heberden nodes) or the proximal interphalangeal joints (Bouchard nodes).

Rheumatoid arthritis is an inflammatory arthritis most often affecting the small joints of the hands (wrist, metacarpophalangeal and proximal interphalangeal joints) and feet (metatarsophalangeal joints) in a symmetric pattern. Stiffness in rheumatoid arthritis usually lasts more than 1 hour, and synovial swelling, tenderness, and warmth are apparent on examination.

de Quervain tenosynovitis is an inflammation of the abductor pollicis longus and extensor pollicis brevis tendons. Pain is present on palpation of the distal aspect of the radial styloid. This point is more proximal than the first carpometacarpal joint. Pain elicited by flexing the thumb into the palm, closing the fingers over the thumb, and then bending the wrist in the ulnar direction (Finkelstein test) is confirmatory.

Carpal tunnel syndrome will often present with pain, numbness, and tingling in the thumb and first two fingers of the hand. Tapping the flexor retinaculum (Tinel sign) or flexing the wrists against each other (Phalen sign) may exacerbate symptoms. Symptoms are often worse at night or with repetitive movements or continuous pressure on the wrist such as typing on a keyboard.

Crystal-induced arthritis in the hands is usually associated with evidence of joint inflammation such as redness and warmth. Additionally, the chronicity of this patient's symptoms argues against crystal-induced arthropathy. Secondary osteoarthritis, however, can develop in the setting of chronic inflammation from crystal-induced arthritis.

KEY POINT

Chronic pain at the base of the thumb is suggestive of osteoarthritis.

Bibliography

Hunter DJ. In the clinic. Osteoarthritis. Ann Intern Med. 2007;147(3): ITC8-1-ITC8-16. [PMID: 17679702]

Item 18   Answer: A
Educational Objective: *Manage acute osteoarthritis of the knee with nonsteroidal anti-inflammatory drugs.*

The best management for this patient is to begin a nonsteroidal anti-inflammatory drug (NSAID). This patient most likely has acute osteoarthritis of the knee. Classic findings of osteoarthritis include pain with activity that is relieved with rest. The patient's radiographic findings of joint space narrowing, subchondral sclerosis and osteophyte formation are consistent with osteoarthritis, and his valgus deformity predisposes him to medial compartment osteoarthritis due to uneven loading forces when ambulating. He has failed treatment with acetaminophen and therefore an oral NSAID such as ibuprofen is the appropriate next management step. Physical therapy, temporary use of a cane and bracing or taping are also reasonable initial interventions. NSAIDs are associated with an increased risk of gastrointestinal bleeding and cardiovascular disease. The American College of Rheumatology guidelines recommend that physicians and patients weigh the potential risks and benefits of treatment with NSAIDs, but no evidence-based guidelines yet exist to indicate which patients can safely use these agents.

Intra-articular corticosteroid or hyaluronan injections may be considered in patients with mono- or pauciarticular osteoarthritis in whom NSAIDs are either contraindicated or do not provide adequate pain relief. Referral to an orthopedic surgeon for consideration of total joint arthroplasty (replacement) of the knee is warranted only when no further medical therapy is available and the patient decides that the impairment caused by his or her condition warrants this intervention. This patient has not had a sufficient trial of more conservative measures to warrant either of these therapies.

Magnetic resonance imaging would be indicated if there were features on history or physical exam that suggested another etiology for the pain. Meniscal tears are seen almost universally in patients with osteoarthritis of the knee and are not necessarily a cause of increased symptoms. Removal of menisci should be avoided unless symptoms of knee locking or the inability to extend the knee are present.

Antibiotic treatment is not indicated because arthrocentesis does not suggest septic arthritis. In noninflammatory arthritis, the synovial fluid leukocyte count is usually less than $2000/\mu L$ ($2.0 \times 10^9/L$). Septic arthritis usually has leukocyte counts greater than $50,000/\mu L$ ($50 \times 10^9/L$) and a predominance of polymorphonuclear cells.

KEY POINT

In patients with osteoarthritis not adequately controlled with acetaminophen, the next pharmacological intervention is usually a nonsteroidal anti-inflammatory drug.

Bibliography

Hunter DJ. In the clinic. Osteoarthritis. Ann Intern Med. 2007;147: ITC8-1-ITC8-16. [PMID: 17679702]

Item 19   Answer: D
Educational Objective: *Diagnose rheumatoid arthritis with characteristic radiographic findings.*

A radiograph showing marginal joint erosions would most likely support a diagnosis of rheumatoid arthritis (RA). Plain radiographs of the hands and feet should be performed at the time of diagnosis in patients with rheumatoid arthritis to detect erosions and joint-space narrowing. Erosions of cartilage and bone are cardinal features of RA. Erosions and joint-space narrowing may develop as early as 2 to 3 months, and are often present 6 months after the onset of rheumatoid arthritis. Progression is more rapid early in the disease. In a patient with symmetrical synovitis of the small joints of the hand and prolonged morning stiffness, x-rays showing joint erosions is most supportive of rheumatoid arthritis.

The results of initial laboratory studies in patients with rheumatoid arthritis may be normal but can reveal thrombocytosis, leukocytosis, mild anemia (normochromic, normocytic, or microcytic), an elevated erythrocyte sedimentation rate, or an elevated C-reactive protein level. Normochromic, normocytic anemia is a nonspecific response to chronic inflammation and is not specific for RA. An elevated erythrocyte sedimentation rate does not always indicate inflammation, just as a normal result does not exclude it. Serologic markers for rheumatoid arthritis, including rheumatoid factor and anti–cyclic citrullinated peptide (CCP) antibodies, have been found in the serum of patients years before the onset of clinically apparent disease. Approximately 75% of patients with rheumatoid arthritis are rheumatoid factor positive, but the prevalence rate may be as low as 50% in early disease. Rheumatoid factor positivity is not specific for rheumatoid arthritis and frequently occurs in other autoimmune disorders and chronic infections, most notably chronic active hepatitis C virus infection.

KEY POINT

Erosions of cartilage and bone are cardinal x-ray features of rheumatoid arthritis.

Bibliography

Huizinga TW, Pincus T. In the clinic. Rheumatoid arthritis. Ann Intern Med. 2010;153(1):ITC1-1-ITC1-15. [PMID: 20621898]

Item 20   Answer: D

Educational Objective: *Screen for latent tuberculosis prior to initiating tumor necrosis factor-α inhibitor therapy.*

A tuberculin skin test should be performed prior to initiating therapy with adalimumab. When adequate disease control is not achieved with oral disease modifying antirheumatic drugs (DMARDs) such as methotrexate, biologic therapy should be initiated. The initial biologic therapy should be a TNF-α inhibitor. This agent generally should be added to the baseline methotrexate therapy, because the rate of radiographic progression has been shown to decrease with combination therapy. Rarely, serious infections have occurred in patients treated with these agents; among these infectious complications, reactivation tuberculosis is the most common. Tuberculin skin testing is indicated before beginning treatment with these agents, and positive results on this test warrant treatment for latent tuberculosis. Furthermore, periodic tuberculin skin testing for tuberculosis is now recommended during treatment with a TNF-α inhibitor. A chest CT scan is not necessary prior to initiating therapy with a TNF-α inhibitor. If the patient has a positive tuberculin skin test (>5 mm induration), a chest x-ray will be required to exclude active pulmonary tuberculosis but neither this test nor a chest CT scan is indicated in an asymptomatic person with a negative tuberculin skin test.

Rare cases of multiple sclerosis or demyelinating conditions such as optic neuritis have been reported as a potential complication of TNF-α inhibitor therapy but usually remit upon discontinuation of therapy. There is no value in screening asymptomatic patients for multiple sclerosis with a brain MRI. Numerous other conditions, such as migraine, cerebrovascular disease, hypertension, smoking, diabetes mellitus, hyperlipidemia, and head trauma, are also associated with white matter abnormalities on brain MRI. Misinterpretation of white matter abnormalities discovered incidentally in a patient with nonspecific symptoms is a leading cause of multiple sclerosis misdiagnosis

Many drugs can interfere with thyroid hormone production, release, transport and activity; however drugs to treat rheumatoid arthritis do not usually fall into this category. Corticosteroids, for example, can interfere with TSH release and decrease thyroid binding globulin, but TNF-α inhibitors do not interfere with thyroid function and there is no need to obtain a TSH measurement in this patient prior to initiating therapy.

KEY POINT

The most common infectious complication of TNF-α inhibitors is reactivation tuberculosis.

Bibliography

Huizinga TW, Pincus T. In the clinic. Rheumatoid arthritis. Ann Intern Med. 2010;153(1):ITC1-1-ITC1-15; quiz ITC1-16. [PMID: 20621898]

Item 21   Answer: D

Educational Objective: *Diagnose rheumatoid arthritis.*

This patient most likely has rheumatoid arthritis, which is the most common cause of chronic, inflammatory polyarthritis in premenopausal women. Rheumatoid arthritis commonly affects the metacarpophalangeal, proximal interphalangeal, and wrist joints. This patient's swelling, prolonged morning stiffness, and elevated erythrocyte sedimentation rate are consistent with this diagnosis. Furthermore, women are three times more likely to develop rheumatoid arthritis than men and have a slightly increased risk of developing this condition during the first 3 months postpartum.

Gout may involve the hand and wrist and is associated with inflammatory features. However, gout usually has an asymmetric presentation and is unlikely to develop in a premenopausal woman.

Osteoarthritis may manifest as chronic arthritis involving the proximal interphalangeal joints but would not affect the metacarpophalangeal joints or the wrists. Secondary osteoarthritis related to trauma or a metabolic condition such as hemochromatosis may explain this patient's pattern of joint involvement, but this condition would be unlikely in a 26-year-old woman. Osteoarthritis also would not have an inflammatory presentation.

Viral arthritis usually is self-limited except when associated with hepatitis B and C virus infection. Parvovirus B19 infection in adults may induce an acute rheumatoid factor–positive oligo- or polyarthritis. Most adult patients with parvovirus B19 infection also develop rash, but only rarely in adults does rash manifest as the classic rash seen in childhood erythema infectiosum, the "slapped cheek" rash. Diagnosis of acute parvovirus B19 infection may be established by detecting circulating IgM antibodies against parvovirus B19.

Viral arthritis usually resolves within 3 weeks, although a minority of patients may develop persistent arthritis. The arthritis associated with acute parvovirus B19 infection does not cause joint destruction, and supportive analgesic therapy with NSAIDs is appropriate as tolerated. Parvovirus B19 infection is unlikely in this patient considering the duration of her symptoms, absence of rash, and negative titers of IgM antibodies against parvovirus B19.

KEY POINT

Rheumatoid arthritis is the most common cause of chronic, inflammatory polyarthritis in premenopausal women.

Bibliography

Huizinga TW, Pincus T. In the clinic. Rheumatoid arthritis. Ann Intern Med. 2010;153(1):ITC1-1-ITC1-15; quiz ITC1-16. [PMID: 20621898]

Item 22 Answer: A

Educational Objective: *Treat early rheumatoid arthritis.*

This patient has rheumatoid arthritis, and the most appropriate treatment patient is the addition of hydroxychloroquine, 400 mg/d. Prominent morning stiffness that usually lasts for more than 1 hour and fatigue are consistent with early presentations of rheumatoid arthritis. This condition most often involves the small joints of the hands and feet in a symmetric pattern, but involvement of the large joints also may occur. The presence of both rheumatoid factor and anti–cyclic citrullinated peptide antibodies is highly specific for rheumatoid arthritis, and radiographic manifestations of affected patients include periarticular osteopenia and, eventually, articular erosions.

In patients with rheumatoid arthritis, early, aggressive disease control is critical and should be instituted as soon as the diagnosis is established. Experts recommend that affected patients begin disease-modifying antirheumatic drug (DMARD) therapy within 3 months of the onset of this condition. Hydroxychloroquine is warranted in a patient with early, mild, and nonerosive rheumatoid arthritis and is well tolerated.

Methotrexate is often used as an initial DMARD in the treatment of rheumatoid arthritis. However, this agent is associated with hepatotoxicity, and risk for this condition is increased in patients who regularly consume alcoholic beverages; therefore, methotrexate is not indicated for these patients. The amount of alcohol that can safely be consumed in patients who use methotrexate has not yet been determined, but daily consumption of alcoholic beverages while using this agent is not recommended and most experts advise against the use of methotrexate for patients who regularly consume alcohol.

The biologic DMARD etanercept would be an appropriate adjunct medication in a patient with rheumatoid arthritis in whom oral DMARD therapy has not provided adequate disease control. Etanercept and other tumor necrosis factor α inhibitors have greater efficacy when used in combination with methotrexate. However, there is currently insufficient evidence showing that single-agent use of a biologic DMARD is an appropriate initial treatment for this condition.

Combination therapy with an NSAID and a DMARD has been shown to reduce joint pain and swelling in patients with rheumatoid arthritis. However, increasing this patient's ibuprofen dosage in the absence of DMARD therapy would not help to control her disease progression or prevent radiographic damage.

KEY POINT

In patients with rheumatoid arthritis, disease-modifying antirheumatic drug therapy should be initiated as soon as the diagnosis is established.

Bibliography

Huizinga TW, Pincus T. In the clinic. Rheumatoid arthritis. Ann Intern Med. 2010;153(1):ITC1-1-ITC1-15; quiz ITC1-16. [PMID: 20621898]

Item 23 Answer: B

Educational Objective: *Diagnose HIV-related psoriatic arthritis.*

The most appropriate diagnostic approach is testing for the presence of HIV infection. HIV-infected patients with a CD4 cell count less than 200/μL who are not taking antiretroviral therapy commonly have psoriasis or other skin conditions, including photodermatitis, prurigo nodularis, molluscum contagiosum, and drug reactions. Psoriasis in patients with a low CD4 cell count can be severe, affect more than 50% of the body surface area, and present in an atypical fashion (more severe, explosive onset). In patients with psoriasis, 20% to 40% develop arthritis. A diagnosis of HIV-related psoriatic arthritis should be suspected in patients with explosive onset, widespread psoriasis and the occurrence of dactylitis; marked distal interphalangeal (DIP) joint involvement; asymmetric joint involvement; symptoms of enthesitis; or joint ankylosis.

No confirmatory laboratory tests for psoriatic arthritis are available. In patients with psoriatic arthritis, low titer antinuclear antibody tests and rheumatoid factor are found in less 50% and 10% of patients, respectively. HLA-B27 antigen testing is neither sensitive nor specific for psoriatic arthritis and is not helpful in establishing the diagnosis.

KEY POINT

Untreated HIV infection is associated with the occurrence of explosive-onset, widely distributed psoriasis and 20% to 40% of patients with psoriasis may go on to develop psoriatic arthritis.

Bibliography

Cantini F, Niccoli L, Nannini C, Kaloudi O, Bertoni M, Cassarà E. Psoriatic arthritis: a systematic review. Int J Rheum Dis. 2010;13(4):300-17. [PMID:21199465]

Item 24   Answer: B
Educational Objective: *Diagnose enteropathic arthritis.*

This patient's joint symptoms are most likely caused by enteropathic arthritis. She has a 6-week history of crampy abdominal pain and the recent onset of bloody diarrhea and rectal urgency. She also has had weight loss. This clinical presentation raises suspicion for inflammatory bowel disease.

For the past 3 weeks, this patient also has had acute arthritis of the right knee and ankle accompanied by inflammatory features such as tenderness and swelling; her synovial fluid findings confirm the presence of an inflammatory process. The presence of acute oligoarticular arthritis involving the lower extremities in a patient with an inflammatory diarrheal illness is suggestive of enteropathic arthritis; enteropathic arthritis also may manifest as axial arthritis, such as a spondyloarthropathy.

Crystal-induced arthritis typically manifests as acute monoarticular arthritis and would be unlikely in a premenopausal woman.

Gonococcal arthritis may be associated with oligoarticular arthritis, and joint manifestations in this condition may be migratory. However, patients with gonococcal arthritis commonly have tenosynovitis and cutaneous involvement, which are not present in this patient. Furthermore, neither gonococcal nor crystal-induced arthritis would explain this patient's diarrhea and abdominal pain.

Whipple disease is an extremely rare infectious syndrome caused by *Tropheryma whippelii*. The most common presenting symptom in affected patients is arthritis; other symptoms include diarrhea, malabsorption, and central nervous system and constitutional symptoms. Joint involvement is usually migratory and follows a chronic course.

KEY POINT
The presence of acute oligoarticular arthritis involving the lower extremities in a patient with inflammatory bowel disease is suggestive of enteropathic arthritis.

Bibliography
Holden W, Orchard T, Wordsworth P. Enteropathic arthritis. Rheum Dis Clin North Am. 2003;29(3):513-530, viii. [PMID: 12951865]

Item 25   Answer: A
Educational Objective: *Diagnose ankylosing spondylitis in a patient with anterior uveitis.*

The patient has anterior uveitis with a hypopyon, and the associated systemic disease is most likely ankylosing spondylitis. The classic triad for acute anterior uveitis is pain, sensitivity to light, and blurred vision; headache, tenderness, and tearing may also occur. Photophobia during penlight examination has a positive predictive value of 60% for severe eye disease and a negative predictive value of 90%.

Prospective studies have documented systemic illness in 53% of patients with anterior uveitis. Patients with uveitis associated with systemic disease usually have a history or physical examination findings that suggest an underlying disorder. The most commonly diagnosed systemic illnesses in this setting are reactive arthritis, ankylosing spondylitis, and sarcoidosis.

Acute anterior uveitis, particularly unilateral presentations that fluctuate between both eyes over time, is strongly associated with the HLA-B27–related arthropathies, including ankylosing spondylitis. In addition, this patient's chronic back stiffness is highly suggestive of ankylosing spondylitis. Furthermore, in up to 65% of patients with uveitis, spondyloarthropathy remains undiagnosed until these patients present with uveitis.

Posterior uveitis may be related to sarcoidosis or vasculitis but is not typically associated with pain or redness of the eye. Patients with posterior uveitis also often have decreased visual acuity and floaters, which is not consistent with this patient's presentation. Furthermore, sarcoidosis is an unlikely cause of this patient's chronic low back pain.

Sicca syndrome manifests as dryness of the mouth, eyes, and vagina and variable enlargement of the parotid glands in association with concomitant redness and gritty irritation of the eyes. This condition is suggestive of primary or secondary Sjögren syndrome. However, Sjögren syndrome would not cause anterior uveitis and also would not explain the presence of chronic low back pain in a young man.

Anterior uveitis is associated with psoriasis and, in rare cases, Whipple disease, systemic lupus erythematosus, and the systemic vasculitides. However, the patient's long history of back pain in the absence of cutaneous and other manifestations of systemic lupus erythematosus makes this diagnosis unlikely.

KEY POINT
The most commonly diagnosed systemic illnesses in patients with anterior uveitis are reactive arthritis, ankylosing spondylitis, and sarcoidosis.

Bibliography
Sampaio-Barros PD, Conde RA, Bonfiglioli R, Bértolo MB, Samara AM. Characterization and outcome of uveitis in 350 patients with spondyloarthropathies. Rheumatol Int. 2006;26(12):1143-1146. [PMID: 16957887]

Item 26   Answer: D
Educational Objective: *Diagnose ankylosing spondylitis with an MRI of the sacroiliac joints.*

This patient most likely has ankylosing spondylitis, and MRI of the sacroiliac joints is most likely to establish a diagnosis. Radiographic evidence of sacroiliitis is required for definitive diagnosis and is the most consistent finding associated with this condition. Onset of ankylosing spondylitis usually occurs in the teenage years or 20s and manifests as persistent pain and morning stiffness involving the low back that are alleviated with activity. This condition also may be associated with tenderness of the pelvis. Typically, the earliest radiographic changes in affected patients involve the sacroiliac joints, but these changes may not be visible for several years; therefore, this patient's normal radiographs of the pelvis do not exclude sacroiliitis. MRI, especially with gadolinium enhancement, is considered a sensitive method for detecting early erosive inflammatory changes in the sacroiliac joints and spine and can assess sites of active disease and response to effective therapy.

Anti–cyclic citrullinated peptide antibodies are highly specific for rheumatoid arthritis. However, rheumatoid arthritis does not involve the sacroiliac joints or lumbar spine, and testing for this condition in this patient is therefore not indicated.

An elevated erythrocyte sedimentation rate would raise suspicion for an inflammatory process but would not help to establish a specific diagnosis. In addition, the erythrocyte sedimentation rate does not correlate with disease activity in patients with ankylosing spondylitis, and measurement of this value is therefore not useful in diagnosing or monitoring patients with this condition.

HLA-B27 positivity is a strong risk factor for ankylosing spondylitis. However, less than 5% of patients who have this allele develop this condition. In addition, not all patients who have ankylosing spondylitis have this allele. Therefore, it is neither 100% sensitive nor 100% specific for the diagnosis of ankylosing spondylitis.

KEY POINT

MRI, especially with gadolinium enhancement, is a sensitive method for detecting early erosive inflammatory changes in the sacroiliac joints and spine.

Bibliography

Maksymowych WP. MRI in ankylosing spondylitis. Curr Opin Rheumatol. 2009;21(4):313-7. [PMID: 19496307]

Item 27   Answer: A
Educational Objective: *Diagnose systemic lupus erythematosus with anti–double-stranded DNA antibody.*

The next, most helpful serologic test for this patient is the anti–double-stranded DNA antibody. This patient with pleuritic chest pain, symmetric synovitis of the hand and wrist joints, leukopenia, proteinuria, and a positive ANA likely has systemic lupus erythematosus (SLE). Patients with a high pretest probability of SLE and ANAs (titer ≥1:160) should undergo confirmatory testing, such as measurement of compliment levels C3, C4, and total hemolytic compliment (CH50) and more specific autoantibody testing, such as anti–double-stranded DNA antibody testing (specificity, 75%-100%).

The antiribonucleoprotein antibody is strongly associated with mixed connective tissue disease but also can be seen in patients with SLE and myositis, but is neither very sensitive nor specific for SLE. Anti–SS-A and anti–SS-B antibodies (sometimes

referred to as anti-Ro and anti-La, respectively) are neither sensitive nor specific for SLE; they are seen in Sjögren syndrome. In patients with SLE, a positive anti–SS-A antibody is often associated with subacute cutaneous lupus erythematosus. Two antibodies are associated with systemic sclerosis: anti-topoisomerase I (anti–Scl-70) and anticentromere. The anti–Scl-70 antibody is seen in approximately half of the patients with diffuse systemic sclerosis and is associated with the development of interstitial lung disease. The anticentromere antibody is associated with limited cutaneous systemic sclerosis. Approximately 75% of patients with rheumatoid arthritis are rheumatoid factor positive, but the prevalence rate of rheumatoid arthritis may be as low as 50% in early disease. Rheumatoid factor positivity is not specific for rheumatoid arthritis and frequently occurs in other autoimmune disorders, including SLE, and chronic infections, most notably chronic active hepatitis C virus infection.

KEY POINT

The anti–double-stranded DNA antibody is very specific for systemic lupus erythematosus.

Bibliography

Cabral AR, Alarcón-Segovia D. Autoantibodies in systemic lupus erythematosus. Curr Opin Rheumatol. 1997;9(5):387-92. [PMID: 9309193]

Item 28   Answer: B
Educational Objective: *Treat drug-induced lupus.*

This patient most likely has drug-induced lupus caused by the tumor necrosis factor α inhibitor infliximab. The most appropriate next step in this patient's management is to discontinue infliximab and begin prednisone.

Many patients who use tumor necrosis factor α inhibitors develop autoantibodies, including antinuclear, anti–double-stranded DNA, and anti–Smith antibodies; rarely, these patients develop drug-induced lupus. Patients with this condition may present with typical manifestations of systemic lupus erythematosus but are particularly likely to have cutaneous and pleuropericardial involvement. Renal and neurologic manifestations are extremely rare.

The most appropriate management of a patient with drug-induced lupus caused by a tumor necrosis factor α inhibitor is discontinuation of the offending agent, which usually resolves this condition. Prednisone also should be added to this patient's medication regimen to control pleuritis and synovitis associated with drug-induced lupus.

Although this patient's worsening joint symptoms may be related to her underlying rheumatoid arthritis, her rheumatoid arthritis had been well controlled on her current medication regimen. If her flare were related to active rheumatoid arthritis, her symptoms would most likely be alleviated by initiation of sulfasalazine or an increase in her infliximab dosage. However, her musculoskeletal features, fever, malar rash, photosensitivity, purpura, symptoms of pleuritis, antinuclear and anti–double-stranded DNA antibody positivity, and findings on chest radiography also raise strong suspicion for drug-induced lupus. Therefore, progressive rheumatoid arthritis is a less likely explanation for this patient's current symptoms than is drug-induced lupus, and initiation of sulfasalazine or an increase in her infliximab dosage would not be indicated.

Hydroxychloroquine may be useful for the treatment of systemic lupus erythematosus and drug-induced lupus and could be added to this patient's existing medication regimen, but discontinuing methotrexate would not be appropriate.

KEY POINT

The most appropriate management of a patient with drug-induced lupus caused by a tumor necrosis factor α inhibitor is discontinuation of the offending agent.

Bibliography

Ramos-Casals M, Brito-Zerón P, Muñoz S, et al. Autoimmune diseases induced by TNF-targeted therapies: analysis of 233 cases. Medicine (Baltimore). 2007;86(4):242-251. [PMID: 17632266]

Item 29   Answer: B
Educational Objective: *Treat suspected lupus glomerulonephritis.*

This patient's hypertension, ankle edema, hematuria, proteinuria, hypoalbuminemia, and erythrocyte casts on urinalysis are highly suggestive of lupus nephritis despite the absence of renal insufficiency. To prevent irreversible renal damage, early treatment with a high-dose corticosteroid such as prednisone is indicated for patients whose condition raises strong suspicion for lupus nephritis. Whether renal biopsy is necessary in this clinical situation in order to establish a diagnosis remains uncertain, and treatment with high-dose corticosteroids would not significantly alter subsequent biopsy results.

Initiation of antihypertensive therapy would benefit this patient but is not the most appropriate next step in the management of her condition; treatment of her nephritis takes precedence and may itself help to control her hypertension. Instead of a calcium channel blocker such as amlodipine, angiotensin-converting enzyme inhibitors are the antihypertensive drugs of choice in patients with lupus nephritis because these agents help to control proteinuria.

Ibuprofen may help to control this patient's arthralgia. However, NSAIDs can significantly worsen renal function in patients with lupus nephritis and are therefore contraindicated in this patient population.

Low-dose prednisone may help to alleviate this patient's arthralgia and rash but would not treat her lupus nephritis.

KEY POINT

Early treatment with high-dose corticosteroids is indicated in patients whose condition raises strong suspicion for lupus nephritis.

Bibliography

Buhaescu I, Covic A, Deray G. Treatment of proliferative lupus nephritis—a critical approach. Semin Arthritis Rheum. 2007;36(4):224-237. [PMID:17067659]

Item 30   Answer: D
Educational Objective: *Diagnose the malar skin rash of systemic lupus erythematosus.*

This woman most likely has systemic lupus erythematosus (SLE). Patients with SLE have sun sensitivity, and their disease is triggered or exacerbated by light in the ultraviolet A and ultraviolet B spectrums. The facial rash, seen in the figure, is a classic presentation, involving the bridge of the nose, malar areas, and forehead (not seen), with erythematosus plaques and a fine scale. The nasolabial folds are relatively protected from the sun, and the absence of the rash in this area helps to distinguish it from other common rashes of the face, including rosacea and seborrheic dermatitis. The rash may last for hours or days and has a tendency to recur.

Rosacea is a chronic inflammatory skin disorder that begins in early to middle adulthood and is characterized by central telangiectasis, flushing, and acneiform papules and pustules. Many patients with rosacea are misdiagnosed as having SLE. However, the nasolabial folds are not typically spared in rosacea, acne-like pustules are more prominent, and rosacea is not associated with other systemic symptoms, such as arthritis.

Patients with dermatomyositis have pronounced proximal muscle weakness and elevated serum concentrations of muscle enzymes such as creatine kinase. Patients with dermatomyositis may have a facial rash that extends up to the eyelids, giving them a purplish (heliotrope) hue. Another characteristic finding is red to purplish plaques on the dorsal hands, more prominent over the joints, and known as Gottron papules.

The lesions of seborrheic dermatitis are ill defined (lack a distinct border), yellowish-red, and of varying size, and are usually associated with a greasy or dandruff-like scale. It occurs most commonly on the scalp, central face, upper mid-chest, and other oily areas of the body, and is not related to sun exposure or associated with systemic symptoms.

KEY POINT

The characteristic facial rash of systemic lupus erythematosus involves the bridge of the nose, malar areas, and forehead with erythematosus plaques and a fine scale.

Bibliography

Rothfield N, Sontheimer RD, Bernstein M. Lupus erythematosus: systemic and cutaneous manifestations. Clin Dermatol. 2006;24:348-62. [PMID: 16966017]

Item 31   Answer: C
Educational Objective: *Diagnose dermatomyositis-related interstitial lung disease.*

The most likely diagnosis is interstitial lung disease (ILD). ILD with progressive pulmonary fibrosis and secondary pulmonary arterial hypertension is one of the leading causes of death in patients with polymyositis and dermatomyositis. ILD may be prominent at the onset of myopathy or develop over the course of the disease. The presence of anti–Jo-1 antibodies is associated with an increased risk for ILD. Patients with ILD have progressive dyspnea, basilar crackles, bibasilar infiltrates on chest radiographs, and restrictive changes on pulmonary function studies, including a decreased forced vital capacity, total lung capacity, and diffusing capacity of the lungs for carbon monoxide. Chest radiographs demonstrate an interstitial pattern, and high-resolution CT scans of the chest most commonly suggest a diagnosis of nonspecific interstitial pneumonia. Lung biopsy is generally not needed for diagnosis, but bronchoscopy may be needed to exclude infection.

Typical community-acquired pneumonia is characterized by rapid onset of high fever, productive cough, and pleuritic chest pain, all of which are absent in this patient. Cardiac involvement in patients with an inflammatory myopathy is rare and includes arrhythmias and cardiomyopathy. Furthermore, this patient has no findings to support heart failure, including an S_3, jugular venous distention, or peripheral edema. Approximately 1% to 2% of patients with rheumatic diseases can develop pneumocystis pneumonia, usually in patients taking combination immunosuppressant therapy that includes corticosteroids. The risk may be higher in patients with dermatomyositis or polymyositis compared with other rheumatic diseases. Most patients with rheumatic disease and pneumocystis pneumonia have an abrupt onset of acute respiratory failure and fever. This patient's 6-week course of progressive dyspnea and absence of fever make pneumocystis pneumonia an unlikely diagnosis.

KEY POINT

Interstitial lung disease with progressive pulmonary fibrosis and secondary pulmonary arterial hypertension is one of the leading causes of death in patients with polymyositis and dermatomyositis.

Bibliography

Fathi M, Lundberg IE, Tornling G. Pulmonary complications of polymyositis and dermatomyositis. Semin Respir Crit Care Med. 2007;28(4):451-8. [PMID: 17764062]

Item 32   Answer: A
Educational Objective: *Treat Raynaud phenomenon associated with systemic sclerosis.*

This patient has Raynaud phenomenon, which is present in more than 95% of patients with systemic sclerosis and is particularly likely to develop in patients with limited cutaneous disease. The most appropriate treatment for this patient is amlodipine.

Systemic sclerosis is classified according to the degree of skin involvement. Systemic sclerosis with limited cutaneous involvement, or CREST syndrome (calcinosis, Raynaud phenomenon, esophageal dysmotility, sclerodactyly, and telangiectasia), manifests as skin thickening distal to the elbows and knees. Conversely, systemic sclerosis with diffuse cutaneous involvement is associated with skin thickening proximal to the elbows and knees. Diffuse and limited cutaneous systemic sclerosis may affect the face.

Episodes of Raynaud phenomenon are often precipitated by cold exposure or stress and usually involve the extremities. In patients with Raynaud phenomenon, cigarette smoking is contraindicated and avoidance of cold is recommended; pharmacologic therapy is warranted for patients in whom these interventions do not provide sufficient relief. Dihydropyridine calcium channel blockers such as amlodipine have been shown to reduce the frequency and severity of attacks in patients with both primary and secondary Raynaud phenomenon, and these agents are frequently used as first-line treatment in this condition. Other agents used to manage Raynaud phenomenon include peripherally acting α-1 blockers, phosphodiesterase inhibitors, and endothelin receptor antagonists.

Topical nitrates applied to the finger webs are often used in the treatment of Raynaud phenomenon but are usually used as second-line therapy. Oral therapy with nitroglycerin is less effective and less well tolerated than amlodipine and is not indicated as a first-line drug for this condition.

Raynaud phenomenon is caused by microvascular involvement in patients with systemic sclerosis and is characterized by intimal proliferation and progressive luminal obliteration, as well as digital spasm. This process does not respond to anti-inflammatory agents; therefore, prednisone is not indicated in the treatment of Raynaud phenomenon.

β-Blockers such as propranolol are not indicated in the treatment of Raynaud phenomenon and may actually worsen symptoms by preventing β-adrenergic–mediated vasodilation.

KEY POINT

Use of a dihydropyridine calcium channel blocker is warranted in patients with Raynaud phenomenon in whom cold avoidance does not provide sufficient relief.

Bibliography

Henness S, Wigley FM. Current drug therapy for scleroderma and secondary Raynaud's phenomenon: evidence-based review. Curr Opin Rheumatol. 2007;19(6):611-618. [PMID: 17917543]

Item 33   Answer: A
Educational Objective: *Diagnose fibromyalgia.*

This patient most likely has fibromyalgia. This condition is characterized by diffuse pain on both sides of the body and above and below the waist as well as axial skeletal pain, or, according to the original American College of Rheumatology criteria, the presence of pain in at least 11 of 18 specified potential tender points. However, expert opinion now states that these tender points are arbitrary and not essential in the diagnosis of fibromyalgia.

Most patients with this condition have fatigue and sleep disturbance. Fibromyalgia also may be associated with dry eyes and mouth. Studies that have assessed the comorbidity of fibromyalgia with other symptom-defined syndromes have found high rates of chronic fatigue syndrome, migraine, irritable bowel syndrome, pelvic pain, and temporomandibular joint pain in patients with fibromyalgia.

Polymyositis may manifest as muscle pain and fatigue but is unlikely in the absence of significant proximal muscle weakness or an elevated creatine kinase level.

Up to 25% of patients with systemic inflammatory conditions, such as systemic lupus erythematosus (SLE) and rheumatoid arthritis, have symptoms consistent with fibromyalgia in the initial stages of their illness. This patient's fatigue, polyarthralgia, dry eyes and mouth, and strongly positive titers of antinuclear antibodies are consistent with SLE and Sjögren syndrome. However, patients with SLE usually have anemia, leukopenia, or lymphopenia. Similarly, joint involvement in Sjögren syndrome typically manifests as inflammatory arthritis. Furthermore, patients with SLE and Sjögren syndrome may have systemic manifestations, including cutaneous, neurologic, and renal involvement, which are absent in this patient.

The presence of antinuclear antibodies is not diagnostic of SLE or Sjögren syndrome. These antibodies are often present in the general population and particularly in patients with autoimmune thyroid disease or in first-degree relatives of patients with SLE. In addition, high titers of antinuclear antibodies do not necessarily indicate the presence of autoimmune disease.

KEY POINT

Fibromyalgia is characterized by diffuse pain on both sides of the body and above and below the waist as well as axial skeletal pain.

Bibliography

Chakrabarty S, Zoorob R. Fibromyalgia. Am Fam Physician. 2007; 76(2):247-254. [PMID:17695569]

Item 34   Answer: C
Educational Objective: *Diagnose Sjögren syndrome.*

This patient has Sjögren's syndrome. Sjögren's syndrome is an autoimmune disease characterized by keratoconjunctivitis sicca, xerostomia, and the presence of multiple autoantibodies. This condition may occur as a primary disease process or may be associated with another autoimmune disease. Primary Sjögren's syndrome usually is diagnosed in patients between 40 and 60 years of age, and this condition has a 9:1 female predominance. The characteristic manifestations of Sjögren's syndrome are symptomatic oral and ocular dryness. Lymphocytic inflammation of the lacrimal glands causes an aqueous tear deficiency with resultant keratoconjunctivitis sicca, whereas lymphocytic inflammation of the major and minor salivary glands is associated with salivary gland enlargement and xerostomia. A cardinal feature of Sjögren's syndrome is the presence of autoantibodies, which may include antibodies to Ro/SSA and La/SSB. These autoantibodies are not specific for Sjögren's syndrome; they may also occur in subsets of patients with systemic lupus erythematosus and in asymptomatic women. Antinuclear antibodies and rheumatoid factor also frequently are present in patients with this condition, as is hypergammaglobulinemia.

Hodgkin disease is an aggressive lymphoid malignancy that typically presents with rapidly progressive, symptomatic disease, often initially localized to one organ or compartment (for example, bone marrow).

Sarcoidosis is a multisystem, granulomatous inflammatory disease of unknown cause. It occurs most commonly in young and middle-aged adults, with a peak incidence in the third decade. The most common presenting manifestations involve the lymphatic and pulmonary systems, along with the eyes and skin.

Systemic lupus erythematosus (SLE) is a chronic multisystem autoimmune disease of unknown cause. Manifestations of this heterogeneous syndrome range from mild to severe and life threatening and most commonly involve the skin and joints. Other manifestations include cytopenias, hemolytic anemia, serositis, aphthous ulcers, and kidney disease.

The syndrome of dry eyes, parotid gland enlargement and arthritis is not found in systemic lupus erythematosus, lymphoma, or sarcoidosis.

KEY POINT

Sjögren syndrome is an autoimmune disease characterized by keratoconjunctivitis sicca, xerostomia, and the presence of multiple autoantibodies.

Bibliography

Tzioufas AG, Voulgarelis M. Update on Sjögren's syndrome autoimmune epithelitis: from classification to increased neoplasias. Best Pract Res Clin Rheumatol. 2007;21:989-1010. [PMID: 18068857]

Item 35   Answer: B

Educational Objective: *Diagnose polyarteritis nodosa as a cause of kidney failure.*

This patient most likely has polyarteritis nodosa, which is characterized by a necrotizing inflammation of the medium-sized or small arteries without glomerulonephritis or vasculitis of the arterioles, capillaries, or venules. Clinical manifestations of this condition include fever; musculoskeletal symptoms; and vasculitis involving the nervous system, gastrointestinal tract, heart, and nonglomerular renal vessels that is associated with hypertension, kidney insufficiency, proteinuria, and hematuria.

Polyarteritis nodosa most commonly affects the kidneys and may cause significant hypertension, kidney insufficiency, and renal vasculitis associated with proteinuria and hematuria. Prompt immunosuppressive therapy is critical to reduce the risk of irreversible kidney failure, but a definitive diagnosis must be established before beginning this treatment.

Sural nerve biopsy may establish the diagnosis of polyarteritis nodosa, and kidney angiography can support this diagnosis. After exclusion of other causes of medium- or small-vessel vasculitis, angiography of the renal arteries is often performed when there is no appropriate tissue to biopsy. Specific angiographic findings in patients with polyarteritis nodosa include microaneurysms or a beaded pattern with areas of arterial narrowing and dilation.

Abdominal fat pad aspiration may help to diagnose AL amyloidosis, but this condition is unlikely in a patient with normal results on serum and urine immunoelectrophoreses.

Kidney biopsy may yield a false-negative result for polyarteritis nodosa and is associated with an increased risk for bleeding secondary to transsection of an intrarenal aneurysm. Biopsy of normal skin has a low diagnostic yield for polyarteritis nodosa because of the minimal histologic abnormalities associated with this condition.

KEY POINT

Polyarteritis nodosa most commonly affects the kidneys and may cause significant hypertension, kidney insufficiency, and renal vasculitis with classic angiographic findings.

Bibliography

Schmidt WA. Use of imaging studies in the diagnosis of vasculitis. Curr Rheumatol Rep. 2004;6(3):203-211. [PMID:15134599]

Item 36   Answer: D

Educational Objective: *Diagnose Wegener granulomatosis.*

This patient most likely has Wegener granulomatosis, a necrotizing vasculitis that typically affects the upper- and lower-respiratory tract and the kidneys. This patient's purpura is consistent with vasculitis. His diffuse pulmonary infiltrates (generally associated with alveolar hemorrhage), history of refractory otitis media, renal failure, and urinalysis findings that suggest glomerulonephritis particularly raise suspicion for Wegener granulomatosis.

Wegener granulomatosis may be associated with inflammatory arthritis involving the small and large joints and joint effusions. The presence of c-ANCA and antiproteinase-3 antibodies is approximately 90% specific for this condition. The presentation of Wegener granulomatosis is highly nonspecific and evolves slowly over a period of months; therefore, diagnosis of this condition is often delayed by several months.

Patients with severe, long-standing rheumatoid arthritis may develop interstitial pneumonitis, and this condition is particularly likely to develop in men. Radiographs of patients with this condition usually show bibasilar interstitial markings. Interstitial lung disease associated with rheumatoid arthritis most characteristically has an insidious onset and is associated with seropositive, erosive joint disease. In most patients, the lung disease appears 5 years or more after the diagnosis of rheumatoid arthritis.

Methotrexate-induced pneumonitis can occur at any time in the course of therapy with this agent, regardless of the dosage or duration of treatment. However, this condition would not explain this patient's entire clinical picture, including c-ANCA positivity, vasculitis, renal failure, and his urinalysis findings.

Pneumocystis pneumonia may manifest as fever, dyspnea, tachypnea, and crackles heard on pulmonary examination. However, dyspnea is typically progressive and not acute and would not result in rapid pulmonary failure. Chest radiography in patients with this condition may show diffuse infiltrates. *Pneumocystis* pneumonia also usually develops in patients who are significantly immunosuppressed, whereas this patient has received only a short course of low-dose methotrexate. Furthermore, *Pneumocystis* pneumonia would not explain this patient's additional findings.

KEY POINT

Wegener granulomatosis should be considered in patients with upper- and lower-airway manifestations, renal involvement, and inflammatory arthritis.

Bibliography

Bosch X, Guilabert A, Font J. Antineutrophil cytoplasmic antibodies. Lancet. 2006;368(9533):404-418. [PMID: 16876669]

Item 37   Answer: B

Educational Objective: *Manage giant cell arteritis.*

This patient's headache, temporal artery tenderness, acute visual loss, fever, and mild anemia are strongly suggestive of giant cell arteritis (GCA). Immediate high-dose intravenous methylprednisolone is indicated for this patient. Pain in the shoulder and hip girdle accompanied by a significant elevation in the erythrocyte sedimentation rate is consistent with polymyalgia rheumatica, which is present in approximately 33% of patients with GCA. Anterior ischemic optic neuropathy usually causes acute and complete visual loss in patients with GCA, and funduscopic examination of these patients typically reveals a pale, swollen optic nerve.

Rarely, patients with GCA regain vision if treated immediately with high doses of an intravenous corticosteroid such as methylprednisolone (1 g/d or 100 mg every 8 hours for 3 days) followed by oral prednisone (1 to 2 mg/kg/d). More importantly, this aggressive regimen helps to prevent blindness in the contralateral eye. Therefore, although temporal artery biopsy is the gold standard for diagnosing GCA, diagnostic testing should not precede treatment in patients whose clinical presentation is suspicious for this condition.

Even in the absence of visual loss, GCA is a medical emergency. In a patient whose condition is suspicious for GCA but who does not have visual loss, immediate initiation of high-dose oral prednisone before diagnostic testing is performed also is indicated. Whether intravenous corticosteroid therapy is more effective than oral administration of prednisone for patients with GCA and visual loss remains uncertain. Nevertheless, intravenous therapy seems reasonable in this circumstance and is recommended by many experts, even though rigorous studies have not validated this approach. However, it is clear that low-dose oral prednisone, which is an adequate treatment for isolated polymyalgia rheumatica, does not sufficiently treat GCA.

A process in the brain is unlikely to cause monocular visual loss, and patients with GCA typically have normal findings on brain MRI. Therefore, this study would most likely be unhelpful in this patient.

In patients whose condition raises a strong suspicion of GCA, temporal artery biopsy should be performed after corticosteroid therapy is begun. Corticosteroid therapy will not affect the results of temporal artery biopsy as long as biopsy is performed within 2 weeks of initiating this therapy; positive biopsy results have been seen as late as 6 weeks after institution of high-dose corticosteroid therapy, but the yield of biopsy is higher when this study is performed sooner.

KEY POINT

In patients whose clinical presentation is suspicious for giant cell arteritis, corticosteroid therapy should be instituted immediately, before diagnostic testing is performed.

Bibliography

Fraser JA, Weyand CM, Newman NJ, Biousse V. The treatment of giant cell arteritis. Rev Neurol Dis. 2008;5(3):140-152. [PMID: 18838954]

NORMAL LABORATORY VALUES
MKSAP® for Students 5

U.S. traditional units are followed in parentheses by equivalent values expressed in S.I. units.

Hematology

Activated partial thromboplastin time — 25-35 s
Bleeding time — less than 10 min
Erythrocyte count — $4.2\text{-}5.9 \times 10^6/\mu L$ ($4.2\text{-}5.9 \times 10^{12}/L$)
Erythrocyte sedimentation rate
　Male — 0-15 mm/h
　Female — 0-20 mm/h
Erythropoietin — less than 30 mU/mL (30 U/L)
D-Dimer — less than 0.5 µg/mL (0.5 mg/L)
Ferritin, serum — 15-200 ng/mL (15-200 µg/L)
Haptoglobin, serum — 50-150 mg/dL (500-1500 mg/L)
Hematocrit
　Male — 41%-51%
　Female — 36%-47%
Hemoglobin, blood
　Male — 14-17 g/dL (140-170 g/L)
　Female — 12-16 g/dL (120-160 g/L)
Leukocyte alkaline phosphatase — 15-40 mg of phosphorus liberated/h per 10^{10} cells; score = 13-130/100 polymorphonuclear neutrophils and band forms
Leukocyte count — 4000-10,000/µL ($4.0\text{-}10 \times 10^9/L$)
Mean corpuscular hemoglobin — 28-32 pg
Mean corpuscular hemoglobin concentration — 32-36 g/dL (320-360 g/L)
Mean corpuscular volume — 80-100 fL
Platelet count — 150,000-350,000/µL ($150\text{-}350 \times 10^9/L$)
Prothrombin time — 11-13 s
Reticulocyte count — 0.5%-1.5% of erythrocytes; absolute: 23,000-90,000/µL ($23\text{-}90 \times 10^9/L$)

Blood, Plasma, and Serum Chemistry Studies

Albumin, serum — 3.5-5.5 g/dL (35-55 g/L)
Alkaline phosphatase, serum — 36-92 U/L
α Fetoprotein, serum — 0-20 ng/mL (0-20 µg/L)
Aminotransferase, alanine (ALT) — 0-35 U/L
Aminotransferase, aspartate (AST) — 0-35 U/L
Ammonia, plasma — 40-80 µg/dL (23-47 µmol/L)
Amylase, serum — 0-130 U/L
Bicarbonate, serum — see Carbon dioxide
Bilirubin, serum
　Total — 0.3-1.2 mg/dL (5.1-20.5 µmol/L)
　Direct — 0-0.3 mg/dL (0-5.1 µmol/L)
Blood gases, arterial (ambient air)
　pH — 7.38-7.44
　P_{CO_2} — 35-45 mm Hg (4.7-6.0 kPa)
　P_{O_2} — 80-100 mm Hg (10.6-13.3 kPa)
　Oxygen saturation — 95% or greater
Blood urea nitrogen — 8-20 mg/dL (2.9-7.1 mmol/L)
C-reactive protein — 0.0-0.8 mg/dL (0.0-8.0 mg/L)
Calcium, serum — 9-10.5 mg/dL (2.2-2.6 mmol/L)
Carbon dioxide content, serum — 23-28 meq/L (23-28 mmol/L)
Chloride, serum — 98-106 meq/L (98-106 mmol/L)
Cholesterol, plasma
　Total — 150-199 mg/dL (3.88-5.15 mmol/L), desirable
　Low-density lipoprotein (LDL) — less than or equal to 130 mg/dL (3.36 mmol/L), desirable
　High-density lipoprotein (HDL) — greater than or equal to 40 mg/dL (1.04 mmol/L), desirable
Complement, serum
　C3 — 55-120 mg/dL (550-1200 mg/L)
　Total (CH_{50}) — 37-55 U/mL (37-55 kU/L)
Creatine kinase, serum — 30-170 U/L
Creatinine, serum — 0.7-1.3 mg/dL (61.9-115 µmol/L)
Electrolytes, serum
　Sodium — 136-145 meq/L (136-145 mmol/L)
　Potassium — 3.5-5.0 meq/L (3.5-5.0 mmol/L)

Chloride — 98-106 meq/L (98-106 mmol/L)
Carbon dioxide — 23-28 meq/L (23-28 mmol/L)
Fibrinogen, plasma — 150-350 mg/dL (1.5-3.5 g/L)
Folate, red cell — 160-855 ng/mL (362-1937 nmol/L)
Folate, serum — 2.5-20 ng/mL (5.7-45.3 nmol/L)
Glucose, plasma — fasting, 70-100 mg/dL (3.9-5.6 mmol/L)
γ-Glutamyltransferase, serum — 0-30 U/L
Homocysteine, plasma
　Male — 0.54-2.16 mg/L (4-16 µmol/L)
　Female — 0.41-1.89 mg/L (3-14 µmol/L)
Immunoglobulins
　Globulins, total — 2.5-3.5 g/dL (25-35 g/L)
　　IgG — 640-1430 mg/dL (6.4-14.3 g/L)
　　IgA — 70-300 mg/dL (0.7-3.0 g/L)
　　IgM — 20-140 mg/dL (0.2-1.4 g/L)
　　IgD — less than 8 mg/dL (80 mg/L)
　　IgE — 0.01-0.04 mg/dL (0.1-0.4 mg/L)
Iron studies
　Ferritin, serum — 15-200 ng/mL (15-200 µg/L)
　Iron, serum — 60-160 µg/dL (11-29 µmol/L)
　Iron-binding capacity, total, serum — 250-460 µg/dL (45-82 µmol/L)
　Transferrin saturation — 20%-50%
Lactate dehydrogenase, serum — 60-100 U/L
Lactic acid, venous blood — 6-16 mg/dL (0.67-1.8 mmol/L)
Lipase, serum — less than 95 U/L
Magnesium, serum — 1.5-2.4 mg/dL (0.62-0.99 mmol/L)
Methylmalonic acid, serum — 150-370 nmol/L
Osmolality, plasma — 275-295 mosm/kg H_2O
Phosphatase, alkaline, serum — 36-92 U/L
Phosphorus, serum — 3-4.5 mg/dL (0.97-1.45 mmol/L)
Potassium, serum — 3.5-5.0 mg/L (3.5-5.0 mmol/L)
Prostate-specific antigen, serum – less than 4 ng/mL (4 µg/L)
Protein, serum
　Total — 6.0-7.8 g/dL (60-78 g/L)
　Albumin — 3.5-5.5 g/dL (35-55 g/L)
　Globulins, total — 2.5-3.5 g/dL (25-35 g/L)
Rheumatoid factor — less than 40 U/mL (40 kU/L)
Sodium, serum — 136-145 meq/L (136-145 mmol/L)
Transferrin saturation — 20%-50%
Triglycerides — less than 150 mg/dL (1.69 mmol/L), desirable
Troponins, serum
　Troponin I — 0-0.5 ng/mL (0-0.5 µg/L)
　Troponin T — 0-0.10 ng/mL (0-0.10 µg/L)
Urea nitrogen, blood — 8-20 mg/dL (2.9-7.1 mmol/L)
Uric acid, serum — 2.5-8 mg/dL (0.15-0.47 mmol/L)
Vitamin B_{12}, serum — 200-800 pg/mL (148-590 pmol/L)

Endocrine

Adrenocorticotropic hormone (ACTH), serum — 9-52 pg/mL (2-11 pmol/L)
Aldosterone, serum
　Supine — 2-5 ng/dL (55-138 pmol/L)
　Standing — 7-20 ng/dL (194-554 pmol/L)
Aldosterone, urine — 5-19 µg/24 h (13.9-52.6 nmol/24 h)
Catecholamines
　Epinephrine, plasma (supine) — less than 75 ng/L (410 pmol/L)
　Norepinephrine, plasma (supine) — 50-440 ng/L (296-2600 pmol/L)
　Catecholamines, 24-hour, urine — less than 100 µg/m² per 24 h (591 nmol/m² per 24 h)
Cortisol, free, urine – less than 50 µg/24 h (138 nmol/24 h)
Dehydroepiandrosterone sulfate (DHEA), plasma
　Male — 1.3-5.5 µg/mL (3.5-14.9 µmol/L)
　Female — 0.6-3.3 µg/mL (1.6-8.9 µmol/L)
Epinephrine, plasma (supine) — less than 75 ng/L (410 pmol/L)

Estradiol, serum
Male — 10-30 pg/mL (37-110 pmol/L);
Female — day 1-10, 14-27 pg/mL (50-100 pmol/L); day 11-20, 14-54 pg/mL (50-200 pmol/L); day 21-30, 19-41 pg/mL (70-150 pmol/L)

Follicle-stimulating hormone, serum
Male (adult) — 5-15 mU/mL (5-15 U/L)
Female — follicular or luteal phase, 5-20 mU/mL (5-20 U/L); midcycle peak, 30-50 mU/mL (30-50 U/L); postmenopausal, greater than 35 mU/mL (35 U/L)

Growth hormone, plasma — after oral glucose: less than 2 ng/mL (2 μg/L); response to provocative stimuli: greater than 7 ng/mL (7 μg/L)

Luteinizing hormone, serum
Male — 3-15 mU/mL (3-15 U/L)
Female — follicular or luteal phase, 5-22 mU/mL (5-22 U/L); midcycle peak, 30-250 mU/mL (30-250 U/L); postmenopausal, greater than 30 mU/mL (30 U/L)

Metanephrine, urine — less than 1.2 mg/24 h (6.1 mmol/24 h)
Norepinephrine, plasma (supine) — 50-440 ng/L (296-2600 pmol/L)
Parathyroid hormone, serum — 10-65 pg/mL (10-65 ng/L)
Prolactin, serum
Male — less than 15 ng/mL (15 μg/L)
Female — less than 20 ng/mL (20 μg/L)

Testosterone, serum
Male (adult) — 300-1200 ng/dL (10-42 nmol/L)
Female — 20-75 ng/dL (0.7-2.6 nmol/L)

Thyroid function tests
Thyroid iodine (^{131}I) uptake — 10%-30% of administered dose at 24 h
Thyroid-stimulating hormone (TSH) — 0.5-5.0 μU/mL (0.5-5.0 mU/L)
Thyroxine (T_4), serum
Total — 5-12 μg/dL (64-155 nmol/L)
Free — 0.9-2.4 ng/dL (12-31 pmol/L)
Free T_4 index — 4-11
Triiodothyronine, free (T_3) — 3.6-5.6 ng/L (5.6-8.6 pmol/L)
Triiodothyronine, resin (T_3) — 25%-35%
Triiodothyronine, serum (T_3) — 70-195 ng/dL (1.1-3.0 nmol/L)

Vanillylmandelic acid, urine — less than 8 mg/24 h (40.4 μmol/24 h)
Vitamin D
1,25-dihydroxy, serum — 25-65 pg/mL (60-156 pmol/L)
25-hydroxy, serum — 25-80 ng/mL (62-200 nmol/L)

Urine

Albumin-creatinine ratio — less than 30 mg/g
Calcium — 100-300 mg/24 h (2.5-7.5 mmol/24 h) on unrestricted diet
Creatinine — 15-25 mg/kg per 24 h (133-221 mmol/kg per 24 h)

Glomerular filtration rate (GFR)
Normal
Male — 130 mL/min/1.73 m²
Female — 120 mL/min/1.73 m²
Stages of Chronic Kidney Disease
Stage 1 — greater than or equal to 90 mL/min/1.73 m²
Stage 2 — 60-89 mL/min/1.73 m²
Stage 3 — 30-59 mL/min/1.73 m²
Stage 4 — 15-29 mL/min/1.73 m²
Stage 5 — less than 15 mL/min/1.73 m²

5-Hydroxyindoleacetic acid (5-HIAA) — 2-9 mg/24 h (10.4-46.8 μmol/24 h)
Protein–creatinine ratio – less than or equal to 0.2 mg/mg
Sodium — 100-260 meq/24 h (100-260 mmol/24 h) (varies with intake)
Uric acid — 250-750 mg/24 h (1.48-4.43 mmol/24 h) (varies with diet)

Gastrointestinal

Gastrin, serum — 0-180 pg/mL (0-180 ng/L)
Stool fat — less than 5 g/d on a 100-g fat diet
Stool weight — less than 200 g/d

Pulmonary

Forced expiratory volume in 1 second (FEV$_1$) — greater than 80% of predicted
Forced vital capacity (FVC) — greater than 80% of predicted
FEV$_1$/FVC — greater than 75%

Cerebrospinal Fluid

Cell count — 0-5/μL (0-5 × 10⁶/L)
Glucose — 40-80 mg/dL (2.2-4.4 mmol/L); less than 40% of simultaneous plasma concentration is abnormal
Pressure (opening) — 70-200 mm H$_2$O
Protein — 15-60 mg/dL (150-600 mg/L)

Hemodynamic Measurements

Cardiac index — 2.5-4.2 L/min/m²
Left ventricular ejection fraction — greater than 55%
Pressures
Pulmonary artery
Systolic — 20-25 mm Hg
Diastolic — 5-10 mm Hg
Mean — 9-16 mm Hg
Pulmonary capillary wedge — 6-12 mm Hg
Right atrium — mean 0-5 mm Hg
Right ventricle
Systolic — 20-25 mm Hg
Diastolic — 0-5 mm Hg

American College of Physicians
190 N. Independence Mall West, Philadelphia, PA 19106-1572

Color Plates

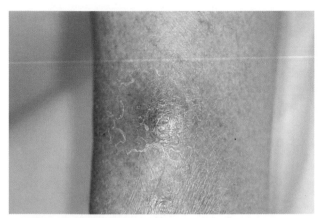

Plate 1
Gastroenterology and Hepatology, Item 46

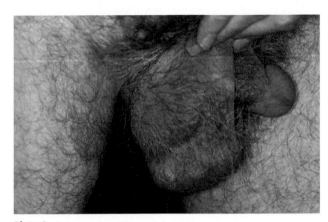

Plate 4
General Internal Medicine, Item 57

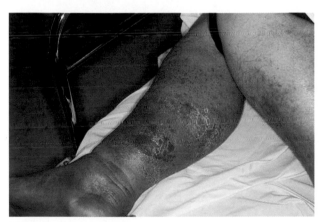

Plate 2
General Internal Medicine, Item 55

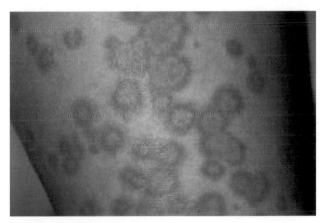

Plate 5
General Internal Medicine, Item 59

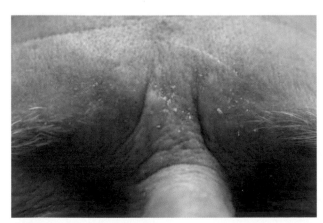

Plate 3
General Internal Medicine, Item 56

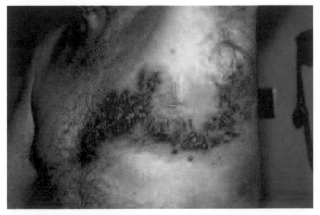

Plate 6
General Internal Medicine, Item 60

1

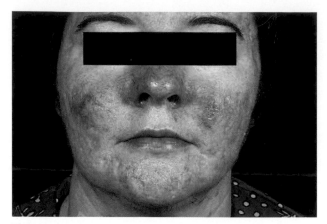

Plate 7
General Internal Medicine, Item 61

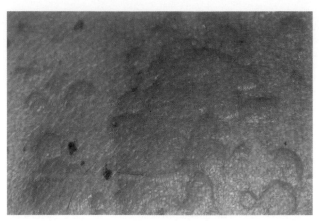

Plate 10
General Internal Medicine, Item 64

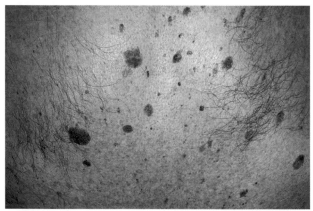

Plate 8
General Internal Medicine, Item 62

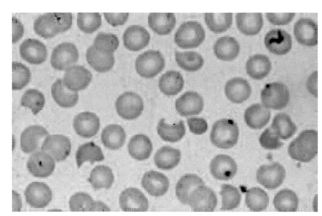

Plate 11
Hematology, Item 4

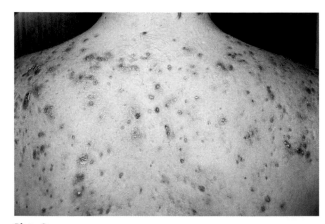

Plate 9
General Internal Medicine, Item 63

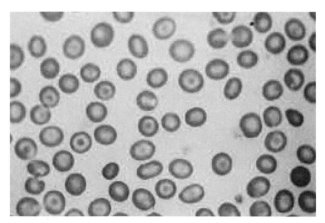

Plate 12
Hematology, Item 5

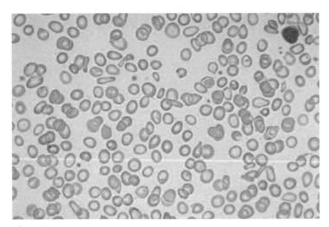

Plate 13
Hematology, Item 8

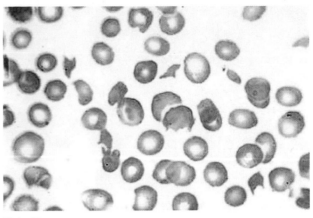

Plate 16
Hematology, Item 20

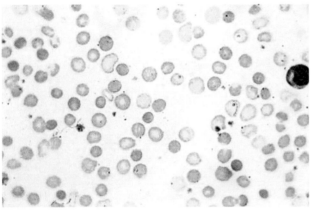

Plate 14
Hematology, Item 9

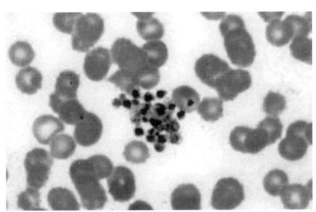

Plate 17
Hematology, Item 21

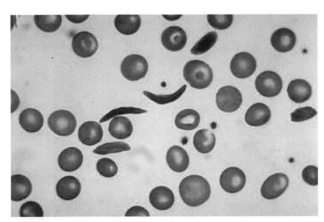

Plate 15
Hematology, Item 18

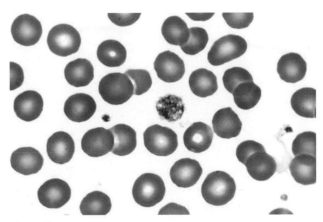

Plate 18
Hematology, Item 22

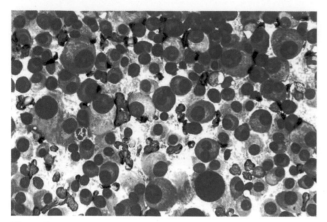

Plate 19
Hematology, Item 27

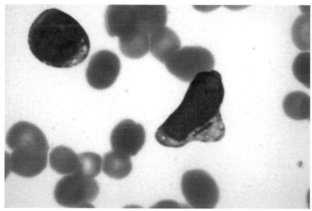

Plate 20
Hematology, Item 30

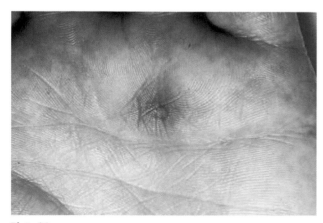

Plate 21
Infectious Disease Medicine, Item 21

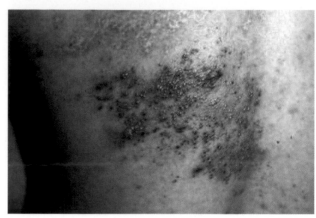

Plate 22
Infectious Disease Medicine, Item 26

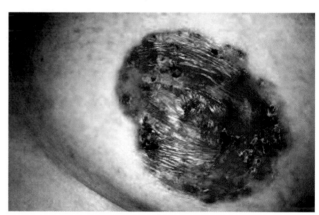

Plate 23
Oncology, Item 2

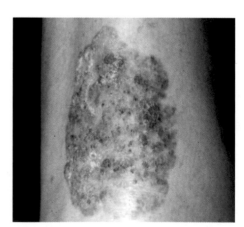

Plate 24
Oncology, Item 22

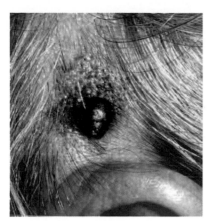

Plate 25
Oncology, Item 23

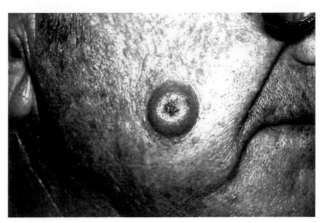

Plate 28
Oncology, Item 26

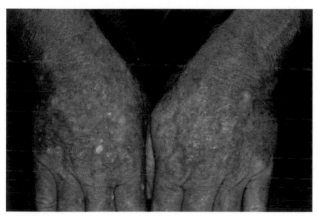

Plate 26
Oncology, Item 24

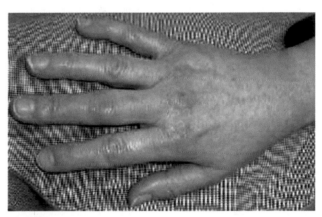

Plate 29
Rheumatology, Item 2

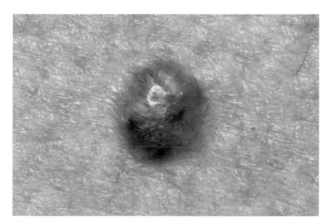

Plate 27
Oncology, Item 25

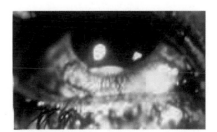

Plate 30
Rheumatology, Item 25

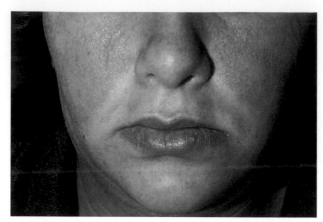

Plate 31
Rheumatology, Item 30

Question

WqqqqqqqqqqqqCbqqqqqqqqqqqqqqqqqqq,'b Dqqqqq?

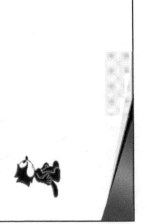